NOW THAT ONE-THIRD OF ALL THE PRODUCTS
ON SUPERMARKET SHELVES ARE
CHOLESTEROL- OR FAT-REDUCED, BE SURE YOU
HAVE THE INFORMATION YOU NEED ABOUT THE
FOODS YOU EAT . . .

What cuts of meat have the least cholesterol?
How many eggs can you eat every week?
Does pasta have much cholesterol?

The Cholesterol Counter supplies the most up-to-date
information on cholesterol—how much you should eat,
where to cut down, and how to calculate your cholesterol intake. And most important, it provides the cholesterol content of the most common—and uncommon—
foods you and your loved ones eat.

ANNETTE B. NATOW, Ph.D., R.D., and JO-ANN HESLIN, M.A., R.D.,
are the authors of nineteen books on nutrition. Both are former
faculty members of Adelphi University and the State University
of New York, Downstate Medical Center. They are editors of the
Journal of Nutrition for the Elderly, serve as editorial board
members for the *Environmental Nutrition Newsletter*, and are
frequent contributors to magazines and journals.

LOOK FOR
THE POCKET FAT COUNTER
AVAILABLE FROM POCKET BOOKS

Books by Annette B. Natow and Jo-Ann Heslin

The Antioxidant Vitamin Counter
The Cholesterol Counter
The Diabetes Carbohydrate and Calorie Counter
The Fast-Food Nutrition Counter
The Fat Attack Plan
The Fat Counter
The Iron Counter
Megadoses
No-Nonsense Nutrition for Kids
The Pocket Encyclopedia of Nutrition
The Pocket Fat Counter
The Pregnancy Nutrition Counter
The Sodium Counter
The Supermarket Nutrition Counter

Published by POCKET BOOKS

THE
CHOLESTEROL
COUNTER

FOURTH EDITION

REVISED AND UPDATED

Annette B. Natow, Ph.D., R.D.

and

Jo-Ann Heslin, M.A., R.D.

POCKET BOOKS

New York   London   Toronto   Sydney   Tokyo   Singapore

An *Original* Publication of POCKET BOOKS

POCKET BOOKS, a division of Simon & Schuster Inc.
1230 Avenue of the Americas, New York, NY 10020

ISBN: 0-671-89472-2

First Pocket Books printing of this revised edition June 1996

10 9 8 7 6 5 4 3 2 1

POCKET and colophon are registered trademarks of
Simon & Schuster Inc.

Cover design by Tom McKeveny

Printed in the U.S.A.

To our families, who support us through every project:
Harry, Allen, Irene, Sarah, Meryl, Marty, Laura, George,
Emily, Steven, Joseph, Kristen and Karen.

ACKNOWLEDGMENTS

———◇———

Without the tireless cooperation of Steven and Stephen, *The Cholesterol Counter* would never have been completed. A special thanks to our agent, Nancy Trichter, and our editor, Julie Rubenstein, and her assistant, Leslie Stern. Our thanks go also to all the food manufacturers who graciously shared their data.

SOURCES OF DATA

◇

Values in this counter have been obtained from the Composition of Foods, United States Department of Agriculture, Agricultural Handbooks: No. 8-1, Dairy and Egg Products; No. 8-2, Spices and Herbs; No. 8-3, Baby Foods; No. 8-4, Fats and Oils; No. 8-5, Poultry Products; No. 8-6, Soups, Sauces and Gravies; No. 8-7, Sausages and Luncheon Meats; No. 8-8, Breakfast Cereals; No. 8-9, Fruit and Fruit Juices; No. 8-10, Pork Products; No. 8-11, Vegetables and Vegetable Products; No. 8-12, Nut and Seed Products; No. 8-13, Beef Products; No. 8-14, Beverages; No. 8-15, Finfish and Shellfish Products; No. 8-16, Legumes and Legume Products; No. 8-17, Lamb, Veal and Game Products; No. 8-19, Snacks and Sweets; No. 8-20, Cereal Grains and Pasta; No. 8-21, Fast Foods; Supplements 1989, 1990, 1991.

"Nutritive Value of Foods," United States Department of Agriculture, Home and Garden Bulletin No. 72.

J. Davies and J. Dickerson, *Nutrient Content of Food Portions.* Cambridge, UK: The Royal Society of Chemistry, 1991.

G. A. Leveille, M. E. Zabik, K. J. Morgan, *Nutrients in Foods.* Cambridge, Mass.: The Nutrition Guild, 1983.

A. Moller, E. Saxholt, B. E. Mikkelsen, Food Composition Table: Amino Acids, Carbohydrates and Fatty Acids in Danish Foods, 1991.

Souci, Fachmann, Kraut, Food Composition and Nutrition Tables. Stuttgart: Wissenschaftliche Verlagsgesellschaft MbH, 1989.

Information from food labels, manufacturers and processors. The values are based on research conducted through 1995. Manufactures' ingredients are subject to change, so current values may vary from those listed in the book.

"If only half a dozen foods were available, the matter would be quickly settled."

MARY SWARTZ ROSE, PH.D.
Feeding the Family
The Macmillan Company, 1919

INTRODUCTION

◇

What Is Cholesterol?

High Cholesterol is a major risk factor for heart disease.

High Cholesterol is a major risk factor for stroke.

High Cholesterol increases your risk of colon and rectal cancer.

High Cholesterol plus high blood pressure may cause hearing loss.

High Cholesterol, fat-rich diets may cause gallstones.

Did you know that every year 600,000 Americans die from coronary heart disease—heart attack and stroke? Heart attack and stroke disable even more people than they kill, more than the number of people who die from all forms of cancer! Coronary heart disease is a disease not only of the old. One out of five men has a heart attack before he is fifty. Often, a heart attack or stroke that causes death or disability is the first sign that something is wrong.

Research in the United States and many other countries shows that a high cholesterol level in the blood is one of the most important risk factors for heart disease. Lowering your cholesterol lowers your risk.

What is cholesterol?

Cholesterol is a white, waxy, fatlike substance that is part of every cell in your body. Cholesterol is important to body function. Hormones, nerve coverings, vitamin D, bile (used for digestion), and the fat that keeps your skin soft (sebum) are all made from cholesterol. Cholesterol makes up a major part of your brain. Cholesterol is needed by the body, but when the level of cholesterol in your blood gets too high, it's not healthy. Some of that extra cholesterol can be deposited on the walls of the arteries, narrowing them and interfering with normal blood flow.

Where does cholesterol come from?

We get some cholesterol every time we eat any animal foods. Meat, poultry, fish, eggs, milk, yogurt, cheese and butter are all animal foods and contain cholesterol. Egg yolk is a major source of cholesterol. An average yolk contains about 213 milligrams. The egg white does not have any cholesterol. Caviar and organ meats like liver, heart and brains are very high in cholesterol.

There is no cholesterol in any food that grows in the ground. Vegetable oils, peanut butter, vegetables, fruits, cereals and grains contain no cholesterol.

Cholesterol is also made in the body. In fact most people make three times as much cholesterol as they get in the food they eat.

How do I know if my blood cholesterol is too high?

Surveys show that the percentage of Americans who have had their cholesterol level checked rose from 35 percent in 1983 to 65 percent in 1990. The National Cholesterol Education Program recommends that all adults over age twenty have their total and high-density lipoprotein (HDL) cholesterol level measured at least once every five years and keep track of their numbers.

Blood cholesterol is measured in milligrams. A milligram is one thousandth of a gram. The number of milligrams of cholesterol in a deciliter (dL), which is a little less than one-half cup, is the ratio used to measure the cholesterol level in the blood. When describing the cholesterol level of the blood, usually just the number is given, such as 180, rather than the more complete 180 milligrams per dL. For simplicity, all cholesterol measurements in the following pages are given as numbers without the mg/dL abbreviation.

For adults, a range from 150 to 200 milligrams is best. A cholesterol level over 200 is considered too high. If your cholesterol is above 200, your risk for heart disease and other problems is increased. The Centers for Disease Control of the National Center for Health Statistics reports that average blood cholesterol levels have declined from 1978 to 1990, with the average falling from 213 to 205. The average low-density lipoprotein (LDL) cholesterol levels fell from 136 to 128. Even so, 20 percent of Americans have very high cholesterol levels—over 240. And as many as 29 percent need diet changes to lower their cholesterol.

CLASSIFICATIONS OF CHOLESTEROL VALUES IN ADULTS*

Total Cholesterol

less than 200 mg/dl	Desirable Blood Cholesterol
200 to 239 mg/dl	Borderline High Blood Cholesterol
240 mg/dl and over	High Blood Cholesterol

HDL Cholesterol

less than 35 mg/dl	Low HDL Cholesterol

*National Institutes of Health, National Heart, Lung and Blood Institute, Detection, Evaluation, and Treatment of High Blood Cholesterol in Adults, 1993 Publication No. 93-3095.

What is the difference between good cholesterol and bad cholesterol?

Cholesterol is coated with protein so it can travel in the blood. These packages of protein, cholesterol and other fats are called "lipoproteins." Two kinds of lipoproteins are low-density lipoprotein (LDL) and high-density lipoprotein (HDL).

LDLs contain large amounts of cholesterol and may deposit this cholesterol on the artery walls. That is why LDL cholesterol is called "bad" cholesterol. Levels of LDL cholesterol above 130 milligrams are considered unhealthy.

HDLs contain small amounts of cholesterol and are believed to take the cholesterol away from the cells in the artery walls and carry it to the liver, where it is processed and removed from the body. That is why HDL cholesterol is called "good" cholesterol. People with higher levels of HDL cholesterol have less heart disease. Levels of HDL cholesterol under 35 milligrams are considered too low.

We are often asked, "What foods contain 'good cholesterol'?" Cholesterol in foods is simply cholesterol and is converted to LDL cholesterol (bad cholesterol) and HDL cholesterol (good cholesterol) after it is eaten. LDL cholesterol and HDL cholesterol refer to forms of cholesterol in your body, not the form of cholesterol in the food you eat.

If my cholesterol is higher than 200, what should I do?

In late 1987 the federal government, along with more than twenty health organizations, issued guidelines to help identify and treat people whose blood cholesterol levels were too high. This affected one in four Americans.

People with desirable cholesterol levels, under 200, were advised to recheck their level every five years.

People with levels above 200 milligrams were advised to go

on a cholesterol-lowering diet that is low in cholesterol, fats and saturated fats.

Many foods are high in all three—cholesterol, fats and saturated fats. By lowering your intake of high cholesterol foods, you reduce your intake of other fats as well and lower your risk of heart disease.

For each 1 percent decrease in blood cholesterol level, you reduce your risk of heart disease by 2 percent. Even the smallest change is to your benefit.

The ratio of total cholesterol to HDL cholesterol has been found to be the best predictor of increased coronary risk, especially in those under age sixty. You can figure your own risk level by dividing your total cholesterol (TC) value by your HDL cholesterol. For example, if your TC is 250 and HDL is 50, the average ratio of TC/HDL is 5. This is considered average risk but is actually not very healthy. A ratio of 9.6 indicates twice the average risk of coronary heart disease, while a ratio of 2.5 signals half the risk.

How much cholesterol should I eat each day?

The National Cholesterol Education Program recommends no more than 300 milligrams of cholesterol a day for everyone over the age of two. In the government guidelines for lowering cholesterol, the Step 1 diet for those whose cholesterol level is 200 to 239 recommends eating less than 300 milligrams of cholesterol a day. Those people whose cholesterol level is 240 or higher are advised to restrict their cholesterol intake to less than 200 milligrams per day.

GUIDELINES FOR CHOLESTEROL INTAKE*

Cholesterol Level In the Blood	MG of Cholesterol You Can Eat Each Day
less than 200 mg/dl	300 mg or less
200 to 239 mg/dl	less than 300 mg
240 mg and over/dl	less than 200 mg

*Adapted from material provided by the National Cholesterol Education Program, Second Report, National Heart, Lung and Blood Institute, National Institutes of Health 1993.

What about taking drugs to lower my cholesterol?

Some people who have a high cholesterol level may not be able to lower it enough by diet changes alone. They may need to use a drug in addition to making changes in the way they eat. Drugs used most often are cholestyramine, colestipol, niacin and lovastatin. The following are some blood cholesterol-lowering drugs.

Cholestyramine (Questran) and colestipol (Colestid) are resins that increase the excretion of cholesterol from the body. Major side effects are constipation, bloating and gas. They are unpleasant to take.

Niacin (nicotinic acid, a B vitamin) causes intense flushing and itching of the skin right after you take it. Major side effects are rashes and upset stomach. It can worsen diabetes and gout.

Statins, a family of drugs, are considered effective and safe.

Lovastatin (Mevacor) a drug, approved by the FDA in 1987, the more recently approved Sinvostatin (Zocor) and Pravastatin (Pravachol) are well tolerated by most people. The most common side effects are mild gastrointestinal disturbances which subside as therapy continues.

Probucol (Lorelco) and gemfibrozil (Lopid) are reserved for use when diet and other medications are not effective.

What about cholesterol levels in children?

It is recommended that children and adolescents be screened for their blood cholesterol levels if there is a family history of heart disease. If parents have high blood cholesterol levels or if grandparents had heart disease before age fifty-five, children should be checked.

CLASSIFICATIONS OF VALUES FOR CHOLESTEROL IN CHILDREN*

Acceptable	less than 170
Borderline	170 to 199
High	equal to or greater than 200

*Report of the Expert Panel on Blood Cholesterol Levels in Children and Adolescents, US Department of Health and Human Services, Public Health Service, National Institutes of Health, Sept. 1991, Publication N. 91-2732.

According to the 1987–88 Nationwide Food Consumption Survey children and adolescents eat 193 to 296 milligrams of cholesterol daily. This is in line with the recommendation of less than 300 milligrams daily.

FACTS ON FIBER

While you are eating less cholesterol to lower its level in your blood, try eating more fiber. Besides helping to fill you up with fewer calories, fiber itself helps cholesterol levels go down. And that's not all. Fiber is believed to help prevent breast and colon cancer, normalize blood sugar levels and help your digestive tract function by preventing constipation.

Animal foods like meat, chicken, milk and cheese do not contain any fiber. Fiber is found in food plants like whole grains, beans, brown rice, dried fruit, vegetables and fruits. Because fiber is not digested and absorbed, it interferes with fat absorption in the intestine. The result is that there is less fat available to raise your blood cholesterol level. There is also less fat available to make you fat!

There are actually two types of fiber: soluble and insoluble. The first dissolves in water and the second doesn't. Both types fill you up, but each one has special health benefits. Soluble fiber helps lower cholesterol, other blood fats and blood sugar. The best food sources of soluble fiber are apples, barley, beans, carrots, grapefruit, oats, oranges, peas, rice bran and strawberries.

Insoluble fiber comes from the hard outer shell of grains and some is found in most fruits and vegetables. It bulks up your stools, helping to prevent or cure constipation, and also is believed to help prevent breast and colon cancer. Wheat bran, celery, corn bran, green beans, green leafy vegetables, potato skins and whole grains are all good sources of insoluble fiber.

The American Dietetic Association, National Cancer Institute and other experts recommend fiber intake of 20 to 30 or even 35 grams a day. To reach this level you would need to eat 3 to 5 servings of whole grain bread and cereals, 3 servings of fruit, and 3 servings of vegetables a day. Most Americans are not eating that much; fiber intake averages only 10 to 20 grams a day.

Start adding more fiber to your diet slowly so that your body can adjust to it. And don't go overboard. Excess intake of fiber—50 to 60 grams a day—can displace other non-fiber foods that contain needed nutrients and may block the absorption of vital minerals like iron, zinc, calcium and magnesium.

Children, too, benefit from fiber in their diet. The American Academy of Pediatrics Committee on Nutrition recommends 0.5 gram of fiber for each kilogram (2.2 pounds) of body weight, not to exceed 35 grams a day. A forty-pound child would need 10 grams of fiber a day, while 15 to 20 grams is right for teens.

Add Some Fiber to Your Life

1. Bran or fiber pills are not necessary. It's healthier to get fiber in your food.
2. Eat whole fruits and vegetables instead of drinking their juices.
3. Enjoy the fiber-rich skins of apples, pears and potatoes.
4. Choose whole grains like whole wheat spaghetti and bread, brown rice, oats and cracked wheat whenever you can.
5. Enjoy beans, lentils and dried split peas. They are beginning to appear on restaurant menus and salad bars.
6. Try soybeans or one of its forms—soynuts or tempeh—for an interesting food or snack.
7. Dried fruits and raisins are favorites, and you'll enjoy some of the more unusual kinds like papaya and persimmon.
8. If you still need an occasional laxative, try a psyllium seed type like Metamucil. Psyllium seeds are rich in fiber.

Count Up Your Cholesterol

Most of us eat too much cholesterol each day. We eat on the run and pick foods high in fat. By the end of the day we've eaten too much cholesterol.

You know that you shouldn't be eating a lot of cholesterol. You want to cut back. But it's not easy since you are not really sure which foods are high in cholesterol and which foods are not. With *The Cholesterol Counter* it's simple to find out which foods have cholesterol and to reduce the amount you eat.

Let's look at a typical day. Are the food choices familiar? Let's see just how much cholesterol this sample day contains and how we can reduce the amount with better food choices.

CHOLESTEROL COUNTING

A SAMPLE DAY OF FOOD CHOICES

Breakfast	CHOLESTEROL (MG)
Orange juice (½ cup)	0
Scrambled egg (w/ milk & margarine)	215
Bacon (2 slices)	27
Toast (1 slice)	0
Butter (1 tsp)	11
Coffee &	0
Half & half (1 tbsp)	6

Lunch	
Double cheeseburger with bun	110
Ketchup	0
French fries	0
Vanilla shake (10 oz)	32

Snack	
Pound cake (1 slice)	25
Coffee &	0
Half & half (1 tbsp)	6

Dinner	
Batter dipped fried chicken w/ skin (½ breast)	119
Baked potato &	0
Sour cream (2 tbsp)	10
Tossed salad &	0
Blue cheese dressing (2 tbsp.)	10
Chocolate pudding cup	5
Tea &	0
Sugar	0

TV Snack	
Rich vanilla ice cream (1 cup)	90
TOTAL CHOLESTEROL	666

This is too much cholesterol for one day—more than twice the recommended level of 300 milligrams a day. Now you can see how easy it is to take in more cholesterol than you need.

CHOLESTEROL COUNTING

A SAMPLE DAY OF BETTER FOOD CHOICES

	CHOLESTEROL (MG)
Breakfast	
Orange juice (½ cup)	0
All Bran &	0
Lowfat milk, 1% (½ cup)	5
Toast (1 slice) &	0
Jelly	0
Coffee &	0
Lowfat milk (2 tbsp)	1
Lunch	
Hamburger with bun	71
Ketchup	0
French fries	0
Cola	0
Snack	
Fat-free pound cake (1 slice)	0
Coffee &	0
Lowfat milk (1 tbsp)	tr
Dinner	
Roasted chicken breast, no skin (½ breast)	73
Baked potato &	0
Plain lowfat yogurt (2 tbsp or 1 oz)	2
Tossed salad &	0
Oil & vinegar dressing (2 tbsp)	0
Lemon pudding cup	0
Tea &	0
Sugar	0
TV Snack	
Vanilla light (1 cup)	18
TOTAL CHOLESTEROL	**170**

Better food choices! A much healthier intake of cholesterol for the day. Check your fiber values regularly. Aim for 20 to 30 grams a day.

Now it's your turn to *count your cholesterol*. Note everything you eat today, then look up the amount of cholesterol in each food you have eaten and see how much cholesterol you had. While you're at it, jot down the calories too! Don't forget to count up your fiber at least once a week.

CHOLESTEROL COUNTING:
A SAMPLE WORKSHEET FOOD AMOUNT

FOOD	PORTION	CALS.	FIB.	CHOL.

Breakfast

Snack

Lunch

Snack

Dinner

Snack

Total   Cholesterol ____ Calories ____ Fiber ____

Did your cholesterol total more than 300 milligrams for the day? If it did, you need to start counting cholesterol and making better food choices. What about fiber? Did you reach the target of 20 to 30 grams?

Ten Steps to Lower Cholesterol

1. Use liquid vegetable oils. Choose olive, canola, corn, soybean, sunflower, safflower and cottonseed oils.
2. Limit amount of meat eaten. Do not use liver, brains, or other organ meats. Poultry, shellfish and other fish also should be eaten in small portions.
3. Use lean cuts of meat; trim off all visible fat. Cook without added fat. Bake, broil or roast to further reduce fat. Remove skin from poultry and fish.
4. Use more beans, grains, pasta, rice and vegetables to make up for the smaller portions of meat, fish and poultry.
5. Avoid coffee whiteners (nondairy creamers) and whipped toppings.
6. Limit eggs to four a week, including those used in cooking and desserts. Two egg whites can be substituted for one egg.
7. Use lowfat or nonfat milk and cheese, yogurt, ice cream and fat-free sour cream. Avoid butter, cream, rich ice cream, regular sour cream and whole milk.
8. When using margarine, salad dressing or gravy, use a teaspoon or tablespoon to measure out a portion.
9. Eat fiber-rich foods: beans, whole grains, bran, brown rice, dried fruits, fruits and vegetables.
10. Substitute soy foods—soynuts, tofu, soymilk, soy yogurt—often. Soy protein lowers cholesterol.

Using Your Cholesterol Counter

This book lists the cholesterol and calorie content of over 18,000 foods. For the first time, cholesterol and fiber values are at your fingertips. Now you will find it easy to follow a low-cholesterol diet.

Before *The Cholesterol Counter* it was impossible to compare how much cholesterol there was in foods. Fresh foods like meat, chicken, fish and cheese do not even have a label. The same goes for take-out items like potato salad, coleslaw, quiche, or foods bought at the bakery. How could you tell how much cholesterol there is in a burger or taco that you enjoy at the local fast-food restaurant? *The Cholesterol Counter* lists them all!

The fourth edition is divided into two main sections. Part I, Brand-Name and Generic Foods, lists foods alphabetically. For each group, you will find brand-name foods listed first in alphabetical order, followed by an alphabetical listing of non-branded foods. Large categories are divided into subcategories—canned, fresh, frozen, ready-to-use—to make it even easier to find what you are looking for.

If you want to know how much cholesterol is in the hamburger you are having for lunch: look under HAMBURGER, where you will find all kinds of hamburgers listed, or, if you are making a homemade hamburger, look under ROLL, where you will find the hamburger roll listed alphabetically, and under BEEF, where you will find a cooked chopped beef patty. For foods like FRENCH TOAST, HONEY or SALAD DRESSING, simply look for the specific food alphabetically in the complete listing. For example, FRENCH TOAST is listed alphabetically between FRENCH BEANS and FROG'S LEGS. One slice has about 75 milligrams of cholesterol.

If you are eating at home, simply look up the individual foods you are eating and total the cholesterol for the meal. For example, your dinner may consist of:

	CHOLESTEROL (MG)
2 rib lamb chops, broiled	156
Broccoli w/Cheese Sauce, ½ cup (Birds Eye)	6
Long Grain & Wild Rice, ½ cup (Minute Rice)	10

Pecan Pie (Mrs. Smith's), 1 slice	30
Glass of red wine	0
TOTAL CHOLESTEROL FOR THE MEAL	202

If you are eating out, most food categories will have a take-out subcategory. Items found in the take-out subcategory will help you estimate the cholesterol, fiber and calories in similar restaurant or take-out menu items. For example, if you order spaghetti and meatballs look under PASTA DINNERS.

Most foods are listed alphabetically. But in some cases, foods are grouped by category. For example, all pasta dishes, like spaghetti and meat balls, lasagna and fettucini are found under the category PASTA DINNERS.

Other group categories include:

DINNER	page 174
includes all frozen dinners by brand name	
ICE CREAM AND FROZEN DESSERTS	page 233
includes all dairy and nondairy ice cream and frozen novelties, except ices, sherbet and sorbet	
LIQUOR/LIQUEUR	page 262
includes all alcoholic beverages except beer, champagne, malt and wine	
LUNCHEON MEATS/COLD CUTS	page 264
includes all sandwich meats except chicken, ham and turkey	
NUTRITIONAL SUPPLEMENTS	page 290
includes all meal replacements, diet aids and fortified drinks	
ORIENTAL FOOD	page 302
includes all Oriental-type foods	
SAUCE	page 397
includes all varieties from Alfredo to Worcestershire	

Part II, Restaurant, Take-Out and Fast-Food Chains, contains an alphabetical listing of over 60 popular chains. Fast foods like BURGER KING, DOMINO'S PIZZA, TACO BELL and WENDY'S are listed alphabetically under the chain's name.

We have tried to include all foods for which cholesterol values are known. There will be some foods, however, that are not listed in *The Cholesterol Counter* because the cholesterol values are not available for that particular food.

When you can't locate your favorite brand, look at similar foods. You will probably find a brand-name food, a generic product or a take-out item that is like your favorite food.

With *The Cholesterol Counter* as your guide, you will never again wonder how much cholesterol is in food. You will always be able to tell if a food is high, moderate, or low in cholesterol. *Your goal is to pick low cholesterol foods each time you eat.*

Finding cholesterol in the foods you eat

When you know the ingredients in a food you can tell if that food contains cholesterol. Read the ingredient list on the label or, if you are using a home recipe, read through the recipe ingredients. To find cholesterol-containing ingredients you need only remember these two simple rules:

If it grows in the ground, the food does not contain cholesterol.

If it has feet, fins, wings or claws and can walk, swim or fly, the food does contain cholesterol.

Try out the rules. Which of the following foods have cholesterol?

Hamburger
Sardines
Lobster

> Chicken leg
> Cheddar cheese
> Milk
> Egg
> Peanut butter
> Apple
> Olive oil

The first seven foods all contain cholesterol. Hamburger comes from a steer. Sardines and lobster are seafood. Chicken leg comes from a chicken. All of these have either feet, fins, wings or claws. Therefore, they all contain cholesterol. Cheddar cheese, milk and egg have cholesterol because they all come from an animal that has feet.

Peanut butter, apples and olive oil are all from plants that grow in the ground. Therefore, they have no cholesterol.

Now you know why all of the ingredients on the following list have cholesterol. These are the ingredients to look for on a label or in a recipe.

Ingredients that Contain Cholesterol

whole eggs	bacon or bacon fat
egg yolks	butter
whole milk	lard
lowfat milk	chicken fat
cream	beef suet or tallow
ice cream	liver
sour cream (unless labeled fat-free)	kidney
	brains
yogurt (unless labeled nonfat)	meat (any variety)
	fish (any variety)
cheese (unless labeled nonfat)	poultry (any variety)

Some packaged foods that do not contain any cholesterol suggest adding ingredients that do contain cholesterol when you prepare the food. For example, instant mashed potatoes made with potato granules do not contain any cholesterol. The package directions, however, tell you to add butter and milk. *Both are sources of cholesterol.* By adding butter and milk, you add cholesterol to the mashed potatoes, so each one-half-cup serving contains over 10 milligrams of cholesterol. To cut down on the cholesterol in the instant mashed potatoes, use margarine and skim milk.

DEFINITIONS

———◇———

as prep (as prepared): refers to food that has been prepared according to package directions.

home recipe: describes homemade dishes; those included can be used as a guide to the cholesterol and calorie values of similar products you may prepare or take-out food you buy ready-to-eat

lean and fat: describes meat with some fat on its edges that is not cut away before cooking or poultry prepared with skin and fat as purchased

lean only: lean portion, trimmed of all visible fat

shelf stable: refers to prepared products found on the supermarket shelf that are ready to be heated and do not require refrigeration

take-out: describes prepared dishes that you purchase ready-to-eat; those included serve as a guide to the cholesterol and calorie values of similar products you may purchase

trace (tr): value used when a food contains less than one calorie, less than one milligram of cholesterol, or less than 1 gram of fiber.

ABBREVIATIONS

—◇—

avg	=	average
diam	=	diameter
frzn	=	frozen
g	=	gram
in	=	inch
lb	=	pound
lg	=	large
med	=	medium
mg	=	milligram
oz	=	ounce
pkg	=	package
pt	=	pint
prep	=	prepared
qt	=	quart
reg	=	regular
sm	=	small
sq	=	square
tbsp	=	tablespoon
tr	=	trace
tsp	=	teaspoon
w/	=	with
w/o	=	without
<	=	less than

EQUIVALENT MEASURES

—◇—

Dry

3 teaspoons	=	1 tablespoon
4 tablespoons	=	¼ cup
8 tablespoons	=	½ cup
12 tablespoons	=	¾ cup
16 tablespoons	=	1 cup
1000 milligrams	=	1 gram
28 grams	=	1 ounce
4 ounces	=	¼ pound
8 ounces	=	½ pound
12 ounces	=	¾ pound
16 ounces	=	1 pound

Liquid

2 tablespoons	=	1 ounce
2 ounces	=	¼ cup
4 ounces	=	½ cup
6 ounces	=	¾ cup
8 ounces	=	1 cup
2 cups	=	1 pint
4 cups	=	1 quart

NOTES

—◇—

Discrepancies in figures are due to rounding, product reformulation and reevaluation.

Throughout the *Counter* portion of this book Cal indicates calories, Chol indicates cholesterol and Fib indicates fiber.

ALL CHOLESTEROL VALUES ARE GIVEN IN MILLIGRAMS (MG)

ALL FIBER VALUES ARE GIVEN IN GRAMS (G)

A DASH (—) INDICATES DATA NOT AVAILABLE

PART · I

BRAND-NAME

AND

GENERIC FOODS

FOOD	PORTION	CALS.	FIB.	CHOL.
ABALONE				
fresh fried	3 oz	161	—	80
raw	3 oz	89	—	72
ACEROLA				
FRESH				
acerola	1	2	—	0
ACEROLA JUICE				
juice	1 cup	51	—	0
ADZUKI BEANS				
CANNED				
Eden				
Organic	½ cup (4.1 oz)	100	5	0
sweetened	1 cup	702	—	0
DRIED				
cooked	1 cup	294	—	0
READY-TO-USE				
yokan sliced	3¼ in slices	112	—	0
AKEE				
fresh	3½ oz	223	—	0
ALE				
(see BEER AND ALE, AND MALT)				
ALFALFA				
sprouts	1 tbsp	1	—	0
sprouts	1 cup	40	—	0
ALLIGATOR				
tail cooked	3½ oz	143	—	65
ALLSPICE				
ground	1 tsp	5	—	0
ALMONDS				
Beer Nuts				
Almonds	1 pkg (1 oz)	180	—	0
Dole				
Blanched Slivered	1 oz	170	—	0
Blanched Whole	1 oz	170	—	0
Chopped Natural	1 oz	170	—	0
Sliced Natural	1 oz	170	—	0
Whole Natural	1 oz	170	—	0
Erewhon				
Almond Butter	1 tbsp (16 g)	90	—	0

FOOD	PORTION	CALS.	FIB.	CHOL.
Hain				
Almond Butter Natural Raw	2 tbsp	190	—	0
Almond Butter Toasted	2 tbsp	220	—	0
Lance				
Smoked	1 pkg (0.7 oz)	120	—	0
Nutella	1 tbsp (0.5 oz)	85	—	0
Planters				
Almonds	1 oz	170	—	0
Honey Roasted	1 oz	170	—	0
Sliced	1 oz	170	—	0
Slivered	1 oz	170	—	0
almond butter honey & cinnamon	1 tbsp	96	—	0
almond butter w/ salt	1 tbsp	101	—	0
almond butter w/o salt	1 tbsp	101	—	0
almond meal	1 oz	116	—	0
almond paste	1 oz	127	—	0
dried blanched	1 oz	166	—	0
dried unblanched	1 oz	167	—	0
dry roasted unblanched	1 oz	167	—	0
dry roasted unblanched salted	1 oz	167	—	0
oil roasted blanched	1 oz	174	3	0
oil roasted blanched salted	1 oz	174	—	0
oil roasted unblanched	1 oz	176	—	0
toasted unblanched	1 oz	167	3	0

AMARANTH

(see also CEREAL, COOKIES)

FOOD	PORTION	CALS.	FIB.	CHOL.
Arrowhead				
Seeds	¼ cup (1.6 oz)	170	3	0
Health Valley				
Amaranth Cereal With Bananas	½ cup (1 oz)	110	4	0
Amaranth Crunch With Raisins	¼ cup (1 oz)	110	3	0
Amaranth Flakes 100% Organic	½ cup (1 oz)	90	3	0
Fast Menu Amaranth With Garden Vegetables	7½ oz	140	8	0
cooked	½ cup	59	—	0
uncooked	½ cup	366	—	0

ANASAZI BEANS

DRIED

FOOD	PORTION	CALS.	FIB.	CHOL.
Arrowhead	¼ cup (1.5 oz)	150	9	0
Bean Cuisine	½ cup	115	5	0

ANISE

FOOD	PORTION	CALS.	FIB.	CHOL.
seed	1 tsp	7	—	0

FOOD	PORTION	CALS.	FIB.	CHOL.
ANTELOPE				
roasted	3 oz	127	—	107
APPLE				
CANNED				
White House				
Escalloped Apples	4 oz	120	1	0
Sliced	4 oz	55	1	0
Spiced Apple Rings	1 ring	25	tr	0
sliced sweetened	1 cup	136	—	0
DRIED				
Del Monte				
Sliced	⅓ cup (1.4 oz)	80	5	0
Mariani	¼ cup	150	—	0
cooked w/ sugar	½ cup	116	—	0
cooked w/o sugar	½ cup	172	—	0
rings	10	155	—	0
FRESH				
Dole	1	80	5	0
apple	1	81	3	0
w/o skin sliced	1 cup	62	2	0
w/o skin sliced & cooked	1 cup	91	—	0
w/o skin sliced & microwaved	1 cup	96	—	0
FROZEN				
Mrs. Paul's				
Apple Fritters	2	270	—	5
sliced w/o sugar	½ cup	41	—	0
APPLE JUICE				
Apple & Eve	6 fl oz	80	—	0
Cider	6 fl oz	80	—	0
Nothin' But Juice	6 fl oz	78	—	0
Bruce				
Lite	½ cup	88	—	0
Hi-C				
Jammin' Apple	8 fl oz	130	—	0
Hood				
Select Cider	1 cup (8 oz)	120	—	0
Juice Works	6 oz	100	—	0
Minute Maid				
Box	8.45 fl oz	120	—	0
Jucies To Go	1 bottle (16 fl oz)	110	—	0
Juices To Go	1 can (11.5 fl oz)	160	—	0
Juices To Go	1 bottle (10 fl oz)	140	—	0
Naturals	8 fl oz	110	—	0

FOOD	PORTION	CALS.	FIB.	CHOL.
Mott's				
From Concentrate as prep	8 fl oz	120	0	0
Fruit Basket Cocktail as prep	8 fl oz	120	0	0
Natural	8 fl oz	120	0	0
Ocean Spray	8 fl oz	110	0	0
Odwalla				
Live Apple	8 fl oz	140	0	0
Red Cheek				
From Concentrate	8 fl oz	120	0	0
Natural	8 fl oz	120	0	0
S&W				
100% Unsweetened	6 oz	85	—	0
Seneca				
Clarifed frzn, as prep	8 fl oz	120	0	0
Granny Smith frzn as prep	8 fl oz	120	0	0
Natural frzn as prep	8 fl oz	120	0	0
Sippin' Pak				
100% Pure	8.45 fl oz	110	—	0
Sipps	8.45 oz	130	—	0
Snapple				
Apple Crisp	10 fl oz	140	—	0
Tree Of Life				
East Coast Apple	8 fl oz	120	—	0
Tree Top				
Cider	6 oz	90	—	0
Cider frzn as prep	6 oz	90	—	0
Frzn, as prep	6 oz	90	—	0
Sparkling Juice	6 oz	90	—	0
Unfiltered	6 oz	90	—	0
Unfiltered frzn as prep	6 oz	90	—	0
w/ Vitamin C	6 oz	90	—	0
Tropicana				
Season's Best	1 container (10 fl oz)	140	—	0
Season's Best	1 bottle (7 fl oz)	100	—	0
Season's Best	8 fl oz	110	—	0
Season's Best	1 bottle (10 fl oz)	140	—	0
Season's Best	1 container (6 fl oz)	80	—	0
Season's Best	1 container (8 fl oz)	110	—	0
Season's Best	1 can (11.5 fl oz)	160	—	0
Veryfine				
100%	8 oz	107	—	0

FOOD	PORTION	CALS.	FIB.	CHOL.
White House	6 oz	90	0	0
frzn as prep	1 cup	111	—	0
frzn not prep	6 oz	349	—	0
juice	1 cup	116	tr	0

APPLESAUCE

FOOD	PORTION	CALS.	FIB.	CHOL.
Eden	½ cup (4.3 oz)	50	2	0
Mott's				
Chunky	5 oz	110	2	0
Cinnamon	5 oz	120	1	0
Fruit Snacks Apple Spice	4 oz	70	1	0
Fruit Snacks Cinnamon	4 oz	90	1	0
Fruit Snacks Strawberry	4 oz	80	1	0
Fruit Snacks Sweetened	4 oz	90	1	0
Sweetened	5 oz	110	1	0
S&W				
Diet	½ cup	55	—	0
Gravenstein Sweetened	½ cup	90	—	0
Gravenstein Unsweetened	½ cup	55	—	0
Sweetened	½ cup	55	—	0
Seneca				
Cinnamon	½ cup	100	3	0
Golden Delicious	½ cup	100	3	0
McIntosh	½ cup	100	3	0
Natural	½ cup	60	3	0
Regular	½ cup	100	3	0
Tree Of Life	½ cup (4.3 oz)	50	2	0
Tree Top				
Cinnamon	½ cup	80	—	0
Natural	½ cup	60	—	0
Original	½ cup	80	—	0
White House				
Chunky	4 oz	800	1	0
Cinnamon	4 oz	100	1	0
Natural Packed w/ Apple Juice	4 oz	60	1	0
Regular	4 oz	80	1	0
Unsweetened	4 oz	50	2	0
sweetened	½ cup	97	2	0
unsweetened	½ cup	53	2	0

APRICOT JUICE

FOOD	PORTION	CALS.	FIB.	CHOL.
Del Monte				
Nectar	8 fl oz	140	1	0
Kern's				
Nectar	6 fl oz	110	—	0

FOOD	PORTION	CALS.	FIB.	CHOL.
Libby				
Nectar	1 can (11.5 fl oz)	220	—	0
S&W				
Nectar	6 oz	35	—	0
nectar	1 cup	141	2	0

APRICOTS
CANNED
Del Monte

FOOD	PORTION	CALS.	FIB.	CHOL.
Halves Unpeeled In Heavy Syrup	½ cup (4.5 oz)	100	1	0
Halves Unpeeled Lite	½ cup (4.3 oz)	60	1	0
Libby				
Halves Unpeeled Lite	½ cup (4.4 oz)	60	1	0
S&W				
Halves Diet	½ cup	35	—	0
Halves Unpeeled In Heavy Syrup	½ cup	110	—	0
Halves Unsweetened	½ cup	35	—	0
Whole Peeled Diet	½ cup	28	—	0
Whole Peeled In Heavy Syrup	½ cup	100	—	0
halves heavy syrup pack w/ skin	1 cup (9.1 oz)	214	—	0
halves water pack w/ skin	1 cup (8.5 oz)	65	—	0
halves water pack w/o skin	1 cup (8 oz)	51	—	0
heavy syrup w/ skin	3 halves	70	—	0
juice pack w/ skin	3 halves	40	—	0
light syrup w/ skin	3 halves	54	—	0
puree juice pack w/ skin	1 cup (8.7 oz)	119	—	0
puree from heavy syrup pack w/ skin	¾ cup (9.1 oz)	214	—	0
puree from light pack w/ skin	¾ cup (8.9 oz)	160	—	0
puree from water pack w/ skin	¾ cup (8.5 oz)	65	—	0
water pack w/ skin	3 halves	22	—	0
water pack w/o skin	4 halves	20	—	0

DRIED
Del Monte

FOOD	PORTION	CALS.	FIB.	CHOL.
Sun Dried	⅓ cup (1.4 oz)	80	6	0
Mariani				
halves	¼ cup	140	—	0
halves	10	83	3	0
halves cooked w/o sugar	½ c	106	—	0

FRESH

FOOD	PORTION	CALS.	FIB.	CHOL.
apricots	3	51	—	0

FROZEN

FOOD	PORTION	CALS.	FIB.	CHOL.
sweetened	½ cup	119	—	0

FOOD	PORTION	CALS.	FIB.	CHOL.
ARROWHEAD				
fresh boiled	1 med (⅓ oz)	9	—	0
ARROWROOT				
flour	1 cup	457	4	0
ARTICHOKE				
CANNED				
S&W				
Hearts Marinated	½ cup	225	—	0
FRESH				
Dole	1 lg	23	3	0
boiled	1 med (4 oz)	60	—	0
hearts cooked	½ cup	42	—	0
sunchoke raw sliced	½ cup	57	—	0
FROZEN				
Birds Eye				
Hearts Deluxe	½ cup	30	3	0
cooked	1 pkg (9 oz)	108	—	0
ARUGULA				
raw	½ cup	2	—	0
ASPARAGUS				
CANNED				
Del Monte				
Salad Tips Tender Green	½ cup (4.4 oz)	20	1	0
Spears Cut Tender Green	½ cup (4.4 oz)	20	1	0
Spears Extra Long Tender Green	½ cup (4.4 oz)	20	1	0
Spears Tender Green	½ cup (4.4 oz)	20	1	0
Tips Tender Green	½ cup (4.4 oz)	20	1	0
Owatonna				
Spears Cut	½ cup	20	—	0
S&W				
Points Water Pack	½ cup	17	—	0
Spears Colossal Fancy	½ cup	20	—	0
Spears Fancy	½ cup	18	—	0
Seneca	½ cup	20	2	0
spears	½ cup	24	—	0
FRESH				
Dole	5 spears	18	2	0
cooked	4 spears	14	—	0
cooked	½ cup	22	—	0
raw	4 spears	14	—	0
raw	½ cup	16	—	0

FOOD	PORTION	CALS.	FIB.	CHOL.
FROZEN				
Big Valley	5-6 spears (3 oz)	20	1	0
Birds Eye				
Cut	½ cup	23	—	0
Spears	½ cup	25	—	0
Green Giant				
Harvest Fresh Cuts	½ cup	25	2	0
cooked	1 pkg (10 oz)	82	—	0
cooked	4 spears	17	—	0

AVOCADO

FOOD	PORTION	CALS.	FIB.	CHOL.
FRESH				
California				
Avocado	½	153	—	0
Avocado, mashed	1 cup	407	—	0
avocado	1	324	—	0
puree	1 cup	370	—	0

BABY FOOD

(Nutritional guidelines for infants are different from those recommended for older children and adults. Check with a pediatrician for advice on feeding children under the age of 2.)

FOOD	PORTION	CALS.	FIB.	CHOL.
CEREAL				
Earth's Best				
Brown Rice	5 tbsp (0.5 oz)	60	—	0
Mixed Grain	5 tbsp (0.5 oz)	60	—	0
Peach Oatmeal Banana	1 jar (4.5 fl oz)	60	—	0
Prunes & Oatmeal	1 jar (4.5 fl oz)	100	—	0
Gerber				
2nd Foods Rice With Applesauce & Bananas	1 jar (4 oz)	90	—	0
Health Valley				
Brown Rice 100% Organic	1 tbsp (0.5 oz)	60	1	0
Sprouted Baby Cereal 100% Organic	1 tbsp (0.5 oz)	60	—	0
DESSERT				
Gerber				
2nd Foods Banana Apple Dessert	1 jar (4 oz)	80	—	0
2nd Foods Cherry Vanilla Pudding	1 jar (4 oz)	80	—	0
2nd Foods Fruit Dessert	1 jar (4 oz)	100	—	0
DINNER				
Earth's Best				
Corn Rice & Cheese Dinner	1 jar (4.5 fl oz)	120	—	10

FOOD	PORTION	CALS.	FIB.	CHOL.
Earth's Best (CONT.)				
Macaroni & Cheese	1 jar (4.5 oz)	100	—	13
Pasta Dinner	1 jar (4.5 fl oz)	90	—	0
Potato & Green Bean Dinner	1 jar (4.5 fl oz)	100	—	10
Rice & Lentil Dinner	1 jar (4.5 fl oz)	80	—	7
Summer Vegetable Dinner	1 jar (4.5 oz)	90	—	0
FRUIT				
Beech-Nut				
Stage 1 Bananas Chiquita	1 jar (2.5 oz)	70	1	0
Stage 1 Peaches Yellow Cling	1 jar (2.5 oz)	45	2	0
Stage 1 Pears Bartlett	1 jar (2.5 oz)	50	2	0
Earth's Best				
Apples	1 jar (4.5 oz)	70	—	0
Apples & Apricots	1 jar (4.5 fl oz)	70	—	0
Apples & Blueberries	1 jar (4.5 fl oz)	70	—	0
Bananas	1 jar (4.5 oz)	90	—	0
Pear	1 jar (4.5 fl oz)	60	—	0
Plums Bananas & Rice	1 jar (4.5 fl oz)	90	—	0
Gerber				
1st Foods Applesauce	1 jar (2.5 oz)	25	—	0
1st Foods Bananas	1 jar (2.5 oz)	70	—	0
1st Foods Peaches	1 jar (2.5 oz)	30	—	0
1st Foods Pears	1 jar (2.5 oz)	40	—	0
1st Foods Prunes	1 jar (2.5 oz)	70	—	0
2nd Foods Apple Blueberry	1 jar (4 oz)	50	—	0
2nd Foods Applesauce	1 jar (4 oz)	60	—	0
2nd Foods Applesauce Apricot	1 jar (4 oz)	60	—	0
JUICE				
Beech-Nut				
Stage 2 Apple Banana	4 fl oz	70	0	0
Stage 2 Apple Cherry	4 fl oz	70	0	0
Stage 2 Apple Cranberry	4 fl oz	60	0	0
Stage 2 Apple Grape	4 fl oz	70	0	0
Stage 2 Juice Plus Grape	4 fl oz	100	0	0
Stage 2 Mango Nectar (Spanish label)	4 fl oz	80	0	0
Stage 2 Mixed Fruit	4 fl oz	70	0	0
Stage 2 Papaya Nectar (Spanish label)	4 fl oz	80	0	0
Stage 2 Tropical Blend	4 fl oz	90	0	0
Stage 2 Tropical Blend Nectar (Spanish label)	4 fl oz	90	0	0
Stage 3 Orange	4 fl oz	60	0	0

FOOD	PORTION	CALS.	FIB.	CHOL.
Earth's Best				
Apple	1 bottle (4.2 fl oz)	60	—	0
Apple Banana	1 bottle (4.2 fl oz)	60	—	0
Apple Grape	1 bottle (4.2 fl oz)	60	—	0
Apples & Bananas	1 jar (4.5 fl oz)	80	—	0
Pear	1 bottle (4.2 fl oz)	60	—	0
Gerber				
1st Foods Apple	4 fl oz	60	—	0
1st Foods Pear	4 fl oz	60	—	0
1st Foods Red Grape	4 fl oz	80	—	0
1st Foods White Grape	4 fl oz	80	—	0
2nd Foods Apple Banana	4 fl oz	60	—	0
2nd Foods Apple Cherry	4 fl oz	60	—	0
2nd Foods Apple Grape	4 fl oz	60	—	0
2nd Foods Apple Peach	4 fl oz	60	—	0
2nd Foods Apple Plum	4 fl oz	60	—	0
2nd Foods Apple Prune	4 fl oz	60	—	0
3rd Foods Apple Carrot	4 fl oz	50	—	0
3rd Foods Apple Sweet Potato	4 fl oz	60	—	0
3rd Foods Orange Carrot	4 fl oz	50	—	0
3rd Foods Pineapple Carrot	4 fl oz	60	—	0
Tropical Foods Guava With Mixed Fruit	4 fl oz	70	—	0
Tropical Foods Mango With Mixed Fruit	4 fl oz	70	—	0
Tropical Foods Papaya With Mixed Fruit	4 fl oz	70	—	0
VEGETABLE				
Beech-Nut				
Stage 1 Carrots Tender Sweet	1 jar (2.5 oz)	30	2	0
Stage 1 Green Beans (Spanish Label)	1 jar (2.5 oz)	20	2	
Earth's Best				
Carrots	1 jar (4.5 fl oz)	40	—	0
Carrots & Parsnips	1 jar (4.5 fl oz)	60	—	0
Corn & Butternut Squash	1 jar (4.5 fl oz)	90	—	0
Garden Vegetables	1 jar (4.5 fl oz)	70	—	0
Green Beans & Rice	1 jar (4.5 fl oz)	40	—	0
Peas & Brown Rice	1 jar (4.5 fl oz)	80	—	0
Spinach & Potatoes	1 jar (4.5 fl oz)	60	—	0
Sweet Potatoes	1 jar (4.5 fl oz)	60	—	0
Winter Squash	1 jar (4.5 fl oz)	50	—	0
Gerber				
1st Foods Carrots	1 jar (2.5 oz)	25	—	0

FOOD	PORTION	CALS.	FIB.	CHOL.
Gerber (CONT.)				
1st Foods Green Beans	1 jar (2.5 oz)	25	—	0
1st Foods Peas	1 jar (2.5 oz)	30	—	0
1st Foods Squash	1 jar (2.5 oz)	25	—	0
1st Foods Sweet Potatoes	1 jar (2.5 oz)	45	—	0
3rd Foods Carrots	1 jar (6 oz)	50	—	0
3rd Foods Mixed Vegetables	1 jar (6 oz)	70	—	0
3rd Foods Sweet Potatoes	1 jar (6 oz)	100	—	0

BACON
(*see also* BACON SUBSTITUTES)

FOOD	PORTION	CALS.	FIB.	CHOL.
Armour				
Lower Salt cooked	1 strip	38	—	6
Star cooked	1 strip	38	—	6
Black Label				
Center Cut cooked	3 slices (0.5 oz)	70	0	15
Cooked	2 slices (0.5 oz)	80	0	15
Low Salt cooked	2 slices (0.5 oz)	80	0	15
Hormel				
Bacon Bits	1 tsp (7 g)	30	0	5
Bacon Pieces	1 tsp (7 g)	25	0	10
Microwave cooked	2 slices (0.5 oz)	70	0	15
Jones				
Sliced	1 slice	130	—	25
Nathan's				
Beef cooked	3 slices	100	—	20
Old Smokehouse				
Cooked	2 slices (0.5 oz)	80	0	15
Oscar Mayer				
Bacon Bits	1 tbsp (7 g)	25	0	5
Center Cut cooked	3 slices (0.5 oz)	70	0	15
Cooked	2 slices (0.4 oz)	60	0	10
Lower Sodium cooked	2 slices (0.5 oz)	60	0	15
Thick Cut cooked	1 slice (0.4 oz)	50	0	10
Range Brand				
Cooked	2 slices (0.7 oz)	100	0	20
Red Label				
Cooked	2 slices (0.5 oz)	80	0	15
breakfast strips cooked	3 strips (34 g)	156	—	36
breakfast strips beef cooked	3 strips (34 g)	153	—	40
cooked	3 strips	109	—	16
grilled	2 slices (1.7 oz)	86	—	27

BACON SUBSTITUTES

FOOD	PORTION	CALS.	FIB.	CHOL.
Bac-Os				
	2 tsp (5 g)	25	—	0

FOOD	PORTION	CALS.	FIB.	CHOL.
Harvest Direct				
Bacon Bits	3.5 oz	320	17	0
Lightlife				
Fakin' Bacon	3 strips (2 oz)	79	—	0
Louis Rich				
Turkey Bacon	1 slice (0.5 oz)	30	0	10
McCormick				
Bac'n Pieces	2 tsp	20	—	0
Mr. Turkey	1 slice	25	—	10
bacon substitute	1 strip	25	—	0

BAGEL

(*see also* CRACKER)

FRESH

Alvarado St. Bakery				
Sprouted Wheat	1 (3.3 oz)	260	2	0
Sprouted Wheat Cinnamon/ Raisin	1 (3.3 oz)	280	3	0
Sprouted Wheat Onion/ Poppyseed	1 (3.3 oz)	320	2	0
Sprouted Wheat Sesame	1 (3.3 oz)	320	2	0
cinnamon raisin	1 (3½ in)	194	—	0
cinnamon raisin toasted	1 (3½ in)	194	—	0
egg	1 (3½ in)	197	—	17
egg toasted	1 (3½ in)	197	—	17
oat bran	1 (3½ in)	181	—	0
oat bran toasted	1 (3½ in)	181	—	0
onion	1 (3½ in)	195	2	0
plain	1 (3½ in)	195	2	0
plain toasted	1 (3½ in)	195	2	0
poppy seed	1 (3½ in)	195	2	0
FROZEN				
Lender's				
Cinnamon 'N Raisin	1 (2.5 oz)	200	1	0
Egg	1 (2 oz)	150	—	5
Onion	1 (2 oz)	160	1	0
Plain	1 (2 oz)	150	—	0
Sara Lee				
Cinnamon & Raisin	1 (3 oz)	240	—	0
Cinnamon Raisin	1 (2.5 oz)	200	—	0
Egg	1 (2.5 oz)	200	—	15
Egg	1 (3 oz)	250	—	20
Oat Bran	1 (2.5 oz)	180	—	0
Oat Bran	1 (3 oz)	220	—	0

FOOD	PORTION	CALS.	FIB.	CHOL.
Sara Lee (CONT.)				
Onion	1 (3 oz)	230	—	0
Onion	1 (2.5 oz)	190	—	0
Plain	1 (3 oz)	230	—	0
Plain	1 (2.5 oz)	190	—	0
Poppy Seed	1 (3 oz)	230	—	0
Poppy Seed	1 (2.5 oz)	190	—	0
Sesame Seed	1 (3 oz)	240	—	0
Sesame Seed	1 (2.5 oz)	190	—	0
Tree Of Life				
Onion	1 (3 oz)	210	0	0
Plain	1 (3 oz)	210	0	0
Poppy	1 (3 oz)	210	0	0
Raisin	1 (3 oz)	210	tr	0
Sesame	1 (3 oz)	210	0	0
Weight Watchers				
Bagel Sandwich Ham And Cheese	1 (3 oz)	210	—	15

BAKING POWDER

Calumet	1 tsp	3	—	0
Clabber Girl	1 tsp	0	—	0
Davis	1 tsp	6	—	0
Watkins	¼ tsp (1 g)	0	0	0
baking powder	1 tsp	2	—	0
low sodium	1 tsp	5	—	0

BAKING SODA

Arm & Hammer	1 tsp	0	—	0
baking soda	1 tsp	0	—	0

BALSAM PEAR

leafy tips cooked	½ cup	10	—	0
leafy tips raw	½ cup	7	—	0
pods cooked	½ cup	12	—	0

BAMBOO SHOOTS

CANNED				
Empress				
Sliced	2 oz	14	—	0
Ka-Me				
Sliced	½ cup (4.5 oz)	15	1	0
La Choy	¼ cup	6	tr	0
sliced	1 cup	25	—	0
FRESH				
cooked	½ cup	15	—	0
raw	½ cup	21	—	0

FOOD	PORTION	CALS.	FIB.	CHOL.

BANANA
banana chips	1 oz	147	2	0
DRIED				
powder	1 tbsp	21	—	0
FRESH				
Chiquita	1 (3½ oz)	110	—	0
Dole	1	120	3	0
banana	1	105	2	0
mashed	1 cup	207	4	0

BANANA JUICE
Libby				
Nectar	1 can (11.5 fl oz)	190	—	0

BARBECUE SAUCE
(see also SAUCE)

Bull's Eye				
Original	2 tbsp	50	—	0
Hain				
Honey	1 tbsp	14	—	0
Healthy Choice				
Hickory	2 tbsp (1.1 oz)	25	0	0
Hot & Spicy	2 tbsp (1.1 oz)	25	0	0
Original	2 tbsp (1.1 oz)	25	0	0
Heinz				
Select	1 oz	40	—	0
Select Hickory	1 oz	35	—	0
Thick & Rich Cajun Style	1 oz	35	—	0
Thick & Rich Chunky	1 oz	30	—	0
Thick & Rich Hawaiian Style	1 oz	40	—	0
Thick & Rich Hickory Smoke	1 oz	35	—	0
Thick & Rich Mesquite Smoke	1 oz	30	—	0
Thick & Rich Mushroom	1 oz	30	—	0
Thick & Rich Old Fashioned	1 oz	35	—	0
Thick & Rich Onion	1 oz	30	—	0
Thick & Rich Original	1 oz	35	—	0
Thick & Rich Texas Hot	1 oz	30	—	0
House Of Tsang				
Hong Kong	1 tbsp (0.6 oz)	10	0	0
Hunt's				
Country Style	1 tbsp	20	tr	0
Homestyle	1 tbsp	20	tr	0
Honey Mustard	1 tbsp (1.2 oz)	50	<1	0
Kansas City Style	1 tbsp	20	tr	0
New Orleans Style	1 tbsp	20	tr	0

FOOD	PORTION	CALS.	FIB.	CHOL.
Hunt's (CONT.)				
Original	2 tbsp (1.2 oz)	40	1	0
Southern Style	1 tbsp	20	tr	0
Texas Style	1 tbsp	25	tr	0
Western Style	1 tbsp	20	tr	0
Kraft				
Char-Grill	2 tbsp (1.2 oz)	60	0	0
Extra Rich Original	2 tbsp (1.2 oz)	50	0	0
Garlic	2 tbsp (1.2 oz)	40	0	0
Hickory Smoke	2 tbsp (1.2 oz)	40	0	0
Hickory Smoke Onion Bits	2 tbsp (1.2 oz)	50	tr	0
Honey	2 tbsp (1.2 oz)	50	0	0
Hot	2 tbsp (1.2 oz)	40	0	0
Hot Hickory Smoke	2 tbsp (1.2 oz)	40	0	0
Italian Seasonings	2 tbsp (1.2 oz)	45	0	0
Kansas City Style	2 tbsp (1.2 oz)	45	tr	0
Mesquite Smoke	2 tbsp (1.2 oz)	40	0	0
Onion Bits	2 tbsp (1.2 oz)	50	0	0
Original	2 tbsp (1.2 oz)	40	0	0
Teriyaki	2 tbsp (1.2 oz)	60	0	0
Thick'N Spicy Hickory Smoke	2 tbsp (1.2 oz)	50	0	0
Thick'N Spicy Honey	2 tbsp (1.2 oz)	60	0	0
Thick'N Spicy Kansas City Style	2 tbsp (1.2 oz)	60	tr	0
Thick'N Spicy Mesquite Smoke	2 tbsp (1.2 oz)	50	0	0
Thick'N Spicy Original	2 tbsp (1.2 oz)	50	0	0
Lawry's				
Dijon Honey	¼ cup	203	tr	0
Maull's	3.5 oz	123	—	1
Beer Non-Alcholic	3.5 oz	128	—	1
Smoky	3.5 oz	124	—	1
Sweet-N-Mild	3.5 oz	167	—	1
Sweet-N-Smoky	3.5 oz	160	—	1
With Onion Bits	3.5 oz	126	—	1
Red Wing				
"K" Sauce	2 tbsp (1.2 oz)	45	0	0
Watkins				
Bold	2 tsp (0.4 oz)	25	0	0
Honey	2 tsp (0.4 oz)	25	0	0
Mesquite	2 tsp (0.4 oz)	25	0	1
Original	2 tsp (0.4 oz)	25	0	0
Smokehouse	2 tsp (0.4 oz)	25	0	0
barbecue	1 cup	188	—	0

BARLEY
Arrowhead	¼ cup (1.7 oz)	170	6	0

FOOD	PORTION	CALS.	FIB.	CHOL.
Arrowhead (CONT.)				
Hulless	¼ cup (1.6 oz)	140	6	0
Quaker				
Medium Pearled	¼ cup	172	5	0
Quick Pearled	¼ cup	172	5	0
Scotch				
Medium Pearled	¼ cup	172	5	0
Quick Pearled	¼ cup	172	5	0
pearled cooked	½ cup	97	—	0
pearled uncooked	½ cup	352	16	0
BASIL				
Watkins				
Liquid Spice	1 tbsp (0.5 oz)	120	0	0
fresh chopped	2 tbsp	1	—	0
ground	1 tsp	4	—	0
leaves fresh	5	1	—	0
BASS				
freshwater raw	3 oz	97	—	58
sea cooked	3 oz	105	—	45
sea raw	3 oz	82	—	35
striped baked	3 oz	105	—	87
BAY LEAF				
Watkins				
crumbled	¼ tsp (0.5 g)	0	0	0
	1 tsp	2	—	0
BEAN SPROUTS				
(*see also* INDIVIDUAL BEAN NAMES)				
CANNED				
La Choy	⅔ cup	8	tr	0
BEANS				
(*see also* INDIVIDUAL NAMES)				
CANNED				
Allen				
Baked	½ cup (4.5 oz)	150	8	0
B&M				
Barbeque Baked Beans	8 oz	260	11	5
Honey Baked	8 oz	240	11	0
Hot N Spicy Baked	8 oz	240	12	3
Maple Baked	8 oz	240	11	<5
Tomato Baked Beans	8 oz	230	—	1
Vegetarian Baked	8 oz	230	—	0
Brown Beauty				
Mexican Beans With Jalapeno	½ cup (4.5 oz)	120	7	0

FOOD	PORTION	CALS.	FIB.	CHOL.
Bush's				
Baked	½ cup (4.6 oz)	150	7	<5
Baked With Onions	½ cup (4.6 oz)	150	6	5
Homestyle Baked	½ cup (4.6 oz)	160	8	5
Vegetarian	½ cup (4.6 oz)	140	6	0
Chi-Chi's				
Ranchero Beans	½ cup (4.3 oz)	100	1	0
Refried	½ cup (4.2 oz)	130	4	0
Crest Top				
Pork And Beans	½ cup (4.5 oz)	130	6	0
Friends				
Maple Baked	8 oz	240	11	<5
Gebhardt				
Chili	4 oz	115	5	0
Refried	4 oz	100	7	2
Refried Jalapeno	4 oz	115	7	2
Green Giant				
Pork And Beans In Tomato Sauce	½ cup	90	6	0
Three Bean Salad	½ cup	70	3	0
Hanover				
Four Bean Salad	½ cup	80	—	0
Health Valley				
Boston Baked	7½ oz	190	5	0
Boston Baked No Salt Added	7.5 oz	190	5	0
Fast Menu Honey Baked Organic Beans With Tofu Weiner	7½ oz	150	16	0
Vegetarian With Miso	7½ oz	180	5	0
Hormel				
Beans & Wieners	1 can (7.5 oz)	290	6	45
Hunt's				
Big John's Beans 'n Fixin's	4 oz	170	6	6
Pork And Beans	4 oz	135	8	1
Kid's Kitchen				
Beans & Weiners	1 cup (7.5 oz)	310	8	45
Little Pancho				
Refried & Green Chili	½ cup	80	—	0
McIlhenny				
Spicy	1 oz	7	1	0
Old El Paso				
Mexe-Beans	½ cup	163	13	0
Refried	4 oz	80	5	<5
Refried Fat Free	½ cup	90	—	0

FOOD	PORTION	CALS.	FIB.	CHOL.
Old El Paso (CONT.)				
Refried Vegetarian	4 oz	70	5	0
Refried With Cheese	¼ cup	130	5	5
Rosarita				
Refried	4 oz	100	6	0
Refried Spicy	4 oz	100	6	0
Refried Vegetarian	4 oz	100	6	0
Refried With Bacon	4 oz	110	6	14
Refried With Green Chilies	4 oz	90	6	0
Refried With Nacho Cheese	4 oz	110	6	2
Refried With Onions	4 oz	110	6	0
S&W				
Maple Sugar Beans	½ cup	150	—	0
Mixed Bean Salad Marinated	½ cup	90	—	0
Smokey Ranch	½ cup	130	—	0
Trappey				
Mexi-Beans With Jalapeno	½ cup (4.5 oz)	130	8	0
Pork And Beans	½ cup (4.5 oz)	110	7	0
Pork And Beans With Jalapeno	½ cup (4.5 oz)	130	6	0
Van Camp's				
Baked Beans Fat Free	½ cup (4.6 oz)	130	5	0
Baked Beans Premium	½ cup (4.6 oz)	140	5	0
Beanee Weenee	1 cup (9 oz)	320	8	40
Beanee Weenee Baked Flavor	1 cup (9 oz)	410	10	40
Beanee Weenee Barbeque	1 cup (9 oz)	340	8	40
Brown Sugar Beans	½ cup (4.6 oz)	170	6	5
Mexican Style Chili Beans	½ cup (4.6 oz)	110	8	0
Pork And Beans	½ cup (4.6 oz)	110	6	0
Vegetarian In Tomato Sauce	½ cup (4.6 oz)	110	5	0
Wagon Master				
Pork And Beans	½ cup (4.5 oz)	110	7	0
baked beans plain	½ cup	118	10	0
baked beans vegetarian	½ cup	118	10	0
baked beans w/ beef	½ cup	161	—	29
baked beans w/ franks	½ cup	182	9	8
baked beans w/ pork	½ cup	133	7	9
baked beans w/ pork & sweet sauce	½ cup	140	7	9
baked beans w/ pork & tomato sauce	½ cup	123	7	9
FROZEN				
Hanover				
Romano Bean Medley	½ cup	25	—	0
MIX				
Bean Cuisine				
Florentine Beans With Bow Ties	½ cup	199	—	6

FOOD	PORTION	CALS.	FIB.	CHOL.
Bean Cuisine (CONT.)				
Pasta & Beans Country French With Gemelli	½ cup	214	—	tr
TAKE-OUT				
baked beans	½ cup	190	—	6
barbecue beans	3.5 oz	120	—	0
four bean salad	3.5 oz	100	—	0
refried beans	½ cup	43	—	2
three bean salad	¾ cup	230	1	0

BEECHNUTS

dried	1 oz	164	—	0

BEEF

(*see also* BEEF DISHES, VEAL)

(Beef is graded according to its marbling, the little flecks of fat in the muscle. Beef graded "Prime" has the highest percentage of fat, followed by "Choice" with less fat and "Select" with the least fat.)

FOOD	PORTION	CALS.	FIB.	CHOL.
CANNED				
Armour				
Chopped Beef	2 oz	170	—	49
Corned Beef	2 oz	120	—	45
Corned Beef Hash	1 cup (8.3 oz)	440	—	100
Potted Meat	1 can (3 oz)	120	—	80
Potted Meat	¼ cup (2.2 oz)	90	—	60
Roast Beef Hash	1 cup (8.4 oz)	400	—	95
Roast Beef In Gravy	½ cup (4.6 oz)	150	—	75
Stew	1 cup (8.6 oz)	220	—	30
Tripe	3 oz	90	—	125
Hormel				
Corned Beef	2 oz	120	0	50
Corned Beef Hash	1 cup (8.3 oz)	390	2	70
Potted Meat	4 tbsp (2 oz)	60	0	50
Roast Beef Hash	1 cup (8.3 oz)	390	2	70
Mary Kitchen				
Corned Beef Hash	1 can (7.5 oz)	350	2	60
Roast Beef Hash	1 can (7.5 oz)	348	2	58
Treet				
50% Less Fat	2 oz	120	—	45
Treet	2 oz	150	—	50
Underwood				
Roast Beef	2.08 oz	140	—	45
Roast Beef Mesquite Smoked	2.08 oz	126	—	45
Roast Beef Light	2.08 oz	90	—	30
corned beef	1 oz	71	—	24

FOOD	PORTION	CALS.	FIB.	CHOL.
DRIED				
Hormel				
Pillow Pack	10 slices (1 oz)	45	0	20
Sliced	10 slices (1 oz)	50	0	25
FRESH				

(Note that the values for cooked beef may differ slightly from values for raw beef. When meat is cooked some moisture and fat is lost, changing the nutrition value slightly. As a rule of thumb it can be assumed that a 4 oz raw portion will equal a 3 oz cooked portion of meat.)

FOOD	PORTION	CALS.	FIB.	CHOL.
Dakota Lean				
Chuck Roast raw	3 oz	80	—	48
Eye Round raw	3 oz	80	—	40
Flank Steak raw	3 oz	80	—	40
Ground raw	3 oz	88	—	50
Outside Round raw	3 oz	80	—	40
Ribeye raw	3 oz	90	—	45
Sirloin Tip raw	3 oz	90	—	40
Strip Loin raw	3 oz	90	—	45
Tenderloin raw	3 oz	70	—	45
Top Round raw	3 oz	80	—	40
Double J				
Filet	3.5 oz	130	—	51
NY Strip	3.5 oz	133	—	52
Rib Eye	3.5 oz	134	—	54
Top Butt	3.5 oz	136	—	50
Laura's Lean				
Eye Of Round	4 oz	150	—	60
Flank Steak	4 oz	160	—	65
Ground	4 oz	180	—	60
Ground Round	4 oz	160	—	65
Ribeye Steak	4 oz	150	—	65
Sirloin Tip Round	4 oz	140	—	65
Sirloin Top Butt	4 oz	140	—	60
Strip Steak	4 oz	150	—	50
Tenderloins	4 oz	150	—	75
Top Round	4 oz	140	—	65
bottom round lean & fat trim 0 in Choice roasted	3 oz	172	—	66
bottom round lean & fat trim 0 in Select roasted	3 oz	150	—	66
bottom round lean & fat trim 0 in Select braised	3 oz	171	—	82
bottom round lean & fat trim 0 in braised	3 oz	193	—	82

FOOD	PORTION	CALS.	FIB.	CHOL.
bottom round lean & fat trim ¼ in Choice roasted	3 oz	221	—	68
bottom round lean & fat trim ¼ in Choice braised	3 oz	241	—	81
bottom round lean & fat trim ¼ in Select roasted	3 oz	199	—	68
bottom round lean & fat trim ¼ in Select braised	3 oz	220	—	81
brisket flat half lean & fat trim 0 in braised	3 oz	183	—	81
brisket flat half lean & fat trim ¼ in braised	3 oz	309	—	81
brisket point half lean & fat trim 0 in braised	3 oz	304	—	78
brisket point half lean & fat trim ¼ in braised	3 oz	343	—	79
brisket whole lean & fat trim 0 in braised	3 oz	247	—	79
brisket whole lean & fat trim ¼ in braised	3 oz	327	—	80
chuck arm pot roast lean & fat trim 0 in braised	3 oz	238	—	85
chuck arm pot roast lean & fat trim ¼ in braised	3 oz	282	—	85
chuck blade roast lean & fat trim 0 in braised	3 oz	284	—	88
chuck blade roast lean & fat trim ¼ in braised	3 oz	293	—	88
corned beef brisket cooked	3 oz	213	—	83
eye of round lean & fat trim 0 in Choice roasted	3 oz	153	—	59
eye of round lean & fat trim 0 in Select roasted	3 oz	137	—	59
eye of round lean & fat trim ¼ in Select roasted	3 oz	184	—	61
eye of round lean & fat trim ¼ in Choice roasted	3 oz	205	—	62
flank lean & fat trim 0 in braised	3 oz	224	—	62
flank lean & fat trim 0 in broiled	3 oz	192	—	58
ground extra lean broiled medium	3 oz	217	—	71
ground extra lean broiled well done	3 oz	225	—	84
ground extra lean fried medium	3 oz	216	—	69
ground extra lean fried well done	3 oz	224	—	79

FOOD	PORTION	CALS.	FIB.	CHOL.
ground extra lean raw	4 oz	265	—	78
ground lean broiled medium	3 oz	231	—	74
ground lean broiled well done	3 oz	238	—	86
ground regular broiled medium	3 oz	246	—	76
ground regular broiled well done	3 oz	248	—	86
ground low-fat w/ carrageenan raw	4 oz	160	—	53
porterhouse steak lean & fat trim ¼ in Choice broiled	3 oz	260	—	70
porterhouse steak lean only trim ¼ in Prime broiled	3 oz	185	—	68
rib eye small end lean & fat trim 0 in Choice broiled	3 oz	261	—	70
rib large end lean & fat trim 0 in roasted	3 oz	300	—	72
rib large end lean & fat trim ¼ in broiled	3 oz	295	—	69
rib large end lean & fat trim ¼ in roasted	3 oz	310	—	72
rib small end lean & fat trim 0 in broiled	3 oz	252	—	70
rib small end lean & fat trim ¼ in broiled	3 oz	285	—	71
rib small end lean & fat trim ¼ in roasted	3 oz	295	—	71
rib whole lean & fat trim ¼ in Choice broiled	3 oz	306	—	70
rib whole lean & fat trim ¼ in Choice roasted	3 oz	320	—	72
rib whole lean & fat trim ¼ in Prime roasted	3 oz	348	—	72
rib whole lean & fat trim ¼ in Select roasted	3 oz	286	—	71
rib whole lean & fat trim ¼ in Select broiled	3 oz	274	—	69
shank crosscut lean & fat trim ¼ in Choice simmered	3 oz	224	—	68
short loin top loin lean & fat trim 0 in Choice broiled	1 steak (5.4 oz)	353	—	119
short loin top loin lean & fat trim 0 in Select broiled	1 steak (5.4 oz)	309	—	119
short loin top loin lean & fat trim 0 in Choice broiled	3 oz	193	—	65
short loin top loin lean & fat trim ¼ in Choice braised	3 oz	253	—	68

FOOD	PORTION	CALS.	FIB.	CHOL.
short loin top loin lean & fat trim ¼ in Select broiled	1 steak (6.3 oz)	473	—	140
short loin top loin lean & fat trim ¼ in Choice broiled	1 steak (6.3 oz)	536	—	143
short loin top loin lean & fat trim ¼ in Prime broiled	1 steak (6.3 oz)	582	—	143
short loin top loin lean only trim 0 in Choice broiled	1 steak (5.2 oz)	311	—	113
short loin top loin lean only trim ¼ in Choice broiled	1 steak (5.2 oz)	314	—	112
shortribs lean & fat Choice braised	3 oz	400	—	80
t-bone steak lean & fat trim ¼ in Choice broiled	3 oz	253	—	70
t-bone steak lean only trim ¼ in Choice broiled	3 oz	182	—	68
tenderloin lean & fat trim 0 in Select broiled	3 oz	194	—	72
tenderloin lean & fat trim ¼ in Choice broiled	3 oz	259	—	73
tenderloin lean & fat trim ¼ in Choice roasted	3 oz	288	—	73
tenderloin lean & fat trim ¼ in Choice broiled	3 oz	208	—	72
tenderloin lean & fat trim ¼ in Prime broiled	3 oz	270	—	73
tenderloin lean & fat trim ¼ in Select roasted	3 oz	275	—	73
tenderloin lean only trim 0 in Select broiled	3 oz	170	—	71
tenderloin lean only trim ¼ in Choice broiled	3 oz	188	—	71
tenderloin lean only trim ¼ in Select broiled	3 oz	169	—	71
tip round lean & fat trim 0 in Choice roasted	3 oz	170	—	69
tip round lean & fat trim 0 in Select roasted	3 oz	158	—	69
tip round lean & fat trim ¼ in Choice roasted	3 oz	210	—	70
tip round lean & fat trim ¼ in Prime roasted	3 oz	233	—	70
tip round lean & fat trim ¼ in Select roasted	3 oz	191	—	70

FOOD	PORTION	CALS.	FIB.	CHOL.
top round lean & fat trim 0 in Choice braised	3 oz	184	—	77
top round lean & fat trim 0 in Select braised	3 oz	170	—	77
top round lean & fat trim ¼ in Choice braised	3 oz	221	—	77
top round lean & fat trim ¼ in Choice broiled	3 oz	190	—	72
top round lean & fat trim ¼ in Choice fried	3 oz	235	—	82
top round lean & fat trim ¼ in Prime broiled	3 oz	195	—	72
top round lean & fat trim ¼ in Select braised	3 oz	199	—	77
top round lean & fat trim ¼ in Select braised	3 oz	175	—	72
top sirloin lean & fat trim 0 in Choice broiled	3 oz	194	—	76
top sirloin lean & fat trim 0 in Select broiled	3 oz	166	—	76
top sirloin lean & fat trim ¼ in Choice fried	3 oz	277	—	83
top sirloin lean & fat trim ¼ in Choice broiled	3 oz	228	—	76
top sirloin lean & fat trim ¼ in Select broiled	3 oz	208	—	76
tripe raw	4 oz	111	—	107
FROZEN				
patties broiled medium	3 oz	240	—	80
READY-TO-USE				
Healthy Choice				
Roast Beef	1.9 oz	60	0	25
Oscar Mayer				
Deli-Thin Roast Beef	4 slices (1.8 oz)	60	0	25
Weight Watchers				
Deli Thin Oven Roasted Cured	5 slices (⅓ oz)	10	—	5
TAKE-OUT				
Sara Lee				
Roast Beef Medium	2 oz	70	—	30
Roast Beef Rare	2 oz	70	—	30

BEEF DISHES
CANNED
Dinty Moore

American Classics Beef Stew	1 bowl (10 oz)	260	3	45

FOOD	PORTION	CALS.	FIB.	CHOL.
Dinty Moore (CONT.)				
American Classics Meatloaf With Mashed Potatoes	1 bowl (10 oz)	300	3	40
American Classics Roast Beef With Mashed Potatoes	1 bowl (10 oz)	240	2	35
American Classics Salisbury Steak	1 bowl (10 oz)	310	3	60
Beef Stew	1 can (7.5 oz)	190	2	30
Meatball Stew	1 cup (8.4 oz)	260	3	35
Microwave Cup Beef Stew	1 cup (7.5 oz)	190	2	30
Microwave Cup Corned Beef Hash	1 cup (7.5 oz)	350	2	60
Microwave Cup Hearty Burger Stew	1 cup (7.5 oz)	240	3	40
Microwave Cup Meatball Stew	1 cup (7.5 oz)	240	2	30
Sliced Potatoes & Beef	1 can (7.5 oz)	230	4	25
Hormel				
Beef Goulash	1 can (7.5 oz)	230	3	50
Roast Beef With Gravy	2 oz	60	0	30
Manwich				
Mexican as prep	1 sandwich	310	2	50
Sloppy Joe as prep	1 sandwich	310	1	50
Micro Cup Meals				
Beef Stew	1 cup (7.5 oz)	180	2	30
FROZEN				
Chefwich				
Beef w/ Barbecue Sauce	1	340	—	29
Luigino's				
Creamed Sauce Shaved Cured Beef With Croutons	1 pkg (8 oz)	360	3	60
Egg Noodles Rich Gravy Swedish Meatballs	1 cup (7.5 oz)	280	3	70
Egg Noodles Rich Gravy Swedish Meatballs	1 pkg (9 oz)	340	3	80
Tyson				
Microwave BBQ Sandwich	1 sandwich	200	—	30
MIX				
Casbah				
Gyro as prep	1 patty (2 oz)	145	tr	63
Manwich				
Seasoning Mix as prep	1 sandwich	320	2	50
SHELF-STABLE				
Lunch Bucket				
Beef Stew	1 pkg (7.5 oz)	180	—	40

FOOD	PORTION	CALS.	FIB.	CHOL.
TAKE-OUT				
roast beef sandwich plain	1	346	—	52
roast beef sandwich w/ cheese	1	402	—	77
roast beef submarine sandwich w/ tomato lettuce & mayonnaise	1	411	—	73
steak sandwich w/ tomato lettuce salt & mayonnaise	1	459	—	73
stew w/ vegetables	1 cup	220	—	71
stroganoff	¾ cup	260	—	69
swiss steak	4.6 oz	214	2	61
BEEFALO				
roasted	3 oz	160	—	49
BEER AND ALE				
Amstel				
Light	12 oz	95	—	0
Anheuser Busch				
Natural Light	12 oz	110	—	0
Bud				
Light	12 oz	108	—	0
Coors	12 oz	132	—	0
Extra Gold	12 oz	147	—	0
Light	12 oz	101	—	0
Hamm's	12 oz	137	—	0
Killian's	12 oz	212	—	0
Michelob				
Light	12 oz	134	—	0
Miller				
Lite	12 oz	96	—	0
Molson				
Light	12 oz	109	—	0
Old Milwaukee	12 oz	145	—	0
Light	12 oz	122	—	0
Olympia	12 oz	143	—	0
Pabst	12 oz	143	—	0
Piels				
Light	12 oz	136	—	0
Schaefer	12 oz	138	—	0
Light	12 oz	111	—	0
Schlitz	12 oz	145	—	0
Light	12 oz	99	—	0
Schmidts				
Light	12 oz	96	—	0
Signature	12 oz	150	—	0

FOOD	PORTION	CALS.	FIB.	CHOL.
Stroh	12 oz	142	—	0
Light	12 oz	115	—	0
Winterfest	12 oz	167	—	0
beer light	12 oz can	100	—	0
beer regular	12 oz can	146	—	0
NONALCOHOLIC				
Guiness				
Kaliber	12 oz	43	—	0
Hamm's	12 oz	55	—	0
Kingsbury	12 fl oz	60	—	0
Pabst	12 oz	55	—	0
Spirit	12 oz	80	—	0

BEET JUICE

juice	3½ oz	36	—	0

BEETS
CANNED
Del Monte				
Pickled Crinkle Style Sliced	½ cup (4.5 oz)	80	2	0
Sliced	½ cup (4.3 oz)	35	2	0
Whole	½ cup (4.3 oz)	35	2	0
Whole Tiny	½ cup (4.3 oz)	35	2	0
S&W				
Diced Tender	½ cup	40	—	0
Julienne French Style	½ cup	40	—	0
Pickled Whole Extra Small	½ cup	70	—	0
Pickled w/ Red Wine Vinegar Sliced	½ cup	70	—	0
Sliced Small Premium	½ cup	40	—	0
Sliced Water Pack	½ cup	35	—	0
Whole Small	½ cup	40	—	0
Seneca				
Cut	½ cup	35	2	0
Diced	½ cup	35	2	0
Harvard	½ cup	90	1	0
Pickled	2 tbsp	20	0	0
Pickled With Onions	2 tbsp	20	0	0
Sliced	½ cup	35	2	0
Whole	½ cup	35	2	0
harvard	½ cup	89	—	0
pickled	½ cup	75	—	0
sliced	½ cup	27	—	0

FOOD	PORTION	CALS.	FIB.	CHOL.
FRESH				
greens cooked	½ cup	20	—	0
greens raw	½ cup	4	—	0
greens raw chopped	½ cup	4	—	0
raw sliced	½ cup (2.4 oz)	29	—	0
sliced cooked	½ cup (3 oz)	38	—	0
whole cooked	2 (3.5 oz)	44	—	0
whole raw	2 (5.7 oz)	70	—	0

BEVERAGES

(*see* BEER AND ALE, CHAMPAGNE, COFFEE, DRINK MIXERS, FRUIT DRINKS, MALT, MINERAL WATER/BOTTLED WATER, LIQUOR/LIQUEUR, SODA, TEA/HERBAL TEA, WINE, WINE COOLER)

BISCUIT

FOOD	PORTION	CALS.	FIB.	CHOL.
FROZEN				
Jimmy Dean				
Chicken Twin	2 (3.2 oz)	280	2	25
Sausage Twin	2 (3.4 oz)	330	2	30
Steak Twin	2 (3.2 oz)	270	2	25
Rudy's Farm				
Ham Twin	2 (3 oz)	160	1	20
Sausage & Cheese Twin	2 (3 oz)	290	1	30
Sausage Twin	2 (2.7 oz)	296	1	30
Weight Watchers				
Sausage Biscuit	3 oz	220	—	70
HOME RECIPE				
buttermilk	1 (2 oz)	212	—	2
plain	1 (2 oz)	212	—	2
MIX				
Arrowhead				
Biscuit Mix	¼ cup (1.2 oz)	120	3	0
Bisquick	½ cup (2 oz)	240	—	0
Reduced Fat	½ cup (2 oz)	210	—	0
Health Valley				
Buttermilk Biscuit Mix not prep	1 oz	100	3	0
Jiffy	¼ cup (1.1 oz)	130	1	0
Buttermilk as prep	1	170	tr	5
as prep	1	150	2	3
REFRIGERATED				
1869 Brand				
Baking Powder	1	100	—	0
Buttermilk	1	100	—	0
Butter Tastin'	1	100	—	0

FOOD	PORTION	CALS.	FIB.	CHOL.
Ballard				
Ovenready	1	50	—	0
Ovenready Buttermilk	1	50	—	0
Big Country				
Southern Style	1	100	—	0
Hungry Jack				
Butter Tastin' Flaky	1	90	—	0
Buttermilk Flaky	1	90	—	0
Buttermilk Fluffy	1	90	—	0
Extra Rich Buttermilk	1	50	—	0
Flaky	1	80	—	0
Honey Tastin' Flaky	1	90	—	0
Pillsbury				
Big Country Butter Tastin'	1	100	—	0
Big Country Buttermilk	1	100	—	0
Butter	1	50	—	0
Buttermilk	1	50	—	0
Country	1	50	—	0
Deluxe Heat N' Eat Buttermilk	2	170	—	0
Good'N Buttery Fluffy	1	90	—	0
Hearty Grains Multi-Grain	1	80	—	0
Hearty Grains Oatmeal Raisin	1	90	—	0
Heat N' Eat Big Premium	2	280	—	0
Tender Layer Buttermilk	1	50	—	0
Roman Meal	2 (2.4 oz)	180	1	0
Honey Nut Oat Bran	1 (1.5 oz)	131	1	0
buttermilk	1 (1 oz)	98	—	0
TAKE-OUT				
plain	1 (35 g)	276	—	5
w/ egg	1	315	—	232
w/ egg & bacon	1	457	—	353
w/ egg & sausage	1	582	—	302
w/ egg & steak	1	474	—	272
w/ egg cheese & bacon	1	477	—	261
w/ ham	1	387	—	25
w/ sausage	1	485	—	34
w/ steak	1	456	—	26

BISON
roasted	3 oz	122		70

BLACK BEANS
CANNED
Allen

Seasoned	½ cup (4.5 oz)	120	7	0

FOOD	PORTION	CALS.	FIB.	CHOL.
Eden				
Organic	½ cup (4.3 oz)	100	6	0
Health Valley				
Fast Menu Organic Black Beans With Tofu Weiners	7½ oz	150	15	0
Fast Menu Western Black Beans With Garden Vegetable	7½ oz	160	14	0
Progresso	½ cup	90	7	0
Trappey				
Seasoned	½ cup (4.5 oz)	120	7	0
DRIED				
Bean Cuisine				
Black Turtle	½ cup	115	5	0
cooked	1 cup	227	—	0
MIX				
Bean Cuisine				
Pasta & Beans Black Beans With Fusilli	½ cup	174	—	tr
Mahatma				
Black Beans & Rice	1 cup	200	6	0

BLACKBERRIES
CANNED

FOOD	PORTION	CALS.	FIB.	CHOL.
Allen-Wolco	½ cup (5.3 oz)	60	9	0
in heavy syrup	½ cup	118	—	0
FRESH				
blackberries	½ cup	37	3	0
FROZEN				
Big Valley	⅔ cup (4.9 oz)	70	4	0
unsweetened	1 cup	97	—	0

BLACKEYE PEAS
CANNED

FOOD	PORTION	CALS.	FIB.	CHOL.
Allen	½ cup (4.5 oz)	110	4	0
Fresh Shell	½ cup (4.4 oz)	120	6	0
With Bacon	½ cup (4.5 oz)	105	5	0
With Snaps	½ cup (4.4 oz)	120	5	0
Dorman				
Fresh Shell	½ cup (4.4 oz)	120	6	0
East Texas Fair	½ cup (4.5 oz)	110	4	0
Fresh Shell	½ cup (4.4 oz)	120	6	0
With Snaps	½ cup (4.4 oz)	120	5	0
Homefolks				
Fresh Shell	½ cup (4.4 oz)	120	6	0

FOOD	PORTION	CALS.	FIB.	CHOL.
Homefolks (CONT.)				
With Jalapeno	½ cup (4.4 oz)	120	5	0
With Snaps	½ cup (4.4 oz)	120	5	0
Sunshine				
With Bacon	½ cup (4.5 oz)	105	5	0
Trappey				
With Bacon	½ cup (4.5 oz)	120	5	0
With Bacon & Jalapeno	½ cup (4.4 oz)	110	5	0
w/pork	½ cup	199	—	17
DRIED				
cooked	1 cup	198	16	0
BLINTZE				
Empire				
Apple	2 (4.4 oz)	220	5	<5
Blueberry	2 (4.4 oz)	190	2	10
Cheese	2 (4.4 oz)	200	3	20
Cherry	2 (4.4 oz)	200	3	10
Potato	2 (4.4 oz)	190	3	10
Golden				
Apple Raisin	1 (2.25 oz)	80	—	10
Blueberry	1 (2.25 oz)	90	—	10
Cheese	1 (2.25 oz)	80	—	13
Cherry	1 (2.25 oz)	95	—	5
Potato	1 (2.25 oz)	90	—	5
TAKE-OUT				
cheese	2	186	tr	149
BLUEBERRIES				
CANNED				
S&W				
In Heavy Syrup	½ cup	111	—	0
in heavy syrup	1 cup	225	—	0
FRESH				
blueberries	1 cup	82	—	0
FROZEN				
Big Valley	¾ cup (4.9 oz)	70	4	0
unsweetened	1 cup	78	—	0
BLUEFIN				
fillet baked	4.1 oz	186	—	88
BLUEFISH				
fresh baked	3 oz	135	—	64
BOK CHOY				
Dole				
Shredded	½ cup	5	—	0

FOOD	PORTION	CALS.	FIB.	CHOL.
BORAGE				
fresh chopped cooked	3½ oz	25	—	0
raw chopped	½ cup	9	—	0
BOYSENBERRIES				
CANNED				
in heavy syrup	1 cup	226	—	0
FROZEN				
unsweetened	1 cup	66	—	0
BOYSENBERRY JUICE				
Smucker's	8 oz	120	—	0
BRAINS				
Armour				
Pork Brains In Milk Gravy	⅔ cup (5.5 oz)	150	—	3500
beef pan-fried	3 oz	167	—	1696
beef simmered	3 oz	136	—	1746
lamb braised	3 oz	124	—	1737
lamb fried	3 oz	232	—	2128
pork, braised	3 oz	117	—	2169
veal braised	3 oz	115	—	2635
veal fried	3 oz	181	—	1802
BRAN				
Arrowhead				
Oat Bran	⅓ cup (1.4 oz)	150	7	0
Wheat Bran	¼ cup (0.6 oz)	30	6	0
Good Shepherd				
Wheat Bran	1 oz	80	3	0
H-O				
Super Bran	⅓ cup	110	3	0
Health Valley				
Fast Menu Oat Bran Pilaf With Garden Vegetables	7½ oz	210	15	0
Hodgson Mill				
Oat	¼ cup (1.3 oz)	120	6	0
Wheat	¼ cup (0.5 oz)	30	7	0
Kretschmer				
Toasted Wheat Bran	⅓ cup	57	3	0
Mother's				
Oat Bran	½ cup	150	6	0
Quaker				
Oat Bran	½ cup	150	6	0
Roman Meal				
Oat	1 oz	94	5	0

FOOD	PORTION	CALS.	FIB.	CHOL.
Stone-Buhr				
Oat	⅓ cup (1 oz)	90	4	0
corn	⅓ cup	56	21	0
oat cooked	½ cup	44	—	0
oat dry	½ cup	116	7	0
rice dry	⅓ cup	88	6	0
wheat dry	½ cup	65	13	0

BRAZIL NUTS
dried unblanched	1 oz	186	—	0

BREAD
(see also BAGEL, BISCUIT, BREADSTICK, CROISSANT, ENGLISH MUFFIN, MUFFIN, ROLL, SCONE)

CANNED

B&M				
Brown Bread	½ in slice (1.6 oz)	92	4	0
Brown Bread Raisins	½ in slice (1.6 oz)	94	4	0
Friends				
Brown Bread	1 slice (1.6 oz)	92	2	0
Brown Bread w/ Raisin	1 slice (1.6 oz)	94	2	0
S&W				
Brown Bread New England Recipe	2 slices	76	—	0

FROZEN

Kineret				
Challah	⅛ loaf (2 oz)	150	1	15

HOME RECIPE

banana	1 slice (2 oz)	195	—	26
cornbread as prep w/ 2% milk	1 piece (2.3 oz)	173	—	26
cornbread as prep w/ whole milk	1 piece (2.3 oz)	176	—	28
datenut	½ in slice	92	—	15
irish soda bread	1 slice (2 oz)	174	—	11
pita whole wheat	1-6 in	247	—	0
pumpkin	1 slice (1 oz)	94	—	13
white as prep w/ nonfat dry milk	1 slice	78	—	0
white as prep w/ 2% milk	1 slice	81	—	1
white as prep w/ whole milk	1 slice	82	—	1
whole wheat	1 slice	79	—	0

MIX

Aunt Jemima				
Corn Bread Easy Mix	⅓ cup (1.3 oz)	150	1	0
Natural Ovens				
Cracked Wheat	2 slices (2.4 oz)	140	4	0
English Muffin Bread	2 slices (2.4 oz)	140	2	0

FOOD	PORTION	CALS.	FIB.	CHOL.
Natural Ovens (CONT.)				
Executive Fitness Sunny Millet	2 slices (2.6 oz)	160	4	0
Garden Bread	1 oz	50	1	0
Glorious Cinnamon & Raisin Fat Free	2 slices (2.1 oz)	110	3	0
Honey 'N Flax	2 slices (2.5 oz)	140	4	0
Hunger Filler Bread	2 slices (2.1 oz)	110	5	0
Light Wheat	2 slices (2.2 oz)	84	5	0
Nutty Natural Wheat Bread	2 slices (2.5 oz)	140	6	0
Seven Grain Herb	2 slices (2.5 oz)	140	4	0
Soft Hearth Whole Wheat	2 slices (2 oz)	100	4	0
Soft Sandwich Very Low Fat	2 slices (2.3 oz)	110	2	0
Stay Slim	2 slices (2 oz)	100	4	0
Zia Foods				
Cornbread Blue Cornmeal	1 piece (1.2 oz)	110	—	41
READY-TO-EAT				
Alvarado St. Bakery				
Barley	1 slice (1.2 oz)	70	2	0
California Style	1 slice (1.2 oz)	60	2	0
French	1 slice (1.2 oz)	80	2	0
Multi-Grain	1 slice (1.2 oz)	60	2	0
Multi-Grain No-Salt	1 slice (1.2 oz)	60	2	0
Oat Berry	1 slice (1.2 oz)	70	2	0
Raisin	1 slice (1.1 oz)	80	2	0
Rye Seed	1 slice (1.2 oz)	60	2	0
Sourdough	1 slice (1.2 oz)	80	2	0
Wheat	1 slice (1.3 oz)	90	3	0
America's Own				
Wheat Cottage	1 slice	70	—	0
Arnold				
12 Grain Natural	1 slice (0.8 oz)	60	1	0
Augusto Pan De Aqua	1 oz	80	1	0
Bran'nola Country Oat	1 slice (1.3 oz)	90	3	0
Bran'nola Dark Wheat	1 slice (1.3 oz)	90	3	0
Bran'nola Hearty Wheat	1 slice (1.3 oz)	100	3	0
Bran'nola Nutty Grains	1 slice (1.3 oz)	90	3	0
Bran'nola Original	1 slice (1.3 oz)	90	3	0
Cinnamon Chip	1 slice	80	tr	0
Cinnamon Raisin	1 slice (0.9 oz)	70	1	0
Country Bran Bakery Light	1 slice (0.8 oz)	40	3	0
Cranberry	1 slice (0.9 oz)	70	1	0
French Stick Savoni	1 oz	80	1	0
Italian Bakery Light	1 slice (0.7 oz)	40	2	0
Oatmeal Bakery	1 slice	60	2	0

FOOD	PORTION	CALS.	FIB.	CHOL.
Arnold (CONT.)				
Oatmeal Bakery Light	1 slice	40	2	0
Oatmeal Raisin	1 slice (0.9 oz)	60	2	0
Pumpernickel	1 slice (1.1 oz)	70	1	0
Rye Bakery Soft Light	1 slice (1.1 oz)	40	2	0
Rye Bakery Soft Seeded	1 slice (1.1 oz)	70	1	0
Rye Bakery Soft Unseeded	1 slice (1.1 oz)	70	1	0
Rye Dill	1 slice (1.1 oz)	60	1	0
Rye Real Jewish Dijon	1 slice	70	1	0
Rye Real Jewish Melba Thin	1 slice (0.7 oz)	40	1	0
Rye Real Jewish Unseeded	1 slice	80	1	0
Rye Real Jewish With Caraway	1 slice	80	1	0
Rye Real Jewish Without Seeds	1 slice (1.1 oz)	70	1	0
Sourdough Francisco	1 slice	90	1	0
Wheat Brick Oven	1 slice (0.8 oz)	60	2	0
Wheat Golden Light	1 slice (0.8 oz)	40	2	0
Wheat Natural	1 slice (1.3 oz)	80	2	0
Wheat Berry Honey	1 slice (1.1 oz)	80	2	0
White Brick Oven	1 slice (0.8 oz)	60	1	0
White Country	1 slice (1.3 oz)	100	1	0
White Extra Fiber Brick Oven	1 slice (0.9 oz)	50	2	0
White Light Brick Oven	1 slice (0.8 oz)	40	2	0
White Premium Light	1 slice	40	2	0
White Thin Sliced Brick Oven	1 slice	40	tr	0
Whole Wheat 100% Light Brick Oven	1 slice (0.8 oz)	40	3	0
Whole Wheat 100% Stoneground	1 slice (0.8 oz)	50	2	<5
August Bros.				
Pumpernickel	1 slice	80	1	0
Pumpernickel	1 slice (24 oz loaf)	90	1	0
Rye Onion	1 slice	80	1	0
Rye With Seeds	1 slice (24 oz loaf)	90	1	0
Rye Without Seeds	1 slice	80	1	0
Rye Without Seeds	1 slice (24 oz loaf)	90	1	0
Rye Thin Unseeded	1 slice	40	1	0
Rye With Seeds	1 slice (1 lb loaf)	80	1	0
Rye N' Pump	1 slice	90	1	0
Beefsteak				
Pumpernickel	1 slice (1 oz)	70	1	0
Rye Hearty	1 slice (1 oz)	70	1	0
Rye Light	2 slices (1.6 oz)	70	5	0
Rye Mild	2 slices (1.4 oz)	90	2	0
Rye Soft	1 slice (1 oz)	70	1	0

FOOD	PORTION	CALS.	FIB.	CHOL.
Beefsteak (CONT.)				
Wheat Hearty	1 slice (1 oz)	70	1	0
Wheat Soft	1 slice (1 oz)	70	tr	0
White Robust	1 slice (1 oz)	70	tr	0
Bread Du Jour				
Austrian Wheat	3 in slice (1 oz)	130	2	0
French	3 in slice (1 oz)	130	1	0
Brownberry				
Bran'nola Country Oat	1 slice	90	3	0
Bran'nola Hearty Wheat	1 slice	88	3	0
Bran'nola Nutty Grains	1 slice	85	3	0
Bran'nola Original	1 slice	85	3	0
Health Nut	1 slice	71	3	0
Oatmeal Natural	1 slice	63	1	0
Oatmeal Soft	1 slice	48	2	0
Raisin Bran	1 slice	61	2	0
Raisin Cinnamon	1 slice	66	1	0
Raisin Walnut	1 slice	68	2	0
Wheat Apple Honey	1 slice	69	2	0
Wheat Soft	1 slice	74	1	0
Cedar's				
Mountain Bread Six Grain	1 piece (2.4 oz)	200	4	0
Dicarlo's				
Foccaccia	⅛ bread (2 oz)	130	1	0
French Parisian	2 slices (1 oz)	70	tr	0
Freihofer's				
Country Potato	1 slice (1.3 oz)	100	1	0
Country White	1 slice (1.3 oz)	100	tr	0
Wheat	1½ slices	70	—	0
Wheat Light	1 slice (1.6 oz)	80	4	0
White Light	2 slices (1.6 oz)	80	4	0
Whole Wheat 100%	1 slice (1.3 oz)	90	2	0
Home Pride				
Hearty Buttermilk & Biscuit White	1 slice (1.3 oz)	100	tr	0
Hearty Deli Rye	1 slice (2 oz)	140	3	0
Hearty Golden Honey Wheat	1 slice (1.3 oz)	90	2	0
Hearty Honey Oats & Cracked Wheat	1 slice (1.4 oz)	100	2	0
Hearty Seven Grain Multi Grain	1 slice (1.3 oz)	100	2	0
Honey Wheat	1 slice (1 oz)	70	1	0
Seven Grain	1 slice (0.9 oz)	60	1	0
Wheat	1 slice (0.9 oz)	70	1	0
Wheat Light	3 slices (2.1 oz)	110	6	0

FOOD	PORTION	CALS.	FIB.	CHOL.
Home Pride (CONT.)				
White	1 slice (0.9 oz)	70	0	0
White Light	3 slices (0.9 oz)	110	6	0
White Grain	1 slice (1 oz)	60	2	0
Whole Wheat Hearty 100% Stoneground	1 slice (1.4 oz)	90	3	0
Malsovit	1 slice	66	4	0
Raisin	1 slice	77	3	0
Matthew's				
9 Grain & Nut	1 slice	80	2	0
Cinnamon	1 slice	70	1	0
Golden	1 slice	70	1	0
Oat Bran	1 slice	65	2	0
Pita Whole Wheat	1	210	7	0
Sodium Free	1 slice	70	1	0
Whole Wheat	1 slice	70	2	0
Monks' Bread				
Hi-Fibre	1 slice	50	—	0
Raisin	1 slice	70	—	0
Sunflower & Bran	1 slice	70	2	0
White	1 slice	60	—	0
Whole Wheat 100% Stoneground	1 slice	70	—	0
Pepperidge Farm				
7 Grain Hearty Slice	2 slices	180	2	0
Cinnamon	1 slice	90	2	0
Cracked Wheat	1 slice	70	1	0
Crunchy Oat 1½ lb Loaf	2 slices	190	3	0
Date Walnut	1 slice	90	2	0
French Fully Baked	2 oz	150	1	0
French Twin	1 oz	80	0	0
Honey Bran	1 slice	90	1	0
Italian Brown & Serve	1 oz	80	0	0
Italian Sliced	1 slice	70	—	0
Oatmeal	1 slice	70	1	0
Oatmeal 1½ lb Loaf	1 slice	90	1	0
Oatmeal Light	1 slice	45	1	0
Oatmeal Very Thin Sliced	1 slice	40	1	0
Pumpernickel Family	1 slice	80	2	0
Pumpernickel Party	4 slices	60	1	0
Raisin With Cinnamon	1 slice	90	1	0
Rye Dijon	1 slice	50	1	0
Rye Dijon Thick Sliced	1 slice	70	2	0
Rye Family	1 slice (32 g)	80	2	0

FOOD	PORTION	CALS.	FIB.	CHOL.
Pepperidge Farm (CONT.)				
Rye Party	4 slices	60	1	0
Rye Seedless Family	1 slice	80	2	0
Rye Soft	1 slice	70	—	0
Sesame Wheat	2 slices	190	3	0
Sprouted Wheat	1 slices	70	2	0
Vienna Light	1 slice	45	1	0
Vienna Thick Sliced	1 slice	70	0	0
Wheat 1½ lb Loaf	1 slice	90	2	0
Wheat Family	1 slice	70	2	0
Wheat Light	1 slice	45	1	0
Wheat Very Thin Sliced	1 slice	35	0	0
White Country	2 slices	190	2	0
White Large Family Thin Slice	1 slice	70	0	0
White Sandwich	2 slices	130	0	0
White Thin Slice	1 slice	80	0	0
White Toasting	1 slice	90	1	0
White Very Thin Sliced	1 slice	40	0	0
Whole Wheat Thin Slice	1 slice	60	2	0
Roman Meal				
Brown & Serve Mini Loaf	½ loaf (2 oz)	136	1	0
Cracked Wheat	1 slice (1.4 oz)	92	2	0
Hearty Wheat Light	1 slice (0.8 oz)	42	2	0
Honey Nut Oat Bran	1 slice (1 oz)	72	1	0
Honey Oat Bran	1 slice (1 oz)	70	1	0
Oat	1 slice (1 oz)	69	1	0
Oat Bran	1 slice (1 oz)	68	1	0
Oat Bran Light	1 slice (0.8 oz)	42	2	0
Round Top	1 slice (1 oz)	67	1	0
Sandwich	1 slice (0.8 oz)	55	1	0
Seven Grain	1 slice (1 oz)	67	1	0
Seven Grain Light	1 slice (0.8 oz)	42	3	0
Sourdough Light	1 slice (0.8 oz)	41	3	0
Sourdough Whole Grain Light	1 slice (0.8 oz)	40	3	0
Sun Grain	1 slice (1 oz)	70	1	0
Twelve Grain	1 slice (1 oz)	70	1	0
Twelve Grain Light	1 slice (0.8 oz)	42	3	0
Wheat Light	1 slice (0.8 oz)	41	3	0
Wheatberry Honey	1 slice (1 oz)	67	1	0
Wheatberry Light	1 slice (0.8 oz)	42	2	0
White Light	1 slice (0.8 oz)	41	3	0
Whole Grain 100%	1 slice (1.4 oz)	91	2	0
Whole Grain Sourdough	1 slice (1 oz)	66	1	0
Whole Wheat 100%	1 slice (1 oz)	64	2	0

FOOD	PORTION	CALS.	FIB.	CHOL.
Roman Meal (CONT.)				
Whole Wheat 100% Light	1 slice (0.8 oz)	42	2	0
Sahara				
Pita Oat Bran	½ pocket (1 oz)	66	2	0
Stroehmann				
White Whole Special Recipe	1 slice	70	—	0
White Whole Special Recipe Kids	1 slice	60	—	0
Sunmaid				
Raisin	1 slice	70	1	0
Tree Of Life				
100% Spelt	1 slice (1.8 oz)	130	3	10
Millet	1 slice (1.8 oz)	130	2	0
Rye Sour Dough	1 slice (1.8 oz)	110	5	0
Sprouted Seven Grain	1 slice (1.8 oz)	110	2	0
Weight Watchers				
Italian	1 slice (0.8 oz)	38	2	0
Multi-Grain	1 slice (0.8 oz)	41	2	0
Oat	1 slice (0.8 oz)	42	2	0
Raisin	1 slice (0.9 oz)	55	1	0
Rye	1 slice (0.8 oz)	38	2	0
Wheat	1 slice (0.8 oz)	40	2	0
White	1 slice (0.8 oz)	40	2	0
Wonder				
Calcium Enriched	1 slice (1 oz)	70	tr	0
Cinnamon Raisin	1 slice (1 oz)	70	tr	0
Cracked Wheat	1 slice (1 oz)	70	1	0
French	1 slice (1 oz)	80	tr	0
French Light	2 slices (1.6 oz)	80	5	0
Granola	1 slice (1.5 oz)	100	2	0
Honey Bran Light	2 slices (1.6 oz)	80	6	0
Italian	1 slice (1.1 oz)	80	tr	0
Italian Family	1 slice (1 oz)	70	tr	0
Italian Light	2 slices (1.6 oz)	80	5	0
Kid	1 slice (0.9 oz)	70	tr	0
Light Calcium Enriched	2 slices (1.6 oz)	80	5	<5
Nine Grain Light	2 slices (1.6 oz)	80	6	0
Oatmeal Light	2 slices (1.6 oz)	90	4	0
Rye	1 slice (1 oz)	70	1	0
Rye Light	2 slices (1.6 oz)	70	5	0
Sourdough	1 slice (1.2 oz)	90	tr	0
Sourdough Light	2 slices (1.6 oz)	80	5	0
Texas Toast	1 slice (1.4 oz)	100	1	0
Vienna	1 slice (1 oz)	70	tr	0

FOOD	PORTION	CALS.	FIB.	CHOL.
Wonder (CONT.)				
Wheat Calcium Light	2 slices (1.6 oz)	80	6	0
Wheat Family	1 slice (0.9 oz)	70	tr	0
Wheat Golden Country Style	2 slices (1.4 oz)	100	1	0
Wheat Light	2 slices (1.6 oz)	80	6	0
White	1 slice (0.9 oz)	70	tr	0
White Calcium	2 slices (1.6 oz)	100	1	0
White Calcium Light	2 slices (1.6 oz)	80	5	0
White Light	2 slices (1.6 oz)	80	5	0
White With Buttermilk	1 slice (1 oz)	80	tr	0
Whole Wheat 100%	1 slice (1 oz)	70	2	0
Whole Wheat 100% Soft	2 slices (1.6 oz)	110	1	0
Whole Wheat 100% Stoneground	1 slice (1.2 oz)	80	2	0
egg	1 slice (1.4 oz)	115	—	20
french	1 loaf (1 lb)	1270	—	0
french	1 slice (1 oz)	78	1	0
gluten	1 slice	47	—	0
italian	1 slice (1 oz)	81	1	0
italian	1 loaf (1 lb)	1255	—	0
navajo fry	1 (10.5 in diam)	527	—	0
navajo fry	1 (5 in diam)	296	—	0
oat bran	1 slice	71	1	0
oat bran reduced calorie	1 slice	46	—	0
oatmeal reduced calorie	1 slice	48	—	0
pita	1 reg (2 oz)	165	1	0
pita	1 sm (1 oz)	78	1	0
pita whole wheat	1 reg (2 oz)	170	5	0
pita whole wheat	1 sm (1 oz)	76	2	0
protein	1 slice	47	—	0
pumpernickel	1 slice	80	2	0
raisin	1 slice	71	—	0
rice bran	1 slice	66	—	0
rye	1 slice	83	2	0
rye reduced calorie	1 slice	47	—	0
seven grain	1 slice	65	2	0
sourdough	1 slice (1 oz)	78	1	0
vienna	1 slice (1 oz)	78	1	0
wheat berry	1 slice	65	1	0
wheat bran	1 slice	89	3	0
white	1 slice	67	—	0
white reduced calorie	1 slice	48	2	0
white toasted	1 slice	67	—	0
white cubed	1 cup	80	—	0

FOOD	PORTION	CALS.	FIB.	CHOL.
REFRIGERATED				
Pillsbury				
Crusty French Loaf	1 in slice	60	—	0
Hearty Grains Cracked Wheat Twists	1	80	—	0
Pipin'Hot Wheat Loaf	1 in slice	70	—	0
Roman Meal				
Loaf	1 slice (1 oz)	85	1	0
Stefano's				
Stuffed Bread Broccoli & Cheese	½ bread (6 oz)	450	7	25
TAKE-OUT				
cornbread	2 in x 2 in (1.4 oz)	107	—	28
cornstick	1 (1.3 oz)	101	tr	30
focaccia onion	1 piece (4.6 oz)	282	2	0
focaccia rosemary	1 piece (3.5 oz)	251	2	0
focaccia tomato olive	1 piece (4.7 oz)	270	2	0
BREAD COATING				
Don's Chuck Wagon				
All Purpose Mix	¼ cup (1 oz)	100	1	0
Fish & Chips Mix	¼ cup (1 oz)	100	1	0
Fish Mix	¼ cup (1 oz)	95	1	0
Frying Mix Chicken	¼ cup (1 oz)	95	1	0
Frying Mix Seafood Seasoned	¼ cup (1 oz)	95	1	0
Mushroom Mix	¼ cup (1 oz)	95	1	0
Onion Ring Mix	¼ cup (1 oz)	100	1	0
Golden Dipt				
Breading Frying Mix	1 oz	90	—	0
Chicken Frying Mix	1 oz	90	—	0
Onion Ring Mix	1 oz	100	—	0
Ka-Me				
Tempura Batter Mix	1 oz	100	0	0
Little Crow				
Fryin' Magic	0.5 oz	43	—	0
Mrs. Dash				
Crispy Coating	0.5 oz	63	—	0
Shake 'N Bake				
Extra Crispy Oven Fry For Pork	¼ pkg (1 oz)	120	—	0
Italian Herb Recipe	¼ pkg (½ oz)	77	—	1
Original Barbecue For Chicken	¼ pkg (½ oz)	93	—	0
Original Barbecue For Pork	¼ pkg (½ oz)	38	—	0
Original Country Mild	¼ pkg (½ oz)	76	—	0
Original For Chicken	¼ pkg (½ oz)	75	—	0

FOOD	PORTION	CALS.	FIB.	CHOL.
Shake 'N Bake (CONT.)				
Original For Fish	¼ pkg (½ oz)	73	—	0
Original For Pork	¼ pkg (½ oz)	41	—	0
BREAD MACHINE MIX				
Dromedary				
Country White	½ in slice (2 oz)	140	1	0
Italian Herb	½ in slice (1.8 oz)	140	1	0
Stoneground Wheat	½ in slice (1.8 oz)	140	2	0
Pillsbury				
Cracked Wheat	1/12 pkg (1.3 oz)	130	2	0
Wanda's				
Dried Tomato Cheddar	¼ cup mix per serv (1.2 oz)	140	3	0
European White	¼ cup mix per serv (1.2 oz)	130	1	0
Oatmeal	¼ cup mix per serv (1.2 oz)	120	1	0
Oatmeal Cinnamon	¼ cup mix per serv (1.2 oz)	120	1	0
Old World Rye	¼ cup mix per serv (1.9 oz)	90	3	0
Onion	¼ cup mix per serv (1.2 oz)	120	1	0
Orange Cinnamon	¼ cup mix per serv (1.3 oz)	130	1	0
Oregano Garlic	¼ cup mix per serv (1.2 oz)	130	2	0
Rosemary Basil	¼ cup mix per serv (1.2 oz)	130	1	0
Rye	¼ cup mix per serv (1.2 oz)	120	1	0
Rye Caraway	¼ cup mix per serv (1.2 oz)	120	1	0
Sourdough	¼ cup mix per serv (1.2 oz)	120	1	0
Sunflower Sesame Poppyseed	¼ cup mix per serv (1.2 oz)	120	2	0
Ten Grain	¼ cup mix per serv (1.4 oz)	140	3	0
Wheat	¼ cup mix per serv (1.2 oz)	130	2	0
White	¼ cup mix per serv (1.2 oz)	130	1	0

FOOD	PORTION	CALS.	FIB.	CHOL.
Wanda's (CONT.)				
Whole Wheat	¼ cup mix per serv (1.3 oz)	130	4	0
BREADCRUMBS				
Arnold				
Italian	½ oz	50	tr	0
Plain	½ oz	50	tr	0
Devonsheer				
Italian Style	1 oz	104	1	0
Plain	1 oz	108	1	0
Friday's				
Seasoned	1 oz	56	—	0
Jaclyn's				
Organic Whole Wheat Plain	½ oz	28	—	0
Organic Whole Wheat Italian Style	½ oz	28	—	0
Progresso				
Italian Style	2 tbsp	60	—	0
Plain	2 tbsp	60	—	0
fresh	⅔ cup	76	1	0
BREADFRUIT				
breadfruit	3.5 oz	109	—	0
fresh	¼ small	99	—	0
seeds cooked	1 oz	48	—	0
seeds raw	1 oz	54	—	0
seeds roasted	1 oz	59	—	0
BREADNUTTREE SEEDS				
dried	1 oz	104	—	0
BREADSTICKS				
Angonoa				
Cheese	5 (1 oz)	120	1	0
Cheese Mini	16 (1 oz)	120	1	0
Garlic	6 (1 oz)	120	1	0
Italian Style Plain	5 (1 oz)	120	1	0
Low Sodium With Sesame Seed	6 (1 oz)	130	2	0
Onion	6 (1 oz)	120	2	0
Pizza Mini	26 (1 oz)	120	1	0
Sesame Mini	16 (1 oz)	130	2	0
Sesame Royale	6 (1 oz)	130	2	0
Whole Wheat Mini	14 (1 oz)	130	3	0
Bread Du Jour				
Italian	1 (1.9 oz)	130	1	0

FOOD	PORTION	CALS.	FIB.	CHOL.
Bread Du Jour (CONT.)				
Sourdough	1 (1.9 oz)	130	1	0
J.J. Cassone				
Garlic	1 (1.6 oz)	150	2	0
Keebler				
Garlic	2	30	—	0
Onion	2	30	—	0
Plain	2	30	—	0
Sesame	2	30	—	0
Lance				
Cheese	2	20	—	0
Garlic	2	30	—	0
Plain	2	30	—	0
Sesame	2	30	—	0
Pillsbury				
Soft Bread Sticks	1	100	—	0
Roman Meal				
Brown & Serve Soft	1 (2.7 oz)	181	3	0
Refrigerated	1 (1.4 oz)	117	1	0
Stella D'Oro				
Deli Garlic Fat Free	5	60	—	0
Deli Original Fat Free	5	60	—	0
Garlic	1	35	—	0
Grissini Garlic Fat Free	3	60	—	0
Grissini Original Fat Free	3	60	—	0
Onion	1	40	—	0
Regular	1	40	—	0
Regular Sodium Free	2	80	—	0
Sesame Low Fat	2	70	—	0
Sesame Sodium Free	1	50	—	0
Traditional Garlic Fat Free	2	70	—	0
Traditional Original Fat Free	2	70	—	0
Wheat	1	40	—	0
onion poppyseed home recipe	1	64	—	10
plain	1	41	—	0
plain	1 sm	25	—	0

BREAKFAST BAR

(see also BREAKFAST DRINKS, NUTRITIONAL SUPPLEMENTS)

Carnation				
Chewy Chocolate Chip	1 (1.26 oz)	150	tr	0
Chewy Peanut Butter Chocolate Chip	1 (1.26 oz)	140	tr	0
Nutri-Grain				
Apple Cinnamon	1 (1.3 oz)	140	1	0

FOOD	PORTION	CALS.	FIB.	CHOL.
Nutri-Grain (CONT.)				
Blueberry	1 bar (1.3 oz)	140	1	0
Peach	1 (1.3 oz)	140	1	0
Raspberry	1 (1.3 oz)	140	1	0
Strawberry	1 (1.3 oz)	140	1	0

BREAKFAST DRINKS

(*see also* BREAKFAST BAR, NUTRITIONAL SUPPLEMENTS)

FOOD	PORTION	CALS.	FIB.	CHOL.
Carnation				
Instant Breakfast Cafe Mocha	1 pkg + skim milk (9 fl oz)	220	1	6
Instant Breakfast Cafe Mocha	1 pkg	130	1	<5
Instant Breakfast Cafe Mocha	1 can (10 fl oz)	220	0	5
Instant Breakfast Classic Chocolate Malt	1 pkg	130	1	<5
Instant Breakfast Classic Chocolate Malt	1 pkg + skim milk (9 fl oz)	220	1	6
Instant Breakfast Creamy Milk Chocolate	1 pkg	130	1	<5
Instant Breakfast Creamy Milk Chocolate	1 can (10 fl oz)	220	1	5
Instant Breakfast Creamy Milk Chocolate	1 pkg + skim milk (9 fl oz)	220	1	8
Instant Breakfast Creamy Milk Chocolate	8 fl oz	220	1	10
Instant Breakfast French Vanilla	1 pkg + skim milk	220	0	6
Instant Breakfast French Vanilla	1 pkg	130	0	<5
Instant Breakfast No Sugar Added Classic Chocolate	1 pkg + skim milk (9 fl oz)	160	1	6
Instant Breakfast No Sugar Added Classic Chocolate	1 pkg	70	1	<5
Instant Breakfast No Sugar Added Creamy Milk Chocolate	1 pkg	70	1	<5
Instant Breakfast No Sugar Added Creamy Milk Chocolate	1 pkg + skim milk (9 fl oz)	160	1	6
Instant Breakfast No Sugar Added French Vanilla	1 pkg	70	0	<5
Instant Breakfast No Sugar Added French Vanilla	1 pkg + skim milk (9 fl oz)	150	0	6
Instant Breakfast No Sugar Added Strawberry Creme	1 pkg + skim milk (9 fl oz)	150	0	6
Instant Breakfast No Sugar Added Strawberry Creme	1 pkg	70	0	<5

FOOD	PORTION	CALS.	FIB.	CHOL.
Carnation (CONT.)				
Instant Breakfast Strawberry Creme	1 pkg + skim milk	220	0	6
Instant Breakfast Strawberry Creme	1 pkg	130	0	<5
orange drink powder	3 rounded tsp	93	—	0
orange drink powder as prep w/ water	6 oz	86	—	0
BROAD BEANS				
canned	1 cup	183	—	0
fresh cooked	3½ oz	56	—	0
dried cooked	1 cup	186	—	0
BROCCOLI				
FRESH				
Dole				
chopped cooked	1 med spear	40	5	0
chopped cooked	½ cup	22	2	0
raw chopped	½ cup	12	1	0
FROZEN				
Big Valley				
Chopped	¾ cup (3 oz)	25	2	0
Cuts	¾ cup (3 oz)	25	2	0
Birds Eye				
Baby Spears Deluxe	⅔ cup	30	3	0
Chopped	⅔ cup	25	3	0
Farm Fresh Spears	¾ cup	30	2	0
Florets Deluxe	½ cup	25	3	0
Polybag Cuts	½ cup	25	3	0
Polybag Deluxe Florets	⅔ cup	25	3	0
Spears	⅔ cup	25	3	0
With Cheese Sauce	½ pkg	110	1	15
Green Giant				
Cut	½ cup	16	2	0
Cuts	½ cup	12	2	0
Harvest Fresh Spears	½ cup	20	2	0
In Butter Sauce	½ cup	40	—	5
In Cheese Sauce	½ cup	60	2	2
Mini Spears Select	4-5 spears	18	3	0
One Serve Cuts In Butter Sauce	1 pkg	70	3	5
One Serve Cuts In Butter Sauce	1 pkg	45	3	5
Valley Combinations Broccoli Fanfare	½ cup	80	—	0
Hanover				
Cut	½ cup	25	—	0

FOOD	PORTION	CALS.	FIB.	CHOL.
Hanover (CONT.)				
Florets	½ cup	30	—	0
Tree Of Life	1 cup (3.1 oz)	25	2	0
chopped cooked	½ cup	25	—	0
spears cooked	10 oz pkg	69	4	0
spears cooked	½ cup	25	3	0
BROWNIE				
FROZEN				
Pepperidge Farm				
Monterey Hot Fudge Chocolate Chunk Brownie	1	480	—	65
Newport Hot Fudge Brownie	1	400	—	80
Weight Watchers				
Brownie Ala Mode	1	180	—	5
Chocolate Brownie	1 (1.25 oz)	100	—	5
Mint Frosted	1 (1.23 oz)	100	—	2
HOME RECIPE				
plain	1 (0.8 oz)	112	1	17
w/nuts	1 (0.8 oz)	95	—	18
MIX				
Betty Crocker				
Brownie With Hot Fudge MicroRave Single	1	350	—	0
Frosted MicroRave	1	180	—	0
Fudge Family Size	1	150	—	10
Fudge Light	1	100	—	0
Fudge MicroRave	1	150	—	0
Fudge Regular Size	1	150	—	15
Supreme Caramel	1	120	—	10
Supreme Frosted	1	160	—	10
Supreme German Chocolate	1	160	—	10
Supreme Original	1	140	—	10
Supreme Party	1	160	—	10
Supreme Walnut	1	140	—	10
Walnut MicroRave	1	160	—	0
Estee				
Lite	2	100	1	0
Jiffy				
Fudge as prep	1	160	tr	7
plain	1 (1.2 oz)	139	1	9
plain low calorie	1 (0.8 oz)	84	1	0
READY-TO-EAT				
Frito Lay				
Fudge Nut	3 oz	360	—	8

FOOD	PORTION	CALS.	FIB.	CHOL.
Greenfield				
Brownie HomeStyle	1 (1.4 oz)	120	1	0
Hostess				
Brownie Bites	5 (2 oz)	260	2	50
Brownie Bites Walnut	5 (2 oz)	270	2	50
Lance	1 pkg (78 g)	320	—	5
Little Debbie				
Fudge	1 pkg (2.1 oz)	270	1	15
Fudge	1 pkg (3.6 oz)	450	2	20
Fudge	1 pkg (2.9 oz)	360	1	15
Fudge	1 pkg (2.5 oz)	310	1	15
Pepperidge Farm				
Charlotte Fudgey Brownie	1	220	2	25
Tahoe Milk Chocolate Pecan	1	210	1	25
Westport Fudgey Brownies w/ Walnuts	1	220	2	25
Tastykake				
Brownie	1 (85 g)	340	5	20
plain	1 lg (2 oz)	227	1	10
plain	1 sm (1 oz)	115	1	5
w/ nuts	1 (1 oz)	100	—	14
w/o nuts	1 (2 oz)	243	—	9
BRUSSELS SPROUTS				
FRESH				
Dole	½ cup	19	2	0
cooked	½ cup	30	3	0
cooked	1 sprout	8	—	0
raw	½ cup	19	—	0
raw	1 sprout	8	1	0
FROZEN				
Big Valley				
Whole	5-8 pieces (3 oz)	35	1	0
Birds Eye				
Brussels Sprouts	½ cup	35	3	0
Green Giant	½ cup	25	2	0
In Butter Sauce	½ cup	40	—	5
Hanover				
Brussels Sprouts	½ cup	40	—	0
cooked	½ cup	33	—	0
BUCKWHEAT				
Wolff's				
Kasha Coarse cooked	¼ cup (1.6 oz)	170	2	0
Kasha Fine cooked	¼ cup (1.6 oz)	170	2	0

FOOD	PORTION	CALS.	FIB.	CHOL.
Wolff's (CONT.)				
Kasha Medium cooked	¼ cup (1.6 oz)	170	2	0
Kasha Whole cooked	¼ cup (1.6 oz)	170	2	0
flour whole groat	1 cup	402	—	0
groats roasted cooked	½ cup	91	—	0
groats roasted uncooked	½ cup	283	—	0

BUFFALO
water roasted	3 oz	111	—	52

BULGUR
Casbah				
Pilaf Mix as prep	1 cup	200	4	0
Salad Mix as prep	⅔ cup	90	1	0
Good Shepherd	¼ cup (43 g)	150	1	0
Hodgson Mill	¼ cup (1.4 oz)	120	1	0
cooked	½ cup	76	—	0
uncooked	½ cup	239	—	0

BURBOT (FISH)
fresh baked	3 oz	98	—	65

BURDOCK ROOT
FRESH				
cooked	1 cup	110	—	0
raw	1 cup	85	—	0

BUTTER
(*see also* BUTTER BLENDS, BUTTER SUBSTITUTES, MARGARINE)

STICK				
Cabot	1 tsp	35	—	11
Unsalted	1 tsp	35	—	11
Crystal				
Salted	1 tbsp (0.5 oz)	102	0	43
Unsalted	1 tbsp (0.5 oz)	102	0	43
Land O'Lakes	1 tbsp (0.5 oz)	100	—	30
Light	1 tbsp	50	—	20
Light Unsalted	1 tbsp	50	—	15
Unsalted	1 tbsp (0.5 oz)	100	—	30
butter	1 pat	36	—	11
butter	1 stick (4 oz)	813	—	248
clarified butter	3½ oz	876	—	256
TUB				
Land O'Lakes	1 tbsp (0.3 oz)	70	—	20
Unsalted	1 tbsp	60	—	20
whipped	1 pat	27	—	8
whipped	4 oz	542	—	165

FOOD	PORTION	CALS.	FIB.	CHOL.

BUTTER BEANS
CANNED
Allen

FOOD	PORTION	CALS.	FIB.	CHOL.
Baby	½ cup (4.5 oz)	120	6	0
Large	½ cup (4.5 oz)	120	7	0
Hanover				
In Sauce	½ cup	80	—	0
In Sauce	½ cup	100	—	0
S&W				
Tender Cooked	½ cup	100	—	0
Sunshine	½ cup (4.5 oz)	120	8	0
Trappey				
Baby White With Bacon	½ cup (4.5 oz)	130	6	0
Large White With Bacon	½ cup (4.5 oz)	110	6	0
Van Camp's	½ cup	110	7	0

BUTTER BLENDS
(*see also* BUTTER, BUTTER SUBSTITUTES, MARGARINE)
STICK
Blue Bonnet

FOOD	PORTION	CALS.	FIB.	CHOL.
Better Blend Unsalted	1 tbsp	90	—	5
Country Morning				
Blend	1 tbsp	100	—	0
Blend Light	1 tbsp (0.5 oz)	50	—	10
Blend Unsalted	1 tbsp	100	—	0
butter blend	1 stick	811	—	99
TUB				
Blue Bonnet				
Better Blend	1 tbsp	90	—	0
Country Morning				
Blend Light	1 tbsp (0.5 oz)	50	—	5
Blend Tub	1 tbsp	100	—	0
Downey's				
Cinnamon Honey-Butter	1 tbsp	52	—	tr
Original Honey-Butter	1 tbsp	52	—	tr
Le Slim Cow	1 tbsp	40	—	7
Touch of Butter	1 tbsp (0.5 oz)	60	0	0

BUTTER SUBSTITUTES
(*see also* BUTTER BLENDS, MARGARINE)
Butter Buds

FOOD	PORTION	CALS.	FIB.	CHOL.
Mix	1 tsp (2 g)	5	—	0
Sprinkles	1 tsp (2 g)	5	—	0
Molly McButter	½ tsp (1g)	3	—	tr
w/ Bacon	½ tsp (1 g)	4	—	tr
w/ Cheese	½ tsp (0.9 g)	4	—	1

FOOD	PORTION	CALS.	FIB.	CHOL.
Molly McButter (CONT.)				
w/ Sour Cream	½ tsp (1.1 g)	4	—	tr
Watkins				
Butter Sprinkles	1 tsp (2 g)	5	0	0
BUTTERBUR				
CANNED				
fuki chopped	1 cup	3	—	0
FRESH				
fuki raw	1 cup	13	—	0
BUTTERFISH				
FRESH				
baked	3 oz	159	—	71
fillet baked	1 oz	47	—	21
BUTTERNUTS				
dried	1 oz	174	—	0
BUTTERSCOTCH				
(*see also* CANDY)				
CABBAGE				
FRESH				
Dole	½ med head	18	2	0
Napa shredded	½ cup	6	tr	0
Fresh Express				
Cole Slaw	1½ cups (3 oz)	25	2	0
chinese pak-choi raw shredded	½ cup	5	—	0
chinese pak-choi shredded cooked	½ cup	10	—	0
chinese pe-tsai raw shredded	1 cup	12	—	0
chinese pe-tsai shredded cooked	1 cup	16	—	0
danish raw	1 head (2 lbs)	228	18	0
danish raw shredded	½ cup (1.2 oz)	9	tr	0
danish shredded cooked	½ cup (2.6 oz)	17	1	0
green raw	1 head (2 lbs)	228	18	0
green raw shredded	½ cup (1.2 oz)	9	tr	0
green shredded cooked	½ cup (2.6 oz)	17	1	0
red raw shredded	½ cup	10	1	0
red shredded cooked	½ cup	16	—	0
savoy raw shredded	½ cup	10	—	0
savoy shredded cooked	½ cup	18	—	0
HOME RECIPE				
coleslaw w/ dressing	¾ cup	147	—	5
TAKE-OUT				
coleslaw w/ dressing	½ cup	42	—	5

FOOD	PORTION	CALS.	FIB.	CHOL.
stuffed cabbage	1 (6 oz)	373	—	95
vinegar & oil coleslaw	3.5 oz	150	—	0

CAKE

(see also BROWNIE, COOKIE, DANISH PASTRY, DOUGHNUT, PIE)

FROSTING/ICING

Betty Crocker

FOOD	PORTION	CALS.	FIB.	CHOL.
Butter Pecan Ready-to-Spread	½ tub	170	—	0
Cherry Ready-to-Spread	½ tub	160	—	0
Chocolate Ready-to-Spread	½ tub	160	—	0
Chocolate Chip Ready-to-Spread	½ tub	170	—	0
Chocolate Fudge as prep	½ mix	180	—	0
Chocolate Light Ready-to-Spread	½ tub	130	—	0
Chocolate With Candy Coated Chocolate Chips Ready-to-Spread	½ tub	160	—	0
Chocolate With Dinosaurs Ready-to-Spread	½ tub	160	—	0
Chocolate With Turbo Racers Ready-to-Spread	½ tub	160	—	0
Coconut Pecan Ready-to-Spread	½ tub	160	—	0
Coconut Pecan as prep	½ mix	180	—	0
Cream Cheese Ready-to-Spread	½ tub	170	—	0
Creamy Milk Chocolate as prep	½ mix	170	—	0
Creamy Vanilla as prep	½ mix	170	—	0
Dark Dutch Fudge Ready-to-Spread	½ tub	160	—	0
Lemon Ready-to-Spread	½ tub	170	—	0
Milk Chocolate Light Ready-to-Spread	½ tub	140	—	0
Milk Chocolate Ready-to-Spread	½ tub	160	—	0
Rainbow Chip Ready-to-Spread	½ tub	170	—	0
Sour Cream Chocolate Ready-to-Spread	½ tub	160	—	0
Sour Cream White Ready-to-Spread	½ tub	160	—	0
Vanilla Ready-to-Spread	½ tub	160	—	0
Vanilla Light Ready-to-Spread	½ tub	140	—	0
Vanilla With Teddy Bears Ready-to-Spread	½ tub	160	—	0

FOOD	PORTION	CALS.	FIB.	CHOL.
Betty Crocker (CONT.)				
White Fluffy as prep	¹⁄₁₂ mix	70	—	0
Duncan Hines				
Chocolate Creamy Homestyle	1 oz	130	2	0
Milk Chocolate Creamy Homestyle	1 oz	130	1	0
Vanilla Creamy Homestyle	1 oz	140	1	0
Estee				
Lite Frosting as prep	3 tbsp (0.7 oz)	100	0	0
Jiffy				
Fudge	¼ cup (1.2 oz)	150	tr	0
White	¼ cup (1.2 oz)	150	0	0
Pillsbury				
Fluffy White Frosting Mix	for ¹⁄₁₂ cake	60	—	0
Frost It Hot Chocolate	for ⅛ cake	50	—	0
Frost It Hot Fluffy White	for ⅛ cake	50	—	0
chocolate as prep w/ butter	¹⁄₁₂ box (1.5 oz)	161	—	10
chocolate as prep w/ butter	1 box (13.7 oz)	1908	—	121
chocolate as prep w/ butter home recipe	¹⁄₁₂ recipe (1.8 oz)	200	—	15
chocolate as prep w/ butter home recipe	1 recipe (21.1 oz)	2409	—	176
chocolate as prep w/ margarine	¹⁄₁₂ box (1.5 oz)	161	—	0
chocolate as prep w/ margarine	1 box (13.7 oz)	1909	—	0
chocolate as prep w/ margarine home recipe	1 recipe (21.1 oz)	2411	—	5
chocolate as prep w/ margarine home recipe	¹⁄₁₂ recipe (1.8 oz)	200	—	0
chocolate ready-to-use	¹⁄₁₂ pkg (1.3 oz)	151	—	0
chocolate ready-to-use	1 pkg (16 oz)	1834	—	0
coconut ready-to-use	1 pkg (16 oz)	1903	—	0
coconut ready-to-use	¹⁄₁₂ pkg (1.3 oz)	157	—	0
cream cheese ready-to-use	¹⁄₁₂ pkg (1.3 oz)	157	—	0
cream cheese ready-to-use	1 pkg (16 oz)	1906	—	0
glaze home recipe	1 recipe (11.5 oz)	1173	—	7
glaze home recipe	¹⁄₁₂ recipe (1 oz)	97	—	1
seven minute home recipe	¹⁄₁₂ recipe (1.1 oz)	102	—	0
seven minute home recipe	1 recipe (13.6 oz)	1231	—	0
vanilla as prep w/ butter	¹⁄₁₂ pkg (1.5 oz)	182	—	10
vanilla as prep w/ butter	1 pkg (14.5 oz)	2188	—	126
vanilla as prep w/ butter home recipe	1 recipe (20.1 oz)	1972	—	67
vanilla as prep w/ butter home recipe	¹⁄₁₂ recipe (1.7 oz)	165	—	6

FOOD	PORTION	CALS.	FIB.	CHOL.
vanilla as prep w/ margarine	1 pkg (14.5 oz)	2190	—	0
vanilla as prep w/ margarine	1/12 pkg (1.5 oz)	182	—	0
vanilla as prep w/ margarine home recipe	1 recipe (20.1 oz)	2326	—	5
vanilla as prep w/ margarine home recipe	1/12 recipe (1.7 oz)	195	—	0
vanilla ready-to-use	1 pkg (16 oz)	1936	—	0
vanilla ready-to-use	1/12 pkg (1.3 oz)	159	—	0
FROZEN				
Pepperidge Farm				
Amhurst Apple Crumb Coffee Cake	1	220	—	20
Apple 'N Spice Bake Dessert Lights	1 piece (4¼ oz)	170	—	10
Berkshire Apple Crisp	1	250	1	40
Boston Cream Supreme	1 piece (2⅞ oz)	290	—	50
Butter Pound	1 slice (1 oz)	130	—	60
Carrot Classic	1 cake	260	—	50
Carrot w/ Cream Cheese Icing	1 slice (1½ oz)	150	—	15
Charleston Peach Melba Shortcake	1	220	—	135
Cherries Supreme Dessert Lights	1 piece (3¼ oz)	170	—	80
Chocolate Supreme	1 piece (2⅞ oz)	300	—	25
Chocolate Fudge Large Layer	1 slice (1⅝ oz)	180	—	20
Chocolate Fudge Strip Large Layer	1 piece (1⅝ oz)	170	—	20
Chocolate Mousse Cake Dessert Lights	1 piece (2½ oz)	190	—	5
Cholesterol Free Pound	1 slice (1 oz)	110	—	0
Coconut Classic	1 cake	230	—	20
Coconut Large Layer	1 slice (1⅝ oz)	180	—	20
Devil's Food Large Layer	1 slice (1⅝ oz)	180	—	20
Double Chocolate Classic	1 cake	250	—	35
Fudge Golden Classic	1 cake	260	—	40
German Chocolate Classic	1 cake	250	—	45
German Chocolate Large Layer	1 slice (1⅝ oz)	180	—	20
Golden Large Layer	1 slice (1⅝ oz)	180	—	20
Lemon Cake Supreme Dessert Lights	1 piece (2¾ oz)	170	—	50
Lemon Coconut Supreme	1 piece (3 oz)	280	—	30
Lemon Cream Supreme	1 piece (1⅝ oz)	170	—	20
Manhattan Strawberry Cheesecake	1	300	—	150

FOOD	PORTION	CALS.	FIB.	CHOL.
Pepperidge Farm (CONT.)				
Peach Melba Supreme	1 (3⅛ oz)	270	—	35
Peach Parfait Dessert Lights	1 piece (4¼ oz)	150	—	10
Pineapple Cream Supreme	1 piece (2 oz)	190	—	20
Raspberry Vanilla Swirl Dessert Lights	1 piece (3¼ oz)	160	—	15
Strawberry Shortcake Dessert Lights	1 piece (3 oz)	170	1	70
Strawberry Cream Supreme	1 piece (2 oz)	190	—	20
Strawberry Strip Large Layer	1 piece (1½ oz)	160	—	20
Vanilla Fudge Swirl Classic	1 cake	250	—	35
Vanilla Large Layer	1 slice (1⅝ oz)	190	—	20
Sara Lee				
Apple Crisp Light	1 (3 oz)	150	—	5
Black Forest Light	1 (3.6 oz)	170	—	10
Carrot Light	1 (2.5 oz)	170	—	5
Carrot Single Layer Iced	1 slice (2.4 oz)	250	—	25
Chocolate Free & Light	1 slice (1.7 oz)	110	—	0
Double Chocolate Light	1 (2.5 oz)	150	—	10
Double Chocolate Three Layer	1 slice (2.2 oz)	220	—	20
French Cheesecake Light	1 slice (3.2 oz)	150	—	15
French Cheese	1 slice (2.9 oz)	250	—	20
Lemon Cream Light	1 (3.2 oz)	180	—	10
Pound Free & Light	1 slice (1 oz)	70	—	0
Strawberry French Cheesecake Light	1 (3.5 oz)	150	—	5
Strawberry Yogurt Dessert Free & Light	1 slice (2.2 oz)	120	—	0
Weight Watchers				
Apple Crisp	1 (3.5 oz)	190	—	0
Brownie Cheesecake	1 (3.5 oz)	200	—	10
Cherries And Cream Cake	1 (3 oz)	150	—	5
Chocolate	1 (2.5 oz)	180	—	5
Chocolate Eclair	1 (2.1 oz)	120	—	15
Double Fudge	1 piece (2.75 oz)	190	—	5
Strawberry Cheesecake	1 piece (3.9 oz)	180	—	20
boston cream pie	1/6 cake (3.2 oz)	232	1	34
eclair w/ chocolate icing & custard filling	1	205	—	35
HOME RECIPE				
angelfood	1/12 cake (1.9 oz)	142	1	0
apple crisp	1 recipe 6 serv (29.6 oz)	1377	—	1
apple crisp	½ cup (5 oz)	230	—	0

FOOD	PORTION	CALS.	FIB.	CHOL.
boston cream pie	1/6 cake (3.3 oz)	293	1	43
carrot w/ cream cheese icing	1/12 cake (3.9 oz)	484	—	60
carrot w/ cream cheese icing	1 cake 10 in diam	6175	—	1183
cheesecake	1/12 cake (4.5 oz)	456	—	155
cheesecake w/ cherry topping	1/12 cake (5 oz)	359	—	106
chocolate cupcake creme filled w/ frosting	1 (1.8 oz)	188	—	9
chocolate w/o frosting	1/12 cake (3.3 oz)	340	—	55
chocolate w/o frosting	2 layers (39.9 oz)	4067	—	661
coffeecake crumb topped cinnamon	1/12 cake (2.1 oz)	240	2	36
cream puff w/ custard filling	1 (4.6 oz)	336	—	174
cream puff shell	1 (2.3 oz)	239	—	129
eclair	1 (3 oz)	262	—	127
fruitcake	1/36 cake (2.9 oz)	302	3	24
fruitcake dark	1 cake 7½ in x 2¼ in	5185	—	640
gingerbread	1/9 cake (2.6 oz)	264	2	24
pineapple upside down	1/9 cake (4 oz)	367	—	25
pound	1 loaf 8½ in x 3½ in	1935	—	1100
pound cake	1 slice (1 oz)	120	—	32
sheet cake w/ white frosting	1 cake 9 in sq	4020	—	636
sheet cake w/ white frosting	1/9 cake	445	—	70
sheet cake w/o frosting	1 cake 9 in sq	2830	—	552
sheet cake w/o frosting	1/9 cake	315	—	61
shortcake	1 (2.3 oz)	225	—	2
sponge	1/12 cake (2.2 oz)	140	—	80
white w/ coconut frosting	1/12 cake (3.9 oz)	399	—	2
white w/o frosting	1/12 cake (2.6 oz)	264	—	2
yellow w/o frosting	1/12 cake (2.4 oz)	245	—	37
yellow w/o frosting	2 layers (28.7 oz)	2947	—	443
MIX				
Aunt Jemima				
Coffee Cake Easy Mix	1/3 cup (1.4 oz)	170	1	0
Betty Crocker				
Angel Food Confetti	1/12 cake	150	—	0
Angel Food Traditional	1/12 cake	130	—	0
Angel Food White	1/12 cake	150	—	0
Angel Food Lemon Custard	1/12 cake	150	—	0
Apple Streusel MicroRave	1/6 cake	240	—	45
Apple Streusel MicroRave No Cholesterol Recipe	1/6 cake	210	—	0
Butter Chocolate	1/12 cake	280	—	75
Butter Pecan SuperMoist	1/12 cake	250	—	55

FOOD	PORTION	CALS.	FIB.	CHOL.
Betty Crocker (CONT.)				
Butter Pecan No Cholesterol Recipe	1/12 cake	220	—	0
Butter Yellow	1/12 cake	260	—	75
Carrot	1/12 cake	250	—	55
Carrot No Cholesterol Recipe	1/12 cake	210	—	0
Cherry Chip	1/12 cake	190	—	0
Chocolate Chocolate Chip	1/12 cake	260	—	55
Chocolate Chip	1/12 cake	290	—	55
Chocolate Chip No Cholesterol Recipe	1/12 cake	220	—	0
Chocolate Fudge	1/12 cake	260	—	55
Cinnamon Pecan Streusel Microwave	1/6 cake	280	—	35
Cinnamon Pecan Streusel Microwave No Cholesterol	1/6 cake	230	—	0
Devil's Food	1/12 cake	260	—	55
Devil's Food Chocolate Frosting MicroRave	1/6 cake	310	—	35
Devil's Food No Cholesterol Recipe	1/12 cake	220	—	0
Devils Food SuperMoist Light	1/12 cake	200	—	55
Devils Food SuperMoist Light No Cholesterol Recipe	1/12 cake	180	—	0
Devils Food With Chocolate Frosting MicroRave Single	1	440	—	50
German Chocolate	1/12 cake	260	—	55
German Chocolate Chocolate Frosting MicroRave	1/6 cake	320	—	35
German Chocolate No Cholesterol Recipe	1/12 cake	220	—	0
Gingerbread Classic Dessert	1/9 cake	22	—	30
Gingerbread Classic Dessert No Cholesterol Recipe	1/9 cake	210	—	0
Golden Pound Classic Dessert	1/12 cake	200	—	35
Golden Vanilla	1/12 cake	280	—	55
Golden Vanilla No Cholesterol Recipe	1/12 cake	220	—	0
Golden Vanilla Rainbow Chip Frosting MicroRave	1/6 cake	320	—	35
Lemon	1/12 cake	260	—	55
Lemon No Cholesterol Recipe	1/12 cake	220	—	0
Marble	1/12 cake	260	—	55
Marble No Cholesterol Recipe	1/12 cake	220	—	0

FOOD	PORTION	CALS.	FIB.	CHOL.
Betty Crocker (CONT.)				
Milk Chocolate	¹⁄₁₂ cake	260	—	55
Milk Chocolate No Cholesterol Recipe	¹⁄₁₂ cake	210	—	0
Pineapple Upsidedown Classic Dessert	¹⁄₉ cake	250	—	40
Rainbow Chip	¹⁄₁₂ cake	250	—	55
Sour Cream Chocolate	¹⁄₁₂ cake	260	—	55
Sour Cream Chocolate No Cholesterol Recipe	¹⁄₁₂ cake	220	—	0
Sour Cream White	¹⁄₁₂ cake	180	—	0
Spice	¹⁄₁₂ cake	260	—	55
Spice No Cholesterol Recipe	¹⁄₁₂ cake	220	—	0
White	¹⁄₁₂ cake	240	—	0
White No Cholesterol Recipe	¹⁄₁₂ cake	220	—	0
White SuperMoist Light	¹⁄₁₂ cake	180	—	0
Yellow	¹⁄₁₂ cake	260	—	55
Yellow SuperMoist Light	¹⁄₁₂ cake	200	—	55
Yellow SuperMoist Light No Cholesterol Recipe	¹⁄₁₂ cake	190	—	0
Yellow Chocolate Frosting MicroRave	¹⁄₆ cake	300	—	35
Yellow No Cholesterol Recipe	¹⁄₁₂ cake	220	—	0
Yellow With Chocolate Frosting MicroRave Single	1	440	—	50
Bisquick	½ cup (2 oz)	240	—	0
Reduced Fat	½ cup (2 oz)	210	—	0
Duncan Hines				
Angel Food	¹⁄₁₂ pkg (1.3 oz)	140	1	0
Cupcake Yellow With Chocolate Frosting	1	180	—	6
Devil's Food Moist Deluxe	¹⁄₁₂ cake (1.5 oz)	290	1	45
French Vanilla Moist Deluxe	¹⁄₁₂ cake (1.5 oz)	250	0	45
Fudge Marble Moist Deluxe	¹⁄₁₂ cake (1.5 oz)	250	0	45
Lemon Supreme Moist Deluxe	¹⁄₁₂ cake (1.5 oz)	250	0	45
Yellow Moist Deluxe	¹⁄₁₂ cake (1.5 oz)	250	—	45
Estee				
Lite White as prep	¹⁄₈ cake (1.7 oz)	200	tr	0
Lite Chocolate	¹⁄₈ cake (1.7 oz)	190	1	0
Lite Pound as prep	¹⁄₈ cake (1.7 oz)	200	tr	0
Jell-O				
Cheesecake	¹⁄₈ cake	277	—	28
Cheesecake New York Style	¹⁄₈ cake	283	—	28
Jiffy				
Devil's Food as prep	¹⁄₅ cake	220	1	42

FOOD	PORTION	CALS.	FIB.	CHOL.
Jiffy (CONT.)				
Golden Yellow as prep	⅓ cake	220	1	36
White as prep	⅓ cake	210	tr	0
Royal				
Cheese Cake Lite No-Bake	⅛ pie	130	—	5
Wanda's				
Double Chocolate	¼ cup mix per serv (1.4 oz)	170	2	0
angelfood	10 in cake (20.9 oz)	1535	9	0
angelfood	1⁄12 cake (1.8 oz)	129	1	0
chocolate w/o frosting	2 layers (26.8 oz)	2393	—	425
chocolate w/o frosting	1⁄12 cake (2.3 oz)	198	—	35
chocolate w/o frosting low sodium	1⁄10 cake (1.3 oz)	116	—	0
coffeecake crumb topped cinnamon	⅛ cake (2 oz)	178	2	28
devil's food w/o frosting	1⁄12 cake (2.3 oz)	198	—	35
devil's food w/ chocolate frosting	1⁄16 cake	235	—	37
devil's food w/ chocolate frosting	1 cake 9 in diam	3755	—	598
fudge w/o frosting	1⁄12 cake (2.3 oz)	198	—	35
german chocolate pudding type w/ coconut nut frosting	1⁄12 cake (3.9 oz)	404	—	53
gingerbread	1 cake 8 in sq	1575	—	6
gingerbread	⅑ cake (2.4 oz)	207	2	24
lemon w/o frosting no sugar low sodium	1⁄10 cake (1.3 oz)	118	—	0
marble pudding type w/o frosting	2 layers (30.6 oz)	3021	—	638
marble pudding type w/o frosting	1⁄12 cake (2.6 oz)	253	—	53
white w/o frosting no sugar low sodium	1⁄10 cake (1.3 oz)	118	—	0
yellow w/ chocolate frosting	1⁄16 cake	235	—	36
yellow w/o frosting	2 layers (26.5 oz)	2415	—	437
yellow w/o frosting	1⁄12 cake (2.2 oz)	202	—	37
yellow w/ chocolate frosting	1 cake 9 in diam	3895	—	609
READY-TO-EAT				
Baker Maid				
Creole Royal Pineapple Apricot	3 slices (5 oz)	270	4	20
Creole Royal Pineapple Apricot	1 slice (1.7 oz)	90	1	5
Dutch Mill				
Dessert Shells Chocolate Covered	1 (0.5 oz)	80	0	0
Freihofer's				
Angel Food	⅕ cake (2 oz)	150	0	0
Cinnamon Swirl Buns	1 (2.8 oz)	290	1	30

FOOD	PORTION	CALS.	FIB.	CHOL.
Freihofer's (CONT.)				
Coffee Cake Cinnamon Pecan	⅛ cake (2 oz)	220	1	25
Crumb	⅛ cake (2 oz)	240	1	15
Homestyle Golden Loaf	⅛ cake (1.8 oz)	200	0	50
Pound	⅕ cake (2.8 oz)	330	0	65
Hostess				
Angel Food Ring	⅙ cake (1.6 oz)	150	0	<5
Fruit Cake Holiday	⅙ cake (5.3 oz)	490	3	10
Pound Cake	⅕ cake (3.2 oz)	350	1	55
Perugira				
Pannettone Au Beurre	⅙ cake (2.9 oz)	310	2	110
Sinbad				
Baklava	1 piece (2 oz)	337	2	10
Thomas'				
Date Nut Loaf	1 oz	90	1	<5
angelfood	1 cake (11.9 oz)	876	5	0
angelfood	1/12 cake (1 oz)	73	1	0
cheesecake	⅙ cake (2.8 oz)	256	2	44
cheesecake	1 cake 9 in diam	3350	—	2053
coffeecake crumb topped cinnamon	⅑ cake (2.2 oz)	263	2	20
fruitcake	1 piece (1.5 oz)	139	—	2
panettone dal forno	⅑ cake (1.9 oz)	212	0	25
pound	⅒ cake (1 oz)	117	—	66
pound fat free	1 oz	80	—	0
pound fat free	1 cake (12 oz)	961	—	0
pound cake	1 cake (8½ x 3½ x 3 in)	1935	—	1100
pound cake	1 slice (1 oz)	110	—	100
sour cream pound	⅒ cake (1 oz)	117	tr	17
sponge	1/12 cake (1.3 oz)	110	—	39
tiramisu	1 piece (5.1 oz)	409	tr	171
tiramisu	1 cake (4.4 lbs)	5732	3	2395
white w/ white frosting	1 cake 9 in diam	4170	—	46
white w/ white frosting	1/16 cake	260	—	3
yellow w/ chocolate frosting	1 cake 9 diam	3895	—	609
yellow w/ chocolate frosting	⅛ cake (2.2 oz)	242	1	35
REFRIGERATED				
Baby Watson				
Cheesecake	1 slice (3.8 oz)	390	2	142
Cheesecake Light	1/16 cake (3.9 oz)	280	3	33
Pillsbury				
Apple Turnovers	1	170	—	0
Cherry Turnovers	1	170	—	0

FOOD	PORTION	CALS.	FIB.	CHOL.
Pillsbury (CONT.)				
Coffee Cake Cinnamon Swirl	⅛ of cake	180	—	0
Coffee Cake Pecan Struesel	⅛ of cake	180	—	0
Pastry Pockets	1	240	—	0
SNACK				
Drake's				
Coffee Cake	1 (1.1 oz)	140	—	10
Coffee Cake Chocolate Crumb	1 (2.5 oz)	245	—	18
Coffee Cake Cinnamon Crumb	½ cake (1.3 oz)	150	—	10
Coffee Cake Small	1 (2 oz)	220	—	15
Devil Dog	1 (1.5 oz)	160	—	0
Funny Bones	1 (1.25 oz)	150	—	0
Light & Fruity Apple	1 (1.2 oz)	90	—	0
Light & Fruity Blueberry	1 (1.2 oz)	90	—	0
Light & Fruity Cinnamon Raisin	1 (1.2 oz)	90	—	0
Pound Cake	1	110	—	25
Ring Ding	1 (1.5 oz)	180	—	0
Ring Ding Mint	1 (1.5 oz)	190	—	0
Sunny Doodle	1 (1 oz)	100	—	10
Yankee Doodle	1 (1 oz)	100	—	0
Greenfield				
Blondie Apple Spice	1 (1.4 oz)	120	0	0
Blondie Chocolate Chip	1 (1.4 oz)	120	0	0
Hostess				
Apple Twist	1 (2.5 oz)	220	tr	15
Baseball Yellow Cakes	1 (1.6 oz)	160	0	<5
Choco Licious	1 (1.5 oz)	170	1	10
Choco-Diles	1 (1.8 oz)	210	1	20
Cinnaminis Original	5 (2.4 oz)	300	2	20
Cinnamon Roll	1 (2.3 oz)	220	1	25
Crumb Cake	1 (1.9 oz)	210	1	15
Crumb Cake Light	1 (1.8 oz)	150	tr	0
Cup Cakes Chocolate	1 (1.6 oz)	170	tr	<5
Cup Cakes Chocolate Light	1 (1.4 oz)	120	tr	0
Cup Cakes Orange	1 (1.5 oz)	160	0	10
Dessert Cups	1 (1 oz)	90	0	10
Ding Dongs	1 (1.3 oz)	160	tr	5
Fruit Loaf	1 (3.8 oz)	350	2	5
Ho Ho's	1 (1 oz)	130	tr	10
Holiday Cakes	1 (1.6 oz)	160	0	<5
Honey Bun Glazed	1 (2.7 oz)	320	2	15
Honey Bun Iced	1 (3.4 oz)	390	2	15
Hopper Cakes	1 (1.6 oz)	160	0	<5
Lil Angels	1 (1 oz)	90	0	<5

FOOD	PORTION	CALS.	FIB.	CHOL.
Hostess (CONT.)				
Pecan Spinners	1 (1 oz)	110	tr	0
Sno Balls	1 (1.6 oz)	160	1	0
Suzy Q's	1 (2 oz)	220	2	10
Suzy Q's Banana	1 (2 oz)	220	tr	25
Swirls Caramel Pecan	1 (2 oz)	140	1	15
Tiger Tails	1 (1.5 oz)	160	tr	15
Twinkies	1 (1.4 oz)	140	0	15
Twinkies Banana	2 (2.7 oz)	300	tr	35
Twinkies Devil Food	2 (2.7 oz)	300	2	15
Twinkies Lights	1 (1.4 oz)	120	0	0
Twinkies Strawberry Fruit 'n Creme	1 (1.6 oz)	150	tr	20
Kellogg's				
Pop-Tarts Apple Cinnamon	1 (1.8 oz)	210	1	0
Pop-Tarts Blueberry	1 (1.8 oz)	210	1	0
Pop-Tarts Brown Sugar Cinnamon	1 (1.8 oz)	220	1	0
Pop-Tarts Cherry	1 (1.8 oz)	200	1	0
Pop-Tarts Chocolate Graham	1 (1.8 oz)	210	1	0
Pop-Tarts Frosted Blueberry	1 (1.8 oz)	200	1	0
Pop-Tarts Frosted Brown Sugar Cinnamon	1 (1.8 oz)	210	1	0
Pop-Tarts Frosted Cherry	1 (1.8 oz)	200	1	0
Pop-Tarts Frosted Chocolate Vanilla Creme	1 (1.8 oz)	200	1	0
Pop-Tarts Frosted Chocolate Fudge	1 (1.8 oz)	200	1	0
Pop-Tarts Frosted Grape	1 (1.8 oz)	200	1	0
Pop-Tarts Frosted Raspberry	1 (1.8 oz)	210	1	0
Pop-Tarts Frosted S'mores	1 (1.8 oz)	200	1	0
Pop-Tarts Frosted Strawberry	1 (1.8 oz)	200	1	0
Pop-Tarts Strawberry	1 (1.8 oz)	200	1	0
Pop-Tarts Minis Frosted Chocolate	1 pkg (1.5 oz)	170	1	0
Pop-Tarts Minis Frosted Grape	1 pkg (1.5 oz)	170	0	0
Pop-Tarts Minis Frosted Strawberry	1 pkg (1.5 oz)	170	0	0
Rice Krispies Treats	1 (0.8 oz)	90	0	0
Lance				
Apple Oatmeal	1 pkg (51 g)	200	—	10
Dunking Sticks	1 (39 g)	190	—	5
Fig Cake	1 pkg (60 g)	210	—	0
Honey Buns	1 (85 g)	330	—	0

FOOD	PORTION	CALS.	FIB.	CHOL.
Lance (CONT.)				
Oatmeal Cake	1 (57 g)	240	—	0
Pecan Twirls	1 pkg (57 g)	220	—	0
Raisin Cake	1 (57 g)	230	—	0
Little Debbie				
Apple Delights	1 pkg (1.2 oz)	140	1	5
Apple-Roos	1 pkg (1.5 oz)	150	1	0
Banana Nut Muffin Loaves	1 pkg (1.9 oz)	210	1	10
Banana Twins	1 pkg (2.2 oz)	250	0	10
Be My Valentine	1 pkg (2.2 oz)	280	1	0
Cherry Cordials	1 pkg (1.3 oz)	160	1	0
Choc-o-Jel	1 pkg (1.2 oz)	150	1	0
Choco-Cakes	1 pkg (2.2 oz)	240	1	0
Choco-Cakes	1 pkg (2.1 oz)	250	1	0
Chocolate	1 pkg (3 oz)	360	1	0
Chocolate Chip	1 pkg (2.4 oz)	290	1	0
Chocolate Twins	1 pkg (2.4 oz)	240	1	20
Christmas Tree Cakes	1 pkg (1.5 oz)	190	0	0
Coconut	1 pkg (2.1 oz)	270	1	5
Coconut	1 pkg (2.4 oz)	300	0	5
Coconut Rounds	1 pkg (1.2 oz)	140	1	0
Coffee Cake Apple	1 pkg (1.9 oz)	220	1	10
Coffee Cake Apple Streusel	1 pkg (2 oz)	220	1	10
Devil Cremes	1 pkg (1.6 oz)	190	1	0
Devil Cremes	1 pkg (3.2 oz)	380	1	5
Devil Squares	1 pkg (2.2 oz)	260	1	0
Easter Basket Cakes	1 pkg (2.5 oz)	310	1	0
Fancy Cakes	1 pkg (2.4 oz)	300	0	0
Fudge Crispy	1 pkg (1.1 oz)	170	1	0
Fudge Round	1 pkg (2.5 oz)	290	2	5
Fudge Round	1 pkg (3 oz)	350	2	5
Fudge Rounds	1 pkg (1.2 oz)	140	1	5
Golden Cremes	1 pkg (1.5 oz)	170	0	0
Golden Cremes	1 pkg (3 oz)	330	0	10
Holiday Cake Chocolate	1 pkg (2.4 oz)	290	1	0
Holiday Cake Vanilla	1 pkg (2.5 oz)	310	1	0
Honey Bun	1 pkg (4 oz)	510	5	0
Honey Bun	1 pkg (3 oz)	380	4	0
Jelly Rolls	1 pkg (2.1 oz)	230	0	15
Lemon Stix	1 pkg (1.5 oz)	210	1	0
Marshmallow Supremes	1 pkg (1.1 oz)	130	1	0
Mint Sprints	1 pkg (1.5 oz)	230	1	0
Nutty Bar	1 pkg (2 oz)	290	1	0
Pecan Twins	1 pkg (2 oz)	220	1	0

FOOD	PORTION	CALS.	FIB.	CHOL.
Little Debbie (CONT.)				
Pumpkin Delights	1 pkg (1.1 oz)	130	1	5
Smiley Faces Cherry	1 pkg (1.2 oz)	140	1	5
Smiley Faces Pumpkin	1 pkg (1 oz)	130	1	0
Snack Cake Chocolate	1 pkg (2.5 oz)	300	1	0
Snack Cake Vanilla	1 pkg (2.6 oz)	320	1	0
Spice	1 pkg (2.5 oz)	300	1	10
Star Crunch	1 pkg (1.1 oz)	140	1	0
Star Crunch	1 pkg (2.6 oz)	330	1	0
Swiss Rolls	1 pkg (2.1 oz)	250	1	15
Swiss Rolls	1 pkg (3.2 oz)	380	1	20
Swiss Rolls	1 pkg (2.7 oz)	320	1	15
Teddy Berries	1 pkg (1.2 oz)	130	1	5
Vanilla	1 pkg (3 oz)	370	0	0
Vanilla Cremes	1 pkg (1.4 oz)	170	0	0
Zebra Cakes	1 pkg (2.6 oz)	150	1	0
Nabisco				
Frosted Strawberry	1 (1.7 oz)	190	1	0
Pepperidge Farm				
Toaster Tart Apple Cinnamon	1	170	—	0
Toaster Tart Cheese	1	190	—	14
Toaster Tart Strawberry	1	190	—	0
Rice Krispies				
Cereal Bar Chocolate Chip	1 (1 oz)	120	1	0
Sweet Rewards				
Fat Free Brownie	1 bar (1 oz)	90	<1	0
Tastykake				
Butter Cream Cream Filled Cupcake	1 (32 g)	120	1	5
Chocolate Cream Filled Cupcake	1 (34 g)	130	1	5
Chocolate Cupcake	1 (30 g)	100	1	5
Honeybun Glazed	1 pkg (92 g)	360	4	0
Honeybun Iced	1 pkg (92 g)	350	1	50
Junior Chocolate	1 pkg (94 g)	340	4	60
Junior Coconut	1 pkg (94 g)	300	3	50
Junior Lemon	1 pkg (94 g)	310	1	75
Junior Orange	1 pkg (94 g)	340	1	50
Kandy Kake Chocolate	1 (19 g)	80	1	0
Kandy Kake Coconut	1 (19 g)	80	1	0
Kandy Kake Peanut Butter	1 (19 g)	90	1	5
Koffee Kake Cream Filled	1 (29 g)	110	0	15
Koffee Kake Junior	1 pkg (71 g)	260	1	40
Kreme Kup	1 (25 g)	90	1	5

FOOD	PORTION	CALS.	FIB.	CHOL.
Tastykake (CONT.)				
Krimpet Butterscotch	1 (28 g)	100	0	19
Krimpet Jelly	1 (28 g)	90	1	20
Krimpet Strawberry	1 (28 g)	100	0	20
Pastry Pocket Apple	1 (85 g)	320	—	10
Pastry Pocket Cheese	1 (85 g)	330	1	10
Pastry Pocket Cherry	1 (85 g)	330	1	10
Royale Chocolate Cupcake	1 (46 g)	170	2	5
Tasty Too Chocolate Cream Filled Cupcake	1 (32 g)	100	1	0
Tasty Too Vanilla Cream Filled Cupcake	1 (32 g)	100	1	0
Toastettes				
Frosted Blueberry	1 (1.7 oz)	190	1	0
Frosted Brown Sugar Cinnamon	1 (1.7 oz)	190	1	0
Frosted Cherry	1 (1.7 oz)	190	1	0
Frosted Fudge	1 (1.7 oz)	190	3	0
Strawberry	1 (1.7 oz)	190	1	0
Well-Bred Loaf				
Banana Bread	1 slice (3.5 oz)	330	tr	60
Banana Nut	1 slice (4.3 oz)	440	2	85
Blueberry	1 slice (4.3 oz)	440	1	110
Carrot	1 slice (4.3 oz)	480	2	125
Carrot Traditional	1 slice (4.3 oz)	440	2	40
Chocolate Chip	1 slice (4.3 oz)	490	2	105
Cinnamon Walnut	1 slice (4.3 oz)	480	1	110
Coconut Rum	1 slice (4.3 oz)	490	tr	95
Cranberry	1 slice (4.3 oz)	460	1	100
Marble	1 slice (4.3 oz)	530	1	115
Pound All Butter	1 slice (4.3 oz)	470	tr	115
Pound Mandarin Orange	1 slice (4 oz)	460	tr	70
Raisin	1 slice (4.3 oz)	460	2	105
Yodel's	1 (1 oz)	150	—	5
devil's food cupcake w/ chocolate frosting	1	120	—	19
devil's food w/ creme filling	1 (1 oz)	105	—	15
sponge w/ creme filling	1 (1.5 oz)	155	—	7
TAKE-OUT				
baklava	1 oz	126	1	23
strudel	1 piece (4.1 oz)	272	3	39
CALZONE				
TAKE-OUT				
Cheese	1 (12 oz)	1020	8	100

FOOD	PORTION	CALS.	FIB.	CHOL.
CANADIAN BACON				
Hormel	2 oz	70	0	30
Jones	1 slice	30	—	7
Oscar Mayer	2 slices (1.6 oz)	50	0	25
unheated	2 slices (1.9 oz)	89	—	28
CANDY				
(see also MARSHMALLOW)				
100 Grand	1 bar (1.5 oz)	200	tr	10
3 Musketeers	2 bars fun size (1.1 oz)	140	0	5
3 Musketeers	1 (2.1 oz)	260	1	5
5th Avenue	1 (2.1 oz)	290	—	5
Almond Joy	1 (1.76 oz)	250	—	0
Bar None	1 (1.5 oz)	240	—	10
Bits O Brickle	1 tbsp (0.5 oz)	80	0	5
Bonus Bar	1 bar (2.1 oz)	290	2	0
Breath Savers				
Sugar Free Cinnamon	1 candy	2	0	0
Sugar Free Peppermint	1 candy	2	0	0
Sugar Free Spearmint	1 candy	2	0	0
Sugar Free Wintergreen	1 candy	2	0	0
Brock				
Butterscotch Discs	3 pieces (0.6 oz)	70	—	0
Candy Corn	21 pieces (1.4 oz)	150	—	0
Candy Rolls	2 rolls (0.5 oz)	50	—	0
Cinnamon Discs	3 pieces (0.6 oz)	70	—	0
Circus Peanuts	11 pieces (2.5 oz)	260	—	0
Fruit Basket	3 pieces (0.6 oz)	60	—	0
Fruit Kisses	3 pieces (0.6 oz)	70	—	0
Glitters	2 pieces (0.5 oz)	50	—	0
Gummy Bears	5 pieces (1.4 oz)	130	—	0
Gummy Squirms	5 pieces (1.3 oz)	120	—	0
Jelly Beans	12 pieces (1.4 oz)	140	—	0
Lemon Drops	3 pieces (0.5 oz)	60	—	0
Orange Slices	4 pieces (1.5 oz)	140	—	0
Party Mints	9 pieces (0.5 oz)	60	—	0
Pops Assorted	2 (0.5 oz)	60	—	0
Sour Balls	3 pieces (0.6 oz)	70	—	0
Spearmint Starlights	3 pieces (0.6 oz)	60	—	0
Spice Drops	12 pieces (1.4 oz)	130	—	0
Starlight Mints	3 pieces (0.6 oz)	60	—	0
Butterfinger	1 bar (2.1 oz)	280	—	0
BB's	1 pkg (1.7 oz)	230	1	0
Butternut Bar	1 bar (1.8 oz)	250	1	0

FOOD	PORTION	CALS.	FIB.	CHOL.
Caramello	1 (1.6 oz)	220	—	10
Cellas				
Chocolate Covered Cherries	2 pieces (1 oz)	110	2	0
Milk Chocolate				
Certs	1 piece (1.67 g)	6	—	0
Mini Sugar Free	1 piece (0.365 g)	1	—	0
Sugar Free	1 piece (1.67 g)	7	—	0
Charms				
Blow Pop	1 (0.7 oz)	80	—	0
Pop	1 (0.6 oz)	70	—	0
Chuckles	4 pieces (1.4 oz)	140	—	0
Chunky	1 bar (1.4 oz)	200	2	<5
Clorets				
Mints	1 piece (1.67 g)	6	—	0
Crunch				
Fun Size	4 bars (1.5 oz)	200	1	5
Dove				
Dark Chocolate	¼ bar (1.5 oz)	230	3	0
Dark Chocolate	1 bar (1.3 oz)	200	2	0
Dark Chocolate Minatures	7 (1.5 oz)	230	2	0
Milk Chocolate	¼ bar (1.5 oz)	230	1	10
Milk Chocolate Miniatures	1 bar (1.3 oz)	200	1	5
Milk Chocolate Miniatures	7 (1.5 oz)	230	1	10
Truffles	3 (1.2 oz)	200	1	5
Estee				
Caramels Chocolate & Vanilla	5 (1.3 oz)	150	0	0
No Sugar Added				
Dark Chocolate	½ bar (1.4 oz)	200	0	10
Gum Drops Assorted Fruit	23 (1.4 oz)	140	0	0
Sugar Free				
Gum Drops Licorice	23 (1.4 oz)	140	0	0
Gummy Bears Sugar Free	16 (1.4 oz)	140	—	0
Hard Candies Assorted Fruit	5 (0.5 oz)	60	0	0
Sugar Free				
Hard Candies Assorted Mint	5 (0.5 oz)	60	0	0
Sugar Free				
Hard Candies Butterscotch	2 (0.4 oz)	50	—	0
Sugar Free				
Hard Candies Peppermint	3 (0.5 oz)	60	—	0
Swirls Sugar Free				
Hard Candies Tropical Fruit	5 (0.5 oz)	60	—	0
Sugar Free				
Lollipops Assorted Fruit Sugar	2 (0.5 oz)	60	—	0
Free				

FOOD	PORTION	CALS.	FIB.	CHOL.
Estee (CONT.)				
Milk Chocolate	½ bar (1.4 oz)	230	0	20
Milk Chocolate With Almonds	½ bar (1.4 oz)	230	0	20
Milk Chocolate With Crisp Rice	1 bar (2.3 oz)	370	0	30
Milk Chocolate With Fruit & Nuts	½ bar (1.4 oz)	220	0	20
Mint Chocolate	½ bar (1.4 oz)	200	0	10
Peanut Brittle No Sugar Added	⅓ box (1.5 oz)	210	1	10
Peanut Butter Cups	1 (0.3 oz)	40	0	0
Peanut Butter Cups	5 (1.3 oz)	200	1	5
Toffee Sugar Free	5 (0.5 oz)	60	—	0
Ferreo Rocher	3 pieces (1.3 oz)	220	1	0
Franklin				
Crunch 'N Munch Candied	1.25 oz	170	1	0
Crunch 'N Munch Caramel	1.25 oz	160	1	13
Crunch 'N Munch Maple Walnut	1.25 oz	160	1	6
Crunch 'N Munch Toffee	1.25 oz	160	1	6
Glenny's				
Brown Rice Treats Toasted Almond With Oat Bran	1 bar (1.75 oz)	200	2	34
Godiva				
Almond Butter Dome	3 pieces (1.5 oz)	240	0	5
Bouchee Au Chocolat	1 piece (1.5 oz)	210	0	5
Bouchee Ivory Raspberry	1 pieces (1 oz)	160	0	5
Gold Ballotin	3 pieces (1.5 oz)	210	0	5
Truffle Amaretto Di Saronno	2 pieces (1.5 oz)	210	0	5
Truffle Deluxe Liqueur	2 pieces (1.5 oz)	210	0	5
Golden Almond	½ bar	260	—	5
Golden III	½ bar	250	—	10
Goldenberg's				
Peanut Chews	3 pieces (1.3 oz)	180	1	0
Geobers	1 pkg (1.38 oz)	210	3	<5
Good & Plenty				
Snacksize	3 boxes (1.5 oz)	140	—	0
Heath	1 bar (1.4 oz)	210	0	20
Hershey				
Amazin'Fruit Gummy Candy	2 snack pkg (1.4 oz)	130	—	0
Bar	1 (1.55 oz)	240	—	10
Bar With Almonds	1 (1.45 oz)	230	—	15
Kisses	9 pieces (1.46 oz)	220	—	10
Special Dark Sweet Chocolate Bar	1 (1.45)	220	—	0

FOOD	PORTION	CALS.	FIB.	CHOL.
Jolly Rancher	3 pieces (0.6 oz)	60	—	0
Joyva				
Halvah	1.5 oz	240	2	0
Halvah Chocolate Covered	1 bar (2 oz)	380	3	0
Jells Raspberry	3 pieces (1.6 oz)	200	tr	0
Joys Raspberry	1 (1.6 oz)	200	1	0
Marshmallow Twists Chocolate Covered	2 (1.5 oz)	190	0	0
Rings Orange & Raspberry	3 pieces (1.5 oz)	190	tr	0
Sesame Crunch	3 pieces (0.5)	80	0	0
Sticks Orange	3 pieces (1.6 oz)	200	tr	0
Twists Vanilla & Cherry	2 (1.5 oz)	190	0	0
Juicefuls	3 pieces (0.5 oz)	60	—	0
Kit Kat	1 (1.625 oz)	250	—	10
Krackel	1 (1.55 oz)	230	—	10
Kraft				
Butter Mints	7 (0.5 oz)	60	0	0
Caramels	5 (1.4 oz)	170	0	<5
Fudgies	5 (1.4 oz)	180	0	0
Party Mints	7 (0.5 oz)	60	0	0
Peanut Brittle	5 pieces (1.3 oz)	170	1	0
Lance				
Chocolaty Peanut Bar	1 (57 g)	320	—	0
Peanut Bar	1 pkg (50 g)	260	—	0
Popscotch	1 pkg (35 g)	160	—	0
Lifesavers				
Christmas Lollipops	1	40	—	0
Easter Pops	1	40	—	0
Fancy Fruits	1 candy	8	—	0
Fruit Juicers Citrus Fruits	1 candy	8	0	0
Fruit Juicers Easter Egg-Sortments	1 candy	10	0	0
Fruit Juicers Fruit Punch	1 candy	8	0	0
Fruit Juicers Grape	1 candy	8	0	0
Fruit Juicers Lollipops	1	40	0	0
Fruit Juicers Mixed Berries	1 candy	8	0	0
Fruit Juicers Strawberry	1 candy	8	0	0
Gummi Savers Grape	1 candy	12	0	0
Gummi Savers Mixed Berry	1 candy	12	0	0
Holes Tangerine	1 candy	2	0	0
Lollipops All Flavors	1	45	—	0
Sugar Free	1 piece	8	—	0
Sunshine Fruits	1 candy	8	—	0
Tropical Fruits	1 candy	8	—	0

FOOD	PORTION	CALS.	FIB.	CHOL.
Lifesavers (CONT.)				
Valentine Pops	1	40	—	0
Wild Cherry	1 candy	8	—	0
M&M's				
Almond	1.5 oz	220	2	5
Almond	1 pkg (1.3 oz)	200	2	5
Mint	1 pkg (1.7 oz)	230	1	10
Mint	1.5 oz	200	1	5
Peanut	½ bag king size (1.6 oz)	240	2	5
Peanut	1.5 oz	220	2	5
Peanut	1 pkg (1.7 oz)	250	2	5
Peanut	1 fun size (0.7 oz)	110	1	5
Peanut Butter	1 fun size (0.7 oz)	110	1	5
Peanut Butter	1 pkg (1.6 oz)	240	2	5
Peanut Butter	1.5 oz	220	2	5
Plain	1 pkg fun size (0.7 oz)	100	0	5
Plain	1.5 oz	200	1	5
Plain	1 pkg (1.7 oz)	230	1	6
Plain	½ pkg king size (1.6 oz)	220	1	5
Semisweet	0.5 oz	70	1	0
Mars				
	1 bar (1.8 oz)	240	1	5
Almond Bar	2 fun size (1.3 oz)	190	1	5
Mayfair				
Mints	5 pieces (1.3 oz)	180	tr	0
Milk Duds	1 box (1.8 oz)	230	0	0
Snack Size	4 boxes (1.3 oz)	160	0	0
Milkshake Bar	1 bar (1.8 oz)	220	0	0
Milky Way	1 bar (2.1 oz)	280	0	5
Dark	1 fun size (0.7 oz)	90	0	0
Dark	1 bar (1.8 oz)	220	1	5
Fun Size	2 (1.4 oz)	180	0	5
Miniature	5 (1.5 oz)	190	0	5
Mounds	1 (1.9 oz)	260	—	5
Mr. GoodBar	1 (1.75 oz)	290	—	15
Munch Bar	1 (1.4 oz)	230	2	10
NECCO				
Mint	1 piece	12	—	0
Nestle				
Areo Bar	1 bar (1.45 oz)	210	2	10
Buncha Crunch	1 pkg (1.4 oz)	90	tr	5
Milk Chocolate	1 bar (1.45 oz)	220	2	10

FOOD	PORTION	CALS.	FIB.	CHOL.
Nestle (CONT.)				
Turtles Pecan Caramel Candy	2 pieces (1.2 oz)	160	1	<5
Nestle Crunch	1 bar (1.55 oz)	230	1	5
Ocean Spray				
Fruit Waves Assorted	3 pieces (0.3 oz)	35	—	0
Oh Henry!	1 bar (1.8 oz)	230	2	<5
PB Max	2 (1.6 oz)	240	1	5
PB Max	2 fun size (1.2 oz)	180	1	0
PayDay	1 bar (1.85 oz)	240	2	0
Pez	1 roll (0.3 oz)	30	—	0
Raisinets	1 pkg (1.58 oz)	200	2	<5
Reese's				
Peanut Butter Cups	1 (1.8 oz)	280	—	10
Pieces	1.85 oz	260	—	5
Riesen	5 pieces (1.4 oz)	180	3	<5
Rolo				
Carmels In Milk Chocolate	8 pieces (1.93 oz)	270	—	15
Skittles				
Original	2 pkg fun size (1.4 oz)	160	0	0
Tart-N-Tangy	1.5 oz	170	0	0
Tart-N-Tangy	2 bags fun size (1.4 oz)	160	0	0
Tart-N-Tangy	1 bag (2.2 oz)	250	0	0
Tropical	1.5 oz	170	0	0
Tropical	2 bags fun size (1.4 oz)	160	0	0
Tropical	1 bag (2.2 oz)	250	0	0
Wild Berry	2 bags fun size (1.4 oz)	160	0	0
Wild Berry	1.5 oz	170	0	0
Wild Berry	1 bag (2.2 oz)	250	0	0
Skor				
Toffee Bar	1 (1.4 oz)	220	—	25
Snickers	1 bar (2.1 oz)	280	1	10
Fun Size	2 bars (1.4 oz)	190	1	5
Miniatures	4 (1.3 oz)	170	1	5
Peanut Butter	1 bar (2 oz)	310	1	5
Solitaires				
With Almonds	½ bag	260	—	5
Sour Punch				
Candy Straws Sour Apple	6 pieces (1.4 oz)	130	—	0
Spice Stix And Drops	14 pieces (1.6 oz)	140	—	0
Starburst				
California Fruits	8 pieces (1.4 oz)	160	0	0

FOOD	PORTION	CALS.	FIB.	CHOL.
Starburst (CONT.)				
California Fruits	1 stick (2.1 oz)	240	0	0
Strawberry Fruits	1 stick (2.1 oz)	240	0	0
Strawberry Fruits	8 pieces (1.4 oz)	160	0	0
Tropical Fruits	8 pieces (1.4 oz)	160	0	0
Tropical Fruits	1 stick (2.1 oz)	240	0	0
Swedish Red Fish	19 pieces (1.4 oz)	150	—	0
Switzer				
Cherry Bites	12 pieces (1.6 oz)	50	—	0
Licorice Bites	12 pieces (1.6 oz)	46	—	0
Symphony				
Milk Chocolate	1 (1.4 oz)	220	—	10
Tootsie Roll				
Dots	12 (1.5 oz)	160	—	0
Pop	1 (0.6 oz)	60	—	0
Twix				
Caramel	2 1 pkg (2 oz)	280	0	5
Caramel	1 fun size (0.6 oz)	80	0	0
Caramel	1 (1 oz)	140	0	0
Cookies-N-Creme	1 (0.8 oz)	130	0	0
Fudge N Crunchy	1 (0.7 oz)	110	1	0
Peanut Butter	1 (0.9 oz)	130	1	0
Twizzlers				
Pull-n-Peel Cherry	1 piece (1.1 oz)	110	—	0
Velamints				
Cocoamint	1 piece (1.7 g)	5	—	0
Peppermint	1 piece (1.7 g)	5	—	0
Spearmint	1 piece (1.7 g)	5	—	0
Wintergreen	1 piece (1.7 g)	5	—	0
Whatchamacallit	1 (1.8 oz)	260	—	10
Whitman's				
Assorted	3 pieces (1.4 oz)	190	0	5
Dark Chocolate	3 pieces (1.4 oz)	200	1	<5
Little Ambassadors	7 pieces (1.4 oz)	190	1	5
Pecan Delight	1 bar (2 oz)	310	2	10
Pecan Roll	1 bar (2 oz)	300	1	5
Sampler	3 pieces (1.4 oz)	200	1	5
Whoppers	1 pkg (1.8 oz)	230	1	0
Y&S				
Bites Cherry	1 oz	100	—	0
York				
Peppermint Patty	1 snack size (0.5 oz)	57	—	0
Peppermint Patty	1 (1.5 oz)	180	—	0

FOOD	PORTION	CALS.	FIB.	CHOL.
butterscotch	1 piece (6 g)	24	—	1
butterscotch	1 oz	112	—	3
candied cherries	1 (4 g)	12	—	0
candied citron	1 oz	89	—	0
candied lemon peel	1 oz	90	—	0
candied orange peel	1 oz	90	—	0
candied pineapple slice	1 slice (2 oz)	179	—	0
candy corn	1 oz	105	—	0
caramels	1 pkg (2.5 oz)	271	—	5
caramels	1 piece (8 g)	31	—	1
caramels chocolate	1 bar (2.3 oz)	231	—	0
caramels chocolate	1 piece (6 g)	22	—	0
crisped rice bar almond	1 bar (1 oz)	130	1	0
crisped rice bar chocolate chip	1 bar (1 oz)	115	1	0
dark chocolate	1 oz	150	—	0
fondant chocolate coated	1 sm (0.4 oz)	40	—	0
fondant chocolate coated	1 lg (1.2 oz)	128	—	0
fondant mint	1 oz	105	—	0
gumdrops	10 lg (3.8 oz)	420	—	0
gumdrops	10 sm (0.4 oz)	135	—	0
hard candy	1 oz	106	—	0
jelly beans	10 sm (0.4 oz)	40	—	0
jelly beans	10 lg (1 oz)	104	—	0
lollipop	1 (6 g)	22	—	0
milk chocolate	1 bar (1.55 oz)	226	—	10
milk chocolate crisp	1 bar (1.45 oz)	203	—	8
milk chocolate w/ almonds	1 bar (1.45 oz)	215	—	8
peanuts chocolate covered	10 (1.4 oz)	208	—	4
peanuts chocolate covered	1 cup (5.2 oz)	773	—	13
sesame crunch	1 oz	146	—	0
sesame crunch	20 pieces (1.2 oz)	181	—	0
sweet chocolate	1 oz	143	—	0
sweet chocolate	1 bar (1.45 oz)	201	—	0
HOME RECIPE				
divinity	1 (11 g)	38	—	0
divinity	1 recipe 48 pieces (19 oz)	1891	—	0
fondant	1 recipe 60 pieces (32.6 oz)	3327	—	0
fondant	1 piece (0.6 oz)	57	—	0
fudge brown sugar w/ nuts	1 piece (0.5 oz)	56	—	1
fudge brown sugar w/ nuts	1 recipe 60 pieces (30.7 oz)	3453	—	49
fudge chocolate	1 piece (0.6 oz)	65	—	2

FOOD	PORTION	CALS.	FIB.	CHOL.
fudge chocolate	1 recipe 48 pieces (29 oz)	3161	—	120
fudge chocolate marshmallow	1 piece (0.7 oz)	84	—	5
fudge chocolate marshmallow	1 recipe (43.1 oz)	5182	—	304
fudge chocolate marshmallow w/ nuts	1 piece (0.8 oz)	96	—	5
fudge chocolate marshmallow w/ nuts	1 recipe 60 pieces (43.1 oz)	5182	—	304
fudge chocolate marshmallow w/ nuts	1 recipe 60 pieces (46.1 oz)	5742	—	291
fudge chocolate w/ nuts	1 piece (0.7 oz)	81	—	3
fudge chocolate w/ nuts	1 recipe 48 pieces (32.7 oz)	3967	—	130
fudge peanut butter	1 recipe 36 pieces (20.4 oz)	2161	—	25
fudge peanut butter	1 piece (0.6 oz)	59	—	1
fudge vanilla	1 piece (0.6 oz)	59	—	3
fudge vanilla	1 recipe 48 pieces (27.5 oz)	2893	—	125
fudge vanilla w/ nuts	1 piece (0.5 oz)	62	—	2
fudge vanilla w/ nuts	1 recipe 60 pieces (31 oz)	3666	—	125
peanut brittle	1 recipe (17.6 oz)	2288	—	66
peanut brittle	1 oz	128	—	4
praline	1 recipe 23 pieces (31.8 oz)	4116	—	0
praline	1 piece (1.4 oz)	177	—	0
taffy	1 piece (0.5 oz)	56	—	1
taffy	1 recipe 48 pieces (25 oz)	2677	—	63
toffee	1 piece (0.4 oz)	65	—	13
toffee	1 recipe 48 pieces (19.4 oz)	2997	—	580
truffles	1 recipe 49 pieces (21.5 oz)	2985	—	318
truffles	1 piece (0.4 oz)	59	—	6

CANTALOUPE
FRESH

FOOD	PORTION	CALS.	FIB.	CHOL.
Chiquita	1 cup	70	—	0
Dole	¼	50	0	0
cubed	1 cup	57	1	0
half	½	94	2	0

FOOD	PORTION	CALS.	FIB.	CHOL.
FROZEN				
Big Valley				
Balls	¾ cup (4.9 oz)	40	0	0
CAPERS				
Reese	1 tsp (5 g)	0	—	0
CARAMBOLA				
fresh	1	42	—	0
CARAWAY				
seed	1 tsp	7	—	0
CARDAMON				
ground	1 tsp	6	—	0
CARDOON				
fresh cooked	3½ oz	22	—	0
raw shredded	½ cup	36	—	0
CARIBOU				
roasted	3 oz	142	—	93
CARISSA				
fresh	1	12	—	0
CAROB				
carob mix	3 tsp	45	—	0
carob mix as prep w/ whole milk	9 oz	195	—	33
flour	1 tbsp	14	—	0
flour	1 cup	185	—	0
CARP				
fresh cooked	3 oz	138	—	72
fresh cooked	1 fillet (6 oz)	276	—	143
raw	3 oz	108	—	56
roe raw	3½ oz	130	—	360
CARROT JUICE				
Hain	6 fl oz	80	—	0
Hollywood	6 fl oz	80	2	0
Odwalla	8 fl oz	70	2	0
canned	6 oz	73	—	0
CARROTS				
CANNED				
Allen				
Sliced	½ cup (4.5 oz)	35	3	0
Crest Top				
Sliced	½ cup (4.5 oz)	35	3	0

FOOD	PORTION	CALS.	FIB.	CHOL.
Del Monte				
Cut	½ cup (4.3 oz)	35	3	0
Sliced	½ cup (4.3 oz)	35	3	0
S&W				
Diced Fancy	½ cup	30	—	0
Julienne French Style Fancy	½ cup	30	—	0
Sliced Fancy	½ cup	30	—	0
Sliced Water Pack	½ cup	30	—	0
Whole Tiny Fancy	½ cup	30	—	0
Seneca				
Diced	½ cup	30	2	0
Sliced	½ cup	30	2	0
slices	½ cup	17	1	0
slices low sodium	½ cup	17	1	0
FRESH				
Dole	1 med	40	1	0
baby raw	1 (½ oz)	6	—	0
raw	1 (2.5 oz)	31	2	0
raw shredded	½ cup	24	2	0
slices cooked	½ cup	35	—	0
FROZEN				
Big Valley				
Carrots	½ cup (3 oz)	35	2	0
Birds Eye				
Baby Whole Deluxe	½ cup	40	2	0
Polybag Sliced	¾ cup	35	1	0
Green Giant				
Harvest Fresh Baby	½ cup	18	2	0
Hanover				
Crinkle Sliced	½ cup	35	—	0
slices cooked	½ cup	26	—	0
CASABA				
cubed	1 cup	45	—	0
fresh	⅒	43	—	0
CASHEWS				
Beer Nuts				
Cashews	1 pkg (1 oz)	170	—	0
Eagle				
Honey Roasted	1 oz	170	—	0
Low Salt	1 oz	170	—	0
Fisher				
Honey Roasted Halves	1 oz	150	—	0
Honey Roasted Whole	1 oz	150	—	0

FOOD	PORTION	CALS.	FIB.	CHOL.
Fisher (CONT.)				
Oil Roasted Halves	1 oz	170	—	0
Oil Roasted Whole	1 oz	170	—	0
Frito Lay	1 oz	170	—	0
Guy's				
Whole Salted	1 oz	170	—	0
Hain				
Cashew Butter Raw	2 tbsp	190	—	0
Cashew Butter Toasted	2 tbsp	210	—	0
Lance	1 pkg (32 g)	190	—	0
Planters				
Fancy	1 oz	170	—	0
Honey Roasted	1 oz	170	1	0
Unsalted Halves	1 oz	170	—	0
cashew butter w/o salt	1 tbsp	94	—	0
dry roasted	1 oz	163	—	0
dry roasted salted	1 oz	163	—	0
oil roasted	1 oz	163	—	0
oil roasted salted	1 oz	163	—	0
CASSAVA				
raw	3½ oz	120	—	0
CATFISH				
channel breaded & fried	3 oz	194	—	69
channel raw	3 oz	99	—	49
CATSUP				
(*see* KETCHUP)				
CAULIFLOWER				
FRESH				
Dole	⅙ med head	18	2	0
Green	⅕ head	35	—	0
cooked	½ cup (2.2 oz)	14	1	0
flowerets cooked	3 (2 oz)	12	1	0
flowerets raw	3 (2 oz)	14	1	0
green cooked	½ cup (2.2 oz)	20	—	0
green raw	½ cup (1.8 oz)	16	1	0
raw	½ cup (1.8 oz)	13	1	0
FROZEN				
Big Valley				
Florets	¾ cup (3 oz)	25	1	0
Birds Eye	⅔ cup	25	2	0
Polybag	½ cup	20	—	0
With Cheese Sauce	½ pkg	90	1	15

FOOD	PORTION	CALS.	FIB.	CHOL.
Green Giant				
Cuts	½ cup	12	1	0
In Cheese Sauce	½ cup	60	2	2
One Serve In Cheese Sauce	1 pkg	80	2	5
Hanover				
Cauliflower	½ cup	20	—	0
Florets	½ cup	20	—	0
cooked	½ cup	17	—	0
JARRED				
Vlasic				
Hot & Spicy	1 oz	4	—	0
Sweet	1 oz	35	—	0
CAVIAR				
black granular	1 tbsp	40	—	94
black granular	1 oz	71	—	165
red granular	1 oz	71	—	165
red granular	1 tbsp	40	—	94
CELERIAC				
fresh cooked	3½ oz	25	—	0
raw	½ cup	31	—	0
CELERY				
DRIED				
seed	1 tsp	8	—	0
FRESH				
Dole				
diced cooked	2 med stalks	20	4	0
diced cooked	½ cup	13	—	0
raw	1 stalk (1.3 oz)	6	1	0
raw diced	½ cup	10	1	0
CELTUCE				
raw	3½ oz	22	—	0
CEREAL				
COOKED				
Albers				
Hominy Quick Grits uncooked	¼ cup	140	1	0
Arrowhead				
4 Grain + Flax	¼ cup (1.6 oz)	150	6	0
7 Grain	⅓ cup (1.4 oz)	140	5	0
Bear Mush	¼ cup (1.6 oz)	160	2	0
Oat Flakes Rolled	⅓ cup (1.2 oz)	130	4	0
Oat Groats	¼ cup (1.5 oz)	160	4	0
Rice & Shine	¼ cup (1.5 oz)	150	2	0

FOOD	PORTION	CALS.	FIB.	CHOL.
Arrowhead (CONT.)				
Wheat Flakes Rolled	⅓ cup (1.2 oz)	110	5	0
Aunt Jemima				
Enriched White Hominy Grits Regular	3 tbsp	101	1	0
Erewhon				
Barley Plus	1 oz	110	1	0
Oat Bran With Toasted Wheat Germ	1 oz	115	3	0
Oatmeal Instant Apple Cinnamon	1.25 oz	145	—	0
Good Shepherd				
Spelt	1 oz	90	3	0
H-O				
Farina Instant	1 pkg	110	3	0
Farina not prep	3 tbsp	120	3	0
Oatmeal Instant	1 pkg	110	3	0
Oatmeal Instant	½ cup	130	3	0
Oatmeal Instant Apple Cinnamon	1 pkg	130	3	0
Oatmeal Instant Maple Brown Sugar	1 pkg	160	3	0
Oatmeal Instant Raisin & Spice	1 pkg	150	3	0
Oatmeal Instant Sweet 'n Mellow	1 pkg	150	3	0
Oats 'n Fiber	1 pkg	110	3	0
Oats 'n Fiber	⅓ cup	100	3	0
Oats 'n Fiber Apple & Bran	1 pkg	130	3	0
Oats 'n Fiber Raisin & Bran	1 pkg	150	3	0
Oats Gourmet	⅓ cup	100	3	0
Oats Quick	½ cup	130	3	0
Health Valley				
Oat Bran Natural Apples & Cinnamon	¼ cup (1 oz)	100	4	0
Oat Bran Natural Raisins & Spice	¼ cup	100	4	0
Little Crow				
Coco Wheat	3 tbsp (36 g)	130	4	0
Maltex	1 oz	105	3	0
Maypo				
30 second	1 oz	100	2	0
Vermont Style	1 oz	105	2	0
With Oat Bran	1 oz	130	4	0
McCann's				
Irish Oatmeal	1 oz	110	3	0

FOOD	PORTION	CALS.	FIB.	CHOL.
Mother's				
Oatmeal Instant	½ cup (1.4 oz)	150	4	0
Whole Wheat Natural	½ cup (1.4 oz)	130	4	0
Nabisco				
Cream of Rice	1 oz	100	—	0
Cream of Wheat Instant	1 oz	100	1	<5
Cream of Wheat Quick	1 oz	100	tr	<5
Cream of Wheat Regular	1 oz	100	1	0
Mix'n Eat Cream Of Wheat Brown Sugar Cinnamon	1 pkg (1¼ oz)	130	1	0
Mix'n Eat Cream of Wheat Apple & Cinnamon	1 pkg (1¼ oz)	130	1	0
Mix'n Eat Cream of Wheat Maple Brown Sugar	1 pkg (1¼ oz)	130	1	0
Mix'n Eat Cream of Wheat Our Original	1 pkg (1¼ oz)	100	1	0
Pritikin				
Apple Raisin Spice	1 pkg (1.6 oz)	170	—	0
Multigrain	1 pkg	160	—	0
Quaker				
Enriched White Hominy Grits Quick	3 tbsp	101	1	0
Enriched Yellow Hominy Quick Grits	3 tbsp	101	1	0
Instant Grits White Hominy	1 pkg	79	1	0
Instant Grits With Imitation Ham Bits	1 pkg	99	2	0
Instant Grits With Real Cheddar Cheese	1 pkg	104	1	0
Multigrain	½ cup	130	5	0
Oatmeal Instant	1 pkg (1.2 oz)	130	3	0
Oatmeal Instant Apples & Cinnamon	1 pkg (1.2 oz)	130	3	0
Oatmeal Instant Cinnamon Graham Cookie	1 pkg (1.4 oz)	150	3	0
Oatmeal Instant Cinnamon Spice	1 pkg (1.6 oz)	170	3	0
Oatmeal Instant Cinnamon Toast	1 pkg (1.2 oz)	130	2	0
Oatmeal Instant Fruit & Cream Blueberry	1 pkg (1.2 oz)	130	2	0
Oatmeal Instant Honey Nut	1 pkg (1.2 oz)	130	2	0
Oatmeal Instant Kids Choice Radical Raspberry	1 pkg (1.4 oz)	150	3	0

FOOD	PORTION	CALS.	FIB.	CHOL.
Quaker (CONT.)				
Oatmeal Instant Maple Brown Sugar	1 pkg (1.5 oz)	160	3	0
Oatmeal Instant Peaches & Cream	1 pkg (1.2 oz)	130	2	0
Oatmeal Instant Raisin & Walnut	1 pkg (1.3 oz)	140	3	0
Oatmeal Instant Raisin Date Walnut	1 pkg (1.3 oz)	130	3	0
Oatmeal Instant Raisin Spice	1 pkg (1.5 oz)	160	3	0
Oatmeal Instant Strawberries & Cream	1 pkg (1.2 oz)	130	2	0
Oatmeal Instant Strawberries 'N Stuff	1 pkg (1.4 oz)	150	3	0
Oats Old Fashion	½ cup	150	4	0
Oats Quick	½ cup	150	4	0
Ralston				
Corn Flakes	1¼ cup (1.1 oz)	120	1	0
Roman Meal				
Apple Cinnamon	1.2 oz	105	6	0
Cream Of Rye	1.3 oz	111	5	0
Oats Wheat Dates Raisins Almonds	1.3 oz	129	3	0
Oats Wheat Honey Coconuts Almonds	1.3 oz	155	3	0
Original	1 oz	83	5	0
Original With Oats	1.2 oz	108	5	0
Stone-Buhr				
4 Grain	½ cup (1.6 oz)	140	5	0
Cracked Wheat	¼ cup (2.4 oz)	210	6	0
Manna Golden	6 tsp (1.6 oz)	160	1	0
Rolled Oats Old Fashion	6 tsp (1.6 oz)	150	5	0
Scotch Oats	¼ cup (1.6 oz)	150	4	0
Uncle Roy's				
Muesli Swiss Style	½ cup (1.6 oz)	170	3	0
Wheatena	⅓ cup (1.4 oz)	150	5	0
corn grits instant	1 pkg (0.8 oz)	82	—	0
corn grits quick	1 cup	146	—	0
corn grits quick not prep	1 cup	579	—	0
corn grits quick not prep	1 tbsp	36	—	0
corn grits regular	1 cup	146	—	0
corn grits regular not prep	1 cup	579	—	0
farina	¾ cup	87	3	0
farina not prep	1 tbsp	40	tr	0

FOOD	PORTION	CALS.	FIB.	CHOL.
oatmeal	1 cup	145	—	0
oatmeal instant cooked w/o salt	1 cup	145	—	0
oatmeal not prep	1 cup	311	9	0
oatmeal quick cooked w/o salt	1 cup	145	—	0
oatmeal regular cooked w/o salt	1 cup	145	—	0
READY-TO-EAT				
Arrowhead				
Amaranth Flakes	1 cup (1.2 oz)	130	3	0
Apple Corns	1 cup (1.5 oz)	150	4	0
Bran Flakes	1 cup (1 oz)	100	4	0
Kamut Flakes	1 cup (1.1 oz)	120	3	0
Maple Corns	1 cup (1.9 oz)	190	6	0
Multi Grain Flakes	1 cup (1.2 oz)	140	3	0
Nature O's	1 cup (1.1 oz)	130	3	0
Oat Bran Flakes	1 cup (1.2 oz)	110	4	0
Puffed Corn	1 cup (0.8 oz)	80	1	0
Puffed Kamut	1 cup (0.6 oz)	50	2	0
Puffed Millet	1 cup (0.9 oz)	90	1	0
Puffed Rice	1 cup (0.8 oz)	90	1	0
Puffed Wheat	1 cup (0.9)	90	2	0
Spelt Flakes	1 cup (1.1 oz)	100	3	0
Chex				
Corn	1¼ cup (1 oz)	110	1	0
Double	1¼ cup (1 oz)	120	0	0
Graham	1 cup (1.8 oz)	210	1	0
Rice	1 cup (1.1 oz)	120	0	0
Wheat	¾ cup (1.8 oz)	190	5	0
Erewhon				
Aztec	1 oz	100	1	0
Crispy Brown Rice	1 oz	110	4	0
Fruit 'n Wheat	1 oz	100	3	0
Raisin Bran	1 oz	100	3	0
Super-O's	1 oz	110	4	0
Wheat Flakes	1 oz	100	4	0
Estee				
Corn Flakes	1 pkg (1 oz)	90	4	0
Raisin Bran	1 pkg (1 oz)	90	3	0
General Mills				
Basic 4	¾ cup	130	2	0
Body Buddies Natural Fruit	1 cup (1 oz)	110	—	0
Booberry	1 cup (1 oz)	110	—	0
Cheerios	1¼ cup (1 oz)	110	2	0
Cheerios Apple Cinnamon	¾ cup (1 oz)	110	2	0
Cheerios Honey Nut	¾ cup (1 oz)	110	2	0

FOOD	PORTION	CALS.	FIB.	CHOL.
General Mills (CONT.)				
Cheerios-to-Go	1 pkg (0.75 oz)	80	2	0
Cheerios-to-Go Apple Cinnamon	1 pkg (1 oz)	110	2	0
Cheerios-to-Go Honey Nut	1 pkg (1 oz)	110	2	0
Cinnamon Toast Crunch	¾ cup (1 oz)	120	1	0
Clusters	½ cup (1 oz)	110	2	0
Cocoa Puffs	1 cup (1 oz)	110	—	0
Count Chocula	1 cup (1 oz)	110	—	0
Country Corn Flakes	1 cup (1 oz)	110	—	0
Crispy Wheats 'N Raisins	¾ cup (1 oz)	100	2	0
Fiber One	½ cup (1 oz)	60	13	0
Frankenberry	1 cup (1 oz)	110	—	0
Fruity Yummy Mummy	1 cup (1 oz)	110	—	0
Golden Grahams	¾ cup (1 oz)	110	—	0
Kaboom	1 cup (1 oz)	110	—	0
Kix	1½ cup (1 oz)	110	—	0
Lucky Charms	1 cup (1 oz)	110	—	0
Oatmeal Crisp	½ cup (1 oz)	110	1	0
Oatmeal Raisin Crisp	½ cup (1.2 oz)	130	2	0
Raisin Nut Bran	½ cup (1 oz)	110	3	0
S'Mores Grahams	¾ cup (1 oz)	120	—	0
Sun Crunchers	1 cup (1.9 oz)	210	3	0
Total	1 cup (1 oz)	100	3	0
Total Corn Flakes	1 cup (1 oz)	110	—	0
Total Raisin Bran	1 cup (1.5 oz)	140	4	0
Triples	¾ cup (1 oz)	110	—	0
Trix	1 cup (1 oz)	110	—	0
Wheaties	1 cup (1 oz)	100	3	0
Good Shepherd				
Millet Rice Flakes Wheat Free	1 oz	95	1	0
Spelt Flakes	1 oz	100	2	0
Grist Mill				
Apple Cinnamon Natural	½ cup (1.9 oz)	260	3	0
Bran	½ cup (1.9 oz)	250	11	0
Oat & Honey Natural	½ cup (1.9 oz)	270	4	0
Oat Honey & Raisin Natural	½ cup (1.9 oz)	260	4	0
Health Valley				
100% Natural Bran With Apples & Cinnamon	¼ cup (1 oz)	100	5	0
Blue Corn Flakes 100% Organic	½ cup (1 oz)	90	3	0
Bran Cereal With Dates 100% Organic	¼ cup (1 oz)	100	5	0
Bran Cereal With Raisins 100% Organic	¼ cup (1 oz)	100	5	0

FOOD	PORTION	CALS.	FIB.	CHOL.
Health Valley (CONT.)				
Fiber 7 Flakes 100% Organic	½ cup (1 oz)	90	5	0
Fiber 7 Flakes With Raisins 100% Organic	½ cup (1 oz)	90	5	0
Fruit & Fitness	1 cup (2 oz)	220	11	0
Fruit Lites Corn	½ cup (0.5 oz)	45	tr	0
Fruit Lites Rice	½ cup (0.5 oz)	45	tr	0
Fruit Lites Wheat	½ cup (0.5 oz)	45	2	0
Healthy Crunch Almond Date	¼ cup (1 oz)	110	4	0
Healthy Crunch Apple Cinnamon	¼ cup (1 oz)	110	4	0
Healthy O's 100% Organic	¾ cup (1 oz)	90	3	0
Lites Puffed Corn	½ cup (1 oz)	50	tr	0
Lites Puffed Rice	½ cup (1 oz)	50	tr	0
Lites Puffed Wheat	½ cup (1 oz)	50	1	0
Oat Bran Flakes 100% Organic	½ cup (1 oz)	100	4	0
Oat Bran Flakes Almonds/Dates 100% Organic	½ cup (1 oz)	100	4	0
Oat Bran Flakes With Raisins 100% Organic	½ cup (1 oz)	100	4	0
Oat Bran O'S 100% Organic	½ cup (1 oz)	110	3	0
Oat Bran O'S Fruit & Nuts	½ cup (1 oz)	110	3	0
Orangeola Almonds & Dates	¼ cup	110	4	0
Orangeola Bananas & Hawaiian Fruit	¼ cup (1 oz)	120	4	0
Raisin Bran Flakes 100% Organic	½ cup (1 oz)	100	6	0
Real Oat Bran Almond Crunch	¼ cup (1 oz)	110	4	0
Real Oat Bran Hawaiian Fruit	¼ cup (1 oz)	130	5	0
Real Oat Bran Raisin Nut	¼ cup (1 oz)	130	5	0
Rice Bran O's	½ cup	110	2	0
Rice Bran With Almonds & Dates	½ cup (1 oz)	110	2	0
Sprouts 7 Bananas & Hawaiian Fruit	¼ cup (1 oz)	90	4	0
Sprouts 7 Raisin	¼ cup	90	5	0
Swiss Breakfast Raisin Nut	¼ cup (1 oz)	100	3	0
Swiss Breakfast Tropical Fruit	¼ cup (1 oz)	100	3	0
Healthy Choice				
Multi-Grain Flakes	1 cup (1 oz)	100	3	0
Multi-Grain Raisins Crunchy Oat Clusters & Almonds	1 cup (1.9 oz)	200	4	0
Multi-Grain Squares	1¼ cup (1.9 oz)	190	6	0
Heartland				
Coconut	1 oz	130	2	0

FOOD	PORTION	CALS.	FIB.	CHOL.
Heartland (CONT.)				
Plain	1 oz	130	2	0
Raisin	1 oz	130	2	0
Kellogg's				
All-Bran	½ cup (1 oz)	80	10	0
All-Bran With Extra Fiber	½ cup (1 oz)	50	15	0
Apple Cinnamon Rice Krispies	¾ cup (1 oz)	110	1	0
Apple Cinnamon Squares	¾ cup (1.9 oz)	180	0	0
Apple Jacks	1 cup (1 oz)	110	1	0
Apple Raisin Crisp	1 cup (1.9 oz)	180	4	0
Blueberry Squares	¾ cup (1.9 oz)	180	5	0
Bran Buds	⅓ cup (1 oz)	70	11	0
Cinnamon Mini Buns	¾ cup (1 oz)	120	1	0
Cocoa Krispies	¾ cup (1 oz)	120	0	0
Common Sense Oat Bran	¾ cup (1 oz)	110	4	0
Complete Bran Flakes	¾ cup (1 oz)	100	5	0
Corn Flakes	1 cup (1 oz)	110	1	0
Corn Pops	1 cup (1 oz)	110	1	0
Cracklin' Oat Bran	¾ cup (1.9 oz)	230	6	0
Crispix	1 cup (1 oz)	110	1	0
Double Dip Crunch	¾ cup (1 oz)	110	0	0
Froot Loops	1 cup (1 oz)	120	1	0
Frosted Mini-Wheats	1 cup (1.9 oz)	190	6	0
Frosted Mini-Wheats Bite Size	1 cup (1.9 oz)	190	6	0
Frosted Bran	¾ cup (1 oz)	100	3	0
Frosted Flakes	¾ cup (1 oz)	120	0	0
Frosted Krispies	¾ cup (1 oz)	110	0	0
Fruitful Bran	1¼ cup (1.9 oz)	170	6	0
Fruity Marshmallow Krispies	¾ cups (1 oz)	110	0	0
Just Right Crunchy Nuggets	1 cup (1.9 oz)	200	3	0
Just Right Fruit & Nut	1 cup (1.9 oz)	210	3	0
Mueslix Golden Crunch	¾ cup (1.9 oz)	210	6	0
Nut & Honey Crunch	1¼ cup (1.9 oz)	220	1	0
Nutri-Grain Almond Raisin	1¼ cup (1.9 oz)	200	4	0
Nutri-Grain Golden Wheat	¾ cup (1 oz)	100	4	0
Oatbake Raisin Nut	⅓ cup (1 oz)	110	3	0
Pop-Tart Crunch Frosted Strawberry	¾ cup (1 oz)	120	0	0
Pop-Tart Crunch Frosted Brown Sugar Cinnamon	¾ cup (1 oz)	120	0	0
Product 19	1 cup (1 oz)	110	1	0
Raisin Bran	1 cup (1.9 oz)	170	7	0
Raisin Squares	¾ cup (1.9 oz)	180	5	0
Rice Krispies	1¼ cup (1 oz)	110	1	0

FOOD	PORTION	CALS.	FIB.	CHOL.
Kellogg's (CONT.)				
Special K	1 cup (1 oz)	110	1	0
Strawberry Squares	¾ cup (1.9 oz)	180	5	0
Temptations French Vanilla Almond	¾ cup (1 oz)	120	1	0
Temptations Honey Roasted Pecan	1 cup (1 oz)	120	0	0
LaLoma				
Ruskets Biscuits	2 biscuits (30 g)	110	—	0
Mueslix				
Crispy Blend	⅔ cup (1.9 oz)	200	4	0
Nabisco				
100% Bran	⅓ cup (1 oz)	70	10	1
Fruit Wheats Apple	1 oz	90	3	0
Shredded Wheat 'n Bran	⅔ cup (1 oz)	90	4	0
Shredded Wheat Spoon Size	⅔ cup (1 oz)	90	3	0
Shredded Wheat With Oat Bran	⅔ cup (1 oz)	100	4	0
Nut & Honey				
Crunch O's	¾ cup (1 oz)	120	2	0
Nutri-Grain				
Golden Wheat & Raisin	1¼ cup (1.9 oz)	180	6	0
Post				
Crispy Critters	1 cup (1 oz)	110	1	0
Grape-Nuts	¼ cup (1 oz)	105	3	0
Grape-Nuts Raisin	¼ cup (1 oz)	102	2	0
Honey Bunches Of Oats Honey Roasted	⅔ cup (1 oz)	111	2	0
Honey Bunches Of Oats With Almonds	⅔ cup (1 oz)	115	2	0
Honeycomb	1⅓ cups (1 oz)	110	1	0
Natural Bran Flakes	⅔ cup (1 oz)	88	6	0
Post Toasties Corn Flakes	1¼ cup (1 oz)	111	1	0
Super Golden Crisp	⅞ cup (1 oz)	104	tr	0
Quaker				
Puffed Rice	1 cup	54	tr	0
Puffed Wheat	1 cup	50	1	0
Ralston				
Almond Delight	1 cup (1.8 oz)	210	4	0
Bran Flakes	¾ cup (1.1 oz)	110	5	0
Chex Multi-Bran	1¼ cup (2 oz)	220	7	0
Cocoa Crispy Rice	1 cup (1.8 oz)	200	tr	0
Cocoa Crunchies	¾ cup (1.1 oz)	120	0	0
Cookie Crisp	1 cup (1 oz)	120	0	0
Crisp Crunch	¾ cup (1.1 oz)	120	tr	0

FOOD	PORTION	CALS.	FIB.	CHOL.
Ralston (CONT.)				
Crisp Rice	1¼ cup (1.2 oz)	130	0	0
Frosted Flakes	¾ cup (1.1 oz)	120	1	0
Fruit Rings	¾ cup (0.9 oz)	100	0	0
Magic Stair	¾ cup (1.1 oz)	120	tr	0
Muesli Blueberry	1 cup (1.9 oz)	200	4	0
Muesli Cranberry	¾ cup (1.9 oz)	200	4	0
Muesli Peach	¾ cup (1.9 oz)	200	4	0
Muesli Raspberry	¾ cup (2 oz)	220	4	0
Muesli Strawberry	1 cup (1.9 oz)	210	4	0
Multi Vitamin Whole Grain Flakes	1 cup (1.1 oz)	120	3	0
Nutty Nuggets	½ cup (1.7 oz)	180	5	0
Raisin Bran	¾ cup (1.9 oz)	190	6	0
Tasteeos	1¼ cup (1.1 oz)	130	3	0
Tasteeos Apple Cinnamon	1 cup (1.2 oz)	130	1	0
Tasteeos Honey Nut	1 cup (1.2 oz)	130	1	0
Rice Krispies				
Treats	¾ cup (1 oz)	120	0	0
Smacks	¾ cup (1 oz)	110	1	0
Stone-Buhr				
7 Grain	⅓ cup (1.6 oz)	140	7	0
Bran Flakes	¼ cup (0.6 oz)	64	2	0
Sunbelt				
Muesli	1.9 oz	210	3	1
Team	1 cup	110	—	0
US Mills				
Uncle Sam	1 oz	110	7	0
all bran	½ cup (1 oz)	76	—	0
bran flakes	¾ cup (1 oz)	90	—	0
corn flakes	1¼ cup (1 oz)	110	—	0
corn flakes low sodium	1 cup	100	—	0
crispy rice	1 cup	111	—	0
puffed rice	1 cup	57	—	0
puffed wheat	1 cup	44	—	0
shredded wheat	1 biscuit	83	—	0
sugar-coated corn flakes	¾ cup (1 oz)	110	—	0

CHAMPAGNE

FOOD	PORTION	CALS.	FIB.	CHOL.
Andre				
Blush	1 fl oz	22	—	0
Brut	1 fl oz	21	—	0
Cold Duck	1 fl oz	25	—	0
Extra Dry	1 fl oz	23	—	0

FOOD	PORTION	CALS.	FIB.	CHOL.
Ballatore				
Spumante	1 fl oz	23	—	0
Eden Roc				
Brut	1 fl oz	21	—	0
Brut Rosé	1 fl oz	22	—	0
Extra Dry	1 fl oz	21	—	0
Tott's				
Blanc de Noir	1 fl oz	22	—	0
Brut	1 fl oz	20	—	0
Extra Dry	1 fl oz	21	—	0
sekt german champagne	3.5 fl oz	84	—	0

CHAYOTE
fresh cooked	1 cup	38	—	0
raw	1 (7 oz)	49	—	0
raw cut up	1 cup	32	—	0

CHEESE
(see also CHEESE DISHES, CHEESE SUBSTITUTES, COTTAGE CHEESE, CREAM CHEESE)

NATURAL

FOOD	PORTION	CALS.	FIB.	CHOL.
Alouette				
Brie Baby	1 oz	110	0	30
Brie Baby With Herbs	1 oz	110	0	30
Alpine Lace				
Cheddar Reduced Fat	1 piece (1 oz)	80	0	15
Colby Reduced Fat	1 piece (1 oz)	80	0	15
Monterey Jack Reduced Fat	1 piece (1 oz)	70	0	15
Mozzarella Reduced Sodium	1 piece (1 oz)	70	0	15
Part Skim Low Moisture				
Muenster Reduced Sodium	1 piece (1 oz)	100	0	25
Provolone Reduced Fat	1 piece (1 oz)	70	0	15
Reduced Fat Baby Swiss	1 piece (1 oz)	90	0	6
Reduced Fat Harvati	1 piece (1 oz)	90	0	8
Swiss Reduced Fat	1 piece (1 oz)	90	0	20
Armour				
Cheddar	1 oz	110	—	30
Cheddar Lower Salt	1 oz	110	—	30
Monterey Jack	1 oz	110	—	30
Monterey Jack Lower Salt	1 oz	110	—	30
BabyBel				
Mini Light	1 (0.7 oz)	45	0	5
Bongrain				
Chavrie	2 tbsp (0.8 oz)	40	0	15
Montrachet	1 oz	70	0	30

FOOD	PORTION	CALS.	FIB.	CHOL.
Bongrain (CONT.)				
Montrachet Chive	1 oz	70	0	30
Montrachet Classic	1 oz	70	0	30
Montrachet Classic Herb	1 oz	70	0	30
Montrachet Herbs & Garlic	1 oz	70	0	30
Montrachet In Oil drained	1 oz	70	0	30
Montrachet With Ash	1 oz	70	0	30
Breakstone				
Ricotta	¼ cup (2.2 oz)	110	0	25
Bresse				
Brie	1 oz	110	0	30
Brie Light	1 oz	70	tr	20
Brie With Herbs	1 oz	110	0	30
Creme De Brie	2 tbsp (1 oz)	90	0	25
Creme De Brie Herb	2 tbsp (1 oz)	90	0	25
Brier Run				
Chevre	1 oz	61	—	18
Quark	1 oz	34	—	10
Bristol Gold				
Cheddar Light	1 oz	70	—	15
French Onion Light	1 oz	70	—	15
Garlic & Herb Light	1 oz	70	—	15
Horseradish Light	1 oz	70	—	15
Smoke Light	1 oz	70	—	15
Wine Light	1 oz	70	—	15
Cabot				
Cheddar	1 oz	110	—	30
Monterey Jack	1 oz	80	—	15
Vitalait	1 oz	70	—	15
Vitalait Jalapeno	1 oz	70	—	15
Churney				
Feta	1 oz	80	0	20
Cracker Barrel				
Cheddar Sharp Reduced Fat	1 oz	80	0	20
Cheddar Sharp Reduced Fat Shredded	¼ cup (0.9 oz)	80	0	20
Delice De France	1 oz	110	0	30
With Herbs	1 oz	110	0	30
Di Giorno				
Parmesan	2 tsp (5 g)	20	0	5
Parmesan Grated	2 tsp (5 g)	20	0	5
Parmesan Shredded	2 tsp (5 g)	20	0	<5
Romano	2 tsp (5 g)	20	0	5
Romano Grated	2 tsp (5 g)	25	0	5

FOOD	PORTION	CALS.	FIB.	CHOL.
Di Giorno (CONT.)				
Romano Shredded	2 tsp (5 g)	20	0	5
Dorman				
Cheda-Jack Reduced Fat Low Sodium	1 oz	80	—	19
Cheddar Reduced Fat Low Sodium	1 oz	80	—	20
Monterey Reduced Fat Low Sodium	1 oz	80	—	20
Mozzarella Reduced Fat Low Sodium	1 oz	80	—	17
Muenster Reduced Fat Low Sodium	1 oz	80	—	20
Provolone Reduced Fat Low Sodium	1 oz	80	—	17
Swiss Reduced Fat Low Sodium	1 oz	90	—	15
Father Time				
Cheddar Extra-Sharp Premium	1 oz	110	0	30
Friendship				
Farmer	2 tbsp (1 oz)	50	0	10
Farmer No Salt Added	2 tbsp (1 oz)	50	0	10
Hoop	2 tbsp (1 oz)	20	0	0
Frigo				
Cheddar	1 oz	110	—	30
Cheddar Lite	1 oz	80	—	17
Impastata	1 oz	60	—	15
Mozzarella Part Skim Low Moisture	1 oz	80	—	10
Mozzarella Whole Milk Low Moisture	1 oz	90	—	15
Mozzarella Lite Whole Milk Low Moisture	1 oz	60	—	8
Pizza Shredded	1 oz	65	—	10
Provolone	1 oz	100	—	20
Provolone Lite	1 oz	70	—	10
Ricotta Low Fat Low Salt	1 oz	30	—	5
Ricotta Part Skim	1 oz	40	—	10
Ricotta Whole Milk	1 oz	60	—	15
Romano Dry Grated	1 oz	130	—	35
Romano Grated	1 oz	110	—	30
Romano Whole	1 oz	110	—	30
String	1 oz	80	—	10
String Lite	1 oz	60	—	8

FOOD	PORTION	CALS.	FIB.	CHOL.
Gerard				
Brie	1 oz	90	0	25
Healthy Choice				
Cheddar Fat Free Shredded	¼ cup (1 oz)	45	0	<5
Cheddar Nonfat Fancy Shredded	¼ cup (1 oz)	45	0	<5
Mexican Nonfat Shredded	¼ cup (1 oz)	45	0	<5
Mozzarella Nonfat	1 oz	45	tr	<5
Mozzarella Nonfat Shredded	¼ cup (1 oz)	45	0	<5
Mozzarella String Cheese Nonfat	1 piece (1 oz)	45	0	<5
Mozzeralla Nonfat Fancy Shredded	¼ cup (1 oz)	45	0	<5
Mozzeralla Nonfat Shredded	¼ cup (1 oz)	45	0	<5
Pizza Nonfat Shredded	¼ cup (1 oz)	45	0	<5
Pizza String Nonfat	1 piece (1 oz)	45	0	<5
Heluva Good Cheese				
Cheddar Curds Snack	1 oz	113	0	28
Cheddar Extra-Sharp	1 oz	110	0	30
Cheddar Mild	1 oz	110	0	30
Cheddar Mild Reduced Fat	1 oz	80	0	15
Cheddar Mild White	1 oz	110	0	30
Cheddar Sharp	1 oz	110	0	30
Cheddar Sharp White	1 oz	110	0	30
Cheddar Shredded	¼ cup (1 oz)	110	0	30
Cheddar Very Low Sodium	1 oz	110	0	25
Cheddar White Extra-Sharp	1 oz	110	0	30
Cheddar White Very Low Sodium	1 oz	110	0	25
Cheddar White Shredded	¼ cup (1 oz)	110	0	30
Colby	1 oz	117	0	30
Colby-Jack	1 oz	110	0	30
Monterey Jack	1 oz	100	0	25
Monterey Jack Shredded	¼ cup (1 oz)	100	0	30
Monterey Jack With Jalapenos	1 oz	100	0	25
Mozzarella Part Skim Low Moisture Shredded	¼ cup (1 oz)	80	0	15
Mozzarella Whole Milk	1 oz	80	0	20
Muenster	1 oz	100	0	25
Swiss	1 oz	112	0	28
Washed Curd Cheese	1 oz	110	0	30
Holland Farm				
Edam	1 oz	97	—	25
Farmer	1 oz	102	—	26

FOOD	PORTION	CALS.	FIB.	CHOL.
Holland Farm (CONT.)				
Gouda	1 oz	103	—	27
Monterey Jack	1 oz	102	—	27
Muenster	1 oz	102	—	27
Hollow Road Farms				
Sheep's Milk	1 oz	45	—	15
Keller's				
Chub	2 tbsp (1 oz)	100	0	35
Kraft				
Baby Swiss	1 oz	110	0	25
Blue	1 oz	100	0	30
Blue Crumbles	1 oz	100	0	30
Brick	1 oz	110	0	30
Cheddar	1 oz	110	0	30
Cheddar Fat Free Shredded	¼ cup (1 oz)	45	0	<5
Cheddar Mild Reduced Fat	1 oz	80	0	20
Cheddar Mild Reduced Fat Shredded	¼ cup (1.1 oz)	90	0	20
Cheddar Nacho Blend With Peppers	1 oz	110	0	30
Cheddar Sharp Reduced Fat	1 oz	80	0	20
Cheddar Shredded Finely	¼ cup (0.8 oz)	90	0	25
Colby	1 oz	110	0	30
Colby Reduced Fat	1 oz	80	0	20
Colby And Monterey Jack	1 oz	110	0	30
Colby And Monterey Jack Shredded	¼ cup (1 oz)	120	0	30
Colby And Monterey Jack Shredded Reduced Fat Light	1 oz	80	—	20
Farmers	1 oz	100	0	25
Gouda	1 oz	110	0	25
Havarti	1 oz	120	0	35
House Italian ⅓ Less Fat Grated	2 tsp (0.2 oz)	25	0	<5
Italian Blend Grated	2 tsp (0.2 oz)	25	0	<5
Limburger	1 oz	90	0	25
Monterey Jack	1 oz	110	0	30
Monterey Jack Reduced Fat	1 oz	80	0	20
Monterey Jack Shredded	¼ cup (1 oz)	110	0	30
Monterey Jack With Jalapeno Peppers	1 oz	110	0	30
Monterey Jack With Peppers Reduced Fat	1 oz	80	0	20
Mozzarella Fat Free Shredded	¼ cup (1 oz)	50	tr	<5
Mozzarella Low Moisture Part Skim Reduced Fat Shredded	¼ cup (1.1 oz)	80	0	15

FOOD	PORTION	CALS.	FIB.	CHOL.
Kraft (CONT.)				
Mozzarella Low Moisture Part Skim Shredded	¼ cup (1 oz)	90	0	20
Mozzarella Low Moisture Part Skim Shredded Finely	¼ cup (0.8 oz)	70	0	15
Mozzarella Low Moisture Whole Milk Shredded	¼ cup (1 oz)	90	0	25
Mozzarella Part Skim Low Moisture	1 oz	80	0	15
Mozzarella String Cheese Low Moisture Part Skim	1 stick (1 oz)	80	0	20
Muenster	1 oz	110	0	30
Parmesan Grated	2 tsp (0.2 oz)	20	0	5
Parmesan Shredded	2 tsp (0.2 oz)	20	0	<5
Pizza Four Cheeses Shredded	¼ cup (0.9 oz)	90	0	20
Pizza Mild Cheddar & Mozzarella Shredded	¼ cup (0.9 oz)	90	0	20
Pizza Mozzarella & Cheddar	¼ cup (0.9 oz)	100	0	25
Pizza Mozzarella & Provolone	¼ cup (0.9 oz)	90	0	20
Provolone Smoke Flavor	1 oz	100	0	25
Romano Grated	2 tsp (0.2 oz)	25	0	5
Shredded	¼ cup (1 oz)	120	0	30
String With Jalapeno Peppers	1 oz	80	—	20
Swiss	1 oz	110	0	30
Swiss Shredded	¼ cup (1 oz)	80	0	30
Taco Cheddar & Monterey Jack Shredded	¼ cup (0.9 oz)	100	0	25
Land O'Lakes				
Baby Swiss	1 oz	110	0	25
Brick	1 oz	100	0	30
Chedarella	1 oz	100	0	25
Cheddar Light	1 oz	70	0	10
Gouda	1 oz	110	—	30
Monterey Jack	1 oz	110	0	30
Mozzarella	1 oz	80	0	15
Muenster	1 oz	100	0	25
Provolone	1 oz	100	0	20
Swiss	1 oz	110	0	25
Swiss Light	1 oz	80	0	15
Laughing Cow				
Babybel	1 oz	90	0	10
Babybel Mini	1 (0.7 oz)	70	0	15
Bonbel	1 oz	100	0	25
Bonbel Mini	1 (0.7 oz)	70	0	15

FOOD	PORTION	CALS.	FIB.	CHOL.
Laughing Cow (CONT.)				
Gouda Mini	1 (0.7 oz)	80	0	20
MayBud				
Edam	1 oz	100	0	25
Gouda	1 oz	100	0	25
Gouda Round	1 oz	100	0	25
New Holland				
Garlic	1 oz	90	0	30
	1 oz	90	0	30
Havarti Lower Fat Garden Vegetable	1 oz	80	0	25
Jalapeno	1 oz	80	0	25
Natural Vegetable	1 oz	80	0	25
Northfield				
Naturally Slender	1 oz	90	—	10
Polly-O				
Mozzarella Free	1 oz	35	—	<5
Mozzarella Lite	1 oz	60	—	10
Mozzarella Part Skim	1 oz	70	—	15
Mozzarella Part Skim Shredded	¼ cup	80	—	15
Mozzarella Shredded Free	¼ cup	45	—	<5
Mozzarella Shredded Lite	¼ cup	60	—	15
Mozzarella Whole Milk	1 oz	80	—	20
Mozzarella Whole Milk Shredded	¼ cup	90	—	20
Ricotta Free	¼ cup	50	—	<5
Ricotta Lite	¼ cup	70	—	10
Ricotta Part Skim	¼ cup	90	—	20
Ricotta Whole Milk	¼ cup	110	—	25
String	1 oz	80	—	15
Progresso				
Parmesan Grated	1 tbsp	23	0	4
Romano Grated	1 tbsp	23	0	6
Quaker				
Chub	2 tbsp (1 oz)	100	0	35
Sargento				
4 Cheese Mexican Recipe Blend Shredded	¼ cup (1 oz)	110	0	25
6 Cheese Italian Recipe Blend Shredded	¼ cup (1 oz)	90	0	20
Blue Crumbled	¼ cup (1 oz)	100	0	20
Cheddar	1 slice (1 oz)	110	0	30
Cheddar Mild Shredded Classic Supreme	¼ cup (1 oz)	110	0	30
Cheddar Mild Shredded Fancy Supreme	¼ cup (1 oz)	110	0	30

FOOD	PORTION	CALS.	FIB.	CHOL.
Sargento (CONT.)				
Cheddar Mild Shredded Preferred Light	¼ cup (1 oz)	70	0	10
Cheddar Mild White Shredded Classic Supreme	¼ cup (1 oz)	110	0	30
Cheddar New York Sharp Shredded Classic Supreme	¼ cup (1 oz)	110	0	30
Cheddar Sharp Shredded Classic Supreme	¼ cup (1 oz)	110	0	30
Cheddar Sharp Shredded Fancy Supreme	¼ cup (1 oz)	110	0	30
Cheese For Nachos & Tacos Shredded	¼ cup (1 oz)	110	0	25
Cheese For Pizza Shredded	¼ cup (1 oz)	90	0	20
Cheese For Tacos Shredded	¼ cup (1 oz)	110	0	25
Cheese For Tacos Shredded Preferred Light	¼ cup (1 oz)	70	0	15
Colby	1 slice (1 oz)	110	0	30
Colby-Jack Shredded Fancy Supreme	¼ cup (1 oz)	110	0	25
Gourmet Parm	1 tbsp	20	—	5
Jarlsberg	1 slice (1.2 oz)	120	0	20
Monterey Jack	1 slice (1 oz)	100	0	30
MooTown Snacker Cheese & Sticks	1 pkg (1 oz)	100	0	10
MooTown Snacker String	1 piece (0.8 oz)	70	0	15
MooTown Snackers Cheddar	1 piece (0.8 oz)	100	0	25
MooTown Snackers Cheese & Pretzels	1 pkg (1 oz)	90	0	10
MooTown Snackers Colby-Jack	1 piece (0.8 oz)	90	0	20
MooTown Snackers Pizza Cheese & Sticks	1 pkg (1 oz)	100	0	10
Mozzarella	1 slice (1.5 oz)	130	0	25
Mozzarella Preferred Light	1 slice (1.5 oz)	100	0	15
Mozzarella Shredded Classic Supreme	¼ cup (1 oz)	80	0	15
Mozzarella Shredded Fancy Supreme	¼ cup (1 oz)	80	0	15
Mozzarella Shredded Preferred Light	¼ cup (1 oz)	70	0	10
Muenster	1 slice (1 oz)	100	0	25
Parmesan Fresh	1 oz	111	—	19
Parmesan Shredded	¼ cup (1 oz)	110	0	25
Parmesan & Romano Shredded	¼ cup (1 oz)	110	0	25

FOOD	PORTION	CALS.	FIB.	CHOL.
Sargento (CONT.)				
Pizza Double Cheese Shredded	¼ cup (1 oz)	90	0	20
Provolone	1 slice (1 oz)	100	0	25
Ricotta Light	¼ cup (2.2 oz)	60	0	15
Ricotta Old Fashioned	¼ cup (2.2 oz)	90	0	25
Ricotta Part Skim	¼ cup (2.2 oz)	80	0	20
Swiss	1 slice (0.7 oz)	80	0	20
Swiss Preferred Light	1 slice (1 oz)	80	0	15
Swiss Shredded Fancy Supreme	¼ cup (1 oz)	110	0	30
Swiss Wafer Thin	2 slices (1 oz)	110	0	25
Treasure Cave				
Blue Crumbled	1 oz	110	0	25
Feta Crumbled	1 oz	80	0	20
Tree Of Life				
Cheddar 33% Reduced Fat Organic Milk	1 oz	90	—	15
Cheddar Low Sodium Raw Milk	1 oz	110	—	24
Cheddar Mild Organic Milk	1 oz	110	—	25
Cheddar Mild Raw Milk	1 oz	110	—	25
Cheddar Razor Sharp Raw Milk	1 oz	110	—	25
Cheddar Sharp Organic Milk	1 oz	110	—	25
Cheddar Sharp Raw Milk	1 oz	110	—	25
Colby Organic Milk	1 oz	120	—	30
Colby Raw Milk	1 oz	110	—	30
Farmer Part-Skim Organic Milk	1 oz	90	—	15
Jalapeno Jack Organic Milk	1 oz	110	—	20
Jalapeno Jack Semi-Soft Organic Milk	1 oz	110	—	25
Monterey Jack 35% Reduced Fat Organic Milk	1 oz	80	—	15
Monterey Jack Organic Milk	1 oz	100	—	20
Monterey Jack Semi-Soft Raw Milk	1 oz	110	—	25
Mozzarella Low Moisture Part Skim	1 oz	80	—	15
Mozzarella Low Moisture Part Skim Organic Milk	1 oz	80	—	16
Muenster Organic Milk	1 oz	100	—	25
Muenster Semi-Soft Raw Milk	1 oz	100	—	30
Provolone	1 oz	100	—	20
Swiss Raw Milk	1 oz	110	—	25
Weight Watchers				
Cheddar Mild Shredded	1 oz	80	—	15

FOOD	PORTION	CALS.	FIB.	CHOL.
Weight Watchers (CONT.)				
Cheddar Mild White	1 oz	80	—	15
Cheddar Mild White Low Sodium	1 oz	80	—	15
Cheddar Mild Yellow	1 oz	80	—	15
Cheddar Mild Yellow Low Sodium	1 oz	80	—	15
Cheddar Sharp Cup	1½ tbsp (1 oz)	70	—	10
Cheddar Sharp White	1 oz	80	—	15
Cheddar Sharp Yellow	1 oz	80	—	15
Colby	1 oz	80	—	15
Monterey Jack	1 oz	80	—	15
Mozzarella	1 oz	70	—	15
Mozzarella Shredded	1 oz	80	—	15
White Clover				
Cheddar Light With Simplesse	1 oz	80	—	15
Colby Light With Simplesse	1 oz	80	—	15
Monterey Jack Light With Simplesse	1 oz	70	—	15
Muenster Light With Simplesse	1 oz	70	—	15
blue	1 oz	100	—	21
blue crumbled	1 cup	477	—	102
brick	1 oz	105	—	27
brie	1 oz	95	—	28
camembert	1 oz	85	—	20
camembert	1 wedge (1⅓ oz)	114	—	27
cheddar	1 oz	114	—	30
cheddar low fat	1 oz	49	—	6
cheddar low sodium	1 oz	113	—	28
cheddar shredded	1 cup	455	—	119
cheshire	1 oz	110	—	29
colby	1 oz	112	—	27
colby low fat	1 oz	49	—	6
colby low sodium	1 oz	113	—	28
edam	1 oz	101	—	25
emmentaler	3½ oz	403	—	92
feta	1 oz	75	—	25
fontina	1 oz	110	—	33
goat hard	1 oz	128	—	30
goat semi-soft	1 oz	103	—	22
goat soft	1 oz	76	—	13
gouda	1 oz	101	—	32
gruyere	1 oz	117	—	31
limburger	1 oz	93	—	26

FOOD	PORTION	CALS.	FIB.	CHOL.
mozzarella	1 lb	1276	—	356
mozzarella	1 oz	80	—	22
mozzarella low moisture	1 oz	90	—	25
mozzarella low moisture part skim	1 oz	79	—	15
mozzarella part skim	1 oz	72	—	16
muenster	1 oz	104	—	27
parmesan grated	1 oz	129	—	22
parmesan grated	1 tbsp	23	—	4
parmesan hard	1 oz	111	—	19
port du salut	1 oz	100	—	35
provolone	1 oz	100	—	20
quark 20% fat	3½ oz	116	—	17
quark 40% fat	3½ oz	167	—	37
quark made w/ skim milk	3½ oz	78	—	1
queso anego	1 oz	106	—	30
queso asadero	1 oz	101	—	30
queso chichuahua	1 oz	106	—	30
ricotta	1 cup	428	—	124
ricotta	½ cup	216	—	63
ricotta part skim	1 cup	340	—	76
ricotta part skim	½ cup	171	—	38
romano	1 oz	110	—	29
roquefort	1 oz	105	—	26
swiss	1 oz	107	—	26
tilsit	1 oz	96	—	29
yogurt cheese	1 oz	20	—	7
PROCESSED				
Alouette				
French Onion	2 tbsp (0.8 oz)	70	0	30
Garlic	2 tbsp (0.8 oz)	70	0	30
Light Dill	2 tbsp (0.8 oz)	50	0	20
Light Garlic	2 tbsp (0.8 oz)	50	1	20
Light Herb	2 tbsp (0.8 oz)	50	0	20
Light Herbs & Garlic	2 tbsp (0.8 oz)	50	0	20
Light Spring Vegetable	2 tbsp (0.8 oz)	50	0	20
Salmon	2 tbsp (0.8 oz)	60	0	15
Scallions	2 tbsp (0.8 oz)	70	0	30
Spinach	2 tbsp (0.8 oz)	60	0	25
Alpine Lace				
American	1 piece (1 oz)	80	0	20
American	1 slice (0.66 oz)	50	0	10
American Fat Free	1 piece (1 oz)	45	0	3
Cheddar Fat Free	1 piece (1 oz)	45	0	3
Fat Free For Parmesan Lovers	2 tsp (5 g)	10	0	0

FOOD	PORTION	CALS.	FIB.	CHOL.
Alpine Lace (CONT.)				
Fat Free Mexican Macho	2 tbsp (1 oz)	30	0	3
Fat Free Singles	1 slice (0.66 oz)	25	0	<5
Hot Pepper	1 piece (1 oz)	80	0	6
Mozzarella Fat Free	1 piece (1 oz)	45	0	3
Borden				
American Slices	1 oz	110	—	25
American Very Sharp	1 oz	110	—	25
Swiss Slices	1 oz	100	—	20
Cheez Whiz				
Light	2 tbsp (1.2 oz)	80	0	15
Spread	2 tbsp (1.2 oz)	90	0	20
Spread Hot Salsa	2 tbsp (1.2 oz)	90	0	25
Spread Jalapeno Peppers	2 tbsp (1.2 oz)	90	0	25
Spread Mild Salsa	2 tbsp (1.2 oz)	90	0	25
Squeezable	2 tbsp (1.2 oz)	100	0	15
Zap-A-Pack Cheese Sauce	2 tbsp (1.2 oz)	90	0	20
Zap-A-Pack Cheese Sauce With	2 tbsp (1.2 oz)	90	0	20
Mild Salsa				
Churney				
Diet Snack Cheddar Flavored	1 oz	70	—	10
Diet Snack Port Wine Flavored	1 oz	70	—	10
Cracker Barrel				
Cheddar Extra Sharp	2 tbsp (1.1 oz)	100	0	25
Cheddar Sharp	2 tbsp (1.1 oz)	100	0	25
Delico				
Alouette Cajun	2 tbsp (0.8 oz)	70	0	30
Alouette French Onion	2 tbsp (0.8 oz)	70	0	30
Alouette Garden Vegetable	2 tbsp (0.8 oz)	60	0	30
Alouette Garlic	2 tbsp (0.8 oz)	70	0	30
Alouette Horseradish & Chive	2 tbsp (0.8 oz)	60	0	30
Alouette Spinach	2 tbsp (0.8 oz)	60	0	25
Dorman's				
Lo-Chol Cheddar	1 oz	100	—	<5
Lo-Chol Colby	1 oz	100	—	<5
Lo-Chol Mozzarella	1 oz	90	—	<5
Lo-Chol Muenster	1 oz	100	—	<5
Lo-Chol Swiss	1 oz	100	—	<5
Easy Cheese				
Spread American	2 tbsp (1.2 oz)	100	0	25
Spread Cheddar	2 tbsp (1.2 oz)	100	0	25
Spread Cheddar'n Bacon	2 tbsp (1.2 oz)	100	0	25
Spread Nacho	2 tbsp (1.2 oz)	100	0	25
Spread Sharp Cheddar	2 tbsp (1.2 oz)	100	0	25

FOOD	PORTION	CALS.	FIB.	CHOL.
Formagg				
Formaggio D'Oro	1 oz	70	0	15
Handi-Snacks				
Cheez'n Breadsticks	1 pkg (1.1 oz)	130	0	14
Cheez'n Pretzels	1 pkg (1 oz)	110	tr	15
Cheez'n Crackers	1 pkg (1.1 oz)	130	0	15
Mozzarella String Cheese	1 stick (1 oz)	80	0	20
Harvest Moon				
American	1 slice (0.7 oz)	70	0	20
American	0.7 oz	50	0	10
Spread American	0.7 oz	60	0	15
Healthy Choice				
Fat Free	1 oz	35	tr	<5
Fat Free American Singles	1 slice (0.67 oz)	25	tr	<5
Fat Free American Singles	1 slice (0.75 oz)	30	tr	<5
Heluva Good Cheese				
American	1 slice (0.7)	45	0	15
Cold Pack Cheddar Sharp	2 tbsp (1 oz)	90	0	20
Cold Pack Cheddar Sharp With Bacon	2 tbsp (1 oz)	90	0	20
Cold Pack Cheddar Sharp With Horseradish	2 tbsp (1 oz)	90	0	20
Cold Pack Cheddar Sharp With Jalapenos	2 tbsp (1 oz)	90	0	20
Cold Pack Cheddar Sharp With Port Wine	2 tbsp (1 oz)	90	0	20
Hoffman				
American Yellow	1 oz	110	0	25
Hot Pepper	1 oz	90	0	20
Super Sharp	1 oz	110	0	25
Kraft				
American Grated	1 tbsp (0.2 oz)	25	0	<5
American Shredded	¼ cup (0.9 oz)	110	0	30
Cheese With Garlic	1 oz	90	0	20
Cheese With Jalapeno Peppers	1 oz	60	0	20
Deluxe 25% Less Fat American	0.7 oz	70	0	15
Deluxe American	1 oz	100	0	25
Deluxe American	1 slice (0.7 oz)	70	0	15
Deluxe American	1 slice (1 oz)	110	0	25
Deluxe American White	1 oz	100	0	25
Deluxe American White	1 slice (0.7 oz)	70	0	15
Deluxe American White	1 slice (1 oz)	110	0	25
Deluxe Pimento	1 slice (1 oz)	100	0	25
Deluxe Swiss	1 slice (1 oz)	90	0	25

FOOD	PORTION	CALS.	FIB.	CHOL.
Kraft (CONT.)				
Deluxe Swiss	1 slice (0.7 oz)	70	0	20
Free Singles	1 slice (0.7 oz)	30	0	<5
Free Singles Sharp Cheddar	1 slice (0.7 oz)	30	0	<5
Free Singles Swiss	1 slice (0.7 oz)	30	0	<5
Free Singles White	1 slice (0.7 oz)	30	0	<5
Singles ⅓ Less Fat American	0.7 oz	40	0	10
Singles ⅓ Less Fat American White	0.7 oz	50	0	10
Singles ⅓ Less Fat Sharp Cheddar	0.7 oz	50	0	10
Singles ⅓ Less Fat Swiss	0.7 oz	50	0	10
Singles American	1 slice (0.7 oz)	70	0	15
Singles American	1 slice (1.2 oz)	110	0	30
Singles American White	1 slice (0.7 oz)	70	0	15
Singles Mild Mexican Jalapeno Peppers	1 slice (0.7 oz)	70	0	15
Singles Monterey	1 slice (0.7 oz)	70	0	15
Singles Pimento	1 slice (0.7 oz)	60	0	15
Singles Sharp	1 slice (0.7 oz)	70	0	20
Singles Swiss	1 slice (0.7 oz)	70	0	15
Spread Jalapeno Pepper	1 oz	80	0	20
Spread Olive & Pimento	2 tbsp (1.1 oz)	70	0	20
Spread Pimento	2 tbsp (1.1 oz)	80	0	20
Spread Pineapple	2 tbsp (1.1 oz)	70	0	15
Lactaid				
American	3.5 oz	328	0	64
Land O'Lakes				
American	2 slices (1 oz)	100	0	25
American	1 oz	110	0	30
American	1 slice (0.75 oz)	80	0	20
American Less Salt	1 oz	110	0	30
American Light	1 oz	70	0	20
American Sharp	1 oz	110	0	30
American & Swiss	1 oz	100	0	35
Jalapeno Light	1 oz	70	0	15
Laughing Cow				
Assorted Wedge	1 (1 oz)	70	0	20
Cheesebits	6 pieces (1 oz)	70	0	20
Original Wedge	1 (1 oz)	70	0	20
Wedge Light	1 (1 oz)	50	0	10
Light N'Lively				
Singles 50% Less Fat American	0.7 oz	50	0	10
Singles 50% Less Fat	0.7 oz	50	0	10

FOOD	PORTION	CALS.	FIB.	CHOL.
Light N'Lively (CONT.)				
American White				
Mohawk Valley				
Spread Limburger	2 tbsp (1.1 oz)	80	0	20
Old English				
American Sharp	1 oz	100	0	25
Spread Sharp	2 tbsp (1.1 oz)	70	0	25
Price's				
Cheese & Bacon Spread	2 tbsp (1.1 oz)	90	0	15
Jalapeno Nacho Dip Hot	2 tbsp (1.1 oz)	80	0	15
Jalapeno Nacho Dip Mild	2 tbsp (1.1 oz)	80	0	15
Pimento Cheese Spread	2 tbsp (1.1 oz)	80	0	15
Pimiento Cheese Spread Light	2 tbsp (1.1 oz)	60	0	10
Vegetable Garden	2 tbsp (1.1 oz)	70	0	15
Roka				
Spread Blue	2 tbsp (1.1 oz)	80	0	20
Rondele				
Light Soft Spreadable Garlic & Herb	2 tbsp (0.9 oz)	60	0	10
Soft Spreadable Garlic & Herbs	2 tbsp (1 oz)	100	0	25
Smart Beat				
American	1 slice (0.6 oz)	35	—	0
Low Sodium	1 slice (0.6 oz)	35	—	0
Sharp	1 slice (0.6 oz)	35	—	0
Spreadery				
Medium Cheddar	2 tbsp (1.1 oz)	80	0	15
Pimento Spread	2 tbsp (1.1 oz)	100	0	20
Sharp Cheddar	2 tbsp (1.1 oz)	80	0	15
Vermont Sharp White Cheddar	2 tbsp (1.1 oz)	80	0	15
Squeez-A-Snak				
Spread Sharp	2 tbsp (1.1 oz)	90	0	25
Velveeta	1 slice (0.8 oz)	70	0	15
Hot Mexican With Jalapeno Peppers Shredded	¼ cup (1.3 oz)	130	0	30
Light	1 oz	60	0	10
Mild Mexican With Jalapeno Peppers Shredded	¼ cup (1.3 oz)	130	0	30
Shredded	¼ cup (1.3 oz)	130	0	30
Spread	1 oz	80	0	20
Spread Hot Mexican Jalapeno Pepper	1 oz	80	0	20
Spread Italiana	1 oz	60	0	20
Spread Mild Mexican With Jalapeno Pepper	1 oz	80	0	20

FOOD	PORTION	CALS.	FIB.	CHOL.
Weight Watchers				
American Slices Low Sodium White	2 slices (⅔ oz)	35	—	5
American Slices Low Sodium Yellow	2 slices (⅔ oz)	35	—	5
American Slices White	2 slices (⅔ oz)	35	—	5
American Slices Yellow	2 slices (⅔ oz)	35	—	5
Port Wine Cup	1½ tbsp (1 oz)	70	—	10
Sharp Cheddar Slices	2 slices (⅔ oz)	35	—	5
Swiss Slices	2 slices (⅔ oz)	35	—	5
WisPride				
Chunk	1 oz	110	0	20
Garlic & Herb Cup	2 tbsp (1.1 oz)	100	0	20
Hickory Smoked Cup	2 tbsp (1.1 oz)	100	0	20
Port Wine Ball	2 tbsp (1.1 oz)	100	0	20
Port Wine Cup	2 tbsp (1.1 oz)	100	0	20
Port Wine Light Cup	2 tbsp (1.1 oz)	80	0	10
Sharp Ball	2 tbsp (1.1 oz)	100	0	20
Sharp Cheddar Ball	2 tbsp (1.1 oz)	100	0	20
Sharp Cup	2 tbsp (1.1 oz)	100	0	20
Sharp Light Cup	2 tbsp (1.1 oz)	80	0	10
Swiss Ball	2 tbsp (1.1 oz)	110	0	20
american	1 oz	93	—	18
american cheese food	1 pkg (8 oz)	745	—	145
american cheese spread	1 oz	82	—	16
american cheese spread	1 jar (5 oz)	412	—	78
american cold pack	1 pkg (8 oz)	752	—	144
pimento	1 oz	106	—	27
swiss	1 oz	95	—	24
swiss cheese food	1 pkg (8 oz)	734	—	186

CHEESE DISHES
FROZEN
Stouffer's

Welsh Rarebit	¼ cup (1.1 oz)	120	—	20
TAKE-OUT				
fondue	1 cup (7.5 oz)	492	—	97
fondue	½ cup (3.8 oz)	247	—	49

CHEESE SUBSTITUTES
Borden

Taco-Mate	1 oz	100	—	10
Cheese Two	1 oz	90	—	<5
Formagg				
American White	1 slice (0.66 oz)	60	0	0

FOOD	PORTION	CALS.	FIB.	CHOL.
Formagg (CONT.)				
American Yellow	1 slice (0.66 oz)	60	0	0
Caesar's Italian Garden American	1 oz	60	0	0
Cheddar	1 slice (0.66 oz)	60	0	0
Cheddar Shredded	1 oz	60	0	0
Classic American	1 oz	60	0	0
Macaroni And Cheese Sauce	⅔ cup (5 oz)	190	0	0
Mozzarella Shredded	1 oz	60	0	0
Old World Mozzarella	1 oz	60	0	0
Parmesan Grated	2 tsp (5 g)	15	tr	0
Swiss	1 oz	60	0	0
Swiss White	1 slice (0.66 oz)	60	0	0
Zesty Jalapeno American	1 oz	60	0	0
Vintage Provolone	1 oz	60	0	0
Georgio's				
Imitation Cheddar Shredded	¼ cup (1 oz)	90	0	0
Imitation Mozzarella Shredded	¼ cup (1 oz)	90	0	0
Golden Image				
American	0.7 oz	70	0	5
Harvest Moon				
American Shredded	¼ cup (1.3 oz)	120	0	0
Cheddar Shredded	¼ cup (1.3 oz)	120	0	0
Mozzarella Shredded	¼ cup (1.3 oz)	110	1	0
Lunchwagon				
American	1 slice (0.7 oz)	70	0	0
Sargento				
Classic Supreme Cheddar Shredded	¼ cup (1 oz)	90	0	0
Classic Supreme Mozzarella Shredded	¼ cup (1 oz)	80	0	0
Fancy Supreme Cheddar Shredded	¼ cup (1 oz)	90	0	0
White Wave				
Soy A Melt Cheddar	1 oz	80	—	0
Soy A Melt Fat Free Cheddar	1 oz	40	—	0
Soy A Melt Fat Free Mozzarella	1 oz	40	—	0
Soy A Melt Garlic Herb	1 oz	80	—	0
Soy A Melt Jalapeno Jack	1 oz	80	—	0
Soy A Melt Monterey Jack	1 oz	80	—	0
Soy A Melt Mozzarella	1 oz	80	—	0
Soy A Melt Singles American	1 slice (¾ oz)	60	—	0
Soy A Melt Singles Mozzarella	1 slice (¾ oz)	60	—	0
mozzarella	1 oz	70	—	0

FOOD	PORTION	CALS.	FIB.	CHOL.
CHERIMOYA				
fresh	1	515	—	0
CHERRIES				
CANNED				
Del Monte				
Dark Pitted In Heavy Syrup	½ cup (4.2 oz)	120	tr	0
Sweet Dark Whole Unpitted In Heavy Syrup	½ cup (4.2 oz)	120	tr	0
sour in heavy syrup	½ cup	232	—	0
sour in light syrup	½ cup	189	—	0
sour water packed	1 cup	87	—	0
sweet in heavy syrup	½ cup	107	—	0
sweet in light syrup	½ cup	85	—	0
sweet juice pack	½ cup	68	—	0
sweet water pack	½ cup	57	—	0
DRIED				
Chukar				
Bing	2 oz	160	—	0
Rainer	2 oz	160	—	0
Tart	2 oz	170	—	0
Tart 'n Sweet	2 oz	180	—	0
FRESH				
Dole	1 cup	90	3	0
sour	1 cup	51	—	0
sweet	10	49	—	0
FROZEN				
Big Valley				
Dark Sweet	¾ cup (4.9 oz)	90	3	0
sour unsweetened	1 cup	72	—	0
sweet sweetened	1 cup	232	—	0
CHERRY JUICE				
Hi-C	8 fl oz	130	—	0
Box	8.45 fl oz	140	—	0
Juice Works	6 oz	100	—	0
Juicy Juice	1 box (8.45 fl oz)	130	—	0
Juicy Juice	1 bottle (6 fl oz)	90	—	0
Kool-Aid	8 oz	98	—	0
Black Cherry	8 oz	98	—	0
Sugar Free	8 oz	3	—	0
Sipps				
Wild Cherry	8.45 oz	130	—	0
Smucker's				
Black Cherry	8 oz	130	—	0

FOOD	PORTION	CALS.	FIB.	CHOL.
Tang				
Fruit Box	8.45 oz	121	—	0
Tree Of Life				
Concentrate	8 tsp (1.4 oz)	110	—	0
Wyler's				
Drink Mix Unsweetened Cherry	8 oz	2	—	0
Drink Mix Wild Cherry	8 oz	81	—	0
CHERVIL				
seed	1 tsp	1	—	0
CHESTNUTS				
chinese cooked	1 oz	44	—	0
chinese dried	1 oz	103	—	0
chinese raw	1 oz	64	—	0
chinese roasted	1 oz	68	—	0
cooked	1 oz	37	—	0
dried peeled	1 oz	105	—	0
japanese cooked	1 oz	16	—	0
japanese dried	1 oz	102	—	0
japanese raw	1 oz	44	—	0
japanese roasted	1 oz	57	—	0
raw peeled	1 oz	56	—	0
roasted	1 cup	350	—	0
roasted	1 oz	70	—	0
CHEWING GUM				
Bazooka	1 piece (6 g)	25	—	0
Bazooka	1 piece (4 g)	15	—	0
Fruit Chunk	1 piece (6 g)	25	—	0
Fruit Soft	1 piece (6 g)	25	—	0
Beech-Nut				
Cinnamon	1 piece	10	—	0
Fruit	1 piece	10	—	0
Peppermint	1 piece	10	—	0
Spearmint	1 piece	10	—	0
Big Red	1 stick	10	—	0
Brock				
Bubble Gum	1 piece (0.2 oz)	20	—	0
Bubble Yum				
Fruit Juice Variety	1 piece	20	1	0
Luscious Lime	1 piece	25	1	0
Bubblicious	1 piece (7.9 g)	25	—	0
*Care*Free*				
Sugarless All Flavors	1 piece	8	—	0

FOOD	PORTION	CALS.	FIB.	CHOL.
Care*Free (CONT.)				
Sugarless Bubble Gum All Flavors	1 piece	10	—	0
Chiclets	1 piece (1.59 g)	6	—	0
Tiny Size	8 pieces (0.13 g)	tr	—	0
Clorets	1 piece (1.59 g)	6	—	0
Dentyne	1 piece (1.88 g)	6	—	0
Cinn-A-Burst	1 piece (3.2 g)	9	—	0
Sugar Free	1 piece (1.88 g)	5	—	0
Doublemint	1 piece	10	—	0
Extra Sugar Free				
Cinnamon	1 piece	8	—	0
Spearmint & Peppermint	1 stick	8	—	0
Winter Fresh	1 piece	8	—	0
Freedent				
Spearmint Peppermint & Cinnamon	1 stick	10	—	0
Freshen-Up	1 piece (4.2 g)	13	—	0
Fruit Stripe	1 piece	8	1	0
Bubble Gum	1 piece	8	—	0
Variety Pack	1 piece	8	0	0
Hubba Bubba				
Bubble Gum Cola	1 piece	23	—	0
Bubble Gum Sugarfree Grape	1 piece	13	—	0
Bubble Gum Sugarfree Original	1 piece	14	—	0
Original	1 piece	23	—	0
Strawberry Grape Raspberry	1 piece	23	—	0
Juicy Fruit	1 stick	10	—	0
Rain-Blo				
Bubble Gum Balls	1 piece (2 g)	5	—	0
Swell				
Bubble Gum	1 piece (3 g)	10	—	0
Trident	1 piece (1.88 g)	5	—	0
Soft Bubble Gum	1 piece (3.3 g)	9	—	0
Wrigley's				
Spearmint	1 stick	10	—	0
bubble gum	1 block (8 g)	27	—	0
stick	1 (3 g)	10	—	0
CHIA SEEDS				
dried	1 oz	134	—	0
CHICKEN				
(*see also* CHICKEN DISHES, CHICKEN SUBSTITUTES, DINNER, HOT DOGS)				
CANNED				
Hormel				
Chunk	2 oz	70	0	35

FOOD	PORTION	CALS.	FIB.	CHOL.
Hormel (CONT.)				
Chunk Breast	2 oz	60	0	25
No Salt Chunk Breast	2 oz	60	0	30
Underwood				
Chunky	2.08 oz	150	—	40
Chunky Light	2.08 oz	80	—	30
Smoky	2.08 oz	150	—	40
FRESH				
Perdue				
Breast Oven Stuffer Roaster w/ Skin cooked	1 oz	42	—	20
Breast Quarters Fresh Young w/ Skin cooked	1 oz	48	—	22
Breast Skinless & Boneless Oven Stuffer Roaster cooked	1 oz	31	—	17
Breast Skinless Boneless cooked	1 oz	30	—	17
Breast Split Fresh Young w/ Skin cooked	1 oz	45	—	19
Breast Thin- Sliced Skinless & Boneless Oven Stuffer cooked	1 oz	31	—	17
Breast Whole Fresh Young w/ Skin cooked	1 oz	45	—	19
Breast Whole Oven Stuffer Meat Only cooked	3 oz	169	—	72
Cornish Hen Dark Meat w/ Skin cooked	1 oz	43	—	26
Cornish Hen White Meat w/ Skin cooked	1 oz	42	—	22
Drumsticks Fresh Young w/ Skin cooked	1 oz	42	—	27
Drumsticks Oven Stuffer Roaster w/ Skin cooked	1 oz	41	—	26
Fresh Young Ground cooked	1 oz	49	—	34
Fresh Young Legs w/ Skin cooked	1 oz	51	—	26
Fresh Young Whole Dark Meat w/ Skin cooked	1 oz	47	—	24
Leg Quarters Fresh Young w/ Skin cooked	1 oz	49	—	24
Skinless & Boneless Oven Stuffer Roaster Thighs cooked	1 oz	34	—	24

FOOD	PORTION	CALS.	FIB.	CHOL.
Perdue (CONT.)				
Skinless & Boneless Breast Tenders cooked	1 oz	29	—	17
Soup & Stew Baking Hen Dark Meat w/ Skin cooked	1 oz	41	—	20
Soup & Stew Baking Hen White Meat w/ Skin cooked	1 oz	41	—	16
Thighs Fresh Young w/ Skin cooked	1 oz	57	—	27
Thighs Skinless & Boneless cooked	1 oz	30	—	25
Whole Fresh Young White Meat w/ Skin cooked	1 oz	43	—	21
Whole Oven Stuffer Roaster Dark Meat w/ Skin cooked	1 oz	49	—	22
Whole Oven Stuffer Roaster White Meat w/ Skin cooked	1 oz	44	—	20
Wing Drumettes Fresh Young w/ Skin cooked	1 oz	50	—	26
Wingettes Oven Stuffer Roaster w/ Skin cooked	1 oz	52	—	27
Wings Fresh Young w/ Skin cooked	1 oz	54	—	28
Tyson				
Breast	3 oz	116	—	72
Cornish Hen	3.5 oz	250	—	155
Drumstick	3 oz	131	—	79
Thigh	3 oz	152	—	81
Whole	3 oz	134	—	76
Wing	3 oz	147	—	72
Wampler Longacre				
Ground raw	1 oz	50	—	30
broiler/fryer back w/ skin batter dipped & fried	½ back (2.5 oz)	238	—	63
broiler/fryer back w/ skin floured & fried	1.5 oz	146	—	39
broiler/fryer back w/ skin roasted	1 oz	96	—	28
broiler/fryer back w/ skin stewed	½ back (2.1 oz)	158	—	48
broiler/fryer back w/o skin fried	½ back (2 oz)	167	—	54
broiler/fryer breast w/ skin batter dipped & fried	2.9 oz	218	—	72
broiler/fryer breast w/ skin batter dipped & fried	½ breast (4.9 oz)	364	—	119
broiler/fryer breast w/ skin roasted	2 oz	115	—	49

FOOD	PORTION	CALS.	FIB.	CHOL.
broiler/fryer breast w/ skin roasted	½ breast (3.4 oz)	193	—	83
broiler/fryer breast w/ skin stewed	½ breast (3.9 oz)	202	—	83
broiler/fryer breast w/o skin fried	½ breast (3 oz)	161	—	78
broiler/fryer breast w/o skin roasted	½ breast (3 oz)	142	—	73
broiler/fryer breast w/o skin stewed	2 oz	86	—	44
broiler/fryer dark meat w/ skin batter dipped & fried	5.9 oz	497	—	149
broiler/fryer dark meat w/ skin floured & fried	3.9 oz	313	—	101
broiler/fryer dark meat w/ skin roasted	3.5 oz	256	—	92
broiler/fryer dark meat w/ skin stewed	3.9 oz	256	—	90
broiler/fryer dark meat w/o skin fried	1 cup (5 oz)	334	—	135
broiler/fryer dark meat w/o skin roasted	1 cup (5 oz)	286	—	130
broiler/fryer dark meat w/o skin stewed	3 oz	165	—	76
broiler/fryer dark meat w/o skin stewed	1 cup (5 oz)	269	—	123
broiler/fryer drumstick w/ skin batter dipped & fried	1 (2.6 oz)	193	—	62
broiler/fryer drumstick w/ skin floured & fried	1 (1.7 oz)	120	—	44
broiler/fryer drumstick w/ skin roasted	1 (1.8 oz)	112	—	48
broiler/fryer drumstick w/ skin stewed	1 (2 oz)	116	—	48
broiler/fryer drumstick w/o skin fried	1 (1.5 oz)	82	—	40
broiler/fryer drumstick w/o skin roasted	1 (1.5 oz)	76	—	41
broiler/fryer drumstick w/o skin stewed	1 (1.6 oz)	78	—	40
broiler/fryer leg w/ skin batter dipped & fried	1 (5.5 oz)	431	—	142
broiler/fryer leg w/ skin floured & fried	1 (3.9 oz)	285	—	105
broiler/fryer leg w/ skin roasted	1 (4 oz)	265	—	105
broiler/fryer leg w/ skin stewed	1 (4.4 oz)	275	—	105

FOOD	PORTION	CALS.	FIB.	CHOL.
broiler/fryer leg w/o skin fried	1 (3.3 oz)	195	—	93
broiler/fryer leg w/o skin roasted	1 (3.3 oz)	182	—	89
broiler/fryer leg w/o skin stewed	1 (3.5 oz)	187	—	90
broiler/fryer light meat w/ skin batter dipped & fried	4 oz	312	—	94
broiler/fryer light meat w/ skin floured & fried	2.7 oz	192	—	68
broiler/fryer light meat w/ skin roasted	2.8 oz	175	—	67
broiler/fryer light meat w/ skin stewed	3.2 oz	181	—	66
broiler/fryer light meat w/o skin fried	1 cup (5 oz)	268	—	125
broiler/fryer light meat w/o skin roasted	1 cup (5 oz)	242	—	118
broiler/fryer light meat w/o skin stewed	1 cup (5 oz)	223	—	107
broiler/fryer neck w/ skin stewed	1 (1.3 oz)	94	—	27
broiler/fryer neck w/o skin stewed	1 (.6 oz)	32	—	14
broiler/fryer skin batter dipped & fried	4 oz	449	—	84
broiler/fryer skin batter dipped & fried	from ½ chicken (6.7 oz)	748	—	140
broiler/fryer skin floured & fried	1 oz	166	—	24
broiler/fryer skin floured & fried	from ½ chicken (2 oz)	281	—	41
broiler/fryer skin roasted	from ½ chicken (2 oz)	254	—	46
broiler/fryer skin stewed	from ½ chicken (2.5 oz)	261	—	45
broiler/fryer thigh w/ skin batter dipped & fried	1 (3 oz)	238	—	80
broiler/fryer thigh w/ skin floured & fried	1 (2.2 oz)	162	—	60
broiler/fryer thigh w/ skin roasted	1 (2.2 oz)	153	—	58
broiler/fryer thigh w/ skin stewed	1 (2.4 oz)	158	—	57
broiler/fryer thigh w/o skin fried	1 (1.8 oz)	113	—	53
broiler/fryer thigh w/o skin roasted	1 (1.8 oz)	109	—	49
broiler/fryer thigh w/o skin stewed	1 (1.9 oz)	107	—	49
broiler/fryer w/ skin floured & fried	½ breast (3.4 oz)	218	—	88
broiler/fryer w/ skin floured & fried	½ chicken (11 oz)	844	—	283

FOOD	PORTION	CALS.	FIB.	CHOL.
broiler/fryer w/ skin fried	½ chicken (16.4 oz)	1347	—	404
broiler/fryer w/ skin roasted	½ chicken (10.5 oz)	715	—	263
broiler/fryer w/ skin stewed	½ chicken (11.7 oz)	730	—	262
broiler/fryer w/ skin neck & giblets batter dipped & fried	1 chicken (2.3 lbs)	2987	—	1054
broiler/fryer w/ skin neck & giblets roasted	1 chicken (1.5 lbs)	1598	—	730
broiler/fryer w/ skin neck & giblets stewed	1 chicken (1.6 lbs)	1625	—	726
broiler/fryer w/o skin fried	1 cup	307	—	131
broiler/fryer w/o skin roasted	1 cup (5 oz)	266	—	125
broiler/fryer w/o skin stewed	1 cup (5 oz)	248	—	116
broiler/fryer w/o skin stewed	1 oz	54	—	22
broiler/fryer wing w/ skin batter dipped & fried	1 (1.7 oz)	159	—	39
broiler/fryer wing w/ skin floured & fried	1 (1.1 oz)	103	—	26
broiler/fryer wing w/ skin roasted	1 (1.2 oz)	99	—	29
broiler/fryer wing w/ skin stewed	1 (1.4 oz)	100	—	28
capon w/ skin neck & giblets roasted	1 chicken (3.1 lbs)	3211	—	1458
cornish hen w/o skin & bone roasted	1 hen (3.8 oz)	144	—	113
cornish hen w/o skin & bone roasted	½ hen (2 oz)	72	—	57
cornish hen w/skin roasted	1 hen (8 oz)	595	—	299
cornish hen w/skin roasted	½ hen (4 oz)	296	—	149
roaster dark meat w/o skin roasted	1 cup (5 oz)	250	—	104
roaster light meat w/o skin roasted	1 cup (5 oz)	214	—	105
roaster w/ skin neck & giblets roasted	1 chicken (2.4 lbs)	2363	—	1003
roaster w/ skin roasted	½ chicken (1.1 lbs)	1071	—	365
roaster w/o skin roasted	1 cup (5 oz)	469	—	160
stewing dark meat w/o skin stewed	1 cup (5 oz)	361	—	132
stewing w/ skin neck & giblets stewed	1 chicken (1.3 lbs)	1636	—	603
stewing w/ skin stewed	½ chicken (9.2 oz)	744	—	205
stewing w/ skin stewed	6.2 oz	507	—	140
FROZEN				
Tyson				
Boneless Breasts	3.5 oz	210	—	80

FOOD	PORTION	CALS.	FIB.	CHOL.
Tyson (CONT.)				
Boneless Skinless Breast	3.5 oz	130	—	55
Boneless Skinless Thighs	3.5 oz	200	—	105
Drums & Thighs	3.5 oz	270	—	130
Skinless Breast Tenders	3.5 oz	120	—	50
FROZEN PREPARED				
Country Skillet				
Chicken Chunks	3 oz	260	—	25
Chicken Nuggets	3 oz	250	—	40
Chicken Patties	3 oz	230	—	40
Southern Fried Chicken Chunks	3 oz	270	—	30
Southern Fried Chicken Patties	3 oz	240	—	35
Empire				
Nuggets	5 (3 oz)	180	1	15
Stix	4 (3.1 oz)	180	2	25
Healthy Balance				
Baked Boneless Breast Nuggets	2.25 oz	120	—	30
Baked Boneless Breast Patties	2.25 oz	120	—	30
Baked Boneless Breast Tenders	2.25 oz	120	—	30
Tyson				
BBQ Breast Fillets	3 oz	110	—	50
Breast Chunks	3 oz	240	—	30
Breast Fillets	3 oz	190	—	25
Breast Patties	2.6 oz	220	—	35
Chick'n Cheddar	2.6 oz	220	—	40
Chick'n Chunks	2.6 oz	220	—	35
Cordon Blue Mini	1	90	—	17
Diced	3 oz	130	—	70
Grilled Sandwich	3.5 oz	200	—	32
Hors D'Oeuvres Mesquite Chunks	3.5 oz	100	—	45
Hot BBQ Breast Tenders	2.75 oz	110	—	45
Mesquite Breast Fillets	2.75 oz	100	—	50
Mesquite Breast Strips	2.75 oz	100	—	50
Mesquite Breast Tenders	2.75 oz	110	—	55
Microwave Chunks BBQ Sandwich	4 oz	230	—	30
Roasted Breast Fillets	1 oz	50	—	15
Roasted Breasts	1 oz	50	—	15
Roasted Drumsticks	1 oz	50	—	40
Roasted Half Chicken	1 oz	60	—	30
Roasted Thighs	1 oz	70	—	40
Roasted Whole Chicken	1 oz	60	—	30
Southern Fried Breast Fillets	3 oz	220	—	25

FOOD	PORTION	CALS.	FIB.	CHOL.
Tyson (CONT.)				
Southern Fried Breast Patties	2.6 oz	220	—	35
Southern Fried Chick'n Chunks	2.6 oz	220	—	35
Thick & Crispy Patties	2.6 oz	220	—	40
Weight Watchers				
Chicken Nuggets	5.9 oz	220	—	40
READY-TO-USE				
Carl Buddig	1 oz	50	0	20
Chicken By George				
Cajun	1 breast (4 oz)	120	0	55
Caribbean Grill	1 breast (4 oz)	150	0	55
Garlic & Herb	1 breast (4 oz)	120	0	50
Italian Bleu Cheese	1 breast (4 oz)	130	0	60
Lemon Herb	1 breast (4 oz)	120	0	50
Lemon Oregano	1 breast (4 oz)	130	0	50
Mesquite Barbecue	1 breast (4 oz)	120	0	50
Mustard Dill	1 breast (4 oz)	140	0	65
Roasted	1 breast (4 oz)	110	0	55
Teriyaki	1 breast (4 oz)	130	0	50
Tomato Herb With Basil	1 breast (4 oz)	140	0	60
Empire				
Barbarcue Whole	5 oz	280	0	110
Battered & Breaded Cutlets	1 (3.3 oz)	200	2	25
Battered & Breaded Nuggets	5 (3 oz)	200	1	30
Battered & Breaded Fried Breasts	3 oz	170	tr	45
Bologna	3 slices (1.8 oz)	200	0	40
Fried Drum & Thigh	3 oz	240	2	80
Falls				
BBQ	3 oz	150	—	75
Healthy Choice				
Oven Roasted Breast	1.9 oz	60	0	25
Hebrew National				
Deli Thin Oven Roasted	1.8 oz	45	—	20
Louis Rich				
Deli-Thin Oven Roasted Breast	4 slices (1.8 oz)	60	0	25
Deluxe Oven Roasted Breast	1 slice (1 oz)	40	0	15
Hickory Smoked Breast	1 slice (1 oz)	30	0	15
Oven Roasted Breast	1 slice (1 oz)	40	0	15
Mr. Turkey				
Deli Cuts Hardwood Smoked	3 slices	30	—	13
Deli Cuts Oven Roasted	3 slices	25	—	15
Oscar Mayer				
Deli-Thin Honey Glazed Breast	4 slices (1.8 oz)	60	0	25

FOOD	PORTION	CALS.	FIB.	CHOL.
Oscar Mayer (CONT.)				
Free Oven Roasted Breast	4 slices (1.8 oz)	45	—	25
Healthy Favorites Oven Roasted Breast	4 slices (1.8 oz)	40	0	25
Lunchables Chicken/Monterey Jack	1 pkg (4.5 oz)	350	1	75
Lunchables Deluxe Chicken/ Turkey	1 pkg (5.1 oz)	380	1	70
Lunchables Dessert Chocolate Pudding/Chicken/Jack	1 pkg (6.2 oz)	370	0	55
Perdue				
BBQ Breast Half	1 oz	46	—	28
BBQ Drumsticks	1 oz	53	—	34
BBQ Half Dark Meat	1 oz	57	—	31
BBQ Half White Meat	1 oz	40	—	22
BBQ Thighs	1 oz	59	—	37
BBQ Wings	1 oz	62	—	35
Cornish Hen Roasted Dark Meat	1 oz	45	—	26
Cornish Hen Roasted While Meat	1 oz	39	—	18
Nuggets Fun Shaped	1 (.73 oz)	54	—	8
Nuggets Cheese	1 (.67 oz)	54	—	8
Perdue Done It! Cutlets	3.5 oz	250	—	39
Perdue Done It! Nuggets Original	1 (.67 oz)	48	—	7
Perdue Done It! Tenders	1 oz	62	—	10
Perdue Done It! Wings Hot & Spicy	1 oz	60	—	37
Roasted Drumsticks	1 oz	40	—	33
Roasted Thighs	1 oz	46	—	32
Roasted Breast	1 oz	45	—	22
Whole Or Half Roasted Dark Meat	1 oz	51	—	27
Whole Or Half Roasted White Meat	1 oz	37	—	21
Wings Garlic & Herb	1 oz	61	—	40
Wampler Longacre				
Breast	1 oz	35	—	15
Chef's Select Breast	1 oz	35	—	15
Premium Oven Roasted Breast	1 oz	50	—	20
Roll	1 oz	65	—	25
Roll Sliced	1 slice (0.8 oz)	50	—	20

FOOD	PORTION	CALS.	FIB.	CHOL.
Weaver				
Roasted Wings	1 oz	70	—	45
Weight Watchers				
Raosted Ham	2 slices (¾ oz)	25	—	10
Roasted & Smoked Breast	2 slices (¾ oz)	25	—	15
chicken roll light meat	2 oz	90	—	28
chicken roll light meat	1 pkg (6 oz)	271	—	85
poultry salad sandwich spread	1 oz	238	—	9
poultry salad sandwich spread	1 tbsp (13 g)	109	—	4
TAKE-OUT				
Sara Lee				
Oven Roasted Breast Of Chicken	2 oz	60	—	25
boneless breaded & fried w/ barbecue sauce	6 pieces (4.6 oz)	330	—	61
boneless breaded & fried w/ honey	6 pieces (4 oz)	339	—	61
boneless breaded & fried w/ mustard sauce	6 pieces (4.6 oz)	323	—	62
boneless breaded & fried w/ sweet & sour sauce	6 pieces (4.6 oz)	346	—	61
breast & wing breaded & fried	2 pieces (5.7 oz)	494	—	149
drumstick breaded & fried	2 pieces (5.2 oz)	430	—	165
thigh breaded & fried	2 pieces (5.2 oz)	430	—	165

CHICKEN DISHES

(*see also* CHICKEN SUBSTITUTES, DINNER)

FOOD	PORTION	CALS.	FIB.	CHOL.
CANNED				
Dinty Moore				
American Classics Chicken & Noodles	1 bowl (10 oz)	260	2	80
American Classics Chicken With Mashed Potatoes	1 bowl (10 oz)	220	2	25
Chicken Stew	1 cup (7.5 oz)	180	2	30
Microwave Cup Chicken & Dumpling	1 cup (7.5 oz)	190	1	25
Stew	1 cup (8.5 oz)	220	2	40
Top Shelf				
Chicken Cacciatore	1 bowl (10 oz)	210	3	45
Chicken Acapulco Fiesta Chicken	1 bowl (10 oz)	420	2	70
Chicken Ala King	1 bowl (10 oz)	380	2	45
Glazed Breast Of Chicken	1 bowl (10 oz)	200	2	50
FROZEN				
Jimmy Dean				
Grilled Breast Sandwich	1 (5.5 oz)	330	1	70

FOOD	PORTION	CALS.	FIB.	CHOL.
Luigino's				
Chicken A La King With Noodles	1 pkg (8 oz)	240	2	60
Noodles With Chicken Peas & Carrots	1 pkg (8 oz)	300	2	50
Noodles With Chicken Peas & Carrots	1 cup (6.3 oz)	260	2	40
Sweet & Sour Chicken With Rice	1 pkg (8 oz)	300	2	20
MicroMagic				
Chicken Sandwich	1 pkg (4.5 oz)	390	—	35
Weight Watchers				
Chicken & Broccoli Pita	1 (5.4 oz)	190	—	5
Grilled Chicken Sandwich	1 (4 oz)	210	—	20
READY-TO-USE				
Spreadables				
Chicken Salad	¼ can	100	—	16
Wampler Longacre				
Cacciatore	1 serv (4 oz)	118	—	40
Salad	1 oz	70	—	15
Salad Lite	1 oz	45	—	10
Smokey Barbecue	1 serv (4 oz)	175	—	65
Sweet N Sour	1 serv (4 oz)	106	—	25
Szechwan With Peanuts	1 serv (4 oz)	112	—	22
SHELF-STABLE				
Lunch Bucket				
Light'n Healthy Chicken Fiesta	1 pkg (7.5 oz)	170	—	10
TAKE-OUT				
chicken cacciatore	¾ cup	394	2	99
chicken paprikash	1½ cups	296	—	90
chicken & dumplings	¾ cup	256	tr	109
chicken & noodles	1 cup	365	—	103
chicken a la king	1 cup	470	—	221
fillet sandwich plain	1	515	—	60
fillet sandwich w/ cheese lettuce mayonnaise & tomato	1	632	—	76

CHICKEN SUBSTITUTES

Harvest Direct				
TVP Poultry Chunks	3.5 oz	280	18	0
TVP Poultry Ground	3.5 oz	280	18	0
Jaclyn's				
Salsa Chicken Style Dinner	11.5 oz	325	—	0
Sesame Chicken Style Dinner	11.5 oz	345	—	0

FOOD	PORTION	CALS.	FIB.	CHOL.
LaLoma				
Chicken Supreme not prep	¼ cup (16 g)	50	—	0
Chik Nuggets	5 nuggets (85 g)	270	—	0
Fried Chicken	1 piece (57 g)	180	—	0
Fried Chicken w/ Gravy	2 piece (85 g)	140	—	0
White Wave				
Meatless Sandwich Slices	2 slices (1.6 oz)	80	0	0

CHICKPEAS
CANNED
Allen				
Garbanzo	½ cup (4.4 oz)	120	8	0
East Texas Fair				
Garbanzo	½ cup (4.4 oz)	120	8	0
Eden				
Organic	½ cup (4.1 oz)	110	4	0
Goya				
Spanish Style	7.5 oz	150	9	0
Green Giant				
Garbanzo	½ cup	90	5	0
Hanover	½ cup	100	—	0
Progresso	½ cup	110	6	0
S&W				
Garbanzo Lite 50% Less Salt	½ cup	110	—	0
Garbanzo Premium Large	½ cup	110	—	0
Garbanzo Water Pack	½ cup	105	—	0
chickpeas	1 cup	285	—	0
DRIED				
Bean Cuisine				
Garbanzo	½ cup	115	5	0
cooked	1 cup	269	—	0

CHICORY
greens raw chopped	½ cup	21	—	0
root raw	1 (2.1 oz)	44	—	0
roots raw cut up	½ cup (1.6 oz)	33	—	0
witloof head raw	1 (1.9 oz)	9	—	0
witloof raw	½ cup (1.6 oz)	8	—	0

CHILI
CANNED
Allen				
Mexican Chili Beans	½ cup (4.5 oz)	120	8	0
Armour				
Chili No Beans	1 cup (8.7 oz)	470	—	85

FOOD	PORTION	CALS.	FIB.	CHOL.
Armour (CONT.)				
Chili With Beans	1 cup (8.9 oz)	440	—	50
Chili With Beans Hot	1 cup (8.9 oz)	440	—	50
Chili With Beans Western Style	1 cup (8.8 oz)	460	—	60
Brown Beauty				
Mexican Chili Beans	½ cup (4.5 oz)	120	8	0
Chi-Chi's				
San Antonio	1 cup (8.5 oz)	240	6	60
Del Monte				
Sauce	1 tbsp (0.6 oz)	20	0	0
Gebhardt				
Hot With Beans	1 cup	470	6	65
Plain	1 cup	530	1	70
With Beans	1 cup	495	6	92
Hain				
Spicy Tempeh	7½ oz	160	—	0
Spicy Vegetarian	7½ oz	160	—	0
Spicy Vegetarian Reduced Sodium	7½ oz	170	—	0
Spicy With Chicken	7½ oz	130	—	40
Health Valley				
Mild Vegetarian With Beans	5 oz	160	12	0
Mild Vegetarian With Beans No Salt Added	5 oz	160	12	0
Mild Vegetarian With Lentils No Salt Added	5 oz	140	7	0
Spicy Vegetarian With Beans	5 oz	160	12	0
Hormel				
Chili Mac	1 can (7.5 oz)	200	2	25
Chili No Beans	1 cup (8.3 oz)	410	3	75
Chili With Beans	1 cup (8.7 oz)	340	9	60
Chunky Chili With Beans	1 cup (8.7 oz)	330	8	60
Hot Chili No Beans	1 cup (8.3 oz)	410	3	75
Hot Chili With Beans	1 cup (8.7 oz)	340	9	60
Hot With Beans	1 can (7.5 oz)	250	6	50
No Beans	1 can (7.5 oz)	390	2	65
Turkey Chili With Beans	1 cup (8.7 oz)	220	7	55
Turkey Chili No Beans	1 cup (8.3 oz)	190	3	70
With Beans	1 can (7.5 oz)	250	6	50
Hunt's				
Chili Beans	4 oz	100	6	0
Just Rite				
Hot With Beans	4 oz	195	1	33
With Beans	4 oz	200	1	33

FOOD	PORTION	CALS.	FIB.	CHOL.
Just Rite (CONT.)				
Without Beans	4 oz	180	tr	41
Manwich				
Chili Fixin's as prep	8 oz	290	5	65
Micro Cup Meals				
Chili Mac	1 cup (7.5 oz)	200	2	25
Chili No Beans	1 cup (7.5 oz)	290	3	65
Chili With Beans	1 cup (10.4 oz)	410	12	75
Chili With Beans	1 cup (7.5 oz)	250	6	50
Hot Chili With Beans	1 cup (7.5 oz)	250	6	50
Old El Paso				
Chili With Beans	1 cup	217	6	32
S&W				
Chili Beans	½ cup	130	—	0
Chili Makin's Original	½ cup	100	—	0
Van Camp's				
Chilee Beanee Weenee	1 can (8 oz)	240	9	35
Chili With Beans	1 cup (8.9 oz)	350	7	45
chili w/ beans	1 cup	286	—	43
DRIED				
Gebhardt				
Chili Powder	1 tsp	15	tr	0
Chili Quik Seasoning	1 tsp	10	tr	0
Hain				
Hot Chili	¼ pkg	30	—	0
Medium Chili	¼ pkg	30	—	0
Mild Chili	¼ pkg	30	—	0
Nile Spice				
Chili'n Beans Original	1 pkg	150	6	0
Chili'n Beans Spicy	1 pkg	150	6	0
Old El Paso				
Chili Seasoning Mix	⅛ pkg	21	1	0
Watkins				
Chili Seasoning	1¼ tsp (4 g)	15	—	0
Powder	¼ tsp (0.5 g)	0	—	0
powder	1 tsp	8	—	0
FROZEN				
Lean Cuisine				
Three Bean	1 pkg (9 oz)	210	7	10
Lightlife	4.3 oz	110	—	0
Luigino's				
Chili-Mac	1 pkg (8 oz)	230	3	25
Stouffer's				
With Beans	1 pkg (8.75 oz)	270	8	35

FOOD	PORTION	CALS.	FIB.	CHOL.
Tabatchnick				
Vegetarian	7.5 oz	210	10	0
SHELF-STABLE				
Lunch Bucket				
Chili With Beans	1 pkg (7.5 oz)	300	—	45
TAKE-OUT				
con carne w/ beans	8.9 oz	254	—	133

CHINESE CABBAGE
(see CABBAGE)

CHINESE FOOD
(see ORIENTAL FOOD)

CHINESE PRESERVING MELON

FOOD	PORTION	CALS.	FIB.	CHOL.
cooked	½ cup	11	—	0

CHIPS
(see also POPCORN, PRETZELS, SNACKS)
CORN

FOOD	PORTION	CALS.	FIB.	CHOL.
Energy Food Factory				
Corn Pops Fat Free	½ oz	50	1	0
Corn Pops Nacho	½ oz	50	1	0
Corn Pops Original	½ oz	50	1	0
Fritos	34 pieces (1 oz)	150	1	0
Chili Cheese	34 pieces (1 oz)	160	1	0
Crisp 'N Thin	18 pieces (1 oz)	160	1	0
Dip Size	13 pieces (1 oz)	150	1	0
Non-Stop Nacho Cheese	34 pieces (1 oz)	150	1	tr
Rowdy Rustlers Bar-B-Q	34 pieces (1 oz)	150	1	0
Wild 'N Mild	32 pieces (1 oz)	160	1	0
Health Valley	1 oz	160	1	0
No Salt Added	1 oz	160	1	0
With Cheddar Cheese	1 oz	160	1	2
Lance	1 pkg (50 g)	270	—	0
BBQ	1 pkg (50 g)	260	—	0
Snyder's	1 oz	160	2	0
BBQ	1 oz	160	2	0
Wise	1 oz	160	—	0
Corn Crunchies	1 oz	160	—	0
Crispy Corn	1 oz	160	—	0
Crispy Corn Nacho Cheese	1 oz	160	—	0
barbecue	1 oz	148	1	0
barbecue	1 bag (7 oz)	1036	10	0
cones plain	1 oz	145	—	0
onion	1 oz	142	—	0

FOOD	PORTION	CALS.	FIB.	CHOL.
plain	1 oz	153	1	0
plain	1 bag (7 oz)	1067	9	0
puffs cheese	1 bag (8 oz)	1256	2	9
puffs cheese	1 oz	157	tr	1
twists cheese	1 bag (8 oz)	1256	2	9
twists cheese	1 oz	157	tr	1
MULTIGRAIN				
Sunchips	12 pieces (1 oz)	150	—	0
French Onion	12 pieces (1 oz)	140	—	tr
POTATO				
Barrel O' Fun	1 oz	150	0	0
Barbeque	1 oz	145	0	0
Sour Cream & Onion	1 oz	150	0	0
Butterfield				
Sticks	⅔ cup (1 oz)	150	2	0
Sticks	1 pkg (1.7 oz)	250	3	1
Cape Cod	19 chips (1 oz)	150	1	0
Cottage Fries				
No Salt Added	1 oz	160	—	0
Eagle				
BBQ Thins	1 oz	150	—	0
Kettle Fry BBQ Crunchy	1 oz	150	—	0
Kettle Fry Cape Cod	1 oz	150	—	0
Kettle Fry Cape Cod No Salt	1 oz	150	—	0
Kettle Fry Cape Cod Waves	1 oz	150	—	0
Kettle Fry Cape Cod Waves No Salt	1 oz	150	—	0
Kettle Fry Dill & Sour Cream	1 oz	150	—	0
Kettle Fry Dill & Sour Cream No Salt	1 oz	150	—	0
Kettle Fry Extra Crunchy	1 oz	150	—	0
Kettle Fry Idaho Russet	1 oz	150	—	0
Kettle Fry Louisiana BBQ	1 oz	150	—	0
Ranch Ridged	1 oz	160	—	0
Ridged	1 oz	150	—	0
Sour Cream & Onion	1 oz	150	—	0
Thins	1 oz	150	—	0
Energy Food Factory				
Potato Pops Au Gratin	½ oz	60	1	<5
Potato Pops Fat Free	½ oz	50	1	0
Potato Pops Herb & Garlic	½ oz	50	1	0
Potato Pops Mesquite	½ oz	50	1	0
Potato Pops Original	½ oz	50	1	0
Potato Pops Salt N' Vinegar	½ oz	50	1	0

FOOD	PORTION	CALS.	FIB.	CHOL.
Health Valley				
Country Ripple	1 oz	160	1	0
Country Ripple No Salt Added	1 oz	160	1	0
Dip Chips	1 oz	160	1	0
Dip Chips No Salt Added	1 oz	160	1	0
Natural	1 oz	160	1	0
Natural No Salt Added	1 oz	160	1	0
Kelly's	1 oz	150	2	0
Bar-B-Q	1 oz	150	1	0
Crunchy	1 oz	150	2	0
Rippled	1 oz	150	2	0
Sour Cream n' Onion	1 oz	150	1	0
Unsalted	1 oz	150	—	0
Lance	1 pkg (32 g)	190	—	0
BBQ	1 pkg (32 g)	190	—	0
Cajun Style	1 pkg (32 g)	160	—	0
Hot Fries	1 pkg (28 g)	160	—	0
Ripple	1 pkg (32 g)	190	—	0
Sour Cream & Onion	1 pkg (32 g)	190	—	0
Lay's	17 pieces (1 oz)	150	1	0
Bar-B-Q	17 pieces (1 oz)	150	1	0
Cheddar Cheese	17 pieces (1 oz)	150	1	tr
Crunch Tators	16 pieces (1 oz)	150	1	0
Crunch Tators Amazin' Cajun	16 pieces (1 oz)	150	—	0
Crunch Tators Hoppin' Jalapeno	16 pieces (1 oz)	140	1	0
Crunch Tators Mighty Mesquite	16 pieces (1 oz)	150	—	0
Crunch Tators Supreme Sour Cream	16 pieces (1 oz)	150	—	0
Flamin' Hot	17 pieces (1 oz)	150	1	0
Kansas City Style Bar-B-Q	17 pieces (1 oz)	150	1	0
Salt & Vinegar	17 pieces (1 oz)	150	1	0
Sour Cream & Onion	17 pieces (1 oz)	160	1	tr
Tangy Ranch	17 pieces (1 oz)	160	1	0
Unsalted	17 pieces (1 oz)	150	1	0
Louise's				
"1g" Mesquite BBQ	1 oz	110	2	0
"1g" Original	1 oz	110	2	0
70% Less Fat Mesquite BBQ	1 oz	110	2	0
70% Less Fat Original	1 oz	110	2	0
Fat-Free Maui Onion	1 oz	110	2	0
Fat-Free Mesquite BBQ	1 oz	110	2	0
Fat-Free No Salt	1 oz	110	2	0
Fat-Free Original	1 oz	110	2	0

FOOD	PORTION	CALS.	FIB.	CHOL.
Louise's (CONT.)				
Fat-Free Vinegar & Salt	1 oz	110	2	0
Mr. Phipps				
Tater Crisps Bar-B-Que	21 (1 oz)	130	1	0
Tater Crisps Original	23 (1 oz)	120	1	0
Tater Crisps Sour Cream 'n Onion	22 (1 oz)	130	1	0
New York Deli	1 oz	160	—	0
Pringles				
BBQ	14 chips (1 oz)	150	—	0
Cheez-ums	14 chips (1 oz)	170	—	1
Light BBQ	14 chips (0.9 oz)	130	—	0
Light Original	14 chips (0.9 oz)	130	—	0
Light Ranch	14 chips (0.9 oz)	130	—	0
Light Sour Cream 'N Onion	14 chips (0.9 oz)	130	—	0
Original	14 chips (1 oz)	160	—	0
Ranch	14 chips (1 oz)	150	—	0
Right BBQ	16 chips (1 oz)	140	—	0
Right Original	16 chips (1 oz)	140	—	0
Right Ranch	16 chips (1 oz)	140	—	0
Right Sour Cream 'N Onion	16 chips (1 oz)	140	—	0
Rippled	10 chips (1 oz)	160	—	0
Sour Cream 'N Onion	14 chips (1 oz)	160	—	1
Ruffles	18 chips (1 oz)	150	1	0
Cheddar Cheese & Sour Cream	18 chips (1 oz)	160	1	tr
Light	18 chips (1 oz)	130	1	0
Light Sour Cream & Onion	18 chips (1 oz)	130	1	tr
Mesquite Grille B-B-Q	18 chips (1 oz)	160	1	0
Monterey Jack Cheese Attack	18 chips (1 oz)	160	1	tr
Ranch	18 chips (1 oz)	160	1	0
Sour Cream & Onion	18 chips (1 oz)	160	1	tr
Snyder's	1 oz	150	1	0
BBQ	1 oz	150	1	0
Cheddar Bacon	1 oz	150	1	0
Coney Island	1 oz	150	1	0
Grilled Steak & Onion	1 oz	150	1	0
Hot Buffalo Wings	1 oz	150	1	0
Kosher Dill	1 oz	150	1	0
No Salt	1 oz	150	1	0
Salt & Vinegar	1 oz	150	1	0
Sausage Pizza	1 oz	150	1	0
Sour Cream & Onion	1 oz	150	1	0
Sour Cream & Onion Unsalted	1 oz	150	1	0

FOOD	PORTION	CALS.	FIB.	CHOL.
Suprimos				
Cheddar & Jack	1 oz	140	—	tr
Cool Onion	1 oz	140	—	tr
Weight Watchers				
Great Snackers Barbecue	½ oz	70	—	0
Great Snackers Cheddar Cheese	½ oz	70	—	0
Great Snackers Sour Cream & Onion	½ oz	70	—	0
Wise				
Natural	1 oz	160	—	0
Ridgies Barbecue	1 oz	150	—	0
barbecue	1 oz	139	—	0
barbecue	1 bag (7 oz)	971	—	0
light	1 oz	134	—	0
light	1 bag (6 oz)	801	—	0
potato	1 oz	152	1	0
potato	1 pkg (8 oz)	1217	8	0
sour cream & onion	1 bag (7 oz)	1051	—	14
sour cream & onion	1 oz	150	—	2
sticks	½ cup (0.6 oz)	94	1	0
sticks	1 pkg (1 oz)	148	—	0
sticks	1 oz	148	1	0
sticks	½ cup	94	—	0
TORTILLA				
Barrel O' Fun				
Nacho	1 oz	140	1	0
Tostada Yellow	1 oz	140	0	0
White	1 oz	140	0	0
Doritos				
Lightly Salted	16 chips (1 oz)	150	2	0
Eagle				
Nacho	1 oz	150	—	0
Ranch	1 oz	150	—	0
Restaurant Style	1 oz	150	—	0
Strips	1 oz	150	—	0
Frito Lay				
Salsa 'N Cheese	16 (1 oz)	150	2	0
Guiltless Gourmet				
Baked	22-26 chips (1 oz)	110	1	0
Hain				
Sesame	1 oz	140	—	0
Sesame Cheese	1 oz	160	—	<5
Sesame No Salt Added	1 oz	140	—	0

FOOD	PORTION	CALS.	FIB.	CHOL.
Hain (cont.)				
Taco Style	1 oz	160	—	<5
La FAMOUS	1 oz	140	—	0
No Salt Added	1 oz	140	—	0
Lance				
Jalapeno Cheese	1 pkg (1⅛ oz)	160	—	0
Louise's				
95% Fat-Free	1 oz	120	1	0
Mr. Phipps				
Nacho	28 (1 oz)	130	3	0
Original	28 (1 oz)	130	3	0
Old El Paso				
NACHIPS	9 chips (1 oz)	150	2	0
White Corn	12 chips (1 oz)	150	1	0
Santitas	1 oz	140	2	0
Cantina Style	1 oz	140	2	0
Cantina Style Fajita	1 oz	140	2	0
Strips	1 oz	140	2	0
Snyder's	1 oz	140	2	0
Enchilada	1 oz	140	2	0
Nacho Cheese	1 oz	140	2	0
No Salt	1 oz	140	2	0
Ranch	1 oz	140	2	0
Tostitos	11 pieces (1 oz)	140	2	0
Baked	1 oz	110	2	0
Baked Cool Ranch	1 oz	130	2	0
Baked Unsalted	1 oz	110	2	0
Bite Size	16 pieces (1 oz)	150	2	0
Restaurant Style Lime 'N Chili	7 pieces (1 oz)	150	2	0
Restaurant Style White Corn	7 pieces (1 oz)	150	2	0
Tyson				
Nacho Cheese	1 oz	140	—	0
Ranch Flavor	1 oz	140	—	0
Traditional	1 oz	140	—	0
Unsalted	1 oz	140	—	0
Wise				
Bravos	1 oz	150	—	0
nacho	1 oz	141	2	0
nacho	1 bag (8 oz)	1131	12	0
nacho light	1 oz	126	—	0
nacho light	1 bag (6 oz)	757	—	0
plain	1 oz	142	2	0
plain	1 bag (7.5 oz)	1067	14	0
ranch	1 oz	139	—	0
ranch	1 bag (7 oz)	969	—	1

FOOD	PORTION	CALS.	FIB.	CHOL.
VEGETABLE				
Eden				
Vegetable Chips	50 (1 oz)	130	0	0
Wasabi Chip Hot & Spicy	50 (1 oz)	130	0	0
Hain				
Carrot Chips No Salt Added	1 oz	150	0	0
Health Valley				
Carrot Lites	0.5 oz	75	tr	0
Terra Chips				
Sweet Potato	1 oz	140	1	0
Sweet Potato Spiced	1 oz	140	3	0
Taro Spiced	1 oz	130	2	0
Vegetable	1 oz	140	3	0
Top Banana				
Plantain Chips	1 oz	150	—	0
taro	10 (0.8 oz)	115	—	0
taro	1 oz	141	—	0
CHITTERLINGS				
pork, simmered	3 oz	258	—	122
CHIVES				
freeze-dried	1 tbsp	1	—	0
fresh chopped	1 tbsp	1	—	0
fresh chopped	1 tsp	0	—	0
CHOCOLATE				
(*see also* CANDY, CAROB, COCOA, ICE CREAM TOPPINGS, MILK DRINKS)				
BAKING				
Hershey				
Premium Unsweetened	1 oz	190	—	0
Nestle				
Premier White	½ oz	80	—	<5
baking	1 oz	145	—	0
grated unsweetened	1 cup (4.6 oz)	690	18	0
liquid unsweetened	1 oz	134	—	0
squares unsweetened	1 square (1 oz)	148	4	0
CHIPS				
Baker's				
	1 oz	143	—	5
Big Milk Chocolate	¼ cup	239	—	8
Semi-Sweet	¼ cup	197	—	tr
Hershey				
Milk Chocolate	1 oz	150	—	10
Semi-Sweet	¼ cup (1.5 oz)	220	—	0
Semi-Sweet Miniature	¼ cup (1.5 oz)	220	—	0

FOOD	PORTION	CALS.	FIB.	CHOL.
milk chocolate	1 cup (6 oz)	862	—	38
semisweet	1 cup (6 oz)	804	—	0
semisweet	60 pieces (1 oz)	136	—	0
MIX				
Hershey				
Chocolate Milk Mix	3 tbsp	90	—	0
powder	2-3 heaping tsp	75	—	0
powder as prep w/ whole milk	9 oz	226	—	33
SYRUP				
Crumpy				
Chocolate Hazelnut Spread	1 tbsp (0.5 oz)	80	0	0
Estee				
Choco-Syp	2 tbsp (1.2 oz)	50	—	0
Hershey	2 tbsp	80	—	0
Marzetti	2 tbsp	40	0	0
Red Wing	2 tbsp (1.4 oz)	110	0	0
chocolate	1 cup	653	—	0
chocolate	2 tbsp	82	—	0
chocolate as prep w/ whole milk	9 oz	232	—	33

CHOCOLATE MILK
  (see CHOCOLATE, COCOA, MILK DRINKS)

CHUTNEY
apple cranberry	1 tbsp	16	—	0

CILANTRO
Watkins				
Dried	¼ tsp (0.5 oz)	0	0	0
fresh	¼ cup	1	—	0

CINNAMON
Watkins				
ground	¼ tsp (0.5 g)	0	0	0
ground	1 tsp	6	—	0

CISCO
smoked	3 oz	151	—	27
smoked	1 oz	50	—	9

CLAMS
CANNED				
American Original				
Quahogs	4 oz	66	—	16
Progresso	½ cup	70	—	31
Red Clam Sauce	½ cup	70	—	8
White Clam Sauce	½ cup	110	—	15
meat only	1 cup	236	—	107
meat only	3 oz	126	—	57

FOOD	PORTION	CALS.	FIB.	CHOL.
FRESH				
cooked	3 oz	126	—	57
cooked	20 sm	133	—	60
raw	20 sm (180 g)	133	—	60
raw	9 lg (180 g)	133	—	60
raw	3 oz	63	—	29
FROZEN				
Gorton's				
Microwave Chrunchy Clam Strips	3.5 oz	330	—	30
Mrs. Paul's				
Fried	2½ oz	200	—	15
HOME RECIPE				
breaded & fried	3 oz	171	—	52
breaded & fried	20 sm	379	—	115
TAKE-OUT				
breaded & fried	¾ cup	451	—	87

CLOVES

ground	1 tsp	7	—	0

COCOA
(see also CHOCOLATE)

Carnation				
Hot Cocoa 70 Calorie	3 tsp (21 g)	70	—	2
Hot Cocoa Milk Chocolate	1 pkg or 4 heaping tsp (1 oz)	110	—	2
Hot Cocoa Natural Mint	1 pkg or 4 heaping tsp (1 oz)	110	—	2
Hot Cocoa Rich Chocolate	1 pkg or 4 heaping tsp (1 oz)	110	—	2
Hot Cocoa Rich Chocolate w/ Marshmallows	1 pkg or 4 heaping tsp (1 oz)	110	—	2
Hot Cocoa Sugar Free Mint	1 pkg or 4 heaping tsp (15 g)	50	—	2
Hot Cocoa Sugar Free Rich Chocolate	1 pkg or 4 heaping tsp (15 g)	50	—	2
Hershey	⅓ cup (1 oz)	120	—	0
European Cocoa	1 oz	90	—	0
Hills Bros.				
Hot Cocoa	6 oz	110	—	0
Hot Cocoa Sugar Free	6 oz	60	—	0
Nestle	1 tbsp	15	2	0
Swiss Miss				
Cocoa Diet	6 oz	20	0	1

FOOD	PORTION	CALS.	FIB.	CHOL.
Swiss Miss (CONT.)				
Hot Cocoa Bavarian Chocolate	6 oz	110	0	2
Hot Cocoa Double Rich	6 oz	110	0	0
Hot Cocoa Milk Chocolate	6 oz	110	0	5
Hot Cocoa With Mini Marshmallows	6 oz	110	0	5
Lite as prep	6 oz	70	0	1
Sugar Free With Sugar Free Marshmallows as prep	6 oz	50	0	2
Sugar Free as prep	6 oz	60	0	2
Ultra Slim-Fast				
Hot Cocoa as prep w/ water	8 oz	190	5	8
Weight Watchers	1 pkg	60	—	5
hot cocoa	1 cup	218	—	33
powder unsweetened	1 cup (3 oz)	197	29	0
powder unsweetened	1 tbsp (5 g)	11	2	0

COCONUT

FOOD	PORTION	CALS.	FIB.	CHOL.
Baker's				
Angel Flake Toasted	⅓ cup	212	—	0
Premium Shred	⅓ cup	135	—	0
coconut water	1 cup	46	—	0
coconut water	1 tbsp	3	—	0
cream canned	1 cup	568	—	0
cream canned	1 tbsp	36	—	0
dried sweetened flaked	7 oz pkg	944	—	0
dried sweetened flaked	1 cup	351	—	0
dried sweetened flaked canned	1 cup	341	—	0
dried sweetened shredded	1 cup	466	—	0
dried sweetened shredded	7 oz pkg	997	—	0
dried toasted	1 oz	168	—	0
dried unsweetened	1 oz	187	—	0
fresh	1 piece (1½ oz)	159	4	0
fresh shredded	1 cup	283	7	0
milk canned	1 cup	445	—	0
milk canned	1 tbsp	30	—	0
milk frozen	1 cup	486	—	0
milk frozen	1 tbsp	30	—	0

COD

FOOD	PORTION	CALS.	FIB.	CHOL.
CANNED				
atlantic	3 oz	89	—	47
atlantic	1 can (11 oz)	327	—	171
DRIED				
atlantic	3 oz	246	—	129

FOOD	PORTION	CALS.	FIB.	CHOL.
FRESH				
atlantic raw	3 oz	70	—	37
atlantic cooked	1 fillet (6.3 oz)	189	—	99
atlantic cooked	3 oz	89	—	47
pacific baked	3 oz	95	—	43
roe raw	3½ oz	130	—	360
FROZEN				
Mrs. Paul's				
Light Fillets	1 fillet	240	—	50
Van De Kamp's				
Light Fillets	1 piece	250	—	25
Natural Fillets	4 oz	90	—	25
COFFEE				
(see also COFFEE BEVERAGES, COFFEE SUBSTITUTES)				
INSTANT				
Kava	1 tsp	2	—	0
decaffeinated	1 rounded tsp	4	—	0
	(1.8 g)			
decaffeinated as prep	6 oz	4	—	0
regular	1 rounded tsp	4	—	0
regular as prep	6 oz	4	—	0
regular w/ chicory	1 rounded tsp	6	—	0
regular w/ chicory as prep	6 oz	6	—	0
REGULAR				
brewed	6 oz	4	—	0
TAKE-OUT				
cafe au lait	1 cup (8 fl oz)	77	—	17
cafe brulot	1 cup (4.8 fl oz)	48	—	0
capuccino	1 cup (8 fl oz)	77	—	17
coffee con leche	1 cup (8 fl oz)	77	—	17
espresso	1 cup (3 fl oz)	2	—	0
irish coffee	1 serving (9 fl oz)	107	—	12
mocha	1 mug (9.6 fl oz)	202	—	40
COFFEE BEVERAGES				
(see also COFFEE SUBSTITUTES)				
General Foods				
International Coffee Cafe	6 oz	51	—	tr
Amaretto				
International Coffee Cafe	6 oz	55	—	tr
Francais				
International Coffee Cafe Irish	6 oz	55	—	tr
Creme				
International Coffee Cafe	6 oz	59	—	tr
Vienna				

FOOD	PORTION	CALS.	FIB.	CHOL.
General Foods (CONT.)				
International Coffee Irish Mocha Mint	6 oz	51	—	tr
International Coffee Orange Cappuccino	6 oz	59	—	tr
International Coffee Sugar Free Cafe Francais	6 oz	35	—	tr
International Coffee Sugar Free Cafe Irish Creme	6 oz	31	—	tr
International Coffee Sugar Free Cafe Vienna	6 oz	29	—	tr
International Coffee Sugar Free Irish Mocha Mint	6 oz	28	—	tr
International Coffee Sugar Free Orange Cappuccino	6 oz	29	—	tr
International Coffee Sugar Free Suisse Mocha	6 oz	29	—	tr
International Coffee Suisse Mocha	6 oz	53	—	tr

COFFEE SUBSTITUTES

FOOD	PORTION	CALS.	FIB.	CHOL.
Natural Touch				
Kaffree Roma	1 tsp	6	—	0
Postum				
Instant	6 oz	11	—	0
Instant Coffee Flavored	6 oz	11	—	0
powder	1 tsp	9	—	0
powder as prep	6 oz	9	—	0
powder as prep w/ milk	6 oz	121	—	25

COFFEE WHITENERS
(see also MILK SUBSTITUTES)

FOOD	PORTION	CALS.	FIB.	CHOL.
LIQUID				
Coffee Rich	1 tbsp	20	—	0
Coffee-Mate	1 tbsp (0.5 fl oz)	16	—	0
Hood				
Non Dairy	1 tbsp (0.5 oz)	20	0	0
International Delight				
Amaretto	1 tbsp (0.6 fl oz)	45	0	0
Cinnamon Hazelnut	1 tbsp (0.6 fl oz)	45	0	0
Irish Creme	1 tbsp (0.6 fl oz)	45	0	0
No Fat Amaretto	1 tbsp (0.5 fl oz)	30	0	0
No Fat French Vanilla Royale	1 tbsp (0.5 fl oz)	30	0	0
No Fat Hawaiian Macadamia	1 tbsp (0.5 fl oz)	30	0	0
No Fat Irish Creme	1 tbsp (0.5 fl oz)	30	0	0

FOOD	PORTION	CALS.	FIB.	CHOL.
International Delight (CONT.)				
Suisse Chocolate Mocha	1 tbsp (0.6 fl oz)	45	0	0
Mocha Mix				
Fat-Free	1 tbsp (0.5 fl oz)	10	0	0
Lite	1 tbsp (0.5 fl oz)	10	0	0
Lite	4 fl oz	80	0	0
Original	1 tbsp (0.5 fl oz)	20	0	0
Signature Flavors French Vanilla	1 tbsp (0.5 fl oz)	35	—	0
Signature Flavors Irish Creme	1 tbsp (0.5 fl oz)	35	—	0
Signature Flavors Kahlua	1 tbsp (0.5 fl oz)	35	—	0
Signature Flavors Mauna Loa Macadamia Nut	1 tbsp (0.5 fl oz)	35	—	0
nondairy frzn	1 tbsp	20	—	0
POWDER				
Coffee-Mate	1 tsp (2 g)	10	—	0
N-Rich Creamer	1 tsp	10	0	0
nondairy	1 tsp	11	—	0

COLESLAW
(*see* CABBAGE, SALAD DRESSING)

COLLARDS
CANNED

Allen	½ cup (4.1 oz)	30	3	0
Sunshine	½ cup (4.1 oz)	30	3	0
FRESH				
cooked	½ cup	17	—	0
raw chopped	½ cup	6	—	0
FROZEN				
chopped cooked	½ cup	31	—	0

COOKIES
(*see also* BROWNIE, CAKE, DOUGHNUT, PIE)
HOME RECIPE

chocolate chip as prep w/ butter	1 (0.42 oz)	78	—	11
chocolate chip as prep w/ margarine	1 (0.56 oz)	78	—	5
macaroons	1 (0.8 oz)	97	—	0
oatmeal	1 (0.5 oz)	67	—	5
oatmeal w/ raisins	1 (0.52 oz)	65	—	5
peanut butter	1 (0.7 oz)	95	—	6
shortbread as prep w/ butter	1 (0.38 oz)	60	—	10
shortbread as prep w/ margarine	1 (0.38 oz)	60	—	0
sugar as prep w/ butter	1 (0.49 oz)	66	—	12
sugar as prep w/ margarine	1 (0.49 oz)	66	—	4

FOOD	PORTION	CALS.	FIB.	CHOL.
MIX				
Betty Crocker				
Date Bar Classic Dessert	1	60	—	0
Estee				
Chocolate Chip	3	130	0	0
chocolate chip	1 (0.56 oz)	79	—	7
oatmeal	1 (0.6 oz)	74	tr	7
oatmeal raisin	1 (0.6 oz)	74	tr	7
READY-TO-EAT				
Archway				
Almond Crescents	2 (0.8 oz)	100	tr	<5
Apple N'Raisin	1 (1.1 oz)	130	1	<5
Apricot Filled	1 (1 oz)	110	tr	5
Bells And Stars	3 (1 oz)	150	tr	5
Blueberry Filled	1 (1 oz)	110	tr	5
Carrot Cake	1 (1 oz)	120	0	<5
Cherry Filled	1 (1 oz)	110	tr	10
Cherry Nougat	3 (1 oz)	150	0	0
Chocolate Chip	1 (1 oz)	130	0	tr
Chocolate Chip Bag	3 (0.9 oz)	130	0	10
Chocolate Chip Drop	1 (1 oz)	140	tr	10
Chocolate Chip Ice Box	1 (1 oz)	140	0	5
Chocolate Chip Mini	12 (1.1 oz)	150	0	5
Chocolate Chip & Toffee	1 (1 oz)	140	tr	<5
Cinnamon Snaps	12 (1.1 oz)	150	0	5
Coconut Macaroon	1 (0.8 oz)	90	2	0
Cookie Jar Hermits	1 (1 oz)	110	tr	<5
Dark Chocolate	1 (1 oz)	110	tr	<5
Dutch Chocolate	1 (1 oz)	120	0	<5
Fig Bars Low Fat	2 (1.1 oz)	100	1	0
Frosty Lemon	1 (1 oz)	120	0	0
Frosty Orange	1 (1 oz)	120	1	0
Fruit And Honey Bar	1 (1 oz)	110	tr	5
Fruit Bar No Fat	1 (1 oz)	90	0	0
Fruit Cake	1 (1.1 oz)	140	2	0
Fudge Nut Bar	1 (1 oz)	110	tr	<5
Fun Chip Mini	12 (1.1 oz)	140	0	5
Gingersnaps	5 (1.1 oz)	130	0	0
Granola No Fat	1 (0.5 oz)	50	tr	0
Holiday Pak	3 (1.1 oz)	150	tr	<5
Iced Gingerbread	3 (1.1 oz)	140	0	5
Iced Molasses	1 (1 oz)	110	tr	0
Iced Oatmeal	1 (1 oz)	120	1	<5
Lemon Snaps	12 (1.1 oz)	150	0	5

FOOD	PORTION	CALS.	FIB.	CHOL.
Archway (CONT.)				
New Orleans Cake	1 (1 oz)	110	tr	<5
Nutty Nougat	3 (1.1 oz)	160	0	0
Oatmeal	1 (0.9 oz)	110	tr	<5
Oatmeal Apple Filled	1 (1 oz)	110	0	<5
Oatmeal Date Filled	1 (1 oz)	110	tr	<5
Oatmeal Mini	12 (1.1 oz)	150	1	5
Oatmeal Pecan	1 (1 oz)	120	1	<5
Oatmeal Raisin	1 (1 oz)	110	tr	<5
Oatmeal Raisin Bran	1 (1 oz)	110	tr	<5
Old Fashioned Molasses	1 (1 oz)	120	0	5
Old Fashioned Windmill	1 (0.7 oz)	100	0	0
Party Treats	3 (1.1 oz)	140	0	15
Peanut Butter	1 (1 oz)	140	tr	10
Peanut Butter Nougat	3 (1.1 oz)	160	1	0
Peanut Butter & Chip	3 (0.9 oz)	130	0	10
Peanut Butter n' Chips	1 (1 oz)	140	tr	10
Pecan Crunch	6 (1.1 oz)	150	0	10
Pecan Ice Box	1 (1 oz)	140	0	10
Pecan Malted Nougat	3 (1.1 oz)	160	2	0
Pfeffernusse	2 (1.3 oz)	140	tr	0
Pineapple Filled	1 (0.9 oz)	100	1	5
Raisin Oatmeal	1 (1 oz)	130	1	5
Raisin Oatmeal Bag	3 (1 oz)	130	1	10
Raspberry Filled	1 (1 oz)	110	tr	5
Rocky Road	1 (1 oz)	130	tr	10
Ruth's Golden Oatmeal	1 (1 oz)	120	tr	<5
Select Assortment	3 (0.9 oz)	130	0	10
Soft Molasses Drop	1 (1 oz)	110	1	<5
Soft Sugar	1 (1 oz)	110	0	5
Strawberry Filled	1 (1 oz)	110	tr	<5
Sugar	1 (1 oz)	120	0	<5
Vanilla Wafer	5 (1.1 oz)	130	0	5
Wedding Cakes	3 (1.1 oz)	160	0	0
Bakery Wagon				
Apple Walnut Raisin	1	100	1	0
Cobbler Apple Cranberry Fat Free	1	70	1	0
Cobbler Apple Fat Free	1	70	1	0
Cobbler Mixed Fruit Fat Free	1	70	1	0
Cobbler Raspberry Fat Free	1	70	1	0
Ginger Snaps	5	160	1	0
Honey Fruit Bars	1	100	1	5
Iced Molasses	1	100	1	2

FOOD	PORTION	CALS.	FIB.	CHOL.
Bakery Wagon (CONT.)				
Iced Molasses Mini	3	130	1	0
Oatmeal Apple Filled	1	90	1	0
Oatmeal Chocolate Chunk	1	100	1	0
Oatmeal Date Filled	1	90	1	0
Oatmeal Raspberry Filled	1	100	1	0
Oatmeal Soft	1	100	1	0
Oatmeal Walnut Raisin	1	100	1	0
Vanilla Wafers Cholesterol Free	6	130	1	0
Barnum's				
Animal Crackers	12 (1.1 oz)	140	1	0
Biscos				
Sugar Wafers	8 (1 oz)	140	tr	0
Waffle Cremes	4 (1.2 oz)	180	tr	0
Chip-A-Roos	3 (1.3 oz)	190	1	0
Chips Ahoy!				
Chewy Chocolate Chip	3 (1.3 oz)	170	tr	<5
Chunky Chocolate Chip	1 (0.5 oz)	80	tr	10
Real Chocolate Chip	3 (1.1 oz)	160	1	0
Reduced Fat	3 (1.1 oz)	150	1	0
Sprinkled Real Chocolate Chip	3 (1.3 oz)	170	tr	0
Striped Chocolate Chip	1 (0.5 oz)	80	tr	0
Cookie Lover's				
Blue Ribbon Brownies	1 (0.8 oz)	90	0	11
Classic Shortbread	1 (0.8 oz)	110	0	15
Dutch Chocolate Chip	1 (0.8 oz)	90	0	14
Fancy Peanut Butter	1 (0.8 oz)	100	0	7
Old-Time Raisin	1 (0.8 oz)	90	0	15
Delacre				
Cookie Assortment	4 (1.1 oz)	130	1	8
Drake's				
Chocolate Chip	2 (1 oz)	140	—	0
Chocolate- Chocolate Chip	2 (1 oz)	130	—	0
Coconut	2 (1 oz)	130	—	0
Coconut Macaroon	1 (1 oz)	135	—	0
Hermit	1 (2 oz)	230	—	10
Oatmeal	2 (1 oz)	120	—	0
Oatmeal Creme	1 (2 oz)	240	—	2
Peanut Butter Wafers	1 (2.25 oz)	324	—	0
Dutch Mill				
Chocolate Chip	3 (1.1 oz)	160	1	0
Coconut Macaroons	3 (1 oz)	120	0	0
Oatmeal Raisin	3 (1 oz)	130	1	0

FOOD	PORTION	CALS.	FIB.	CHOL.
Estee				
Chocolate Chip	4 (1.1 oz)	150	tr	0
Coconut	4 (1 oz)	140	tr	0
Creme Wafers Chocolate	7 (1.1 oz)	160	tr	0
Creme Wafers Lemon	5 (1.2 oz)	170	0	0
Creme Wafers Peanut Butter	5 (1.2 oz)	170	0	0
Creme Wafers Triple Decker Banana Split	3 (0.9 oz)	140	0	0
Creme Wafers Triple Decker Chocolate Caramel & Peanut Butter	3 (0.9 oz)	140	0	0
Creme Wafers Vanilla	7 (1.1 oz)	160	0	0
Creme Wafers Vanilla & Strawberry	5 (1.2 oz)	170	0	0
Fig Bars Apple Low Fat	2 (1 oz)	100	3	0
Fig Bars Cranberry Low Fat	2 (1 oz)	100	3	0
Fig Bars Low Fat	2 (1 oz)	100	3	0
Fudge	4 (1 oz)	150	1	0
Lemon	4 (1 oz)	140	tr	0
Oatmeal Raisin	4 (1 oz)	130	1	0
Sandwich Chocolate	3 (1.2 oz)	160	1	0
Sandwich Original	3 (1.2 oz)	160	1	0
Sandwich Peanut Butter	3 (1.2 oz)	160	1	0
Sandwich Vanilla	3 (1.2 oz)	160	tr	0
Shortbread Reduced Fat	4 (1 oz)	130	tr	0
Vanilla	4 (1 oz)	140	tr	0
Freihofer's				
Chocolate Chip	2 (0.9 oz)	120	1	10
Frito Lay				
Peanut Butter Bar	1.75 oz	270	—	0
Frookie				
7-Grain Oatmeal	1	45	—	0
Animal Frackers	6	60	—	0
Apple Cinnamon Oat Bran	1	45	—	0
Apple Cinnamon Oat Bran	1 lg	120	—	0
Apple Fruitins	1	60	—	0
Chocolate Chip	1 lg	120	—	0
Chocolate Chip	1	45	—	0
Chocolate Chip Mint	1	45	—	0
Fig Fruitins	1	60	—	0
Ginger Spice	1	45	—	0
Mandarin Chocolate Chip	1	45	—	0
Oat Bran Muffin	1	45	—	0
Oat Bran Muffin	1 lg	120	—	0

FOOD	PORTION	CALS.	FIB.	CHOL.
Frookie (CONT.)				
Oatmeal Raisin	1	45	—	0
Oatmeal Raisin	1 lg	120	—	0
General Mills				
Dunkaroos	1 pkg (1 oz)	130	—	0
Golden Fruit				
Apple	1 (0.7 oz)	80	tr	0
Cranberry	1 (0.7 oz)	70	tr	0
Cranberry Low Fat	1 (0.7 oz)	70	tr	0
Raisin	1 (0.7 oz)	80	tr	0
Grandma's				
Animal Cookies Candied	5 (1 oz)	140	—	0
Chocolate Chip	2 (2.75 oz)	370	—	5
Chocolate Chip Rich'N Chewy	3 (1 oz)	140	—	5
Fudge Chocolate Chip	2 (2.75 oz)	350	—	5
Grab Cookie Bits Chocolate	8 (1 oz)	140	—	0
Grab Cookie Bits Peanut Butter	8 (1 oz)	140	—	0
Grab Cookie Bits Vanilla	8 (1 oz)	140	—	5
Oatmeal Apple Spice	2 (2.75 oz)	330	—	10
Old Time Molasses	2 (2.75 oz)	320	—	5
Peanut Butter	2 (2.75 oz)	410	—	10
Raisin Soft	2 (2.75 oz)	320	—	10
Health Valley				
Amaranth Cookies	1	70	2	0
Fancy Fruit Chunks Apricot Almond	2	90	2	0
Fancy Fruit Chunks Date Pecan	2	90	2	0
Fancy Fruit Chunks Raisin Oat Bran	2	70	2	0
Fancy Fruit Chunks Tropical Fruit	2	90	2	0
Fancy Peanut Chunks	2	90	2	0
Fat Free Hawaiian Fruit	3	75	3	0
Fat Free Apple Spice	3	75	3	0
Fat Free Apricot Delight	3	75	3	0
Fat Free Date Delight	3	75	3	0
Fat Free Jumbos Apple Raisin	1	70	3	0
Fat Free Jumbos Raisin	1	70	3	0
Fat Free Jumbos Raspberry	1	70	3	0
Fat Free Raisin Oatmeal	3	75	3	0
Fiber Jumbos Blueberry Nut	1	100	3	0
Fiber Jumbos Chunky Pecan	1	100	3	0
Fiber Jumbos Raisin Nut	1	100	3	0
Fruit & Fitness	5	200	6	0

FOOD	PORTION	CALS.	FIB.	CHOL.
Health Valley (CONT.)				
Fruit Jumbos Almond Date	1	70	1	0
Fruit Jumbos Oat Bran	1	70	2	0
Fruit Jumbos Raisin Nut	1	70	1	0
Fruit Jumbos Tropical Fruit	1	70	2	0
Graham Amaranth	7	110	3	0
Graham Honey	7	100	2	0
Graham Oat Bran	7	120	5	0
Honey Jumbos Crisp Cinnamon	1	70	1	0
Honey Jumbos Crisp Peanut Butter	1	70	1	0
Honey Jumbos Fancy Oat Bran	2	130	4	0
Oat Bran Animal Cookies	7	110	3	0
Oat Bran Fruit & Nut	2	110	3	0
The Great Tofu	2	90	4	0
The Great Wheat Free	2	80	3	0
Heyday				
Caramel & Peanut	1 (0.8 oz)	110	tr	0
Fudge	1 (0.8 oz)	110	tr	0
Honey Maid				
Cinnamon Grahams	10 (1.1 oz)	140	1	0
Honey Grahams	8 (1 oz)	120	1	0
Hydrox				
Reduced Fat	3	150	1	0
	3 (1.1 oz)	130	1	0
Keebler				
Buttercup	3	70	—	0
Chocolate Fudge Sandwich	1	80	—	0
Commodore	1	60	—	0
Cookies Mates	2	50	—	0
French Vanilla Creme	1	80	—	0
Graham Honey Fiber Enriched	2	90	—	0
Graham Kitchen Rich	2	60	—	0
Homeplate	1	60	—	1
Keebies	1	80	—	0
Krisp Kreem Wafers	2	50	—	0
Old Fashion Chocolate Chip	1	80	—	0
Old Fashion Double Fudge	1	80	—	0
Old Fashion Oatmeal	1	80	—	0
Old Fashion Peanut Butter	1	80	—	0
Old Fashion Sugar	1	80	—	0
Pitter Patter	1	90	—	0
Vanilla Wafers	4	80	—	1
LU				
Chocolatiers	4 (1.1 oz)	170	2	0

FOOD	PORTION	CALS.	FIB.	CHOL.
LU (CONT.)				
Chocolatiers Dipped	3 (1 oz)	170	1	0
Little Schoolboy Dark Chocolate	2 (0.9 oz)	130	0	5
Little Schoolboy Milk Chocolate	2 (0.9 oz)	130	0	5
Marie Lu	3 (1.2 oz)	170	1	5
Truffle Lu	4 (1.2 oz)	180	1	0
La Choy				
Fortune	1	15	tr	0
Lance				
Choc-O-Lunch	1 pkg (37 g)	180	—	0
Choc-O-Mint	1 pkg (35 g)	180	—	0
Chocolate Chip Fudge	1 (28 g)	130	—	5
Chocolate Chip Soft	1 (28 g)	130	—	5
Coated Graham	1 pkg (50 g)	200	—	0
Fig Bar	1 pkg (42 g)	150	—	0
Lem-O-Lunch	1 pkg (48 g)	240	—	0
Lemon Nekot	1 pkg (42 g)	220	—	5
Malt	1 pkg (35 g)	190	—	0
Nut-O-Lunch	1 oz	140	—	0
Oatmeal	1 (57 G)	130	—	0
Peanut Butter Creme Filled Wafer	1 pkg (50 g)	240	—	0
Van-O-Lunch	1 pkg (37 g)	180	—	0
Little Debbie				
Animal	1 pkg (1.5 oz)	190	0	0
Caramel Cookie Bars	1 pkg (1.2 oz)	160	1	0
Chocolate Chip Chewy	1 pkg (2 oz)	370	1	10
Chocolate Chip Crisp	1 pkg (1.5 oz)	210	1	5
Cookie Wreaths	1 pkg (0.6 oz)	90	0	0
Creme Filled Chocolate	1 pkg (1.8 oz)	260	1	0
Creme Filled Chocolated	1 pkg (1.2 oz)	180	1	0
Easter Puffs	1 pkg (1.2 oz)	140	0	0
Figaroos	1 pkg (1.5 oz)	160	3	0
Figaroos	1 pkg (2 oz)	200	2	0
Fudge Macaroons	1 pkg (1 oz)	140	1	0
Ginger	1 pkg (0.7 oz)	90	1	5
Oatmeal Crisp	1 pkg (1.5 oz)	210	1	5
Oatmeal Lights	1 pkg (1.3 oz)	140	1	0
Oatmeal Raisin	1 pkg (2.7 oz)	320	2	0
Peanut Butter	1 pkg (1.5 oz)	210	1	5
Peanut Butter Bars	1 pkg (1.9 oz)	270	1	0
Peanut Butter & Jelly Sandwiches	1 pkg (1.1 oz)	130	1	0

FOOD	PORTION	CALS.	FIB.	CHOL.
Little Debbie (CONT.)				
Peanut Clusters	1 pkg (1.4 oz)	190	1	0
Pecan Spinwheels	1 pkg (1 oz)	110	1	0
Pecan Shortbread	1 pkg (1.5 oz)	220	0	5
Lorna Doone	4 (1 oz)	140	tr	5
Mallomars	2 (0.9 oz)	120	1	0
Mallopuffs	1 (0.6 oz)	70	tr	0
Manischewitz				
Macaroons Chocolate	2 (0.9 oz)	90	4	0
Mother's				
Almond Shortbread	3	180	1	0
Butter	5	140	—	10
Checkerboard Wafers	8	150	1	0
Chocolate Chip	2	160	0	10
Chocolate Chip Angel	3	180	1	0
Chocolate Chip Bag	4	140	1	2
Chocolate Chip Parade	4	130	1	0
Circus Animals	6	140	0	0
Cocadas	5	150	2	5
Cookie Parade	4	140	2	0
Dinosaur Grrrahams	2	130	—	0
Double Fudge	3	170	2	0
Duplex Creme	3	170	1	0
English Tea	2	180	1	0
Fig Bar	2	130	0	0
Fig Bar Fat Free	1	70	1	0
Fig Bar Whole Wheat	2	130	3	0
Fig Bar Whole Wheat Fat Free	1	70	1	0
Flaky Flix Fudge	2	140	2	0
Flaky Flix Vanilla	2	140	1	0
Frosted Holiday	4	130	0	0
Fudge Bowl Crowns	2	140	1	0
Fudge Bowl Nuggets	2	140	1	0
Gaucho Peanut Butter	2	190	2	0
Gingerbread Man	6	140	1	5
Iced Oatmeal	2	120	1	0
Iced Oatmeal Bag	4	120	1	0
Iced Raisin	2	180	1	0
MLB Double Header Duplex	3	170	1	5
Macaroon	2	150	2	0
Marias	3	170	1	5
North Poles	2	140	0	0
Oatmeal	2	110	1	0
Oatmeal Chocolate Chip	2	120	1	0

FOOD	PORTION	CALS.	FIB.	CHOL.
Mother's (CONT.)				
Oatmeal Raisin	5	150	2	5
Oatmeal Walnut Chocolate Chip	2	130	1	0
Pecan Goldens	2	170	5	0
Rainbow Wafers	8	150	1	0
Striped Shortbread	3	170	1	0
Sugar	2	140	1	0
Taffy	2	180	2	0
Triplet Assortment	2	140	1	0
Vanilla Wafers	6	150	1	4
Walnut Fudge	2	130	1	0
Zoo Pals	14	140	1	0
Mystic Mint	1 (0.5 oz)	90	0	0
Nabisco				
Brown Edge Wafers	5 (1 oz)	140	tr	<5
Bugs Bunny Chocolate Graham	13 (1.1 oz)	140	1	0
Bugs Bunny Cinnamon Graham	13 (1.1 oz)	140	tr	0
Bugs Bunny Granham	13 (1.1 oz)	140	1	0
Cameo	2 (1 oz)	130	tr	0
Chocolate Grahams	3 (1.1 oz)	160	1	0
Chocolate Chip Snaps	7 (1.1 oz)	150	tr	0
Chocolate Snaps	7 (1.1 oz)	140	1	0
Cookie Break	3 (1.1 oz)	160	tr	0
Danish Imported	5 (1.1 oz)	170	1	0
Family Favorites Fudge Covered Grahams	3 (1 oz)	140	1	0
Family Favorites Fudge Striped Shortbread	3 (1.1 oz)	160	1	0
Family Favorites Oatmeal	1 (0.5 oz)	80	tr	0
Family Favorites Vanilla Sandwich	3 (1.2 oz)	170	0	0
Famous Chocolate Wafers	5 (1.1 oz)	140	1	<5
Ginger Snaps Old Fashioned	4 (1 oz)	120	tr	0
Grahams	8 (1 oz)	120	1	0
Marshmallow Puffs	1 (0.75 oz)	90	0	0
Marshmallow Twirls	1 (1 oz)	130	tr	0
Nilla Wafers	8 (1.1 oz)	140	0	5
Pecan Passion	1 (0.5 oz)	90	0	<5
Pinwheels	1 (1 oz)	130	tr	0
National				
Arrowroot	1 (5 g)	20	tr	0
Newtons				
Apple Fat Free	2 (1 oz)	100	1	0
Cranberry Fat Free	2 (1 oz)	100	1	0

FOOD	PORTION	CALS.	FIB.	CHOL.
Newtons (CONT.)				
Fig	2 (1.1 oz)	110	1	0
Fig Fat Free	1 (1 oz)	100	2	0
Raspberry Fat Free	2 (1 oz)	100	tr	0
Strawberry Fat Free	2 (1 oz)	100	tr	0
Nutter Butter				
Peanut Butter Sandwich	2 (1 oz)	130	1	<5
Peanut Creme Patties	5 (1.1 oz)	160	1	0
Oreo	3 (1.2 oz)	160	1	0
Double Stuf	2 (1 oz)	140	tr	0
Fudge Covered	1 (0.75 oz)	110	tr	0
Halloween Treats	2 (1 oz)	140	1	0
Reduced Fat	3 (1.2 oz)	140	1	0
White Fudge Covered	1 (0.75 oz)	110	tr	0
Pally				
Butter	4 (0.88 oz)	100	—	7
Pepperidge Farm				
Beacon Hill Chocolate Chocolate Walnut	1	120	1	5
Blondie Chocolate Chip Fat Free	1 (1.4 oz)	120	tr	0
Bordeaux	2	70	0	0
Brownie Chocolate Nut	2	110	—	<5
Brownie Nut Large	1	140	—	5
Brussels	2	110	0	0
Brussels Mint	2	130	—	0
Butter Chessman	2	90	—	10
Cappucino	1	50	—	<5
Capri	1	80	—	0
Chantilly	1	80	—	<5
Cheasapeake Chocolate Chunk Pecan	1	120	1	5
Cheyenne Peanut Butter Milk Chocolate Chunk	1	110	1	5
Chocolate Chip	2	100	0	5
Chocolate Chip Large	1	130	—	5
Chocolate Chunk Pecan	1	70	—	12
Dakota Milk Chocolate Oatmeal	1	110	1	5
Date Pecan	2	110	—	10
Fruit Filled Apricot- Raspberry	2	100	—	10
Fruit Filled Strawberry	2	100	—	10
Geneva	2	130	—	0
Gingerman	2	70	—	5
Hazelnut	2	110	—	0
Irish Oatmeal	2	90	—	5

FOOD	PORTION	CALS.	FIB.	CHOL.
Pepperidge Farm (CONT.)				
Lemon Nut Crunch	2	110	—	<5
Lido	1	90	—	<5
Linzer	1	120	—	<5
Milano	2	120	—	15
Mint Milano	2	150	—	5
Molasses Crisps	2	70	—	0
Nantucket Chocolate Chunk	1	120	1	5
Nassau	1	80	—	<5
Oatmeal Large	1	120	—	5
Oatmeal Raisin	2	110	—	10
Old Fashioned Chocolate Chip	2	100	0	5
Orange Milano	2	150	—	5
Orleans	3	90	—	0
Orleans Sandwich	2	120	—	0
Pecan Shortbread	1	70	—	0
Pirouettes Chocolate Laced	2	70	—	<5
Pirouettes Original	2	70	—	<5
Raisin Bran	2	110	—	<5
Ripple Milk Chocolate Fat Free	1 (0.6 oz)	60	tr	0
Sante Fe Oatmeal Raisin	1	100	1	<5
Sausalito Milk Chocolate Macadamia	1	120	0	5
Shortbread	2	150	—	<5
Sugar	2	100	—	10
Tahiti	1	90	—	5
Zurich	1	60	—	0
Ritz				
Chocolate Covered	3 (1 oz)	150	1	0
Salerno				
Dinosaur Grrrahams Chocolate	1 pkg (1.25 oz)	167	1	0
Dinosaur Grrrahams Cinnamon	1 pkg (1.25 oz)	165	1	0
Dinosaur Grrrahams Original	1 pkg (1.25 oz)	156	1	0
Sargento				
MooTown Snackers Cookies & Creme Honey Graham Sticks & Vanilla Creme w/Sprinkle	1 pkg (1.1 oz)	140	0	0
MooTown Snackers Cookies & Creme Vanilla Sticks & Chocolate Fudge Creme	1 pkg (1.1 oz)	140	0	0
Snackwell's				
Fat Free Cinnamon Grahams	20 (1 oz)	110	1	0
Fat Free Devil's Food	1 (0.5 oz)	50	tr	0
Fat Free Double Fudge	1 (0.5 oz)	50	tr	0

FOOD	PORTION	CALS.	FIB.	CHOL.
Snackwell's (CONT.)				
Reduced Fat Chocolate Sandwich With Chocolate Creme	2 (0.9 oz)	100	1	0
Reduced Fat Chocolate Chip	13 (1 oz)	130	1	0
Reduced Fat Oatmeal Raisin	2 (1 oz)	110	1	0
Reduced Fat Vanilla Sandwich With Vanilla Creme	2 (0.9 oz)	110	1	0
Social Tea	6 (1 oz)	120	tr	5
Stella D'Oro				
Almond Toast Mandel	1	60	—	tr
Angel Bars	1	80	—	tr
Angel Wings	1	70	—	1
Angelica Goodies	1	110	—	tr
Anginetti	1	30	—	tr
Anisette Sponge	1	50	—	tr
Anisette Toast	1	50	—	tr
Anisette Toast Jumbo	1	110	—	tr
Apple Pastry Low Sodium	1	80	—	>5
Breakfast Treats	1	100	—	tr
Castelets Chocolate	1	60	—	tr
Chinese Dessert Cookies	1	170	—	tr
Como Delight	1	150	—	1
Deep Night Fudge	1	65	—	2
Dutch Apple Bars	1	110	—	1
Egg Biscuits Low Sodium	3	120	—	40
Egg Biscuits Sugared	1	80	—	1
Egg Jumbo	1	50	—	tr
Fruit Delight Apple Cinnamon Fat Free	1	70	—	0
Fruit Delight Peach Apricot Fat Free	1	70	—	0
Fruit Delight Raspberry Fat Free	1	70	—	0
Fruit Slices	1	60	—	tr
Fruit Slices Fat Free	1	50	—	0
Golden Bars	1	110	—	tr
Holiday Rings & Stars	1	47	—	0
Holiday Trinkets	1	40	—	tr
Hostess Assortment	1	40	—	tr
Indulgente Cashew Biscottini	1 (1.1 oz)	150	tr	10
Kichel Low Sodium	21	150	—	80
Lady Stella Assortment	1	40	—	tr
Margherite Chocolate	1	70	—	tr
Margherite Vanilla	1	70	—	tr

FOOD	PORTION	CALS.	FIB.	CHOL.
Stella D'Oro (CONT.)				
Peach Apricot Pastry Sodium Free	1	80	—	>5
Pfeffernusse Spice Drops	1	40	—	tr
Prune Pastry Dietetic	1	90	—	>5
Roman Egg Biscuits	1	140	—	tr
Royal Nuggets	1	2	—	tr
Sesame Regina	1	50	—	tr
Swiss Fudge	1	70	—	tr
Sunshine				
Almond Crescents	4 (1.1 oz)	150	tr	0
Animal Crackers	1 box (2 oz)	260	1	0
Animal Crackers	14 (1.1 oz)	140	1	0
Classics Chocolate Chip With Pecans	1 (0.7 oz)	110	tr	3
Classics Chocolate Chip With Walnuts	1 (0.7 oz)	100	1	5
Classics Premier Chocolate Chip	1 (0.7 oz)	100	—	5
Dixie Vanilla	2 (0.9 oz)	120	tr	0
Fig Bars	2 (1 oz)	110	1	0
Fudge Family Bears Vanilla	2 (1 oz)	140	tr	0
Fudge Mint Patties	2 (0.8 oz)	130	tr	0
Fudge Striped Shortbread	3 (1.1 oz)	160	1	0
Ginger Snaps	7 (1 oz)	130	tr	0
Grahams Cinnamon	2 (1.1 oz) (1.9 oz)	140	tr	0
Grahams Fudge Dipped	4 (1.2 oz)	170	1	0
Grahams Honey	2 (1 oz)	120	1	0
Grahamy Bears	1 pkg (2 oz)	260	2	0
Grahamy Bears	10 (1.1 oz)	140	1	0
Iced Gingerbread	5 (1 oz)	130	tr	5
Iced Oatmeal	2 (0.9 oz)	120	tr	0
Jingles	6 (1.1 oz)	150	tr	0
Lemon Coolers	5 (1 oz)	140	tr	0
Mini Chocolate Chip Cookies	5 (1.1 oz)	160	tr	0
Mini Fudge Royals	15 (1.1 oz)	160	1	0
Oatmeal Chocolate Chip	3 (1.3 oz)	170	2	0
Oatmeal Country Style	3 (1.2 oz)	170	1	0
School House Cookies	20 (1.1 oz)	140	tr	0
Sugar Wafers Chocolate	3 (0.9 oz)	130	tr	0
Sugar Wafers Peanut Butter	4 (1.1 oz)	170	1	0
Sugar Wafers Vanilla	3 (0.9 oz)	130	tr	0
Tru Blu Chocolate	1 (0.6 oz)	80	tr	0
Tru Blu Lemon	1 (0.6 oz)	80	tr	0

FOOD	PORTION	CALS.	FIB.	CHOL.
Sunshine (CONT.)				
Tru Blu Vanilla	1 (0.5 oz)	80	tr	0
Vanilla Wafers	7 (1.1 oz)	150	tr	3
Vienna Fingers	2 (1 oz)	140	tr	0
Tastykake				
Chocolate Chip Bar	1 (43 g)	190	1	5
Chocolate Chunk Macadamia Nut	1 pkg (56 g)	310	2	40
Fudge Bar	1 (50 g)	200	1	5
Oatmeal Raisin Bar	1 (50 g)	210	1	15
Soft'n Chewy Chocolate Chocolate Chip	1 (32 g)	170	1	5
Soft'n Chewy Chocolate Chip	1 (39 g)	170	1	10
Soft'n Chewy Oatmeal Raisin	1 (39 g)	160	1	5
Vanilla Sugar Wafer	1 (6 g)	36	0	0
Teddy Grahams				
Chocolate	24 (1 oz)	140	1	0
Cinnamon	24 (1 oz)	140	1	0
Honey	24 (1 oz)	140	1	0
Tree Of Life				
Creme Supremes	2 (0.9 oz)	120	1	0
Creme Supremes Mint	2 (0.9 oz)	120	1	0
Fat Free Classic Carrot Cake	1 (0.8 oz)	60	1	0
Fat Free Devil's Food Chocolate	1 (0.8 oz)	70	1	0
Fat Free Golden Oatmeal Raisin	1 (0.8 oz)	70	1	0
Fat Free Harvest Fruit & Nut	1 (0.8 oz)	70	1	0
Fat Free Toasted Almond Butter	1 (0.8 oz)	70	1	0
Fruit Bars Apple Spice	2 (1.3 oz)	120	2	0
Fruit Bars Fat Free Fig	1 (0.8 oz)	70	2	0
Fruit Bars Fat Free Peach Apricot	1 (0.8 oz)	70	1	0
Fruit Bars Fat Free Wildberry	1 (0.8 oz)	70	2	0
Fruit Bars Fig	2 (1.3 oz)	120	3	0
Fruit Bars Peach Apricot	2 (1.3 oz)	120	2	0
Honey-Sweet Colossal Carrot Cake	1 (0.8 oz)	110	1	0
Honey-Sweet Lemon Burst	1 (0.8 oz)	110	1	0
Honey-Sweet Oh-So-Oatmeal	1 (0.8 oz)	110	1	0
Honey-Sweet Pecans-A-Plenty	1 (0.8 oz)	125	1	0
Monster Fat Free Carrot Cake	¼ cookie (0.9 oz)	60	1	0
Monster Fat Free Devil's Food Chocolate	¼ cookie (0.9 oz)	80	2	0
Monster Fat Free Gingerbread	¼ cookie (0.9 oz)	80	2	0
Monster Fat Free Maple Pecan	¼ cookie (0.9 oz)	90	2	0

FOOD	PORTION	CALS.	FIB.	CHOL.
Tree Of Life (CONT.)				
Royal Vanilla	2 (0.9 oz)	120	0	0
Small World Animal Grahams	7 (1 oz)	120	3	0
Small World Chocolate Chip	7 (1 oz)	120	3	0
Soft-Bake Chocolate Chip	1 (0.8 oz)	125	1	0
Soft-Bake Double Fudge	1 (0.8 oz)	110	2	0
Soft-Bake Maui Macaroon	1 (0.8 oz)	135	2	0
Soft-Bake Oatmeal	1 (0.8 oz)	115	2	0
Soft-Bake Peanut Butter	1 (0.8 oz)	125	1	0
Wheat-Free American Oatmeal	1 (0.8 oz)	90	1	0
Wheat-Free California Carob	1 (0.8 oz)	105	6	0
Wheat-Free Georgia Peanut Butter	1 (0.8 oz)	95	1	0
Wheat-Free Mountain Maple Walnut	1 (0.8 oz)	100	6	0
Vienna Fingers				
Low Fat	2 (1 oz)	130	tr	0
Weight Watchers				
Chocolate Sandwich	2	90	—	0
Fruit Filled Bar Apple	1	80	—	0
Fruit Filled Bar Raspberry	1	80	—	0
Oatmeal Raisin	2	90	—	0
animal crackers	1 box (2.4 oz)	299	—	11
chocolate chip	1 box (1.9 oz)	233	—	12
chocolate chip low fat	1 (0.25 oz)	45	—	0
chocolate chip low sugar low sodium	1 (0.24 oz)	31	—	0
chocolate chip soft-type	1 (0.5 oz)	69	tr	0
chocolate wafer	1 (0.2 oz)	26	—	0
chocolate wafer cookie crumbs	½ cup (5.9 oz)	728	—	0
gingersnaps	1 (0.24 oz)	29	—	0
graham	1 square (0.24 oz)	30	—	0
graham chocolate covered	1 (0.49 oz)	68	—	0
graham cracker crumbs	½ cup (4.4 oz)	540	3	0
graham honey	1 (0.24 oz)	30	tr	0
ladyfingers	1 (0.38 oz)	40	—	40
molasses	1 (0.5 oz)	65	—	0
oatmeal	1 (0.52 oz)	71	tr	0
oatmeal	1 (0.6 oz)	81	1	0
oatmeal raisin	1 (0.6 oz)	81	1	0
oatmeal raisin low sugar no sodium	1 (0.24 oz)	31	—	0
peanut butter sandwich	1 (0.5 oz)	67	—	0
peanut butter soft-type	1 (0.5 oz)	69	tr	0

FOOD	PORTION	CALS.	FIB.	CHOL.
raisin soft-type	1 (0.5 oz)	60	—	0
shortbread	1 (0.28 oz)	40	—	2
shortbread pecan	1 (0.49 oz)	79	tr	5
sugar	1 (0.52 oz)	72	—	8
sugar low sugar sodium free	1 (0.24 oz)	30	—	0
sugar wafers w/ creme filling	1 (0.12 oz)	18	—	0
sugar wafers w/ creme filling sugar free sodium free	1 (0.14 oz)	20	—	0
vanilla sandwich	1 (0.35 oz)	48	tr	0
REFRIGERATED				
Pillsbury				
Chocolate Chip	1	70	—	5
Oatmeal Raisin	1	60	—	0
Peanut Butter	1	70	—	5
Sugar	1	70	—	5
chocolate chip	1 (0.42 oz)	59	—	3
chocolate chip unbaked	1 oz	126	—	7
oatmeal	1 (0.4 oz)	56	—	3
oatmeal raisin	1 (0.4 oz)	56	—	3
peanut butter	1 (0.4 oz)	60	—	4
peanut butter dough	1 oz	130	—	8
sugar	1 (0.42 oz)	58	—	4
sugar dough	1 oz	124	—	8
TAKE-OUT				
biscotti with nuts chocolate dipped	1 (1.3 oz)	117	1	18

CORIANDER

leaf dried	1 tsp	2	—	0
leaf fresh	¼ cup	1	—	0
seed	1 tsp	5	—	0

CORN

(*see also* BRAN, CEREAL, CORNMEAL, FLOUR)

CANNED				
Del Monte				
Cream Style Golden	½ cup (4.4 oz)	90	2	0
Cream Style Golden 50% Less Salt	½ cup (4.4 oz)	90	2	0
Cream Style Golden No Salt Added	½ cup (4.4 oz)	90	2	0
Cream Style Supersweet Golden	½ cup (4.4 oz)	60	2	0
Cream Style White	½ cup (4.4 oz)	100	2	0
Whole Kernel Golden	½ cup (4.4 oz)	90	3	0

FOOD	PORTION	CALS.	FIB.	CHOL.
Del Monte (CONT.)				
Whole Kernel Golden Supersweet 50% Less Salt	½ cup (4.4 oz)	60	3	0
Whole Kernel Golden Supersweet No Salt Added	½ cup (4.4 oz)	60	3	0
Whole Kernel Golden Supersweet No Sugar	½ cup (4.4 oz)	60	3	0
Whole Kernel Golden Supersweet Vaccum Packed	½ cup (3.7 oz)	70	3	0
Whole Kernel Golden Supersweet Vaccum Packed No Salt Added	½ cup (3.7 oz)	70	3	0
Whole Kernel White Sweet	½ cup (4.4 oz)	80	2	0
Green Giant				
50% Less Salt No Sugar Added	½ cup	50	2	0
Corn	½ cup	70	2	0
Cream Style	½ cup	100	2	0
Deli Corn	½ cup	80	2	0
Golden Kernel 50% Less Salt	½ cup	70	2	0
Golden Vacuum Packed	½ cup	80	2	0
Mexi Corn	½ cup	80	2	0
No Salt No Sugar	½ cup	80	2	0
Sweet Select	½ cup	60	2	0
White Vacuum Packed	½ cup	80	2	0
Ka-Me				
Baby	½ cup (4.5 oz)	20	2	0
Stir Fry	½ cup (4.5 oz)	20	2	0
Owatonna				
Cream Style	½ cup	100	—	0
Whole Kernel In Brine	½ cup	90	—	0
Whole Kernel Vacuum Pack	½ cup	100	—	0
S&W				
Cream Style Premium Homestyle	½ cup	105	—	0
Whole Kernel Tender Young	½ cup	90	—	0
Whole Kernel Water Pack	½ cup	80	—	0
Seneca				
Cream Style	½ cup	80	1	0
Whole Kernel	½ cup	90	2	0
Whole Kernel Natural Pack	½ cup	80	2	0
cream style	½ cup	93	—	0
w/ red & green peppers	½ cup	86	—	0
white	½ cup	66	—	0
yellow	½ cup	66	1	0

FOOD	PORTION	CALS.	FIB.	CHOL.
FRESH				
on-the-cob w/ butter cooked	1 ear	155	—	6
white cooked	½ cup	89	—	0
white raw	½ cup	66	—	0
yellow cooked	1 ear (2.7 oz)	83	—	0
yellow cooked	½ cup	89	—	0
yellow raw	½ cup	66	—	0
yellow raw	1 ear (3 oz)	77	—	0
FROZEN				
Birds Eye				
Big Ears	1 ear	160	—	0
In Butter Sauce	½ cup	90	2	5
Little Ears	2 ears	130	—	0
On The Cob	1 ear	120	—	0
Polybag Cut	½ cup	80	2	0
Polybag Deluxe Tender Sweet	½ cup	80	2	0
Sweet	½ cup	80	2	0
Green Giant				
Cream Style	½ cup	110	3	0
Harvest Fresh Niblets	½ cup	80	2	0
Harvest Fresh White Shoepeg	½ cup	90	2	0
In Butter Sauce	½ cup	100	—	5
Nibblers Corn On The Cob	2 ears	120	2	0
Niblet Ears	1 ear	120	2	0
Niblets	½ cup	90	2	0
One Serve Niblets In Butter Sauce	1 pkg	120	3	5
One Serve On The Cob	1 pkg	120	2	0
Super Sweet Nibblers Corn On The Cob	2 ears	90	2	0
Super Sweet Niblet Ears	1 ear	90	2	0
Super Sweet Niblet Select	½ cup	60	2	0
White In Butter Sauce	½ cup	100	2	5
White Select	½ cup	90	2	0
Hanover				
White Shoepeg	½ cup	80	—	0
White Sweet	½ cup	80	—	0
Yellow Sweet	½ cup	80	—	0
Mrs. Paul's				
Fritters	2	240	—	10
Ore Ida				
Cob Corn	1 ear (6.1 oz)	180	4	0
Cob Corn Mini-Gold	1 ear (3.1 oz)	90	2	0

FOOD	PORTION	CALS.	FIB.	CHOL.
Stouffer's				
Souffle	½ cup (2.4 oz)	170	1	65
Tree Of Life	⅔ cup (3.2 oz)	80	1	0
cooked	½ cup	67	—	0
on-the-cob cooked	1 ear (2.2 oz)	59	—	0
SHELF-STABLE				
Pantry Express				
Golden Whole Kernel	½ cup	60	1	0
TAKE-OUT				
fritters	1 (1 oz)	62	1	12
scalloped	½ cup	258	—	47

CORN CHIPS
(see CHIPS)

CORNISH HENS
(see CHICKEN)

CORNMEAL
(see also POLENTA)

FOOD	PORTION	CALS.	FIB.	CHOL.
Albers				
White	3 tbsp	110	tr	0
Yellow	3 tbsp	110	tr	0
Arrowhead				
Yellow	¼ cup (1.2 oz)	120	3	0
Aunt Jemima				
White	3 tbsp	102	1	0
Yellow	3 tbsp	102	1	0
Quaker				
White	3 tbsp	102	1	0
Yellow	3 tbsp	102	1	0
corn grits cooked	1 cup	146	—	0
corn grits uncooked	1 cup	579	—	0
degermed	1 cup	506	7	0
self-rising degermed	1 cup	489	—	0
whole grain	1 cup	442	13	0
HOME RECIPE				
hush puppies	5 (2.7 oz)	256	4	135
hush puppies	1 (¾ oz)	74	1	10
MIX				
Arrowhead				
Corn Bread	¼ cup (1.2 oz)	120	4	0
Golden Dipt				
Corny Dog Batter Mix	1 oz	100	—	0
Hush Puppy Deluxe Mix	1¼ oz	120	—	0

FOOD	PORTION	CALS.	FIB.	CHOL.
Golden Dipt (CONT.)				
Hush Puppy Jalapeno Mix	1¼ oz	120	—	0
Hush Puppy With Onion	1¼ oz	120	—	0
Hodgson Mill				
Yelllow Self Rising	¼ cup (1 oz)	90	3	0
Yellow	¼ cup (1 oz)	100	3	0
Kentucky Kernal				
White Corn Meal Mix	¼ cup (1 oz)	100	2	0
Miracle Maize				
Complete as prep	1 piece (1.5 oz)	193	2	0
Country Style as prep	1 piece 2 in x 2 in (1.8 oz)	230	2	0
Sweet as prep	1 piece 2 in x 2 in (1.8 oz)	236	1	0
Stone-Buhr				
Yellow Corn Meal	¼ cup (1 oz)	100	1	0
READY-TO-USE				
Aurora				
Polenta	½ cup (5 oz)	110	1	0

CORNSALAD

FOOD	PORTION	CALS.	FIB.	CHOL.
raw	1 cup	12	—	0

CORNSTARCH

FOOD	PORTION	CALS.	FIB.	CHOL.
Argo	1 tbsp (8 g)	30	—	0
Argo	1 cup (128 g)	460	—	0
Hodgson Mill	2 tsp (0.4 oz)	35	—	0
Kingsford's	1 cup (128 g)	460	—	0
Kingsford's	1 tbsp (8 g)	30	—	0
cornstarch	⅓ cup	164	tr	0

COTTAGE CHEESE

FOOD	PORTION	CALS.	FIB.	CHOL.
Axelrod				
Nonfat	½ cup (4.4 oz)	90	0	10
Breakstone				
2% Fat Large Curd	½ cup (4.2 oz)	90	0	15
2% Fat Small Curd	½ cup (4.2 oz)	90	0	15
4% Fat Large Curd	½ cup (4.2 oz)	120	0	25
4% Fat Small Curd	½ cup (4.2 oz)	120	0	25
Dry Curd ½% Fat	¼ cup (1.9 oz)	45	0	5
Cabot	4 oz	120	—	17
Light	4 oz	90	—	5
Friendship				
California Style	½ cup (4 oz)	115	0	25
Lowfat No Salt Added	½ cup (4 oz)	90	0	10

FOOD	PORTION	CALS.	FIB.	CHOL.
Friendship (CONT.)				
Lowfat Pineapple	½ cup (4 oz)	120	0	10
Lowfat 1%	½ cup (4 oz)	90	0	10
Nonfat	½ cup (4 oz)	80	0	0
Nonfat Plus Peach	½ cup (4 oz)	110	0	0
Pot Style	½ cup (4 oz)	90	0	15
With Pineapple	½ cup (4 oz)	140	0	15
Hood				
1% Fat	½ cup (4 oz)	90	0	10
1% Fat Chive & Onion	½ cup (4 oz)	90	0	10
1% Fat No Salt Added	½ cup (4 oz)	90	0	10
1% Fat Pepper & Herb	½ cup (4 oz)	90	0	10
1% Fat Pineapple Cherry	½ cup (4 oz)	110	0	10
4% Fat	½ cup (4 oz)	120	0	25
4% Fat Chive	½ cup (4 oz)	130	0	25
4% Fat Pineapple	½ cup (4 oz)	130	0	20
Nonfat	½ cup (4 oz)	80	0	5
Nonfat Pineapple	½ cup (4 oz)	110	0	<5
Knudsen				
1.5% Fat Peach	4 oz	110	0	10
1.5% Fat Pineapple	4 oz	110	0	15
1.5% Fat Strawberry	4 oz	110	0	10
1.5% Fat Tropical Fruit	4 oz	120	0	10
2% Fat Small Curd	½ cup (4.2 oz)	100	0	15
4% Fat Large Curd	½ cup (4.5 oz)	130	0	30
4% Fat Small Curd	½ cup (4.3 oz)	120	0	25
Free	½ cup (4.3 oz)	80	0	10
Lactaid				
1%	4 oz	72	—	4
Light N'Lively				
1% Fat	½ cup (4 oz)	80	0	15
1% Fat Garden Salad	½ cup (4.2 oz)	90	0	15
1% Fat Peach & Pineapple	½ cup (4.3 oz)	120	0	10
Free	½ cup (4.4 oz)	80	0	10
Sealtest				
2% Fat Small Curd	½ cup (4.2 oz)	90	0	15
4% Fat Large Curd	½ cup (4.2 oz)	120	0	25
4% Fat Small Curd	½ cup (4.2 oz)	120	0	25
Viva				
Nonfat	½ cup	70	—	5
creamed	1 cup	217	—	31
creamed	4 oz	117	—	17
creamed w/ fruit	4 oz	140	—	13
dry curd	4 oz	96	—	8

FOOD	PORTION	CALS.	FIB.	CHOL.
dry curd	1 cup	123	—	10
lowfat 1%	4 oz	82	—	5
lowfat 1%	1 cup	164	—	10
lowfat 2%	1 cup	203	—	19
lowfat 2%	4 oz	101	—	9

COTTONSEED
kernels roasted	1 tbsp	51	—	0

COUGH DROPS
Halls
	1 (3.8 g)	15	—	0
Plus	1 (4.7 g)	18	—	0
With Vitamin C	1 (3.8 g)	14	—	0

COUSCOUS
Casbah
Almond Chicken Vegetarian	1 pkg (1.5 oz)	160	tr	0
Asparagus Au Gratin Organic	1 pkg (1.5 oz)	150	1	<5
Cheddar Broccoli	1 pkg (1.3 oz)	130	tr	<5
Hearty Harvest Zestful Organic as prep	1 pkg (10 fl oz)	180	2	0
Moroccan Stew	1 pkg (2 oz)	180	1	0
Pilaf as prep	1 cup	200	tr	0
Tomato Parmesan	1 pkg (1.8 oz)	170	2	<5
Near East as prep	1¼ cup	260	2	0
cooked	½ cup	101	—	0
dry	½ cup	346	—	0

COWPEAS
catjang dried cooked	1 cup	200	—	0
common canned	1 cup	184	—	0
frozen cooked	½ cup	112	—	0
leafy tips chopped cooked	1 cup	12	—	0
leafy tips raw chopped	1 cup	10	—	0

CRAB
CANNED
blue	3 oz	84	—	76
blue	1 cup	133	—	120
FRESH				
alaska king cooked	1 leg (4.7 oz)	129	—	72
alaska king cooked	3 oz	82	—	45
alaska king raw	1 leg (6 oz)	144	—	72
alaska king raw	3 oz	71	—	35
blue cooked	3 oz	87	—	85
blue cooked	1 cup	138	—	135

FOOD	PORTION	CALS.	FIB.	CHOL.
blue raw	3 oz	74	—	66
blue raw	1 crab (.7 oz)	18	—	16
dungeness raw	3 oz	73	—	50
dungeness raw	1 crab (5.7 oz)	140	—	97
queen steamed	3 oz	98	—	60
FROZEN				
Mrs. Paul's				
Deviled Crab	1 cake	180	—	20
Deviled Crab Miniatures	3½ oz	240	—	20
READY-TO-USE				
crab cakes	1 cake (2.1 oz)	93	—	90
TAKE-OUT				
baked	1 (3.8 oz)	160	—	184
cake	1 (2 oz)	160	—	82
soft-shell fried	1 (4.4 oz)	334	—	45

CRACKER CRUMBS

FOOD	PORTION	CALS.	FIB.	CHOL.
Golden Dipt				
Cracker Meal	1 oz	100	—	0
Honey Maid				
Graham Cracker	0.5 oz	70	tr	0
Keebler				
Cracker Meal	1 cup	100	—	0
Graham Crumbs	1 cup	520	—	0
Zesty Meal	1 cup	85	—	0
Kellogg's				
Corn Flake Crumbs	2 tbsp (0.4 oz)	40	0	0
Lance				
Cracker Meal	1 oz	100	—	0
Nabisco				
Nilla Cookie Crumbs	2 tbsp (0.5 oz)	70	tr	<5
Oreo				
Cookie Crumbs	2 tbsp (0.5 oz)	80	1	0
Premium				
Fat Free Cracker Crumbs	¼ cup (1 oz)	100	1	0
Ritz				
Cracker Crumbs	⅓ cup (1 oz)	140	1	0
Sunshine				
Graham	3 tbsp (0.6 oz)	80	tr	0
cracker meal	1 cup (4 oz)	440	—	0

CRACKERS

(see also CRACKER CRUMBS)

FOOD	PORTION	CALS.	FIB.	CHOL.
Adrienne's				
Gourmet Flatbread Caraway & Rye	2	20	—	<5

FOOD	PORTION	CALS.	FIB.	CHOL.
Adrienne's (CONT.)				
Gourmet Flatbread Classic Island	2	20	—	<5
Gourmet Flatbread Slightly Onion	2	20	—	<5
Gourmet Flatbread Ten Grain	2	20	1	0
American Heritage				
Sesame	9 (1.1 oz) (1.9 oz)	160	1	0
Wheat & Bran	9 (1 oz) (1.9 oz)	140	2	0
Better Cheddars	22 (1 oz)	70	tr	<5
Low Sodium	22 (1 oz)	150	tr	<5
Reduced Fat	24 (1 oz)	140	tr	<5
Burns & Ricker				
Bagel Crisps Garlic	5 (1 oz)	100	1	0
Cheez-It	1 pkg (1.5 oz) (1.9 oz)	220	1	3
Cheez-It	1 pkg (2 oz) (1.9 oz)	290	2	3
Cheez-It	27 (1 oz)	160	tr	0
Hot & Spicy	26 (1 oz) (1.9 oz)	160	1	0
Hot & Spicy	1 pkg (1.5 oz) (1.9 oz)	220	1	0
Low Sodium	27 (1 oz)	160	tr	0
Party Mix	½ cup (1 oz)	140	1	0
Reduced Fat	30 (1 oz) (1.9 oz)	130	tr	0
White Cheddar	26 (1 oz) (1.9 oz)	160	tr	3
White Cheddar	1 pkg (1.5 oz) (1.9 oz)	220	tr	3
Crown Pilot	1 (0.5 oz)	70	tr	0
Devonsheer				
Melba Rounds Garlic	½ oz	56	1	0
Melba Rounds Honey Bran	½ oz	52	1	0
Melba Rounds Onion	½ oz	51	1	0
Melba Rounds Plain	½ oz	53	1	0
Melba Rounds Plain Unsalted	½ oz	52	1	0
Melba Rounds Rye	½ oz	53	1	0
Melba Rounds Sesame	½ oz	57	1	0
Eagle				
Bacon Cheese	1 oz	140	—	0
Cheese	1 oz	130	—	0
Eden				
Brown Rice	5 (1 oz)	120	2	0
Escort	3 (0.5 oz)	70	—	0
Estee				
Unsalted	1 (0.5 oz)	70	0	0

FOOD	PORTION	CALS.	FIB.	CHOL.
Frito Lay				
Cheese Filled	6 (1.5 oz)	210	—	5
Cracker Snacks Cheddar	13-16 (1 oz)	70	—	0
Cracker Snacks Zesty Italian	13-16 (1 oz)	70	—	0
Peanut Butter Filled	6 (1.5 oz)	210	—	0
Harvest Crisps				
5 Grain	13 (1.1 oz)	130	1	0
Oat	13 (1.1 oz)	140	1	0
Health Valley				
Herb Stoned Wheat	13	55	2	0
Herb Stoned Wheat No Salt	13	55	2	0
Rice Bran	7	130	2	0
Sesame Stoned Wheat	13	55	2	0
Sesame Stoned Wheat No Salt Added	13	55	2	0
Seven Grain Vegetable Stoned Wheat	13	55	2	0
Seven Grain Vegetable Stoned Wheat No Salt Added	13	55	2	0
Stoned Wheat	13	55	2	0
Stoned Wheat No Salt Added	13	55	2	0
Hi Ho	9	160	tr	0
Butter Flavored	9 (1.1 oz)	160	tr	3
Cracked Pepper	9 (1.1 oz)	160	tr	3
Low Salt	9 (1.1 oz)	160	tr	0
Multi Grain	9 (1.1 oz)	160	1	0
Reduced Fat	10 (1.1 oz)	140	tr	0
Whole Wheat	9 (1.1 oz)	150	2	0
Ideal Crispbread				
Extra Thin	3	48	1	0
Fiber Thins	2	41	2	0
Oatbran Thins	2	50	2	0
J.J. Flats				
Breadflats Caraway	1	52	1	tr
Breadflats Caraway And Salt	1	51	1	tr
Breadflats Cinnamon	1	53	1	tr
Breadflats Flavorall	1	52	1	tr
Breadflats Garlic	1	52	1	tr
Breadflats Oat Bran	1	49	2	0
Breadflats Onion	1	53	1	tr
Breadflats Plain	1	53	1	tr
Breadflats Poppy	1	53	1	tr
Breadflats Sesame	1	55	1	tr
Kavli	1 piece	40	2	0

FOOD	PORTION	CALS.	FIB.	CHOL.
Keebler				
Club	2	30	—	0
Melba Toast Garlic	2	25	—	0
Melba Toast Long	2	30	—	0
Melba Toast Onion	2	25	—	0
Melba Toast Plain	2	25	—	0
Melba Toast Sesame	2	25	—	0
Oyster Crackers Large	26	80	—	0
Oyster Crackers Small	50	80	—	0
Snack Crackers Toasted Rye	2	30	—	0
Snack Crackers Toasted Sesame	2	30	—	0
Snack Crackers Toasted Wheat	2	30	—	0
Toasted Snack Bacon	2	30	—	0
Toasted Snack Onion	2	30	—	0
Toasted Snack Pumpernickel	2	30	—	0
Wholegrain Wheat	2	30	—	0
Krispy				
Cracked Pepper	5 (0.5 oz)	60	tr	0
Fat Fre	5 (0.5 oz)	60	tr	0
Mild Cheddar	5 (0.5 oz)	60	tr	0
Original	5 (0.5 oz)	60	tr	0
Soup & Oyster Crackers	17 (0.5 oz)	60	tr	0
Unsalted Tops	5 (0.5 oz)	60	tr	0
Whole Wheat	5 (0.5 oz)	60	tr	0
Lance				
Bonnie	1 pkg (34 g)	160	—	5
Captain Wafers	2	30	—	0
Captain Wafers Very Low Sodium	2	30	—	0
Captain Wafers w/ Cream Cheese & Chives	1 pkg (37 g)	170	—	0
Cheese-On-Wheat	1 pkg (37 g)	180	—	5
Lanchee	1 pkg (35 g)	180	—	5
Melba Toast Oblong	2	30	—	0
Melba Toast Plain	2	20	—	0
Melba Toast Round Garlic	2	20	—	0
Melba Toast Round Onion	2	20	—	0
Melba Toast Sesame	2	25	—	0
Nekot	1 pkg (42 g)	210	—	5
Nip-Chee	1 pkg (37 g)	180	—	5
Oyster Crackers	1 pkg (14 g)	70	—	0
Peanut Butter Wheat	1 pkg (37 g)	190	—	0
Rye Twins	2	30	—	0

FOOD	PORTION	CALS.	FIB.	CHOL.
Lance (CONT.)				
Rye-Chee	1 pkg (41 g)	190	—	5
Saltines	2	25	—	0
Saltines Slug Pack	4 crackers	50	—	0
Sesame Twins	2	40	—	0
Toastchee	1 pkg (39 g)	190	—	5
Toasty	1 pkg (35 g)	180	—	0
Wheat Twins	2	30	—	0
Wheatswafer	2	30	—	0
Lavash				
Bread Crisp Original	2 (0.5 oz)	60	—	0
Bread Crisp Sesame	2 (0.5 oz)	60	—	0
Little Debbie				
Cheese Crackers With Peanut Butter	1 pkg (1.4 oz)	210	1	0
Cheese Crackers With Peanut Butter	1 pkg (0.9 oz)	140	1	0
Toasty Crackers With Peanut Butter	1 pkg (0.9 oz)	140	1	0
Toasty Crackers With Peanut Butter	1 pkg (1.4 oz)	200	1	0
Wheat Crackers With Cheddar Cheese	1 pkg (0.9 oz)	140	0	5
Manischewitz				
Tam Tams	10	147	—	0
Tam Tams No Salt	10	138	—	0
Tams Garlic	10	153	—	0
Tams Onion	10	150	—	0
Tams Wheat	10	150	—	0
McCrackens				
Cracker Crisp Country Butter	1 oz	140	—	tr
Cracker Crisp Sour Cream & Chives	1 oz	140	—	tr
Cracker Crisp Tangy Cheddar	1 oz	140	—	tr
Cracker Crisp Toasted Wheat	1 oz	140	—	0
NABS				
Cheese Peanut Butter Sandwich	6 (1.4 oz)	190	1	0
Peanut Butter Toast Sandwich	6 (1.4 oz)	190	1	0
Nabisco				
Bacon Flavored	15 (1.1 oz)	160	tr	0
Chicken In A Biskit	14 (1 oz)	160	tr	0
Garden Crisps	15 (1 oz)	130	1	0
Oat Thins	18 (1 oz)	140	2	0
Royal Lunch	1 (0.4 oz)	50	0	0

FOOD	PORTION	CALS.	FIB.	CHOL.
Nabisco (CONT.)				
Swiss	15 (1 oz)	140	tr	0
Tid-Bit Cheese	32 (1 oz)	150	tr	0
Vegetable Thins	14 (1.1 oz)	160	1	0
Wheat Thins Original	16 (1 oz)	140	2	0
Wheat Thins Reduced Fat	18 (1 oz)	120	2	0
Zings!	1 pkg (1.8 oz)	240	2	0
Nips				
Cheese	29 (1 oz)	150	tr	0
Old London				
Melba Toast Pumpernickel	½ oz	54	1	0
Melba Toast Rye	½ oz	52	—	0
Melba Toast Sesame	½ oz	55	1	0
Melba Toast Sesame Unsalted	½ oz	55	1	0
Melba Toast Wheat	½ oz	51	1	0
Melba Toast White	½ oz	51	1	0
Melba Toast White Unsalted	½ oz	51	1	0
Melba Toast Whole Grain	½ oz	52	1	0
Melba Toast Whole Grain Unsalted	½ oz	53	1	0
Rounds Bacon	½ oz	53	1	0
Rounds Garlic	½ oz	56	1	0
Rounds Onion	½ oz	52	1	0
Rounds Rye	½ oz	52	—	0
Rounds Sesame	½ oz	56	1	0
Rounds White	½ oz	48	1	0
Rounds Whole Grain	½ oz	54	1	0
Oysterettes	19 (0.5 oz)	60	tr	0
Pepperidge Farm				
Butter Thins	4	70	0	<5
Cracked Wheat	3	100	1	0
Crispy Graham	4	70	—	0
English Water Biscuits	4	70	0	0
Flutters Garden Herb	¾ oz	100	—	0
Flutters Golden Sesame	¾ oz	110	—	0
Flutters Original Butter	¾ oz	100	—	5
Flutters Toasted Wheat	¾ oz	110	—	0
Garden Vegetable	5	60	—	0
Goldfish Cheddar Cheese	1 pkg (1½ oz)	190	1	5
Goldfish Cheddar Cheese	1 oz	120	1	5
Goldfish Cheese Thins	4	50	0	0
Goldfish Original	1 oz	130	1	0
Goldfish Parmesan Cheese	1 oz	120	1	<5
Goldfish Pizza Flavored	1 oz	130	1	<5

FOOD	PORTION	CALS.	FIB.	CHOL.
Pepperidge Farm (CONT.)				
Goldfish Pretzel	1 oz	110	1	0
Hearty Wheat	4	100	1	0
Multi Grain	4	70	—	0
Sesame	4	80	2	0
Snack Mix Classic	1 oz	140	1	0
Snack Mix Lightly Smoked	1 oz	150	1	0
Snack Sticks Cheese	8	130	1	0
Snack Sticks Pretzel	8	120	1	0
Snack Sticks Pumpernickel	8	140	1	0
Snack Sticks Sesame	8	140	1	0
Spicy Lightly Smoked	1 oz	140	1	<5
Toasted Rice	4	60	—	0
Toasted Wheat With Onion	4	80	0	0
Premium				
Saltine Fat Free	5 (0.5 oz)	50	0	0
Saltine Low Sodium	5 (0.5 oz)	60	tr	0
Saltine Original	5 (0.5 oz)	60	tr	0
Saltine Unsalted Tops	5 (0.5 oz)	60	tr	0
Saltine Bits	34 (1 oz)	150	tr	0
Soup & Oyster	23 (0.5 oz)	60	tr	0
Ralston				
Oat Bran Krisp	2	60	3	0
Ritz				
	5 (0.5 oz)	80	—	0
Bits	48 (1 oz)	160	1	0
Bits Sandwiches With Peanut Butter	13 (1 oz)	150	1	0
Bits Sanwiches With Real Cheese	14 (1.1 oz)	160	1	5
Low Sodium	5 (0.5 oz)	80	tr	0
Sandwiches With Real Cheese	1 pkg (1.4 oz)	210	1	5
Rykrisp				
Natural	2	40	4	0
Seasoned	2	45	3	0
Seasoned Twindividuals	2	45	3	0
Sesame	2	50	3	0
Ryvita				
Crisp Bread Dark Finn Crisp	2	38	—	0
Crisp Bread Dark Rye	1	26	—	0
Crisp Bread Dark w/ Caraway Seeds Finn Crisp	2	38	—	0
Crisp Bread High Fiber	1	23	—	0
Crisp Bread Light Rye	1	26	—	0
Crisp Bread Toasted Sesame Rye	1	31	—	0

FOOD	PORTION	CALS.	FIB.	CHOL.
Ryvita (CONT.)				
Snackbread High Fiber	1	14	—	0
Snackbread Original Wheat	1	20	—	0
Sesmark				
Brown Rice	15 (1 oz)	120	tr	0
Cheese Thins	15 (1 oz)	130	tr	0
Rice Thins Original	15 (1 oz)	130	tr	0
Rice Thins Teriyaki Flavored	13 (1 oz)	130	tr	0
Savory Thins Original	15 (1 oz)	125	1	0
Sesame Thins Cheddar	9 (1 oz)	150	3	0
Sesame Thins Garlic	9 (1 oz)	150	3	0
Sesame Thins Original	9 (1 oz)	150	2	0
Sesame Thins Unsalted	11 (1 oz)	150	3	0
Snackwell's				
Cracked Pepper	7 (0.5 oz)	60	tr	0
Fat Free Wheat	5 (0.5 oz)	60	1	0
Reduced Fat Cheese	38 (1 oz)	130	1	0
Reduced Fat Classic Golden	6 (0.5 oz)	60	0	0
Snorkles				
Cheddar	56 (1 oz)	140	1	5
Sociables	7 (0.5 oz)	80	tr	0
Sunshine				
Saltines Cracked Pepper	5 (0.5 oz)	60	tr	0
Town House	2	35	—	0
Tree Of Life				
Bite Size Fat Free Corn & Salsa	12	60	0	0
Bite Size Fat Free Cracked Pepper	12	55	0	0
Bite Size Fat Free Garden Vegetable	12	55	0	0
Bite Size Fat Free Garlic & Herb	12	55	0	0
Bite Size Fat Free Soya Nut	12	60	0	0
Bite Size Fat Free Toasted Onion	12	60	0	0
Bite Size Fat Free Whole Wheat	12	60	2	0
Fat Free Oyster	40 (0.5 oz)	60	0	0
Saltine Cracked Pepper Fat Free	4 (0.5 oz)	60	1	0
Saltine Fat Free	4 (0.5 oz)	50	0	0
Triscuit	7 (1.1 oz)	140	4	0
Deli-Style Rye	7 (1.1 oz)	140	4	0
Garden Herb	6 (1 oz)	130	3	0
Low Sodium	7 (1.1 oz)	150	3	0
Reduced Fat	8 (1.1 oz)	130	4	0
Wheat 'n Bran	7 (1.1 oz)	140	4	0

FOOD	PORTION	CALS.	FIB.	CHOL.
Tuscany				
Pita Crisps	1 oz	90	—	0
Pita Crisps Sesame	1 oz	96	—	0
Toast	1 oz	95	—	0
Toast Pepato	1 oz	93	—	0
Toast Pesto	1 oz	96	—	3
Toast Tomato	1 oz	95	—	0
Twigs				
Sesame & Cheese Sticks	15 (1 oz)	150	tr	0
Uneeded Biscuit				
Unsalted Tops	2 (0.5 oz)	60	tr	0
Venus				
Armenian Thin Bread	2 (0.9 oz)	100	—	0
Bran Wafers Salt Free	5 (0.5 oz)	60	2	0
Corn Crackers Salt Free	5 (0.5 oz)	60	2	0
Cracked Wheat Wafers Salt Free	5 (0.5 oz)	60	—	0
Cracker Bread	5 (0.5 oz)	60	—	0
Hors D'oeuvre	3 (0.5 oz)	60	—	0
Oat Bran Wafers	5 (0.5 oz)	60	2	0
Oat Bran Wafers Salt Free	5 (0.5 oz)	60	1	0
Old Brussels Cheddar Waferettes	5 (0.5 oz)	80	—	1
Old Brussels Jalapeno Waferettes	5 (0.5 oz)	80	1	1
Rye Wafers Low Salt	5 (0.5 oz)	60	—	0
Stoned Wheat Wafers Bite Size	7 (0.5 oz)	60	—	0
Water Crackers Fat Free	5 (0.5 oz)	55	—	0
Wheat Wafers Low Salt	5 (0.5 oz)	60	1	0
Waldorf				
Sodium Free	2	30	—	0
Wasa Crispbread				
Breakfast	1	50	1	0
Extra Crisp	1	25	—	0
Falu Rye	1	30	2	0
Fiber Plus	1	35	3	0
Golden Rye	1	30	3	0
Hearty Rye	1	50	1	0
Light Rye	1	25	1	0
Royal	½	26	1	0
Savory Sesame	1	30	2	0
Sesame Rye	1	30	2	0
Sesame Wheat	1	60	1	0
Toasted Wheat	1	50	1	0

FOOD	PORTION	CALS.	FIB.	CHOL.
Waverly	5 (0.5 oz)	70	0	0
Weight Watchers				
Crispbread Garlic	2	30	—	0
Wheat Thins				
Low Salt	16 (1 oz)	140	2	0
Multi-Grain	17 (1 oz)	130	2	0
Wheatworth				
Stone Ground	5 (0.5 oz)	80	1	0
cheese	1 (1 in sq) (1 g)	5	—	0
cheese	14 (½ oz)	71	—	2
cheese low sodium	14 (½ oz)	71	—	2
cheese low sodium	1 (1 in sq) (1 g)	5	—	0
cheese w/ peanut butter filling	1 (0.24 oz)	34	—	0
crispbread rye	1 (0.35 oz)	37	2	0
melba toast plain	1 (5 g)	19	tr	0
melba toast pumpernickel	1 (5 g)	19	tr	0
melba toast rye	1 (5 g)	19	tr	0
melba toast wheat	1 (5 g)	19	tr	0
oyster cracker	1 (1 g)	4	tr	0
rye w/ cheese filling	1 (0.24 oz)	34	—	1
rye wafers plain	1 (0.9 oz)	84	—	0
rye wafers seasoned	1 (0.8 oz)	84	—	0
saltines	1 (3 g)	13	tr	0
saltines fat free low sodium	6 (1 oz)	118	—	0
saltines fat free low sodium	3 (0.5 oz)	59	—	0
saltines low salt	1 (3 g)	13	tr	0
snack cracker	1 (3 g)	15	tr	0
snack cracker low salt	1 (3 g)	15	tr	0
snack cracker w/ cheese filling	1 (7 g)	33	—	0
soup cracker	1 (1 g)	4	tr	0
wheat w/ cheese filling	1 (0.24 oz)	35	—	1
wheat w/ peanut butter filling	1 (0.24 oz)	35	—	0
wheat thins	1 (2 g)	9	—	0
wheat thins	7 (0.5 oz)	67	1	0
wheat thins low salt	7 (0.5 oz)	67	1	0
whole wheat	1 (4 g)	18	—	0
whole wheat low salt	1 (4 g)	18	—	0

CRANBERRIES
CANNED
Ocean Spray

FOOD	PORTION	CALS.	FIB.	CHOL.
CranFruit Cranberry Raspberry Sauce	2 oz	100	—	0
CranFruit Cranberry Strawberry Sauce	2 oz	100	—	0

FOOD	PORTION	CALS.	FIB.	CHOL.
Ocean Spray (CONT.)				
CranFruit Cranberry Orange Sauce	2 oz	100	—	0
Cranberry Sauce Jellied	2 oz	90	—	0
Whole Berry Sauce	2 oz	90	—	0
S&W				
Cranberry Sauce Jellied Old Fashioned	½ cup	90	—	0
Cranberry Sauce Whole Berry Old Fashioned	½ cup	90	—	0
cranberry sauce sweetened	½ cup	209	—	0
FRESH				
Ocean Spray	½ cup	25	—	0
chopped	1 cup	54	—	0

CRANBERRY BEANS
CANNED

cranberry beans	1 cup	216	—	0
DRIED				
Bean Cuisine	½ cup	115	5	0
cooked	1 cup	240	—	0

CRANBERRY JUICE

Apple & Eve	6 fl oz	100	—	0
Ocean Spray				
Cocktail	8 fl oz	140	0	0
Cocktail Reduced Calorie	8 fl oz	50	0	0
Lightstyle Low Calorie Cranberry Juice Cocktail	8 fl oz	40	0	0
Seneca				
Cocktail frzn as prep	8 fl oz	140	0	0
Snapple				
Cranberry Royal	10 fl oz	150	—	0
Tree Of Life				
Concentrate	8 tsp (1.4 oz)	110	—	0
Tropicana				
Twister Ruby Red	8 fl oz	120	—	0
Twister Ruby Red	1 bottle (10 fl oz)	150	—	0
Veryfine	8 oz	160	—	0
cocktail	1 cup	147	—	0
cranberry juice cocktail	6 oz	108	—	0
cranberry juice cocktail low calorie	6 oz	33	—	0
cranberry juice cocktail frzn	12 oz can	821	—	0
cranberry juice cocktail frzn as prep	6 oz	102	—	0

FOOD	PORTION	CALS.	FIB.	CHOL.
CRAYFISH				
(see also LOBSTER)				
cooked	3 oz	97	—	151
raw	3 oz	76	—	118
raw	8	24	—	37
CREAM				
(see also SOUR CREAM, SOUR CREAM SUBSTITUTES, WHIPPED TOPPINGS)				
LIQUID				
Farmland				
Half & Half	2 tbsp	40	0	0
Light Cream	2 tbsp	30	0	0
Hood				
Half & Half	2 tbsp (1 oz)	40	0	15
Heavy	1 tbsp (0.5 oz)	50	0	20
Light	1 tbsp (0.5 oz)	30	0	10
Whipping Cream	1 tbsp (0.5 oz)	45	0	20
Parmalat				
Half & Half	2 tbsp (1 oz)	40	0	15
half & half	1 cup	315	—	89
half & half	1 tbsp	20	—	6
heavy whipping	1 tbsp	52	—	21
light coffee	1 tbsp	29	—	10
light coffee	1 cup	496	—	159
light whipping	1 tbsp	44	—	17
WHIPPED				
heavy whipping	1 cup	411	—	163
light whipping	1 cup	345	—	132
CREAM CHEESE				
Alpine Lace				
Fat Free Garden Vegetable	2 tbsp (1 oz)	30	0	3
Fat Free Garlic & Herbs	2 tbsp (1 oz)	30	0	3
Breakstone				
Temp-Tee Whipped	3 tbsp (1.2 oz)	110	0	30
Fleur De Lait	2 tbsp (1 oz)	100	0	35
Bermuda Onion & Chives	2 tbsp (0.9 oz)	90	0	30
Cinnamon Raisin	2 tbsp (0.9 oz)	90	0	25
Date Nut Rum	2 tbsp (0.9 oz)	90	0	30
Fresh Cut Garden Vegetable	2 tbsp (0.9 oz)	80	0	30
Garden Vegetable	2 tbsp (0.9 oz)	80	0	30
Garlic & Spice	2 tbsp (0.9 oz)	90	0	30
Herb & Spice	2 tbsp (0.9 oz)	90	0	30
Irish Creme	2 tbsp (0.9 oz)	100	0	30
Lemon	2 tbsp (0.9 oz)	90	0	25

FOOD	PORTION	CALS.	FIB.	CHOL.
Breakstone (CONT.)				
Lox	2 tbsp (0.9 oz)	90	0	30
Mandarin Orange	2 tbsp (0.9 oz)	90	0	30
Peach	2 tbsp (0.9 oz)	90	0	25
Pineapple	2 tbsp (0.9 oz)	90	0	30
Strawberry	2 tbsp (0.9 oz)	90	0	30
Toasted Onion	2 tbsp (0.9 oz)	90	0	30
Wildberry	2 tbsp (0.9 oz)	90	0	25
Fresh Cut				
Bac'n & Horseradish	2 tbsp (0.9 oz)	90	0	30
Bermuda Onion & Chives	2 tbsp (0.9 oz)	90	0	30
Date Nut & Rum	2 tbsp (0.9 oz)	90	0	30
Garlic & Spice	2 tbsp (0.9 oz)	90	0	35
Herb & Spice	2 tbsp (0.9 oz)	90	0	30
Lox	2 tbsp (0.9 oz)	90	0	30
Peaches & Cream	2 tbsp (0.9 oz)	90	0	25
Strawberry	2 tbsp (0.9 oz)	90	0	30
Friendship				
NY Style Reduced Fat	2 tbsp (1 oz)	50	0	10
Healthy Choice				
Fat Free Herbs & Garlic	2 tbsp (1 oz)	25	tr	<5
Nonfat	2 tbsp (1 oz)	25	tr	<5
Nonfat With Strawberries	2 tbsp (1 oz)	35	1	<5
Heluva Good Cheese				
Cream Cheese	1 tbsp (1 oz)	100	0	30
Philadelphia				
	1 oz	100	0	30
Free	1 oz	25	0	<5
Free Soft	2 tbsp (1.2 oz)	30	0	<5
Light Soft	2 tbsp (1.1 oz)	70	0	15
Soft	2 tbsp (1 oz)	100	0	30
Soft Herb & Garlic	2 tbsp (1.1 oz)	110	0	30
Soft Olive & Pimento	2 tbsp (1.1 oz)	100	0	30
Soft Pineapple	2 tbsp (1.1 oz)	100	0	30
Soft Smoked Salmon	2 tbsp (1.1 oz)	100	0	30
Soft Strawberries	2 tbsp (1.1 oz)	100	0	30
Soft With Chives & Onions	2 tbsp (1.1 oz)	110	0	30
Whipped	3 tbsp (1.1 oz)	110	0	35
Whipped Smoked Salmon	3 tbsp (1.1 oz)	100	0	30
With Chives	1 oz	90	0	30
With Pimentos	1 oz	90	0	30
Ultra Delight				
Cheddar Cream Cheese	2 tbsp (0.9 oz)	60	1	20
Chive	2 tbsp (0.9 oz)	60	1	20
Garlic	2 tbsp (0.9 oz)	60	1	20

FOOD	PORTION	CALS.	FIB.	CHOL.
Ultra Delight (CONT.)				
Mixed Berry	2 tbsp (0.9 oz)	70	1	20
Nacho	2 tbsp (0.9 oz)	60	1	20
Salsa	2 tbsp (0.9 oz)	60	1	20
Shrimp	2 tbsp (0.9 oz)	60	1	30
Strawberry	2 tbsp (0.9 oz)	60	1	20
Vegetable	2 tbsp (0.9 oz)	50	1	20
cream cheese	1 pkg (3 oz)	297	—	93
cream cheese	1 oz	99	—	31

CREAM CHEESE SUBSTITUTES
Tofutti

Better Than Cream Cheese French Onion	1 oz	80	—	0
Better Than Cream Cheese Herb & Chive	1 oz	80	—	0
Better Than Cream Cheese Plain	1 oz	80	—	0

CREAM OF TARTAR

cream of tartar	1 tsp	8	—	0

CREPES

basic crepe unfilled	1	75	—	55

CRESS
(*see also* WATERCRESS)

garden cooked	½ cup	16	—	0
garden raw	½ cup	8	—	0

CROAKER

atlantic breaded & fried	3 oz	188	—	71
atlantic raw	3 oz	89	—	52

CROISSANT
Rudy's Farm

Ham & Swiss Sandwich	1 (3.4 oz)	310	1	25
TAKE-OUT				
w/ egg & cheese	1	369	—	216
w/ egg cheese & bacon	1	413	—	215
w/ egg cheese & ham	1	475	—	213
w/ egg cheese & sausage	1	524	—	216

CROUTONS
Arnold

Crispy Cheddar Romano	½ oz	64	tr	3
Crispy Cheese Garlic	½ oz	60	tr	0
Crispy Fine Herbs	½ oz	50	1	0

FOOD	PORTION	CALS.	FIB.	CHOL.
Arnold (CONT.)				
Crispy Italian	½ oz	60	tr	0
Crispy Onion & Garlic	½	60	—	0
Crispy Seasoned	½ oz	60	—	0
Brownberry				
Ceasar Salad	½ oz	62	1	tr
Cheddar Cheese	½ oz	63	tr	3
Onion & Garlic	½ oz	60	tr	1
Seasoned	½ oz	59	1	1
Toasted	½ oz	56	tr	1
Pepperidge Farm				
Cheddar & Romano Cheese	½ oz	60	—	0
Cheese & Garlic	½ oz	70	—	0
Onion & Garlic	½ oz	70	—	0
Seasoned	½ oz	70	—	0
Sour Cream & Chive	½ oz	70	—	0
plain	1 cup (1 oz)	122	2	0

CUCUMBER
FRESH

raw	1 (11 oz)	38	3	0
raw sliced	½ cup (1.8 oz)	7	1	0
JARRED				
Rosoff's				
Salad	3 slices (1 oz)	12	—	0
Schorr's				
Cucumber Garden Salad	3 slices (1 oz)	12	—	0
TAKE-OUT				
cucumber salad	3.5 oz	50	—	0

CUMIN

seed	1 tsp	8	—	0

CURRANTS

black fresh	½ cup	36	—	0
zante dried	½ cup	204	—	0

CUSK

fillet baked	3 oz	106	—	50

CUSTARD
HOME RECIPE

baked	½ cup (5 oz)	148	—	123
baked	1 recipe 4 serv (19.8 oz)	549	—	491
flan	½ cup (5.4 oz)	220	—	140

FOOD	PORTION	CALS.	FIB.	CHOL.
flan	1 recipe 10 serv (53.7 oz)	2206	—	1408
MIX				
Jell-O				
Flan	½ cup	151	—	17
Golden Egg Americana as prep	½ cup	160	—	81
as prep w/ 2% milk	½ cup (4.7 oz)	148	—	74
as prep w/ 2% milk	1 recipe 4 serv (18.7 oz)	595	—	297
flan as prep w/ 2% milk	1 recipe 4 serv (18.7 oz)	542	—	57
flan as prep w/ 2% milk	½ cup (4.7 oz)	135	—	9
flan as prep w/ whole milk	1 recipe 4 serv (18.7 oz)	600	—	66
flan as prep w/ whole milk	½ cup (4.7 oz)	150	—	17
TAKE-OUT				
baked	½ cup (5 oz)	148	—	123
zabaione	½ cup (57.2 g)	135	0	213

CUTTLEFISH
steamed	3 oz	134	—	190

DANDELION GREENS
fresh cooked	½ cup	17	—	0
raw chopped	½ cup	13	—	0

DANISH PASTRY
FOOD	PORTION	CALS.	FIB.	CHOL.
FROZEN				
Sara Lee				
Apple Free & Light	1 slice (2 oz)	130	—	0
Apple Danish Twist	1 slice (1.9 oz)	190	—	10
Cheese Danish Twist	1 slice (1.9 oz)	200	—	15
Raspberry Danish Twist	1 slice (1.9 oz)	200	—	15
READY-TO-EAT				
Hostess				
Apple	1 (3.8 oz)	400	2	20
Apple Fruit Roll	1 (2 oz)	180	1	<5
Coffee Cake Raspberry	1 (1.2 oz)	110	tr	<5
almond	1 (4¼ in diam) (2.3 oz)	280	2	30
cheese	1 (3 oz)	353	—	20
cinnamon	1 (3 oz)	349	—	28
cinnamon nut	1 (4¼ in diam) (2.3 oz)	280	2	30
fruit	1 (3.3 oz)	335	—	19

FOOD	PORTION	CALS.	FIB.	CHOL.
plain ring	1 (12 oz)	1305	—	292
raisin nut	1 (4¼ in diam) (2.3 oz)	280	2	30

REFRIGERATED
Pillsbury

Caramel Danish w/ Nuts	1	160	—	0
Cinnamon Raisin Danish w/ Icing	1	150	—	0
Orange Danish w/ Icing	1	150	—	0

DATES
DRIED
Bordo

Diced	2 oz	203	—	0
Dole				
Chopped	½ cup	230	—	0
Pitted	½ cup	280	—	0
Dromedary				
Chopped	¼ cup	130	—	0
Pitted	5	100	—	0
California Deglet Noor	10	240	—	0
chopped	1 cup	489	—	0
whole	10	228	—	0

DEER
(*see* VENISON)

DIETING AIDS
(*see* NUTRITIONAL SUPPLEMENTS)

DILL
Watkins

Liquid Spice	1 tbsp (0.5 oz)	120	0	0
seed	1 tsp	6	—	0
sprigs fresh	5	0	—	0
sprigs fresh	1 cup	4	—	0
weed dry	1 tsp	3	—	0

DINNER
(*see also* BEEF DISHES, PASTA DINNERS, POT PIES, ORIENTAL FOOD,
SPANISH FOODS, VEAL DISHES)
FROZEN
Armour

Classics Chicken Fettucini	11 oz	260	—	50
Classics Chicken Parmigiana	11.5 oz	370	—	75
Classics Chicken & Noodles	11 oz	230	—	50

FOOD	PORTION	CALS.	FIB.	CHOL.
Armour (CONT.)				
Classics Chicken Mesquite	9.5 oz	370	—	55
Classics Chicken w/ Wine & Mushroom Sauce	10.75 oz	280	—	50
Classics Glazed Chicken	10.75 oz	300	—	60
Classics Meat Loaf	11.25 oz	360	—	65
Classics Salisbury Parmigiana	11.5 oz	410	—	60
Classics Salisbury Steak	11.25 oz	350	—	55
Classics Swedish Meatballs	11.25 oz	330	—	80
Classics Turkey w/ Dressing & Gravy	11.5 oz	320	—	50
Classics Veal Parmigiana	11.25 oz	400	—	55
Lite Beef Pepper Steak	11.25 oz	220	—	35
Lite Beef Stroganoff	11.25 oz	250	—	55
Lite Chicken Marsala	10.5 oz	250	—	80
Lite Chicken Ala King	11.25 oz	290	—	55
Lite Chicken Burgundy	10 oz	210	—	45
Lite Chicken Oriental	10 oz	180	—	35
Lite Salisbury Steak	11.5 oz	300	—	40
Lite Shrimp Creole	11.25 oz	260	—	45
Lite Sweet & Sour Chicken	11 oz	240	—	35
Banquet				
Beans & Frankfurters	10 oz	350	—	25
Chicken & Dumplings	10 oz	270	—	30
Chicken w/ Noodles	9 oz	240	—	50
Extra Helping Beef Dinner	15.5 oz	430	—	100
Extra Helping Chicken Nuggets & Barbecue Sauce	10 oz	540	—	80
Extra Helping Chicken Nuggets & Sweet & Sour Sauce	10 oz	540	—	80
Extra Helping Fried Chicken	14.25 oz	790	—	150
Extra Helping Fried Chicken All White Meat	14.25 oz	760	—	120
Extra Helping Meat Loaf	16.25 oz	640	—	85
Extra Helping Mexican Style Dinner	19 oz	680	—	5
Extra Helping Salisbury Steak	16.25 oz	590	—	85
Extra Helping Southern Fried Chicken	13.25 oz	790	—	135
Extra Helping Turkey Dinner	17 oz	460	—	70
Fried Chicken	9 oz	520	—	90
Italian Style Dinner	9 oz	180	—	5
Meat Loaf	9.5 oz	340	—	35
Mexican Style Combination Dinner	11 oz	360	—	15

FOOD	PORTION	CALS.	FIB.	CHOL.
Banquet (CONT.)				
Mexican-Style Dinner	11 oz	410	—	20
Platter Beef	9 oz	230	—	55
Platter Boneless Chicken Drumsnacker	7 oz	290	—	45
Platter Boneless Chicken Nugget	6 oz	340	—	40
Platter Boneless Chicken Pattie	6.75 oz	310	—	50
Platter Fish	8 oz	270	—	30
Platter Ham	8.25 oz	200	—	35
Salisbury Steak	9 oz	280	—	25
Southern Fried Chicken Platter	8.75 oz	400	—	80
Veal Parmagian	9.25 oz	330	—	25
Western Style Dinner	9 oz	300	—	30
White Meat Fried Chicken Platter	8.75 oz	390	—	80
White Meat Hot'n Spicy Fried Chicken Platter	9 oz	440	—	80
Birds Eye				
Easy Recipe Beef Burgundy not prep	½ pkg	120	4	0
Easy Recipe Beef Fajitas not prep	½ pkg	80	3	0
Budget Gourmet				
Beef Cantonese	1 pkg (9.1 oz)	270	—	40
Beef Stroganoff	1 pkg (8.75 oz)	260	—	50
Chicken And Egg Noodles	1 pkg (10 oz)	440	—	90
Chicken Au Gratin	1 pkg (9.1 oz)	230	—	40
Chicken Breast Parmigiana	1 pkg (11 oz)	270	—	50
Chicken Marsala	1 pkg (9 oz)	260	—	90
Chicken With Fettucini	1 pkg (10 oz)	400	—	85
Chinese Style Vegetables & Chicken	1 pkg (10 oz)	280	—	10
French Recipe Chicken	1 pkg (10 oz)	220	—	40
Glazed Turkey	1 pkg (9 oz)	260	—	30
Ham & Asparagus Au Gratin	1 pkg (8.7 oz)	300	—	50
Herbed Chicken Breast With Fettucini	1 pkg (11 oz)	240	—	45
Italian Style Vegetables & Chicken	1 pkg (10.25 oz)	310	—	30
Mandarin Chicken	1 pkg (10 oz)	240	—	40
Mesquite Chicken Breast	1 pkg (11 oz)	250	—	40
Orange Glazed Chicken	1 pkg (9 oz)	270	—	25
Oriental Beef	1 pkg (10 oz)	290	—	30

FOOD	PORTION	CALS.	FIB.	CHOL.
Budget Gourmet (CONT.)				
Oriental Chicken With Vegetables	1 pkg (9 oz)	280	—	20
Pepper Steak With Rice	1 pkg (10 oz)	300	—	35
Pot Roast Beef	1 pkg (10.5 oz)	230	—	60
Roast Chicken With Homestyle Gravy	1 pkg (11 oz)	280	—	35
Roast Sirloin Supreme	1 pkg (9 oz)	320	—	85
Sirloin Salisbury Steak	1 pkg (9 oz)	220	—	25
Sirloin Salisbury Steak	1 pkg (11 oz)	280	—	40
Sirloin Cheddar Melt	1 pkg (9.4 oz)	380	—	85
Sirloin Of Beef In Herb Sauce	1 pkg (9.5 oz)	250	—	30
Sirloin Of Beef In Wine Sauce	1 pkg (11 oz)	280	—	25
Sirloin Tips And Country Vegetables	1 pkg (10 oz)	290	—	40
Special Recipe Sirloin Of Beef	1 pkg (11 oz)	250	—	60
Stuffed Turkey Breast	1 pkg (11 oz)	250	—	35
Swedish Meatballs With Noodles	1 pkg (10 oz)	590	—	145
Sweet And Sour Chicken	1 pkg (10 oz)	340	—	30
Teriyaki Beef	1 pkg (10.75 oz)	260	—	30
Teriyaki Chicken Breast	1 pkg (11 oz)	300	—	30
Dining Light				
Chicken Ala King	9 oz	240	—	40
Salisbury Steak	9 oz	200	—	55
Sauce & Swedish Meatballs	9 oz	280	—	55
Healthy Choice				
Beef & Peppers Cantonese	1 meal (11.5 oz)	270	5	35
Beef Pepper Steak Oriental	1 meal (9.5 oz)	250	3	35
Beef Tips Francais	1 meal (9.5 oz)	280	4	30
Beef Tips With Sauce	1 meal (11 oz)	290	5	40
Chicken Cantonese	1 meal (11.25 oz)	210	5	30
Chicken Parmigiana	1 meal (11.5 oz)	300	6	35
Chicken & Vegetables Marsala	1 meal (11.5 oz)	220	3	30
Chicken Bangkok	1 meal (9.5 oz)	270	5	45
Chicken Broccoli Alfredo	1 meal (12.1 oz)	370	6	45
Chicken Dijon	1 meal (11 oz)	280	9	30
Chicken Imperial	1 meal (9 oz)	230	3	40
Chicken Picante	1 meal (11.25 oz)	220	6	35
Chicken Teriyaki	1 meal (12.25 oz)	270	5	40
Classics Beef Broccoli Beijing	1 meal (12 oz)	330	5	20
Classics Cacciatore Chicken	1 meal (12.5 oz)	260	6	25
Classics Chicken Fransesca	1 meal (12.5 oz)	360	5	30
Classics Country Inn Roast Turkey	1 meal (10 oz)	250	6	30

FOOD	PORTION	CALS.	FIB.	CHOL.
Healthy Choice (CONT.)				
Classics Ginger Chicken Hunan	1 meal (12.6 oz)	350	5	25
Classics Mesquite Beef Barbecue	1 meal (11 oz)	310	6	45
Classics Salisbury Steak	1 meal (11 oz)	260	5	30
Classics Sesame Chicken Shanghai	1 meal (12 oz)	310	5	30
Classics Shrimp & Vegetables Maria	1 meal (12.5 oz)	260	5	35
Country Glazed Chicken	1 meal (8.5 oz)	200	3	30
Country Herb Chicken	1 meal (11.5 oz)	270	6	35
Country Roast Turkey With Mushroom	1 meal (8.5 oz)	220	3	25
Country Turkey & Pasta	1 meal (12.6 oz)	300	6	35
Homestyle Turkey With Vegetables	1 meal (9.5 oz)	260	3	35
Honey Mustard Chicken	1 meal (9.5 oz)	260	4	30
Lemon Pepper Fish	1 meal (10.7 oz)	290	7	25
Mandarin Chicken	1 meal (10 oz)	280	4	25
Mesquite Chicken BBQ	1 meal (10.5 oz)	320	6	35
Shrimp Marinara	1 meal (10.5 oz)	220	5	50
Smoky Chicken Barbecue	1 meal (12.75 oz)	380	7	50
Southwestern Glazed Chicken	1 meal (12.5 oz)	300	6	45
Sweet & Sour Chicken	1 meal (11.5 oz)	310	5	50
Traditional Breast Of Turkey	1 meal (10.5 oz)	280	7	45
Traditional Meatloaf	1 meal (12 oz)	320	7	35
Traditional Beef Tips	1 meal (11.25 oz)	260	6	40
Tradtional Salisbury Steak	1 meal (11.5 oz)	320	7	45
Yankee Pot Roast	1 meal (11 oz)	280	5	45
Kid Cuisine				
Chicken Sandwiches	8.2 oz	470	—	40
Chicken Nuggets	6.8 oz	360	—	55
Fish Sticks	7 oz	360	—	35
Fried Chicken	7.5 oz	430	—	85
Hot Dogs w/ Buns	6.7 oz	450	—	40
Mexican Style	5.7 oz	290	—	20
Le Menu				
Entree LightStyle Chicken A La King	8¼ oz	240	—	30
Entree LightStyle Chicken Dijon	8 oz	240	—	40
Entree LightStyle Empress Chicken	8¼ oz	210	—	30
Entree LightStyle Glazed Turkey	8¼ oz	260	—	35
Entree LightStyle Herb Roast Chicken	7¾ oz	260	—	45

FOOD	PORTION	CALS.	FIB.	CHOL.
Le Menu (CONT.)				
Entree LightStyle Swedish Meatballs	8 oz	260	—	40
Entree LightStyle Traditional Turkey	8 oz	200	—	25
LightStyle Glazed Chicken Breast	10 oz	230	—	55
LightStyle Herb Roasted Chicken	10 oz	240	—	70
LightStyle Salisbury Steak	10 oz	280	—	35
LightStyle Sliced Turkey	10 oz	210	—	30
LightStyle Turkey Divan	10 oz	260	—	60
LightStyle Veal Marsala	10 oz	230	—	75
Lean Cuisine				
Baked Chicken	1 pkg (8 oz)	240	3	35
Beef Pot Roast	1 pkg (9 oz)	210	3	40
Chicken Italiano	1 pkg (9 oz)	270	3	40
Chicken & Vegetables	1 pkg (10.5 oz)	240	5	35
Chicken A L'Orange	1 pkg (8 oz)	260	1	40
Chicken In Peanut Sauce	1 pkg (9 oz)	280	3	45
Chicken In Honey Barbecue Sauce	1 pkg (8.75 oz)	250	6	50
Chicken Marsala	1 pkg (8.1 oz)	180	5	60
Chicken Oriental	1 pkg (9 oz)	260	3	30
Chicken Parmesan	1 pkg (10.9 oz)	220	5	50
Chicken Pie	1 pkg (9.5 oz)	320	3	35
Fiesta Chicken	1 pkg (8.5 oz)	240	3	45
Fish Divan	1 pkg (10.4 oz)	210	3	65
Glazed Chicken	1 pkg (8.5 oz)	240	2	60
Homestyle Turkey	1 pkg (9.4 oz)	230	3	50
Honey Mustard Chicken	1 pkg (7.5 oz)	250	4	32
Meatloaf	1 pkg (9.4 oz)	270	4	55
Oriental Beef	1 pkg (9 oz)	250	4	30
Roasted Turkey Breast	1 pkg (9.75 oz)	290	3	25
Salisbury Steak With Macaroni & Cheese	1 pkg (9.5 oz)	200	2	60
Stuffed Cabbage	1 pkg (9.5 oz)	220	5	25
Swedish Meatballs	1 pkg (9.1 oz)	290	3	55
Sweet & Sour Chicken	1 pkg (10.4 oz)	260	3	45
Turkey Pie	1 pkg (9.5 oz)	300	3	50
Morton				
Beans & Franks w/ Sauce	8.5 oz	300	—	25
Fish w/ Mashed Potatoes & Carrots	9.25 oz	350	—	65

FOOD	PORTION	CALS.	FIB.	CHOL.
Morton (CONT.)				
Glazed Ham	8 oz	230	—	35
Gravy & Charbroiled Beef Patty	9 oz	270	—	30
Gravy & Salisbury Steak	9 oz	270	—	35
Tomato Sauce & Meatloaf	9 oz	280	—	45
Veal Parmigiana	8.75 oz	230	—	30
Stouffer's				
Chicken A La King	1 pkg (9.5 oz)	320	3	55
Chicken Divan	1 pkg (8 oz)	210	1	65
Creamed Chicken	1 pkg (6.5 oz)	280	1	80
Creamed Chipped Beef	½ cup (4.5 oz)	150	1	40
Creamed Chipped Beef Over Country Biscuit	1 pkg (9 oz)	460	3	70
Escalloped Chicken & Noodles	1 pkg (10 oz)	440	2	80
Green Pepper Steak	1 pkg (10.5 oz)	330	3	35
Ham & Asparagus Bake	1 pkg (9.5 oz)	520	2	75
Homestyle Beef Pot Raost	1 pkg (8.9 oz)	270	4	40
Homestyle Breaded Chicken Tenders	1 pkg (6.6 oz)	380	4	50
Homestyle Chicken Parmigiana	1 pkg (10.9 oz)	320	4	75
Homestyle Chicken & Noodles	1 pkg (10 oz)	310	2	80
Homestyle Chicken Monterey	1 pkg (9.4 oz)	410	4	75
Homestyle Fish Filet With Macaroni & Cheese	1 pkg (9 oz)	430	2	70
Homestyle Fried Chicken	1 pkg (7.1 oz)	330	3	55
Homestyle Meatloaf	1 pkg (9.9 oz)	380	3	80
Homestyle Roast Turkey	1 pkg (7.9 oz)	280	1	40
Homestyle Salisbury Steak	1 pkg (9.6 oz)	370	—	50
Homestyle Sliced Beef & Potatoes	1 pkg (8.1 oz)	270	2	45
Homestyle Veal Parmigiana	1 pkg (11.9 oz)	420	6	75
Homestyle Baked Chicken	1 pkg (8.9 oz)	270	2	75
Lunch Express Chicken With Garden Vegetables	1 pkg (9.9 oz)	340	2	30
Lunch Express Mandarin Chicken	1 pkg (9.75 oz)	270	2	30
Lunch Express Mexican Style Rice With Chicken	1 pkg (9 oz)	270	3	20
Lunch Express Oriental Beef	1 pkg (6.2 oz)	260	4	20
Lunch Express Stir-Fry Rice & Chicken	1 pkg (9 oz)	280	3	15
Stuffed Pepper	1 pkg (10 oz)	200	1	25
Swedish Meatballs	1 pkg (9.25 oz)	440	3	85
Tyson				
Beef Champignon	1 pkg (10.5 oz)	370	—	51

FOOD	PORTION	CALS.	FIB.	CHOL.
Tyson (CONT.)				
Chicken Picante	1 pkg (9 oz)	250	—	50
Chicken Supreme	1 pkg (9 oz)	230	—	51
Francais	1 pkg (9.5 oz)	280	—	54
Glazed Chicken With Sauce	1 pkg (9.25 oz)	240	—	44
Grilled Chicken	1 pkg (7.75 oz)	220	—	55
Grilled Italian Chicken	1 pkg (9 oz)	210	—	40
Healthy Portions BBQ Chicken	1 pkg (12.5 oz)	400	—	50
Healthy Portions Chicken Marinara	1 pkg (13.75 oz)	340	—	45
Healthy Portions Herb Chicken	1 pkg (13.75 oz)	340	—	50
Healthy Portions Italian Style Chicken	1 pkg (13.75 oz)	310	—	50
Healthy Portions Mesquite Chicken	1 pkg (13.25 oz)	330	—	45
Healthy Portions Salsa Chicken	1 pkg (13.75 oz)	370	—	45
Healthy Portions Sesame Chicken	1 pkg (13.5 oz)	400	—	45
Honey Roasted Chicken	1 pkg (9 oz)	220	—	48
Kiev	1 pkg (9.25 oz)	450	—	78
Marsala	1 pkg (9 oz)	200	—	52
Mexquite	1 pkg (9 oz)	320	—	55
Picatta	1 pkg (9 oz)	200	—	60
Roasted Chicken	1 pkg (9 oz)	200	—	42
Turkey With Gravy	1 pkg (9.5 oz)	320	—	35
Ultra Slim-Fast				
Beef Pepper Steak	12 oz	270	0	45
Chicken Fettucini	12 oz	380	1	65
Chicken & Vegetable	12 oz	290	4	30
Country Style Vegetable & Beef Tips	12 oz	230	4	45
Mesquite Chicken	12 oz	360	5	65
Roasted Chicken In Mushroom Sauce	12 oz	280	0	55
Shrimp Creole	12 oz	240	5	80
Shrimp Marinara	12 oz	290	0	70
Sweet & Sour Chicken	12 oz	330	0	45
Turkey Medallions In Herb Sauce	12 oz	280	0	40
Weight Watchers				
Barbecue Glazed Chicken	7 oz	200	—	30
Beef Sirloin Tips	7.5 oz	210	—	30
Beef Stroganoff	8.5 oz	280	—	30
Chicken Ala King	9 oz	230	—	30

FOOD	PORTION	CALS.	FIB.	CHOL.
Weight Watchers (CONT.)				
Chicken Cordon Bleu	7.7 oz	170	—	50
Chicken Kiev	7 oz	190	—	15
Homestyle Chicken & Noodles	9 oz	240	—	30
Imperial Chicken	8.5 oz	210	—	25
London Broil	7.5 oz	110	—	25
Oven Baked Fish	7 oz	150	—	10
Southern Baked Chicken	6.3 oz	170	—	45
Stuffed Turkey Breast	8.5 oz	270	—	60
Veal Patty Parmigiana	8.2 oz	150	—	50
SHELF-STABLE				
My Own Meal				
Chicken Mediterranean	1 pkg (10 oz)	270	4	45
Chicken Noodles	1 pkg (10 oz)	270	3	65
Chicken & Black Beans	1 pkg (10 oz)	240	6	40
Old World Stew	1 pkg (10 oz)	310	3	55
DIP				
Breakstone				
Sour Cream Bacon & Onion	2 tbsp (1.1 oz)	60	0	20
Sour Cream Chesapeake Clam	2 tbsp (1.1 oz)	50	0	30
Sour Cream French Onion	2 tbsp (1.1 oz)	50	0	20
Sour Cream Jalapeno Cheddar	2 tbsp (1.1 oz)	60	0	15
Sour Cream Toasted Onion	2 tbsp (1.1 oz)	50	0	20
Chi-Chi's				
Fiesta Bean	2 tbsp (0.9 oz)	35	1	0
Fiesta Cheese	2 tbsp (0.9 oz)	40	1	10
Eagle				
Bean	1 oz	35	—	0
Frito Lay				
Cheddar Cheese	1 oz	45	—	6
French Onion	1 oz	50	—	12
Jalapeno Bean	1 oz	30	—	0
Picante Sauce	1 oz	10	—	0
Guiltless Gourmet				
Black Bean Mild	1 oz	25	1	0
Black Bean Spicy	1 oz	25	1	0
Pinto Bean	1 oz	25	1	0
Hain				
Hot Bean	4 tbsp	70	—	5
Mexican Bean	4 tbsp	60	—	5
Onion Bean	4 tbsp	70	—	5
Taco Dip & Sauce	4 tbsp	25	—	5
Heluva Good Cheese				
Bacon Horseradish	2 tbsp (1.1 oz)	60	0	20

FOOD	PORTION	CALS.	FIB.	CHOL.
Heluva Good Cheese (CONT.)				
Clam	2 tbsp (1.1 oz)	50	0	20
French Onion	2 tbsp (1.1 oz)	50	0	20
Homestyle Onion	2 tbsp (1.1 oz)	60	0	20
Light French Onion	2 tbsp (1.1 oz)	35	0	10
Light Jalapeno Cheddar	2 tbsp (1.1 oz)	40	0	10
Ranch	2 tbsp (1.1 oz)	60	0	20
Knudsen				
Nacho Cheese	2 tbsp (1.1 oz)	60	0	15
Sour Cream Bacon & Onion	2 tbsp (1.1 oz)	60	0	20
Sour Cream French Onion	2 tbsp (1.1 oz)	50	0	20
Kraft				
Avocado	2 tbsp (1.1 oz)	60	0	0
Bacon & Horseradish	2 tbsp (1.1 oz)	60	0	0
Clam	2 tbsp (1.1 oz)	60	0	0
French Onion	2 tbsp (1.1 oz)	60	0	0
Green Onion	2 tbsp (1.1 oz)	60	0	0
Jalapeno	2 tbsp (1.1 oz)	60	0	0
Jalapeno Cheese	2 tbsp (1.1 oz)	60	0	15
Premium Bacon & Horseradish	2 tbsp (1.1 oz)	50	0	15
Premium Bacon & Onion	2 tbsp (1.1 oz)	60	0	15
Premium Blue Cheese	2 tbsp (1.1 oz)	45	0	10
Premium Clam	2 tbsp (1.1 oz)	45	0	10
Premium Creamy Cucumber	2 tbsp (1.1 oz)	50	0	15
Premium Creamy Onion	2 tbsp (1.1 oz)	45	0	10
Premium French Onion	2 tbsp (1.1 oz)	50	0	10
Premium Nacho Cheese	2 tbsp (1.1 oz)	60	0	15
Ranch	2 tbsp (1.1 oz)	60	0	0
Louise's				
Fat Free Honey Mustard	1 oz	40	0	0
Fat Free Sour Cream & Onion	1 oz	25	0	0
Fat Free White Cheese Peppercorn	1 oz	25	0	0
Marzetti				
Blue Cheese Veggie	2 tbsp	200	0	20
Lemon Dill Veggie	2 tbsp	140	0	25
Light Ranch Veggie	2 tbsp	60	1	10
Ranch Veggie	2 tbsp	140	0	10
Sour Cream & Onion	2 tbsp	130	0	25
Southwestern Veggie	2 tbsp	130	0	25
Spinach Veggie	2 tbsp	130	0	20
Old El Paso				
Chunky Salsa Medium	2 tbsp	10	1	0
Chunky Salsa Mild	2 tbsp	10	1	0

FOOD	PORTION	CALS.	FIB.	CHOL.
Old El Paso (CONT.)				
Jalapeno Bean Mild	1 tbsp	14	1	0
Sealtest				
French Onion	2 tbsp (1.1 oz)	50	0	20
Snyder's				
Mustard Pretzel	2 tbsp (1.2 oz)	90	1	20
Wise				
Jalapeno Bean	2 tbsp	25	—	0
Taco	2 tbsp	12	—	0
DOCK				
fresh cooked	3½ oz	20	—	0
raw chopped	½ cup	15	—	0
DOGFISH				
raw	3½ oz	193	—	74
DOLPHINFISH				
fresh baked	3 oz	93	—	80
fresh fillet baked	5.6 oz	174	—	149
DOUGHNUTS				
(*see also* DUNKIN' DONUTS, WINCHELL'S)				
Drake's				
Old Fashion Donuts	1 (1.7 oz)	182	—	10
Powdered Sugar Donut Delites	7 (2.5 oz)	300	—	16
Dutch Mill				
Cider	1 (2.1 oz)	240	1	15
Cinnamon	1 (1.8 oz)	210	1	15
Donut Holes Double-Dipped Chocolate	3 (1.4 oz)	220	0	5
Donut Holes Shootin' Stars	3 (1.4 oz)	190	0	5
Double-Dipped Chocolate	1 (2.1 oz)	280	1	15
Glazed	1 (2.1 oz)	250	0	15
Glazed Chocolate	1 (2.4 oz)	270	1	15
Plain	1 (1.8 oz)	210	1	15
Sugared	1 (1.8 oz)	220	1	15
Earth Grains				
Cinnamon Apple	1	310	—	25
Devil's Food	1	330	—	20
Glazed Old Fashioned	1	310	—	20
Powdered Old Fashioned	1	290	—	20
Freihofer's				
Assorted	1 (2 oz)	270	0	10
Hostess				
Assorted Regular	1 (1.6 oz)	200	tr	10

FOOD	PORTION	CALS.	FIB.	CHOL.
Hostess (CONT.)				
Cinnamon Family Pack	1 (1 oz)	110	tr	5
Cinnamon Swirl	1 (1.6 oz)	180	tr	<5
Crumb Regular	1 (1 oz)	130	tr	5
Frosted Regular	1 (1.4 oz)	180	1	5
Gem Donettes Cinnamon	6 (3 oz)	320	1	10
Gem Donettes Frosted	6 (3 oz)	390	2	10
Gem Donettes Frosted Strawberry Filled	3 (3 oz)	240	1	<5
Gem Donettes Powdered	6 (3 oz)	350	1	10
Gem Donettes Powdered Strawberry Filled	3 (3 oz)	210	tr	<5
Glazed Party	1 (2.3 oz)	260	1	5
Jumbo Frosted	1 (2 oz)	260	1	10
Jumbo Plain	1 (1.1 oz)	140	tr	10
Jumbo Powdered	1 (1.3 oz)	160	tr	5
Mini Chocolate	5 (2 oz)	220	1	35
O's Raspberry Filled Powdered	1 (2.2 oz)	230	tr	5
Old Fashioned Glazed	1 (2.1 oz)	250	tr	15
Old Fashioned Glazed Honey Wheat	1 (2.1 oz)	250	1	25
Old Fashioned Plain	1 (1.5 oz)	170	tr	10
Plain Regular	1 (1 oz)	120	tr	5
Powdered Family Pack	1 (1 oz)	110	1	5
Little Debbie				
Donut Sticks	1 pkg (3 oz)	390	1	10
Donut Sticks	1 pkg (2 oz)	250	1	5
Donut Sticks	1 pkg (2.5 oz)	320	1	10
Donut Sticks	1 pkg (1.6 oz)	210	1	5
Tastykake				
Cinnamon	1 (47 g)	180	1	10
Frosted Rich	1 (57 g)	260	3	10
Frosted Rich Mini	1 (14 g)	44	1	5
Honey Wheat	1 (57 g)	210	1	10
Honey Wheat Mini	1 (12 g)	40	0	5
Orange Glazed	1 (57 g)	210	1	10
Plain	1 (47 g)	190	1	10
Powdered Sugar	1 (46 g)	180	1	24
Powdered Sugar Mini	1 (12 g)	40	0	5
cake type unsugared	1 (1.6 oz)	198	1	18
creme filled	1 (3 oz)	307	—	20
french cruller glazed	1 (1.4 oz)	169	—	5
honey bun	1 (2.1 oz)	242	1	4
jelly	1 (3 oz)	289	—	22

FOOD	PORTION	CALS.	FIB.	CHOL.
old fashioned	1 (1.6 oz)	198	1	18
sugared	1 (1.6 oz)	192	1	14
wheat glazed	1 (1.6 oz)	162	—	9
wheat sugared	1 (1.6 oz)	162	—	9
yeast glazed	1 (2.1 oz)	242	1	4

DRESSING
(*see* STUFFING/DRESSING)

DRINK MIXERS
(*see also* SODA, MINERAL/BOTTLED WATER)

Bacardi

Margarita Mix w/o liquor	8 fl oz	100	—	0
Pina Colada	8 fl oz	140	—	0
Rum Runner	8 fl oz	140	—	0
Strawberry Daiquiri w/o liquor	8 fl oz	140	—	0

Canada Dry

Collins Mixer	8 fl oz	120	0	0
Sour Mixer	8 fl oz	90	0	0

Libby

Bloody Mary Mix	6 oz	40	—	0

McIlhenny

Tabasco Bloody Mary Mix	8 fl oz	56	1	0

Schweppes

Collins Mixer	8 fl oz	100	0	0

Tabasco

Bloody Mary Mix Extra Spicy	8 fl oz	58	2	0
whiskey sour mix	2 oz	55	—	0
whiskey sour mix as prep	3.6 oz	169	—	0

DRUM

freshwater fillet baked	5.4 oz	236	—	126
freshwater baked	3 oz	130	—	70

DUCK
FRESH

w/ skin roasted	½ duck (13.4 oz)	1287	—	320
w/ skin roasted	6 oz	583	—	145
w/o skin roasted	3.5 oz	201	—	89
w/o skin roasted	½ duck (7.8 oz)	445	—	198
wild w/ skin raw	½ duck (9.5 oz)	571	—	216

DURIAN

fresh	3½ oz	141	—	0

EEL

fresh cooked	1 fillet (5.6 oz)	375	—	257

FOOD	PORTION	CALS.	FIB.	CHOL.
fresh cooked	3 oz	200	—	137
raw	3 oz	156	—	107

EGG
(see also EGG DISHES, EGG SUBSTITUTES)
CHICKEN

fried w/ margarine	1	91	—	211
frozen	1 cup	363	—	1033
frozen	1	75	—	213
hard cooked	1	77	—	213
hard cooked chopped	1 cup	210	—	578
poached	1	74	—	212
raw	1	75	—	213
scrambled plain	2	200	—	400
scrambled w/ whole milk & margarine	1 cup	365	—	774
scrambled w/ whole milk & margarine	1	101	—	215
white only	1 cup	121	—	0
white only	1	17	—	0

OTHER POULTRY

duck raw	1	130	—	619
quail raw	1	14	—	76
turkey raw	1	135	—	737

EGG DISHES
FROZEN
Chefwich

Cheese Omelet	5 oz	380	—	130
Ham & Cheese Omelet	5 oz	340	—	140
Sausage & Cheese Omelet	5 oz	400	—	130
Western Style Omelet	5 oz	350	—	100

Quaker

Scrambled Eggs Cheddar Cheese & Fried Potatoes	1 pkg (5.9 oz)	250	—	176
Scrambled Eggs & Sausage With Hash Browns	1 pkg (5.7 oz)	290	—	212
Scrambled Eggs & Sausage With Pancakes	1 pkg (5.2 oz)	270	—	180

TAKE-OUT

deviled	2 halves	145	—	280
salad	½ cup	307	—	562
sandwich w/ cheese	1	340	—	291
sandwich w/ cheese & ham	1	348	—	245

FOOD	PORTION	CALS.	FIB.	CHOL.
EGG SUBSTITUTES				
Egg Beaters				
Omelette Cheese	¼ cup	25	0	0
Omelette Cheese	½ cup	110	—	5
Omelette Vegetable	½ cup	50	—	0
Egg Watchers	2 oz	50	—	0
Healthy Choice				
Cholesterol Free	¼ cup (2 oz)	25	0	0
Second Nature				
No Cholesterol	2 fl oz	60	—	0
No Fat	2 fl oz	40	—	0
No Fat With Garden Vegetables	2.5 fl oz	40	—	0
Simply Eggs	1.75 fl oz	35	1	30
frozen	1 cup	384	—	5
frozen	¼ cup	96	—	1
liquid	1 cup	211	—	3
liquid	1½ oz	40	—	tr
powder	0.7 oz	88	—	113
powder	0.35 oz	44	—	57
EGGNOG				
Hood				
Fat Free	4 fl oz	100	0	<5
Golden	4 fl oz	180	0	65
Light	4 fl oz	120	0	40
Select	4 fl oz	210	0	80
eggnog	1 qt	1368	—	596
eggnog	1 cup	342	—	149
eggnog flavor mix as prep w/ milk	9 oz	260	—	33
EGGPLANT				
CANNED				
Progresso				
Caponata	2 tbsp (1 oz)	30	2	0
FRESH				
cubed cooked	½ cup	13	—	0
raw cut up	½ cup (1.4 oz)	11	—	0
slices, cooked	4 (7 oz)	38	—	0
whole peeled raw	1 (1 lb)	117	—	0
FROZEN				
Mrs. Paul's				
Parmigiana	5 oz	240	—	15
TAKE-OUT				
baba ghannouj	¼ cup	55	—	0
ELDERBERRIES				
fresh	1 cup	105	—	0

FOOD	PORTION	CALS.	FIB.	CHOL.
ELDERBERRY JUICE				
elderberry	3½ oz	38	—	0
ELK				
roasted	3 oz	124	—	62
ENDIVE				
fresh	3½ oz	9	2	0
raw chopped	½ cup	4	—	0
ENGLISH MUFFIN				
FROZEN				
Weight Watchers				
Sandwich With Egg Ham & Cheese	1 (4 oz)	230	—	160
HOME RECIPE				
cinnamon raisin	1	186	—	0
english muffin	1	158	—	0
honey bran	1	153	—	0
whole wheat	1	167	—	1
READY-TO-EAT				
Arnold				
Extra Crisp	1	130	1	0
Sourdough	1	130	1	0
Matthew's				
9 Grain & Nut	1	140	5	0
Cinnamon Raisin	1	160	4	0
Golden White	1	140	1	0
Whole Wheat	1	150	4	0
Pepperidge Farm				
Cinnamon Apple	1	140	—	0
Cinnamon Chip	1	160	—	0
Cinnamon Raisin	1	150	—	0
Plain	1	140	—	0
Sourdough	1	135	—	0
Roman Meal	1 (2.2 oz)	135	3	0
Tastykake	1 (57 g)	130	—	0
Cinnamon Raisin	1 (64 g)	150	—	0
Sourdough	1 (57 g)	130	—	0
Thomas'				
Oat Bran	1	116	3	0
Sandwich Size	1 (92 g)	210	2	0
Wonder	1 (2 oz)	120	1	0
Raisin Rounds	1 (2.1 oz)	150	2	0
Sourdough	1 (2 oz)	120	1	0

FOOD	PORTION	CALS.	FIB.	CHOL.
apple cinnamon	1	138	—	0
granola	1	155	—	0
mixed grain	1	155	—	0
plain	1	134	—	0
plain toasted	1	133	—	0
raisin cinnamon	1	138	—	0
sourdough	1	134	—	0
wheat	1	127	—	0
whole wheat	1	134	4	0
REFRIGERATED				
Roman Meal	½ muffin (1.1 oz)	66	1	0
Honey Nut Oat Bran	½ muffin (1.1 oz)	81	1	0
TAKE-OUT				
w/ butter	1	189	—	13
w/ cheese & sausage	1	394	—	58
w/ egg cheese & bacon	1	487	—	274
w/ egg cheese & canadian bacon	1	383	—	234

EPPAW

FOOD	PORTION	CALS.	FIB.	CHOL.
raw	½ cup	75	—	0

FALAFEL

FOOD	PORTION	CALS.	FIB.	CHOL.
MIX				
Casbah				
as prep	5	130	2	0
Near East				
as prep	2½ patties	230	5	0
TAKE-OUT				
falafel	3 (1.8 oz)	170	—	0
falafel	1 (1.2 oz)	57	—	0

FAST FOODS

(see individual names)

FAT

(see also BUTTER, BUTTER BLENDS, BUTTER SUBSTITUTES, MARGARINE, OIL)

FOOD	PORTION	CALS.	FIB.	CHOL.
Crisco	1 tbsp	110	—	0
Butter Flavor	1 tbsp	110	—	0
Sticks	1 tbsp (0.4 oz)	110	0	0
Sticks Butter Flavor	1 tbsp (0.4 oz)	110	0	0
Empire				
Chicken Fat Rendered	1 tbsp (0.5 oz)	120	0	10
Wesson				
Shortening	1 tbsp	100	0	0
beef cooked	1 oz	193	—	27

FOOD	PORTION	CALS.	FIB.	CHOL.
beef suet	1 oz	242	—	19
beef tallow	1 tbsp (13 g)	115	—	14
chicken	1 tbsp	115	—	11
chicken	1 cup	1846	—	174
cocoa butter	1 tbsp	120	—	0
duck	1 tbsp	115	—	13
goose	1 tbsp	115	—	13
lamb new zealand raw	1 oz	182	—	25
lard	1 tbsp (13 g)	115	—	12
lard	1 cup (205 g)	1849	—	195
pork backfat	1 oz	230	—	16
pork cured	1 oz	164	—	19
pork cured roasted	1 oz	167	—	24
pork, cooked	1 oz	200	—	26
salt pork	1 oz	212	—	25
shortening	1 cup	1812	—	0
shortening	1 tbsp	113	—	0
turkey	1 tbsp	115	—	13

FEIJOA

fresh	1 (1.75 oz)	25	—	0
puree	1 cup	119	—	0

FENNEL

fresh bulb	1 (8.2 oz)	72	—	0
fresh sliced	1 cup	27	—	0
seed	1 tsp	7	—	0

FENUGREEK

seed	1 tsp	12	—	0

FIBER
Delta

Natural Fiber	½ cup (1 oz)	20	20	0

FIGS
CANNED
S&W

Kadota Figs Whole Fancy	½ cup	100	—	0
in heavy syrup	3	75	—	0
in light syrup	3	58	—	0
water pack	3	42	—	0
DRIED				
California	½ cup (3.5 oz)	200	17	0
cooked	½ cup	140	—	0
whole	10	477	17	0

FOOD	PORTION	CALS.	FIB.	CHOL.
FRESH				
fig	1 med	50	—	0
FILBERTS				
dried blanched	1 oz	191	—	0
dried unblanched	1 oz	179	—	0
dry roasted unblanched	1 oz	188	—	0
oil roasted unblanched	1 oz	187	2	0
FISH				
(see also FISH SUBSTITUTES, INDIVIDUAL NAMES, SUSHI)				
CANNED				
Holmes				
Finest Kippered Snacks drained	1 can (3.2 oz)	135	0	60
Port Clyde				
Fish Steaks In Louisiana Hot Sauce	1 can (3.75 oz)	150	0	80
Fish Steaks In Mustard Sauce	1 can (3.75 oz)	140	0	70
Fish Steaks In Soybean Oil With Hot Chilies drained	1 can (3.3 oz)	155	0	80
Fish Steaks In Soybean Oil drained	1 can (3.3 oz)	220	0	115
Progresso				
Mixed Seafood Sauce	½ cup	110	—	11
Seafood	½ cup	190	tr	95
FROZEN				
Gorton's				
Crispy Batter Dipped Fillets	2	290	—	35
Crispy Batter Sticks	4	260	—	25
Crunch Fillets	2	230	—	40
Crunchy Sticks	4	210	—	25
Light Recipe Lightly Breaded Fish Fillets	1 fillet	180	—	30
Light Recipe Tempura Fillets	1 fillet	200	—	30
Microwave Entree Fillets In Herb Butter	1 pkg	190	—	90
Microwave Fillets	2	340	—	30
Microwave Larger Cut Fillets	1	320	—	35
Microwave Sticks	6	340	—	35
Potato Crisp Fillets	2	300	—	30
Potato Crisp Sticks	4	260	—	25
Kineret				
Fish Sticks	5 pieces (4 oz)	280	1	20
Mrs. Paul's				
Entree Light Seafood Dijon	8¾ oz	200	—	60

FOOD	PORTION	CALS.	FIB.	CHOL.
Mrs. Paul's (CONT.)				
Entree Light Seafood Florentine	8 oz	220	—	95
Entrees Light Seafood Mornay	9 oz	230	—	80
Fish Cakes	2	190	—	20
Fish Fillets Batter Dipped	2 fillets	330	—	60
Fish Fillets Crispy Crunchy	2 fillets	220	—	22
Fish Fillets Crunchy Batter	2 fillets	280	—	22
Fish Sticks Crispy Crunchy	4 sticks	190	—	25
In Butter Sauce Light Fillets	1 fillet	140	—	40
Portions Battered Fish	2 portions	300	—	33
Portions Crispy Crunchy Breaded Fish	2 portions	230	—	25
Seafood Platter Combination	9 oz	600	—	85
Sticks Battered Fish	4 sticks	210	—	25
Sticks Crispy Crunchy Breaded Fish	4 sticks	140	—	20
Van De Kamp's				
Crispy Microwave Fillets	1 piece	140	—	15
Crispy Microwave Fish Sticks	3 pieces	130	—	15
Crispy Microwave Large Fillets	1 piece	290	—	25
Fish Fillets Battered	1	170	—	20
Fish Fillets Breaded	2	280	—	35
Fish Sticks Battered	4	160	—	20
Fish Sticks Breaded	4	200	—	20
Fish Sticks Breaded Value Pack	4	170	—	20
breaded fillet	1 (2 oz)	155	—	64
sticks	1 stick (1 oz)	76	—	31
MIX				
Golden Dipt				
Beer Batter Fry	1 oz	100	—	0
Cajun Style Fish Fry	⅔ oz	60	—	0
Fish & Chips Batter Mix	1¼ oz	120	—	0
Fish Fry	⅔ oz	60	—	0
Seafood Frying Mix	⅔ oz	60	—	0
Tempura Batter Mix	1 oz	100	—	0
TAKE-OUT				
sandwich w/ tartar sauce & cheese	1	524	—	68

FISH SUBSTITUTES
LaLoma

Ocean Platter mix not prep	¼ cup (16 g)	50	—	0

FLAXSEED

Arrowhead	3 tbsp (1 oz)	140	6	0
Stone-Buhr	1 tsp (1 oz)	150	5	0

FOOD	PORTION	CALS.	FIB.	CHOL.

FLOUNDER
FRESH
cooked	1 fillet (4.5 oz)	148	—	86
cooked	3 oz	99	—	58

FROZEN
Gorton's
Microwave Entree Stuffed	1 pkg	350	—	120

Mrs. Paul's
Crunchy Batter Fillets	2 fillets	220	—	40
Light Fillets	1 fillet	240	—	50

Van De Kamp's
Light Fillets	1 piece	260	—	45
Natural Fillets	4 oz	100	—	35

TAKE-OUT
battered & fried	3.2 oz	211	—	31
breaded & fried	3.2 oz	211	—	31

FLOUR
Arrowhead
Kamut	¼ cup (1.2 oz)	110	4	0
Pastry	⅓ cup (1.1 oz)	100	3	0
Rye Whole Grain	¼ cup (1.6 oz)	160	6	0
Spelt	¼ cup (1.2 oz)	100	5	0
Teff	¼ cup (1.4 oz)	140	5	0
Unbleached White	⅓ cup (1.6 oz)	160	0	0
Whole Grain Wheat	¼ cup (1.6 oz)	160	7	0
Whole Wheat	¼ cup (1.2 oz)	130	4	0

Aunt Jemima
Self-Rising	3 tbsp	90	1	0

Ballard
All Purpose	1 cup	400	—	0
Self-Rising	1 cup	380	—	0

Ceresota
All Purpose	1 cup	390	—	0
Whole Wheat	1 cup	400	—	0

General Mills
Drifted Snow	1 cup	400	—	0
Softasilk	¼ cup	100	—	0

Gold Medal
La Pina	1 cup	390	—	0

Heckers
All Purpose	1 cup	390	—	0
Whole Wheat	1 cup	400	—	0

Hodgson Mill
50/50 Flour	¼ cup (1 oz)	100	2	0

FOOD	PORTION	CALS.	FIB.	CHOL.
Hodgson Mill (CONT.)				
Best For Bread	¼ cup (1 oz)	100	1	0
Buckwheat	⅓ cup (1.6 oz)	160	2	0
Oat Bran Blend	¼ cup (1 oz)	110	3	0
Oat Bran Flour	¼ cup (1 oz)	110	3	0
Rye	¼ cup (1 oz)	90	5	0
Seasoned Flour	¼ cup (1 oz)	90	0	0
White	¼ cup (1 oz)	100	3	0
Whole Wheat	¼ cup (1 oz)	100	3	0
King Arthur				
All Purpose Unbleached	¼ cup (1 oz)	100	tr	0
Pillsbury				
All Purpose Best	1 cup	400	—	0
Bohemian Style Rye and Wheat Best	1 cup	400	—	0
Bread Best	1 cup	400	—	0
Rye Medium Best	1 cup	400	—	0
Self-Rising Best	1 cup	380	—	0
Shake & Blend Best	2 tbsp	50	—	0
Unbleached Best	1 cup	400	—	0
Whole Wheat Best	1 cup	400	—	0
Red Band				
All-Purpose	1 cup	390	—	0
Self-Rising	1 cup	380	—	0
Stone Ground Mills				
White Unbleached Organic	¼ cup (1.4 oz)	130	1	0
Whole Wheat 100% Stone Ground	3 tbsp (1 oz)	90	3	0
White Deer				
All-Purpose	1 cup	400	—	0
Wondra	1 cup	400	—	0
corn masa	1 cup	416	—	0
corn whole grain	1 cup	422	8	0
cottonseed lowfat	1 oz	94	—	0
peanut defatted	1 cup	196	—	0
peanut defatted	1 oz	92	—	0
peanut lowfat	1 cup	257	—	0
potato	1 cup (6.3 oz)	628	—	0
rice brown	1 cup	574	4	0
rice white	1 cup	578	2	0
rye dark	1 cup	415	—	0
rye light	1 cup	374	7	0
rye medium	1 cup	361	7	0
sesame lowfat	1 oz	95	—	0

FOOD	PORTION	CALS.	FIB.	CHOL.
triticale whole grain	1 cup	440	9	0
white all-purpose	1 cup	455	2	0
white bread	1 cup	495	—	0
white cake	1 cup	395	—	0
white self-rising	1 cup	442	—	0
whole wheat	1 cup	407	8	0

FRANKFURTER
(see HOT DOG)

FRENCH BEANS
dried cooked	1 cup	228	—	0

FRENCH FRIES
(see POTATOES)

FRENCH TOAST
FROZEN
Aunt Jemima	2 pieces (4.1 oz)	240	1	80
Aunt Jemima				
Cinnamon Swirl	2 pieces (4.1 oz)	240	2	90
Downyflake	2	270	—	73
Healthy Starts				
French Toast With LeanLinks	6.5 oz	400	—	0
Quaker				
French Toast Sticks & Syrup	1 pkg (5.2 oz)	400	—	64
French Toast Wedges &	1 pkg (5.3 oz)	360	—	96
Sausage				
Weight Watchers				
French Toast With Cinnamon	2 slices (3 oz)	160	—	4
french toast	1 slice (2 oz)	126	2	48
HOME RECIPE				
as prep w/ 2% milk	1 slice	149	—	75
as prep w/ whole milk	1 slice	151	—	75
TAKE-OUT				
w/ butter	2 slices	356	—	117

FROG'S LEGS
frog leg as prep w/ seasoned flour & fried	1 (0.8)	70	—	12

FROSTING
(see CAKE)

FRUCTOSE
Estee	1 pkg (3 g)	10	—	0
Estee	1 tsp (4 g)	15	—	0

FOOD	PORTION	CALS.	FIB.	CHOL.
FRUIT DRINKS				
(see also LEMONADE)				
FROZEN				
Bright & Early				
Fruit Punch	8 fl oz	130	—	0
Dole				
100% Juice Blend Country Raspberry as prep	8 fl oz	140	0	0
100% Juice Blend Orchard Peach as prep	8 fl oz	140	0	0
Mountain Cherry 100% Juice Blend as prep	8 fl oz	120	0	0
Pineapple Grapefruit as prep	8 fl oz	130	0	0
Pineapple Passion Banana as prep	8 fl oz	120	0	0
Pineapple Orange Banana as prep	8 fl oz	130	0	0
Pineapple Orange Banana as prep	8 fl oz	130	0	0
Pineapple Orange Guava as prep	8 fl oz	120	0	0
Pineapple Orange as prep	8 fl oz	120	0	0
Tropical Fruit as prep	8 fl oz	140	0	0
Five Alive				
Berry Citrus	8 fl oz	120	—	0
Citrus	8 fl oz	120	—	0
Tropical Citrus	8 fl oz	120	—	0
Minute Maid				
Berry Punch	8 fl oz	130	—	0
Citrus Punch	8 fl oz	120	—	0
Fruit Punch	8 fl oz	120	—	0
Limeade	8 fl oz	100	—	0
Pineapple Orange	8 fl oz	120	—	0
Tropical Punch	8 fl oz	120	—	0
Seneca				
Cranberry-Apple Juice Cocktail frzn as prep	8 fl oz	140	0	0
Raspberry-Cranberry Juice Cocktail frzn as prep	8 fl oz	140	0	0
Tree Top				
Apple Citrus as prep	6 oz	90	—	0
Apple Cranberry as prep	6 oz	100	—	0
Apple Grape as prep	6 oz	100	—	0

FOOD	PORTION	CALS.	FIB.	CHOL.
Tree Top (CONT.)				
Apple Pear as prep	6 oz	90	—	0
Apple Raspberry as prep	6 oz	80	—	0
citrus juice drink as prep	1 cup	114	—	0
citrus juice drink not prep	1 can (12 fl oz)	684	—	0
fruit punch as prep w/water	1 cup	113	—	0
fruit punch not prep	1 can (12 fl oz)	678	—	0
limeade	1 can (6 oz)	408	—	0
limeade as prep w/ water	1 cup	102	—	0
MIX				
Crystal Light				
Berry Blend Sugar Free	8 oz	3	—	0
Fruit Punch Sugar Free	8 oz	3	—	0
Lemon-Lime	8 oz	4	—	0
Tropic Quencher	8 oz	5	—	0
Kool-Aid				
Lemon-Lime	8 oz	98	—	0
Purplesaurus Rex	8 oz	98	—	0
Rainbow Punch	8 oz	98	—	0
Raspberry	8 oz	98	—	0
Sharkleberry Fin	8 oz	98	—	0
Strawberry	8 oz	98	—	0
Sugar Free Berry Blue	8 oz	3	—	0
Sugar Free Berry Punch	8 oz	3	—	0
Sugar Free Purplesaurus Rex	8 oz	3	—	0
Sugar Free Rainbow Punch	8 oz	4	—	0
Sugar Free Sharkleberry Fin	8 oz	3	—	0
Sugar Free Tropical Punch	8 oz	3	—	0
Sugar Sweetened Mountain Berry Punch	8 oz	98	—	0
Sugar Sweetened Purplesaurus Rex	8 oz	84	—	0
Sugar Sweetened Rainbow Punch	8 oz	84	—	0
Sugar Sweetened Sharkleberry Fin	8 oz	84	—	0
Sugar Sweetened Sunshine Punch	8 oz	83	—	0
Sugar Sweetened Surfin' Berry Punch	8 oz	79	—	0
Sugar Sweetened Tropical Punch	8 oz	84	—	0
Tropical Punch	8 oz	98	—	0
Unsweetened Berry Blue	8 oz	98	—	0

FOOD	PORTION	CALS.	FIB.	CHOL.
Wylers				
Drink Mix Unsweetened Bunch O' Berries	8 oz	2	—	0
Drink Mix Unsweetened Pink	8 fl oz	3	—	0
Drink Mix Unsweetened Tropical Punch	8 oz	2	—	0
fruit punch as prep w/water	9 oz	97	—	0
READY-TO-DRINK				
Apple & Eve				
Apple Cranberry	6 fl oz	80	—	0
Apple Grape	6 fl oz	120	—	0
Cranberry Grape	6 fl oz	100	—	0
Fruit Punch	6 fl oz	78	—	0
Raspberry Cranberry	6 fl oz	90	—	0
BAMA				
Fruit Punch	8.45 fl oz	130	—	0
Boku				
White Grape Raspberry	16 fl oz	120	—	0
Chiquita				
Orange Banana	6 fl oz	90	—	0
Crystal Geyser				
Juice Squeeze Citrus Grape	1 bottle (12 fl oz)	145	—	0
Juice Squeeze Orange & Passion Fruit	1 bottle (12 fl oz)	130	—	0
Juice Squeeze Passion Fruit & Mango	1 bottle (12 fl oz)	125	—	0
Juice Squeeze Wild Berry	1 bottle (12 fl oz)	130	—	0
Dole				
Pineapple Passion Banana	6 fl oz	100	—	0
Pineapple Orange	6 fl oz	90	—	0
Pineapple Orange Banana	6 fl oz	100	—	0
Pineapple Orange Guava	6 fl oz	100	—	0
Five Alive				
Citrus	1 can (11.5 fl oz)	170	—	0
Citrus	6 fl oz	90	—	0
Citrus	1 bottle (16 fl oz)	120	—	0
Citrus Chilled	8 fl oz	120	—	0
Hawaiian Punch				
Fruit Juicy Red	6 fl oz	90	—	0
Island Fruit Cocktail	6 fl oz	90	—	0
Lite Fruit Juicy Red	6 fl oz	60	—	0
Tropical Fruits	6 fl oz	90	—	0
Very Berry	6 fl oz	90	—	0
Wild Fruit	6 fl oz	90	—	0

FOOD	PORTION	CALS.	FIB.	CHOL.
Hi-C				
Boppin Berry Box	8.45 fl oz	140	—	0
Boppin' Berry	8 fl oz	130	—	0
Double Fruit Box	8.45 fl oz	130	—	0
Double Fruit Cooler	8 fl oz	130	—	0
Ecto Cooler	1 can (11.5 fl oz)	180	—	0
Ecto Cooler	8 fl oz	130	—	0
Ecto Cooler Box	8.45 fl oz	130	—	0
Fruit Punch	8 fl oz	130	—	0
Fruit Punch	1 can (11.5 fl oz)	190	—	0
Fruit Punch Box	8.45 fl oz	140	—	0
Fruity Bubble Gum	8 fl oz	120	—	0
Fruity Bubble Gum Box	8.45 fl oz	130	—	0
Hula Punch	8 fl oz	120	—	0
Hula Punch	1 can (11.5 fl oz)	170	—	0
Hula Punch Box	8.45 fl oz	120	—	0
Jammin' Apple Box	8.45 fl oz	130	—	0
Stompin' Banana Berry	8 fl oz	130	—	0
Stompin' Banana Berry Box	8.45 fl oz	130	—	0
Wild Berry	8 fl oz	120	—	0
Wild Berry Box	8.45 fl oz	130	—	0
Juice Works				
Appleberry	6 fl oz	100	—	0
Juicy Juice				
Apple Grape	1 box (8.45 fl oz)	120	—	0
Berry	1 bottle (6 fl oz)	90	—	0
Berry	1 box (8.45 fl oz)	130	—	0
Punch	1 box (8.45 fl oz)	140	—	0
Punch	1 bottle (6 fl oz)	100	—	0
Tropical	1 bottle (6 fl oz)	110	—	0
Tropical	1 box (8.45 fl oz)	150	—	0
Kern's				
Apple Strawberry Nectar	6 fl oz	110	—	0
Apricot Pineapple Nectar	6 fl oz	110	—	0
Banana Pineapple Nectar	6 fl oz	110	—	0
Coconut Pineapple Nectar	6 fl oz	140	—	0
Orange Banana Nectar	6 fl oz	110	—	0
Strawberry Banana Nectar	6 fl oz	110	—	0
Tropical Nectar	6 fl oz	110	—	0
Kool-Aid				
Koolers Sharkleberry Fin	1 pkg (8.45 fl oz)	140	—	0
Libby				
Strawberry Banana Nectar	1 can (11.5 fl oz)	220	—	0

FOOD	PORTION	CALS.	FIB.	CHOL.
Lifesavers				
Fruit Punch	8 fl oz	140	—	0
Mauna La'i				
Island Guava Hawaiian Guava Fruit Juice Drink	8 fl oz	130	0	0
Mango & Hawaiian Guava Fruit Juice Drink	8 fl oz	130	0	0
Paradise Guava Hawaiian Guava & Passion Fruit Juice Drink	8 fl oz	130	0	0
Minute Maid				
Berry Punch Box	8.45 fl oz	130	—	0
Berry Punch Chilled	8 fl oz	130	—	0
Citrus Punch Chilled	8 fl oz	130	—	0
Fruit Punch Box	8.45 fl oz	120	—	0
Fruit Punch Chilled	8 fl oz	120	—	0
Juices To Go Citrus Punch	1 bottle (10 fl oz)	160	—	0
Juices To Go Citrus Punch	1 can (11.5 fl oz)	180	—	0
Juices To Go Concord Punch	1 can (11.5 fl oz)	180	—	0
Juices To Go Concord Punch	1 bottle (10 fl oz)	160	—	0
Juices To Go Concord Punch	1 bottle (16 fl oz)	130	—	0
Juices To Go Fruit Punch	1 can (11.5 fl oz)	180	—	0
Juices To Go Fruit Punch	1 bottle (10 fl oz)	160	—	0
Juices To Go Fruit Punch	1 bottle (16 fl oz)	120	—	0
Juices To Go Orange Blend	1 bottle (10 fl oz)	150	—	0
Juices To Go Orange Blend	1 can (11.5 fl oz)	170	—	0
Naturals Apple Cranberry	8 fl oz	170	—	0
Naturals Concord Medley	8 fl oz	130	—	0
Naturals Fruit Medley	8 fl oz	120	—	0
Naturals Tropical Medley	8 fl oz	120	—	0
Tropical Punch Box	8.45 fl oz	130	—	0
Tropical Punch Chilled	8 fl oz	120	—	0
Mott's				
Apple Cranberry Blend	10 fl oz	180	0	0
Apple Cranberry From Concentrate as prep	8 fl oz	120	0	0
Apple Grape From Concentrate as prep	8 fl oz	120	0	0
Apple Raspberry Blend	10 fl oz	140	0	0
Apple Raspberry From Concentrate	8.45 fl oz	120	0	0
Fruit Basket Apple Raspberry Juice Cocktail as prep	8 fl oz	130	0	0
Fruit Basket Tropical Blend Juice Cocktail as prep	8 fl oz	120	0	0

FOOD	PORTION	CALS.	FIB.	CHOL.
Mott's (CONT.)				
Fruit Punch From Concentrate	8.45 fl oz	120	0	0
Fruit Punch From Concentrate	10 fl oz	170	0	0
Grape Apple	10 fl oz	170	0	0
Pineapple Orange	10 fl oz	170	0	0
Ocean Spray				
Cran.Blueberry	8 fl oz	160	0	0
Cran.Cherry	6 fl oz	160	0	0
Cran.Grape	8 fl oz	170	0	0
Cran.Raspberry	8 fl oz	140	0	0
Cran.Raspberry Reduced Calorie	8 fl oz	50	0	0
Cran.Strawberry	8 fl oz	140	tr	0
Cranapple	8 fl oz	160	tr	0
Cranapple Reduced Calorie	8 fl oz	50	0	0
Cranicot	8 fl oz	160	0	0
Crantastic	8 fl oz	150	0	0
Fruit Punch	8 fl oz	130	0	0
Lightstyle Low Calorie Cran.Grape	8 fl oz	40	0	0
Lightstyle Low Calorie Cran.Raspberry	8 fl oz	40	0	0
Refreshers Juice Drink Citrus Cranberry	8 fl oz	140	0	0
Refreshers Juice Drink Citrus Peach	8 fl oz	120	0	0
Refreshers Juice Drink Orange Cranberry	8 fl oz	130	0	0
Ruby Red & Tangerine Grapefruit Juice Cocktail	8 fl oz	130	0	0
Odwalla				
Boyzenberry Mango	8 fl oz	140	2	0
C Monster	16 fl oz	300	4	0
Fruitshake Blackberry	8 fl oz	160	3	0
Guanaba Dabba Doo!	8 fl oz	130	0	0
Raspberry Smoothie	8 fl oz	140	2	0
Strawberry Banana Smoothie	8 fl oz	100	2	0
Pek				
Passionate Peach Grapefruit	8 fl oz	110	0	0
S&W				
Apricot Pineapple Nectar	6 fl oz	120	—	0
Apricot Pineapple Nectar Diet	6 fl oz	80	—	0
Sipps				
Fruit Punch	8.45 oz	130	—	0

FOOD	PORTION	CALS.	FIB.	CHOL.
Sipps (CONT.)				
Lemon Lime Cooler	8.45 oz	130	—	0
Mixed Berry	8.45 oz	130	—	0
Sunshine Punch	8.45 oz	130	—	0
Smucker's				
Apple Cranberry	8 oz	120	—	0
Orange Banana	8 oz	120	—	0
Snapple				
Diet Kiwi Strawberry	8 fl oz	13	—	0
Fruit Punch	8 fl oz	120	—	0
Kiwi Strawberry Cocktail	8 fl oz	130	—	0
Melonberry Cocktail	8 fl oz	120	—	0
Vitamin Supreme	10 fl oz	150	—	0
Squeezit				
Berry B. Wild	1 (6.75 fl oz)	90	—	0
Chucklin' Cherry	1 (6.75 fl oz)	90	—	0
Grumpy Grape	1 (6.75 fl oz)	90	—	0
Mean Green Puncher	1 (6.75 fl oz)	90	—	0
Silly Billy Strawberry	1 (6.75 fl oz)	90	—	0
Smarty Arty Orange	1 (6.75 fl oz)	90	—	0
Sunny Delight	6 fl oz	90	—	0
Tang				
Mixed Fruit	8.45 fl oz	137	—	0
Tree Top				
Apple Citrus	6 fl oz	90	—	0
Apple Cranberry	6 fl oz	100	—	0
Apple Grape	6 fl oz	100	—	0
Apple Pear	6 fl oz	90	—	0
Apple Raspberry	6 fl oz	80	—	0
Tropicana				
Berry Punch	8 fl oz	120	—	0
Citrus Punch	1 bottle (10 fl oz)	180	—	0
Citrus Punch	8 fl oz	140	—	0
Cranberry Punch	1 can (11.5 fl oz)	200	—	0
Cranberry Punch	1 bottle (10 fl oz)	170	—	0
Cranberry Punch	8 fl oz	140	—	0
Fruit Punch	1 bottle (10 fl oz)	150	—	0
Fruit Punch	1 can (11.5 fl oz)	170	—	0
Fruit Punch	8 fl oz	130	—	0
Fruit Punch	1 container (10 fl oz)	160	—	0
Orange Pineapple	8 fl oz	110	—	0
Orange Pineapple	8 fl oz	110	—	0
Orange Pineapple	1 bottle (10 fl oz)	130	—	0

FOOD	PORTION	CALS.	FIB.	CHOL.
Tropicana (CONT.)				
Pineapple Punch	8 fl oz	120	—	0
Pineapple Punch	1 bottle (10 fl oz)	160	—	0
Season's Best Cranberry Medley	8 fl oz	120	—	0
Tropics Apple Cranberry Kiwi	8 fl oz	120	—	0
Tropics Orange Strawberry Banana	8 fl oz	110	—	0
Tropics Orange Kiwi Passion	8 fl oz	100	—	0
Tropics Orange Peach Mango	8 fl oz	110	—	0
Tropics Orange Pineapple	8 fl oz	110	—	0
Tropics Pineapple Passion	8 fl oz	120	—	0
Twister Apple Raspberry Blackberry	8 fl oz	120	—	0
Twister Apple Raspberry Blackberry	1 bottle (10 fl oz)	150	—	0
Twister Apple Raspberry Blackberry	1 can (11.5 fl oz)	180	—	0
Twister Cranberry Raspberry Strawberry	8 fl oz	120	—	0
Twister Cranberry Raspberry Strawberry	1 bottle (10 fl oz)	160	—	0
Twister Light Cranberry Raspberry Strawberry	8 fl oz	45	—	0
Twister Light Cranberry Raspberry Strawberry	1 container (10 fl oz)	50	—	0
Twister Light Orange Strawberry Banana	8 fl oz	35	—	0
Twister Light Orange Strawberry Banana	1 container (10 fl oz)	45	—	0
Twister Light Orange Strawberry Banana	1 container (10 fl oz)	45	—	0
Twister Light Orange Cranberry	8 fl oz	30	—	0
Twister Light Orange Cranberry	1 container (10 fl oz)	35	—	0
Twister Light Orange Cranberry	1 container (10 fl oz)	35	—	0
Twister Light Orange Raspberry	8 fl oz	35	—	0
Twister Light Orange Raspberry	1 container (10 fl oz)	45	—	0
Twister Orange Strawberry Banana	1 container (10 fl oz)	140	—	0
Twister Orange Cranberry	1 container (10 fl oz)	140	—	0

FOOD	PORTION	CALS.	FIB.	CHOL.
Tropicana (CONT.)				
Twister Orange Cranberry	1 bottle (10 fl oz)	140	—	0
Twister Orange Cranberry	8 fl oz	120	—	0
Twister Orange Peach	1 can (11.5 fl oz)	160	—	0
Twister Orange Peach	1 bottle (10 fl oz)	140	—	0
Twister Orange Peach	8 fl oz	120	—	0
Twister Orange Raspberry	1 bottle (10 fl oz)	140	—	0
Twister Orange Raspberry	8 fl oz	120	—	0
Twister Strawberry Banana	1 bottle (10 fl oz)	140	—	0
Twister Strawberry Banana	8 fl oz	120	—	0
Twister Strawberry Banana	1 can (11.5 fl oz)	160	—	0
Twister Strawberry Guava	1 bottle (10 fl oz)	140	—	0
Twister Strawberry Guava	8 fl oz	110	—	0
Veryfine				
Apple Cherryberry	8 fl oz	130	—	0
Apple Cranberry	8 fl oz	130	—	0
Apple Raspberry	8 fl oz	110	—	0
Fruit Punch	8 fl oz	130	—	0
Guava Strawberry	8 fl oz	120	—	0
Lemon & Lime	8 fl oz	120	—	0
Papaya Punch	8 fl oz	120	—	0
Passionfruit Orange	8 fl oz	110	—	0
Pineapple Orange	8 fl oz	130	—	0
White House				
Apple Cherry	6 fl oz	90	0	0
cranberry apple drink	6 fl oz	123	—	0
cranberry apricot drink	6 fl oz	118	—	0
fruit punch	6 fl oz	87	—	0
orange grapefruit juice	8 fl oz	107	—	0
orange & apricot	8 fl oz	128	—	0
pineapple & grapefruit	8 fl oz	117	—	0
pineapple & orange drink	8 fl oz	125	—	0

FRUIT MIXED
(see also individual names)
CANNED
Del Monte

FOOD	PORTION	CALS.	FIB.	CHOL.
Fruit Cocktail Fruit Naturals	½ cup (4.4 oz)	60	1	0
Fruit Cocktail In Heavy Syrup	½ cup (4.5 oz)	100	1	0
Fruit Cocktail Lite	½ cup (4.4 oz)	60	1	0
Lite Mixed Fruits Chunky	½ cup (4.4 oz)	60	1	0
Mixed Fruits Chunky Fruit Naturals	½ cup (4.4 oz)	60	1	0
Mixed Fruits Chunky In Heavy Syrup	½ cup (4.5 oz)	100	1	0

FOOD	PORTION	CALS.	FIB.	CHOL.
Del Monte (CONT.)				
Snack Cups Mixed Fruit Fruit Naturals	1 serv (4.5 oz)	60	1	0
Snack Cups Mixed Fruit Fruit Naturals EZ-Open Lid	1 serv (4.5 oz)	60	1	0
Snack Cups Mixed Fruit In Heavy Syrup	1 serv (4.5 oz)	100	1	0
Snack Cups Mixed Fruit In Heavy Syrup EZ-Open Lid	1 serv (4.2 oz)	90	1	0
Snack Cups Mixed Fruit Lite	1 serv (4.5 oz)	60	1	0
Snack Cups Mixed Fruit Lite EZ-Open Lid	1 serv (4.5 oz)	60	1	0
Dole				
Tropical Fruit Salad	½ cup	70	—	0
Hunt's				
Fruit Cocktail	4 oz	90	tr	0
Libby				
Chunky Mixed Lite	½ cup (4.3 oz)	60	1	0
Fruit Cocktail Lite	½ cup (4.3 oz)	60	1	0
S&W				
Chunky Mixed Diet	½ cup	40	—	0
Chunky Mixed Natural Style	½ cup	90	—	0
Chunky Mixed Unsweetened	½ cup	40	—	0
Fruit Cocktail Diet	½ cup	40	—	0
Fruit Cocktail Heavy Syrup	½ cup	90	—	0
Fruit Cocktail Natural Lite	½ cup	60	—	0
Fruit Cocktail Natural Style	½ cup	90	—	0
Fruit Cocktail Unsweetened	½ cup	40	—	0
fruit cocktail in heavy syrup	½ cup	93	—	0
fruit cocktail juice pack	½ cup	56	—	0
fruit cocktail water pack	½ cup	40	—	0
fruit salad in heavy syrup	½ cup	94	—	0
fruit salad in light syrup	½ cup	73	—	0
fruit salad juice pack	½ cup	62	—	0
fruit salad water pack	½ cup	37	—	0
mixed fruit in heavy syrup	½ cup	92	—	0
tropical fruit salad in heavy syrup	½ cup	110	—	0
DRIED				
Del Monte				
Mixed	⅓ cup (1.4 oz)	110	5	0
Planters				
Fruit'n Nut Mix	1 oz	150	—	0
mixed	11 oz pkg	712	—	0

FOOD	PORTION	CALS.	FIB.	CHOL.
FROZEN				
Big Valley				
Burst O' Berries	⅔ cup (4.9 oz)	70	3	0
California Tropics	⅔ cup (4.9 oz)	60	2	0
Cup A Fruit	1 pkg (4 oz)	50	2	0
Mixed	4.9 oz	60	2	0
Birds Eye				
Mixed Fruit	½ cup	120	1	0
Dole				
Applesauce Strawberry	1 pkg (4 oz)	60	1	0
mixed fruit sweetened	1 cup	245	—	0
FRUIT SNACKS				
Betty Crocker				
String Thing Berry 'N Blue	1 pkg (0.7 oz)	80	—	0
String Thing Cherry	1 pkg (0.7 oz)	80	—	0
String Thing Strawberry	1 pkg (0.7 oz)	80	—	0
Brock				
Beauty & The Beast	1 pkg (0.9 oz)	90	—	0
Cinderella	1 pkg (0.9 oz)	90	—	0
Dinosaurs	1 pkg (0.9 oz)	90	—	0
Ninja Trolls	1 pkg (0.9 oz)	90	—	0
Sharks	1 pkg (0.9 oz)	90	—	0
Del Monte				
Sierra Trail Mix	¼ cup (1.2 oz)	150	3	0
Sierra Trail Mix	1 pkg (1 oz)	120	2	0
Sierra Trail Mix	1 pkg (0.9 oz)	110	2	0
Health Valley				
Bakes Apple	1 bar	100	3	0
Bakes Date	1 bar	100	3	0
Bakes Raisin	1 bar	100	3	0
Fat Free Fruit Bars 100% Organic Apple	1 bar	140	4	0
Fat Free Fruit Bars 100% Organic Date	1 bar	140	4	0
Fat Free Fruit Bars 100% Organic Raisin	1 bar	140	4	0
Fat Free Fruit Bars 100% Fruit Organic Apricot	1 bar	140	4	0
Fruit & Fitness Bars	2 bars	200	5	0
Oat Bran Bakes Apricot	1 bar	100	2	0
Oat Bran Bakes Fig & Nut	1 bar	110	2	0
Oat Bran Jumbo Fruit Bar Almond & Date	1 bar	170	7	0

FOOD	PORTION	CALS.	FIB.	CHOL.
Health Valley (CONT.)				
Oat Bran Jumbo Fruit Bars Raisin & Cinnamon	1 bar	160	6	0
Rice Bran Jumbo Fruit Bars Almond & Date	1 bar	160	4	0
Sovex				
Fruit Bites Jungle Pals	1 pkg (0.9 oz)	90	—	0
Stretch Island				
Fruit Leather Berry Blackberry	2 pieces (1 oz)	90	3	0
Fruit Leather Chunky Cherry	2 pieces (1 oz)	90	2	0
Fruit Leather Great Grape	2 pieces (1 oz)	90	2	0
Fruit Leather Organic Apple	2 pieces (1 oz)	90	2	0
Fruit Leather Organic Grape	2 pieces (1 oz)	90	2	0
Fruit Leather Organic Raspberry	2 pieces (1 oz)	90	2	0
Fruit Leather Rare Raspberry	2 pieces (1 oz)	90	2	0
Fruit Leather Snappy Apple	2 pieces (1 oz)	90	3	0
Fruit Leather Tangy Apricot	2 pieces (1 oz)	90	2	0
Fruit Leather Truly Tropical	2 pieces (1 oz)	90	1	0
Sunbelt				
Fruit Booster Strawberry	1 (1.3 oz)	130	0	0
Fruit Boosters Apple	1 (1.3 oz)	130	0	0
Fruit Boosters Blueberry	1 (1.3 oz)	130	1	0
Fruit Jammers	1 (1 oz)	100	0	0
Sunkist				
Fruit Roll Apricot	1	76	0	0
Fruit Roll Cherry	1	75	0	0
Fruit Roll Grape	1	76	0	0
Fruit Roll Raspberry	1	75	0	0
Fruit Roll Strawberry	1	74	0	0
Fun Fruit Animals	0.9 oz	100	0	0
Fun Fruit Dinosaurs Strawberry	0.9 oz	100	0	0
Fun Fruit Spooky Fruit	1 pkg	100	0	0
Fun Fruit Strawberry	0.9 oz	100	—	0
Weight Watchers				
Apple	½ oz	50	—	0
Apple Chips	¾ oz	70	—	0
Cinnamon	½ oz	50	—	0
Peach	½ oz	50	—	0
Strawberry	½ oz	50	—	0
fruit leather	1 bar (0.8 oz)	81	—	0
fruit leather pieces	1 oz	97	—	0
fruit leather pieces	1 pkg (0.9 oz)	92	—	0
fruit leather rolls	1 lg (0.7 oz)	73	—	0
fruit leather rolls	1 sm (0.5 oz)	49	—	0

FOOD	PORTION	CALS.	FIB.	CHOL.
GARBANZO				
(see CHICKPEAS)				
GARLIC				
Watkins				
Garlic & Chive Seasoning	1 tbsp (7 g)	25	0	5
Garlic Lover's Herb Blend	¼ tsp (0.5 oz)	0	0	0
Liquid Spice	1 tbsp (0.5 oz)	120	0	0
clove	1	4	—	0
powder	1 tsp	9	—	0
GEFILTE FISH				
READY-TO-USE				
sweet	1 piece (1.5 oz)	35	—	12
GELATIN				
DRINKS				
Knox				
Orange Flavored Drinking Gelatin w/ Nutrasweet	1 pkg	39	0	0
MIX				
D-Zerta				
Cherry	½ cup	8	—	0
Lemon	½ cup	8	—	0
Lime	½ cup	9	—	0
Orange	½ cup	8	—	0
Raspberry	½ cup	8	—	0
Strawberry	½ cup	8	—	0
Emes				
Kosher-Jel	½ cup (4 fl oz)	60	—	0
Kosher-Jel Plain	1 tbsp (7 g)	21	1	0
Jell-O				
Apricot	½ cup	82	0	0
Black Cherry	½ cup	82	tr	0
Black Raspberry	½ cup	82	tr	0
Blackberry	½ cup	82	tr	0
Cherry Sugar Free	½ cup	9	—	0
Concord Grape	½ cup	82	0	0
Hawaiian Pineapple Sugar Free	½ cup	8	—	0
Lemon	½ cup	82	0	0
Lemon Sugar Free	½ cup	8	—	0
Lime	½ cup	82	tr	0
Lime Sugar Free	½ cup	9	—	0
Mixed Fruit	½ cup	82	tr	0
Mixed Fruit Sugar Free	½ cup	8	—	0

FOOD	PORTION	CALS.	FIB.	CHOL.
Jell-O (CONT.)				
Orange	½ cup	82	tr	0
Orange Sugar Free	½ cup	8	—	0
Peach Sugar Free	½ cup	8	—	0
Raspberry Sugar Free	½ cup	8	—	0
Strawberry Banana Sugar Free	½ cup	9	—	0
Strawberry Sugar Free	½ cup	9	—	0
Triple Berry Sugar Free	½ cup	8	—	0
Wild Strawberry	½ cup	81	tr	0
Royal				
Apple	½ cup	80	—	0
Blackberry	½ cup	80	—	0
Cherry	½ cup	80	—	0
Cherry Sugar Free	½ cup	8	—	0
Concord Grape	½ cup	80	—	0
Fruit Punch	½ cup	80	—	0
Lemon	½ cup	80	—	0
Lemon-Lime	½ cup	80	—	0
Lime	½ cup	80	—	0
Lime Sugar Free	½ cup	8	—	0
Mixed Berry	½ cup	80	—	0
Orange	½ cup	80	—	0
Orange Sugar Free	½ cup	10	—	0
Peach	½ cup	80	—	0
Pineapple	½ cup	80	—	0
Raspberry	½ cup	80	—	0
Raspberry Sugar Free	½ cup	8	—	0
Strawberry	½ cup	80	—	0
Strawberry Banana Sugar Free	½ cup	8	—	0
Strawberry Orange	½ cup	80	—	0
Strawberry Sugar Free	½ cup	8	—	0
Tropical Fruit	½ cup	80	—	0
low calorie	½ cup	8	0	0
mix artificially sweetened as prep	½ cup (4.1 oz)	8	—	0
mix artificially sweetened as prep	1 pkg 4 serv (16.5 oz)	33	—	0
mix as prep	1 pkg 4 serv (19 oz)	319	—	0
mix as prep	½ cup (4.7 oz)	80	—	0
mix not prep	1 pkg (3 oz)	324	—	0
mix w/ fruit as prep	1 pkg 8 serv (19 oz)	588	—	0
mix w/ fruit as prep	½ cup (3.7 oz)	73	—	0
READY-TO-USE				
Del Monte				
Gel Snack Cups Blue Berry	1 serv (3.5 oz)	70	tr	0

FOOD	PORTION	CALS.	FIB.	CHOL.
Del Monte (cont.)				
Gel Snack Cups Cherry	1 serv (3.5 oz)	70	tr	0
Gel Snack Cups Orange	1 serv (3.5 oz)	70	tr	0
Gel Snack Cups Strawberry	1 serv (3.5 oz)	70	tr	0
GIBLETS				
capon simmered	1 cup (5 oz)	238	—	629
chicken floured & fried	1 cup (5 oz)	402	—	647
chicken simmered	1 cup (5 oz)	228	—	570
turkey simmered	1 cup (5 oz)	243	—	606
GINGER				
Ka-Me				
Crystallized Slices	5 pieces (1 oz)	100	1	0
Sliced	20 pieces (0.5 oz)	0	0	0
ground	1 tsp (1.8 g)	6	—	0
root fresh	5 slices	8	—	0
root fresh	¼ cup	17	—	0
root fresh sliced	¼ cup	17	—	0
GINKGO NUTS				
canned	1 oz	32	—	0
dried	1 oz	99	—	0
raw	1 oz	52	—	0
GIZZARDS				
chicken simmered	1 cup (5 oz)	222	—	281
turkey simmered	1 cup (5 oz)	236	—	336
GOAT				
roasted	3 oz	122	—	64
GOOSE				
w/ skin roasted	6.6 oz	574	—	172
w/ skin roasted	½ goose (1.7 lbs)	2362	—	708
w/o skin roasted	5 oz	340	—	138
w/o skin roasted	½ goose (1.3 lbs)	1406	—	569
GOOSEBERRIES				
fresh	1 cup	67	—	0
CANNED				
in light syrup	½ cup	93	—	0
GRANOLA				
BARS				
Carnation				
Honey & Oats	1 (1.26 oz)	130	1	0
Fi-Bar				
Coconut	1	120	6	0

FOOD	PORTION	CALS.	FIB.	CHOL.
Fi-Bar (CONT.)				
Peanut Butter	1	130	6	0
General Mills				
Nature Valley Cinnamon	1	120	1	0
Nature Valley Oat Bran Honey Graham	1	110	1	0
Nature Valley Oats N'Honey	1	120	1	0
Nature Valley Peanut Butter	1	120	1	0
Nature Valley Rice Bran Cinnamon Graham	1	90	1	0
Grist Mill				
Chew Chocolate Chip	1 (1 oz)	130	1	0
Chewy Apple Cinnamon	1 (1 oz)	120	1	0
Chewy Chunky Nut & Raisin	1 (1 oz)	130	1	0
Chewy Peanut Butter	1 (1 oz)	130	1	0
Chewy Peanut Butter Chocolate	1 (1 oz)	130	2	0
Chocolate Snack Chocolate Chip	1 (1.2 oz)	180	1	5
Chocolate Snack Nutty Fudge	1 (1.3 oz)	190	2	5
Crunchy Cinnamon	1 (0.8 oz)	110	1	0
Crunchy Oats 'N Honey	1 (0.8 oz)	110	1	0
Hershey				
Chocolate Covered Cocoa Creme	1 (1.2 oz)	180	—	5
Chocolate Covered Peanut Butter	1 (1.2 oz)	180	—	5
Kellogg's				
Low Fat Crunchy Almond & Brown Sugar	1 (0.7 oz)	80	1	0
Low Fat Crunchy Apple Spice	1 (0.7 oz)	80	1	0
Low Fat Crunchy Cinnamon Raisin	1 (0.7 oz)	80	1	0
Kudos				
Chocolate Chip	1 bar (1 oz)	130	1	5
Milk & Cookies	1 bar (1 oz)	130	1	5
Nutty Fudge	1 bar (1 oz)	130	1	5
Peanut Butter	1 bar (1 oz)	130	1	5
Quaker				
Chewy Chocolate Chip	1	128	1	tr
Chewy Chunky Nut & Raisin	1	131	2	tr
Chewy Cinnamon Raisin	1	128	1	tr
Chewy Honey & Oats	1	125	1	tr
Chewy Peanut Butter	1	128	1	tr
Chewy Peanut Butter Chocolate Chip	1	131	1	tr

FOOD	PORTION	CALS.	FIB.	CHOL.
Quaker (CONT.)				
Dipps Caramel Nut	1	148	1	2
Dipps Chocolate Chip	1	139	1	1
Dipps Peanut Butter	1	170	1	2
Sunbelt				
Chewy Chocolate Chip	1 (1.8 oz)	220	2	0
Chewy Oats & Honey	1 (1.7 oz)	210	2	0
Chewy With Almonds	1 (1.5 oz)	190	2	0
Chewy Chocolate Chip	1 (1.25 oz)	160	2	0
Chewy Oats & Honey	1 (1 oz)	130	1	0
Chewy With Almonds	1 (1 oz)	130	1	0
Chewy With Raisins	1 (1.2 oz)	150	2	0
Fudge Dipped Chewy With Peanuts	1 (2 oz)	270	2	0
Fudge Dipped Chewy Chocolate Chip	1 (1.5 oz)	190	2	0
Fudge Dipped Chewy Macaroo	1 (1.4 oz)	200	2	0
Fudge Dipped Chewy Macaroo	1 bar (2 oz)	280	3	0
Fudge Dipped Chewy With Peanuts	1 bar (1.5 oz)	210	2	0
almond	1 (0.8 oz)	117	—	0
almond	1 (1 oz)	140	—	0
chewy chocolate coated chocoate chip	1 (1 oz)	132	1	1
chewy chocolate coated chocolate chip	1 (1.25 oz)	165	1	2
chewy chocolate coated peanut butter	1 (1.3 oz)	187	—	4
chewy chocolate coated peanut butter	1 (1 oz)	144	—	3
chewy raisin	1 (1.5 oz)	191	2	0
chewy raisin	1 (1 oz)	127	1	0
chocolate chip	1 (0.8 oz)	103	1	0
chocolate chip	1 (1 oz)	124	1	0
chocolate chip chewy	1 (1.5 oz)	178	2	1
chocolate chip chewy	1 (1 oz)	119	1	0
chocolate chip, graham & marshmallow chewy	1 (1 oz)	121	1	0
nut & raisin chewy	1 (1 oz)	129	2	0
peanut	1 (1 oz)	136	—	0
peanut	1 (0.8 oz)	113	1	0
peanut butter	1 (0.8 oz)	114	—	0
peanut butter	1 (1 oz)	137	—	0
peanut butter chewy	1 (1 oz)	121	1	0

FOOD	PORTION	CALS.	FIB.	CHOL.
peanut butter & chocolate chip chewy	1 (1 oz)	122	1	0
plain	1 (0.9 oz)	115	1	0
plain	1 (1 oz)	134	2	0
plain chewy	1 (1 oz)	126	1	0
CEREAL				
Erewhon				
Date Nut	1 oz	130	—	0
Honey Almond	1 oz	130	—	0
Maple	1 oz	130	—	0
Spiced Apple	1 oz	130	—	0
Sunflower Crunch	1 oz	130	—	0
With Bran	1 oz	130	4	0
General Mills				
Nature Valley Cinnamon & Raisin	⅓ cup (1 oz)	120	1	0
Nature Valley Fruit & Nut	⅓ cup (1 oz)	130	1	0
Nature Valley Toasted Oat	⅓ cup (1 oz)	130	1	0
Good Shepard				
Crunchy	1 oz	130	2	0
Honey Almond	1 oz	120	2	0
Organic 5 Grain Muesli	1 oz	160	3	0
Organic Brown Rice	1 oz	130	4	0
Organic Wheat Free	1 oz	90	3	0
Organic Wheat Free Apple Cinnamon	1 oz	125	3	0
Organic Wheat Free Blueberry Amaranth	1 oz	110	2	0
Organic Wheat Free Strawberry Amaranth	1 oz	110	2	0
Grist Mill				
Low-Fat With Raisins	⅔ cup (1.9 oz)	220	3	0
Kellogg's				
Low Fat	½ cup (1.9 oz)	210	3	0
Low Fat With Raisins	⅔ cup (1.9 oz)	210	3	0
Stone-Buhr				
Hot Apple	⅓ cup (1.6 oz)	153	5	0
Sun Country				
100% Natural With Almonds	¼ cup	130	1	0
100% Natural With Raisins & Dates	¼ cup	123	2	0
With Raisins	¼ cup	125	2	0
Sunbelt				
Banana Nut	1.9 oz	250	4	1

FOOD	PORTION	CALS.	FIB.	CHOL.
Sunbelt (CONT.)				
Fruit & Nut	1.9 oz	230	4	1
Low Fat	1.9 oz	200	4	0
Uncle Roy's				
Cashew Raisin	½ cup (1.6 oz)	180	3	0
Fat Free Apple Cinnamon	½ cup (1.6 oz)	175	3	0
Fat Free Wild Cherry	½ cup (1.6 oz)	175	3	0
Fruit & Nut	½ cup (1.6 oz)	175	3	0
Low Fat Berries Jubilee	½ cup (1.6 oz)	175	3	0
Low Fat Crispy	½ cup (1.4 oz)	160	3	0
Low Fat Luscious Raspberry	½ cup (1.6 oz)	175	3	0
Low Fat True Blueberry	½ cup (1.6 oz)	175	3	0
Maple Date Nut	½ cup (1.6 oz)	180	3	0
Nut Butter & Almonds	½ cup (1.6 oz)	195	3	0
Organic Golden Honey	½ cup (1.6 oz)	190	3	0
Organic Maple Nut'N Rice	½ cup (1.4 oz)	170	3	0
Organic Maple Raisin	½ cup (1.6 oz)	190	3	0

GRAPE JUICE

FOOD	PORTION	CALS.	FIB.	CHOL.
BAMA	8.45 fl oz	120	—	0
Bright & Early				
Frozen	8 fl oz	140	—	0
Hawaiian Punch	6 oz	90	—	0
Hi-C	1 can (11.5 fl oz)	180	—	0
Box	8.45 fl oz	130	—	0
Hi-C	8 fl oz	130	—	0
Juice Works	6 oz	100	—	0
Juicy Juice	1 box	130	—	0
Juicy Juice	1 bottle (6 fl oz)	90	—	0
Kool-Aid	8 oz	98	—	0
Sugar Free	8 oz	3	—	0
Sugar Sweetened	8 oz	80	—	0
Lifesavers				
Grape Punch	8 fl oz	150	—	0
Minute Maid				
Chilled	8 fl oz	130	—	0
Grape Punch frzn	8 fl oz	130	—	0
Punch Chilled	8 fl oz	130	—	0
Mott's				
Drink	10 fl oz	170	0	0
Fruit Basket Cocktail as prep	8 fl oz	130	0	0
S&W				
Concord Unsweetened	6 oz	100	—	0
Seneca				
Blush Grape Juice frzn as prep	8 fl oz	170	0	0

FOOD	PORTION	CALS.	FIB.	CHOL.
Seneca (CONT.)				
Fortified With Vitamin C frzn as prep	8 fl oz	170	0	0
Sweetened frzn as prep	8 fl oz	140	0	0
White Grape Juice frzn as prep	8 fl oz	140	0	0
Sippin' Pak				
100% Pure	8.45 fl	130	—	0
Sipps	8.45 oz	130	—	0
Snapple				
Grapeade	8 fl oz	120	—	0
Tang				
Fruit Box	8.45 oz	131	—	0
Tree Top	6 oz	120	—	0
Sparkling Juice	6 oz	120	—	0
Tropicana				
Season's Best	8 fl oz	160	—	0
Veryfine				
100%	8 oz	153	—	0
Grape Drink	8 oz	130	—	0
Wylers				
Drink Mix Unsweetened	8 oz	2	—	0
bottled	1 cup	155	—	0
frzn sweetened as prep	1 cup	128	—	0
frzn sweetened not prep	6 oz	386	—	0
grape drink	6 oz	84	—	0

GRAPE LEAVES

Cedar's

Graped Leaves Stuffed With Rice	6 pieces (4.9 oz)	180	8	0

GRAPEFRUIT

CANNED

S&W

Sections Unsweetened	½ cup	40	—	0
Sections In Light Syrup	½ cup	80	—	0
Sections Natural Style	½ cup	40	—	0
juice pack	½ cup	46	—	0
unsweetened	1 cup	93	—	0
water pack	½ cup	44	—	0

FRESH

Chiquita

Ruby Red	½ fruit	40	—	0
Dole	½	50	6	0

FOOD	PORTION	CALS.	FIB.	CHOL.
Ocean Spray				
Pink	½ med	50	—	0
White	½ med	45	—	0
pink	½	37	1	0
pink sections	1 cup	69	1	0
red	½	37	—	0
red sections	1 cup	69	—	0
white	½	39	1	0
white sections	1 cup	76	1	0

GRAPEFRUIT JUICE

FOOD	PORTION	CALS.	FIB.	CHOL.
Crystal Geyser				
Juice Squeeze	1 bottle (12 fl oz)	150	—	0
Del Monte	8 fl oz	100	1	0
Hood				
Select	1 cup (8 oz)	100	—	0
Minute Maid				
Frozen	8 fl oz	100	—	0
Juices To Go	1 can (11.5 fl oz)	140	—	0
Juices To Go	1 bottle (16 fl oz)	100	—	0
Juices To Go	1 bottle (10 fl oz)	120	—	0
Juices To Go Pink Cocktail	1 bottle (10 fl oz)	140	—	0
Juices To Go Pink Cocktail	1 bottle (16 fl oz)	110	—	0
Juices to Go Pink Cocktail	8 fl oz	160	—	0
Mott's				
From Concentrate as prep	8 fl oz	120	0	0
Ocean Spray				
100% Juice	8 oz	100	tr	0
Lightstyle Low Calorie Pink Cocktail	8 fl oz	40	0	0
Pink Juice Cocktail	8 oz	110	0	0
Ruby Red Drink	8 oz	130	0	0
Odwalla	8 fl oz	90	—	0
S&W				
Unsweetened	6 oz	80	—	0
Snapple				
Pink Grapefruit Cocktail	8 fl oz	120	—	0
Snapple	10 fl oz	110	—	0
Tree Of Life	8 fl oz	100	0	0
Tree Top	6 oz	80	—	0
Tropicana	8 fl oz	90	—	0
Ruby Red	8 fl oz	100	—	0
Ruby Red	1 container (10 fl oz)	120	—	0

FOOD	PORTION	CALS.	FIB.	CHOL.
Tropicana (CONT.)				
Season's Best	8 fl oz	90	—	0
Season's Best	1 can (11.5 fl oz)	120	—	0
Season's Best	1 bottle (7 fl oz)	80	—	0
Season's Best	1 bottle (10 fl oz)	110	—	0
Twister Light Pink	8 fl oz	40	—	0
Twister Light Pink	1 container (10 fl oz)	50	—	0
Twister Pink	1 container (10 fl oz)	140	—	0
Twister Pink	1 can (11.5 fl oz)	160	—	0
Twister Pink	8 fl oz	110	—	0
Veryfine				
100%	8 oz	101	—	0
Pink	8 oz	120	—	0
fresh	1 cup	96	—	0
frzn as prep	1 cup	102	—	0
frzn not prep	6 oz	302	—	0
sweetened	1 cup	116	—	0

GRAPES
CANNED
S&W

Thompson Seedless Premium	½ cup	100	—	0
thompson seedless in heavy syrup	½ cup	94	—	0
thompson seedless water pack	½ cup	48	—	0
FRESH				
Dole	1½ cup	85	2	0
grapes	10	36	tr	0

GRAVY
(see also SAUCE)
CANNED

Gravymaster	¼ tsp	3	—	0
Rudy's Farm				
Sausage Gravy	¼ cup (2 oz)	50	0	10
au jus	1 cup	38	—	1
beef	1 cup	124	—	7
beef	1 can (10 oz)	155	—	9
chicken	1 cup	189	—	5
mushroom	1 cup	120	—	0
turkey	1 cup	122	—	5
DRY				
Hain				
Brown	¼ pkg	16	—	0

FOOD	PORTION	CALS.	FIB.	CHOL.
Pillsbury				
Brown	¼ cup	15	—	0
Home Style	¼ cup	15	—	0
au jus as prep w/ water	1 cup	32	—	1
brown as prep w/ water	1 cup	75	—	2
chicken as prep	1 cup	83	—	3
mushroom as prep	1 cup	70	—	1
onion as prep w/ water	1 cup	77	—	tr
pork as prep	1 cup	76	—	3
turkey as prep	1 cup	87	—	3

GREAT NORTHERN BEANS
CANNED

FOOD	PORTION	CALS.	FIB.	CHOL.
Allen	½ cup (4.5 oz)	100	7	0
Green Giant	½ cup	80	5	0
Hanover	½ cup	110	—	0
Trappey				
With Sausage	½ cup (4.5 oz)	100	7	0
great northern	1 cup	300	14	0
DRIED				
Bean Cuisine	½ cup	115	5	0
cooked	1 cup	210	—	0

GREEN BEANS
CANNED

FOOD	PORTION	CALS.	FIB.	CHOL.
Allen				
Cut	½ cup (4.2 oz)	30	3	0
Cut No Added Salt	½ cup (4.2 oz)	15	2	0
French Style	½ cup (4.2 oz)	25	2	0
Italian	½ cup (4.2 oz)	35	3	0
Shell Outs	½ cup (4.5 oz)	30	2	0
Alma				
Cut	½ cup (4.2 oz)	30	3	0
Crest Top				
Cut	½ cup (4.2 oz)	30	3	0
Del Monte				
Cut	½ cup (4.3 oz)	20	2	0
Cut 50% Less Salt	½ cup (4.3 oz)	20	2	0
Cut Italian	½ cup (4.3 oz)	30	3	0
Cut No Salt Added	½ cup (4.3 oz)	20	2	0
French Style	½ cup (4.3 oz)	20	2	0
French Style 50% Less Salt	½ cup (4.3 oz)	20	2	0
French Style No Salt Added	½ cup (4.3 oz)	20	2	0
French Style Seasoned	½ cup (4.3 oz)	20	2	0
Whole	½ cup (4.3 oz)	20	2	0

FOOD	PORTION	CALS.	FIB.	CHOL.
GaBelle				
Cut	½ cup (4.2 oz)	30	3	0
Green Giant				
Almondine	½ cup	45	2	0
Cut	½ cup	16	1	0
French	½ cup	16	1	0
Kitchen Sliced	½ cup	16	1	0
Hanover				
Cut	½ cup	20	—	0
Owatonna				
Cut	½ cup	20	—	0
French	½ cup	20	—	0
S&W				
Cut Water Pack	½ cup	20	—	0
Cut Premium Blue Lake	½ cup	20	—	0
Dilled	½ cup	60	—	0
French Style Premium Blue Lake	½ cup	20	—	0
Green Beans & Wax Beans	½ cup	20	—	0
Whole Fancy Stringless	½ cup	20	—	0
Whole Vertical Pack	½ cup	20	—	0
Seneca				
Cut	½ cup	20	2	0
Cuts Natural Pack	½ cup	25	2	0
French	½ cup	20	2	0
French Natural Pack	½ cup	25	2	0
Whole	½ cup	20	2	0
Sunshine				
Cut	½ cup (4.2 oz)	30	3	0
Italian	½ cup (4.2 oz)	35	3	0
FROZEN				
Birds Eye				
Cut	½ cup	25	2	0
Farm Fresh Whole	¾ cup	30	2	0
French Cut	½ cup	25	2	0
In Sauce French Green Beans With Toasted Almonds	½ cup	50	2	0
Italian	½ cup	30	3	0
Polybag Cut	½ cup	25	2	0
Polybag Deluxe Whole	½ cup	20	2	0
Polybag French Cut	½ cup	25	2	0
Whole Deluxe	½ cup	45	2	0
Green Giant	½ cup	14	2	0
Cut	½ cup	16	1	0

FOOD	PORTION	CALS.	FIB.	CHOL.
Birds Eye (CONT.)				
Cut In Butter Sauce	½ cup	30	2	5
One Serve In Butter Sauce	1 pkg	60	3	5
Hanover				
Cut	½ cup	20	—	0
French Style Blue Lake	½ cup	25	—	0
Italian Cut	½ cup	35	—	0
Whole Blue Lake	½ cup	30	—	0
Southland				
Cut Beans	3 oz	25	—	0
French	3 oz	25	—	0
Stouffer's				
Green Bean Mushroom Casserole	½ cup (1.9 oz)	130	2	10
Tree Of Life	⅔ cup (2.8 oz)	25	2	0
SHELF-STABLE				
Pantry Express				
Cut	½ cup	12	1	0

GREENS
CANNED
Allen

Mixed	½ cup (4.2 oz)	30	4	0
Sunshine				
Mixed	½ cup (4.2 oz)	30	4	0

GROUNDCHERRIES

fresh	½ cup	37	—	0

GROUPER

cooked	3 oz	100	—	40
cooked	1 fillet (7.1 oz)	238	—	95
raw	3 oz	78	—	31

GUANABANA JUICE
Libby

Nectar	1 can (11.5 fl oz)	210	—	0

GUAVA

fresh	1	45	—	0
guava sauce	½ cup	43	—	0

GUAVA JUICE
Kern's

Nectar	6 fl oz	110	—	0
Libby				
Nectar	6 oz	110	—	0

FOOD	PORTION	CALS.	FIB.	CHOL.
Libby (CONT.)				
Nectar	1 can (11.5 fl oz)	220	—	0
Snapple				
Guava Mania	8 fl oz	110	—	0

GUINEA HEN

w/o skin raw	½ hen (9.3 oz)	292	—	166

HADDOCK

FRESH

cooked	1 fillet (5.3 oz)	168	—	110
cooked	3 oz	95	—	63
raw	3 oz	74	—	49
roe raw	3½ oz	130	—	360

FROZEN

Gorton's

Microwave Entree Haddock In Lemon Butter	1 pkg	360	—	100

Mrs. Paul's

Crunchy Batter Fillets	2 fillets	190	—	25
Light Fillets	1 fillet	220	—	45

Van De Kamp's

Battered	2 pieces	250	—	30
Breaded Fillets	2 pieces	270	—	25
Light Fillets	1 piece	240	—	35
Natural Fillets	4 oz	90	—	20

SMOKED

smoked	1 oz	33	—	21
smoked	3 oz	99	—	65

HALIBUT

FRESH

atlantic & pacific cooked	3 oz	119	—	35
atlantic & pacific cooked	½ fillet (5.6 oz)	223	—	65
atlantic & pacific raw	3 oz	93	—	27
greenland baked	3 oz	203	—	50
greenland baked	5.6 oz	380	—	94

FROZEN

Van De Kamp's

Battered	2 pieces	150	—	10

HALVA

(*see* SESAME)

HAM

(*see also* HAM DISHES, PORK, TURKEY)

Alpine Lace

Boneless Cooked	2 slices (2 oz)	60	0	25

FOOD	PORTION	CALS.	FIB.	CHOL.
Armour				
Chopped Ham canned	2 oz	120	—	35
Deviled Ham canned	1 pkg (3 oz)	200	—	60
Golden Star Boneless	1 oz	33	—	13
Golden Star Canned	1 oz	32	—	11
Lower Salt 93% Fat Free	1 oz	35	—	14
Lower Salt Boneless	1 oz	34	—	13
Star Boneless	1 oz	41	—	15
Star Canned	1 oz	34	—	11
Star Speedy Cut	1 oz	44	—	15
1877 Boneless	1 oz	42	—	42
Black Label				
Chopped	2 oz	140	0	30
Carl Buddig	1 oz	50	0	20
Honey Ham	1 oz	50	—	30
Hansel n' Gretel				
Baked Virginia	1 oz	34	—	12
Black Forest	1 oz	32	—	16
Cappy	1 oz	31	—	11
Cooked Fresh	1 oz	33	—	13
Deluxe	1 oz	31	—	12
Honey Valley	1 oz	31	—	10
Jalapeno	1 oz	25	—	11
Lessalt	1 oz	30	—	13
Lessalt Virginia	1 oz	32	—	13
Light AM	1 oz	27	—	11
Travane	1 oz	31	—	15
Healthy Choice				
Baked With Natural Juice Deli-Thin	1.9 oz	60	0	25
Cooked	3 slices (2.2 oz)	70	0	30
Deli-Thin Variety Pack	2.2 oz	70	0	30
Honey With Natural Juices	1.9 oz	60	0	25
Smoked	3 slices (2.2 oz)	70	0	30
Smoked With Natural Juices	1.9 oz	60	0	25
Hormel				
Black Label Canned (refrigerated)	3 oz	100	0	40
Black Label Canned (shelf stable)	3 oz	110	0	45
Canned Chunk	2 oz	90	0	30
Cure 81 Half Ham	3 oz	100	0	45
Curemaster	3 oz	80	0	40
Deli Cooked	1 oz	29	—	11

FOOD	PORTION	CALS.	FIB.	CHOL.
Hormel (CONT.)				
Deviled Ham	4 tbsp (2 oz)	150	0	40
Ham & Cheese Patties	1 patty (2 oz)	190	0	45
Light & Lean	3 oz	90	0	35
Light & Lean 97	3 oz	90	0	35
Light & Lean 97 Cuts	16 pieces (1 oz)	35	0	15
Light & Lean 97 Sliced	1 slice (1 oz)	25	0	15
Patties	1 patty (2 oz)	180	0	35
Primissimo Proscuitti	1 oz	70	0	25
Spread	4 tbsp (2 oz)	100	0	40
Supreme Cut Canned	1 oz	31	—	14
Jones				
Family Ham	1 slice	40	—	14
Ham Slices	1 slice	30	—	21
Krakus	1 oz	25		25
Louis Rich				
Carving Board Baked With Natural Juices	2 slices (1.6 oz)	45	0	25
Carving Board Carved Thin Honey With Natural Juices	6 slices (2.1 oz)	70	0	35
Carving Board Honey With Natural Juices	2 slices (1.6 oz)	50	0	25
Carving Board Smoked Cooked With Natural Juices	1 slice (1.6 oz)	50	0	25
Dinned Slices Baked	1 slice (3.3 oz)	80	0	40
Mr. Turkey				
Deli Cuts Honey Cured	3 slices	35	—	20
Oscar Mayer				
Baked	3 slices (2.2 oz)	60	0	30
Boiled	3 slices (2.2 oz)	60	0	30
Chopped	1 slice (1 oz)	50	0	15
Deli-Thin Boiled	4 slices (1.8 oz)	50	0	25
Deli-Thin Honey Ham	4 slices (1.8 oz)	60	0	25
Deli-Thin Smoked	4 slices (1.8 oz)	50	0	25
Dinner Slice	3 oz	90	0	45
Dinner Steaks	1 (2 oz)	60	0	30
Ham & Cheese Loaf	1 slice (1 oz)	70	0	20
Healthy Favorites Baked	4 slices (1.8 oz)	50	0	25
Healthy Favorites Honey Ham	4 slices (1.8 oz)	50	0	25
Healthy Favorites Smoked Cooked	4 slices (1.8 oz)	50	0	25
Honey Ham	3 slices (2.2 oz)	70	0	30
Lower Sodium	3 slices (2.2 oz)	70	0	30
Lunchables Cookies/Ham/ Swiss	1 pkg (4.2 oz)	360	tr	50

FOOD	PORTION	CALS.	FIB.	CHOL.
Oscar Mayer (CONT.)				
Lunchables Dessert Chocolate Pudding/Ham/American	1 pkg (6.2 oz)	390	tr	55
Lunchables Ham/Cheddar	1 pkg (4.5 oz)	340	0	75
Lunchables Ham/Garden Vegetable Cheese	1 pkg (4.5 oz)	380	1	45
Lunchables Honey Ham/Herb & Chive Cheese	1 pkg (4.5 oz)	390	1	45
Smoked Cooked	3 slices (2.2 oz)	60	0	30
Russer				
Baked	2 oz	70	—	30
Canadian Brand Maple	2 oz	70	—	30
Chopped	2 oz	130	—	30
Cooked Ham	2 oz	60	—	30
Ham & Cheese Loaf	2 oz	120	—	30
Honey & Maple Cured	2 oz	70	—	30
Honey Cured	2 oz	60	—	30
Hot	2 oz	70	—	30
Light Cooked	2 oz	60	—	30
Light Smoked	2 oz	60	—	30
Smoked Virginia	2 oz	70	—	30
Spiced	2 oz	160	—	30
Sara Lee				
Bavarian Brand Baked	2 oz	80	—	40
Bavarian Brand Baked Honey	2 oz	80	—	40
Honey Roasted	2 oz	90	—	30
Spreadables				
Ham Salad	¼ can	100	—	24
Underwood				
Deviled	2.08 oz	220	—	50
Deviled Light	2.08 oz	120	—	35
Deviled Smoked	2.08 oz	190	—	65
Weight Watchers				
Deli Thin Oven Roasted	5 slices (⅓ oz)	12	—	5
Deli Thin Oven Roasted Honey Ham	5 slices (⅓ oz)	12	—	5
Deli Thin Premium Smoked	5 slices (⅓ oz)	12	—	5
Oven Roasted Honey Ham	2 slices (¾ oz)	25	—	15
Oven Roasted Smoked	2 slices (¾ oz)	25	—	15
Premium Cooked	2 slices (¾ oz)	25	—	15
boneless 11% fat	3 oz	151	—	50
boneless extra lean roasted	3 oz	140	—	48
canned 13% fat	3 oz	192	—	52
canned 13% fat	1 oz	54	—	11

FOOD	PORTION	CALS.	FIB.	CHOL.
canned extra lean	3 oz	142	—	34
canned extra lean	1 oz	41	—	11
canned extra lean 4% fat	3 oz	116	—	25
center slice lean & fat	4 oz	229	—	61
chopped	1 oz	65	—	15
chopped canned	1 oz	68	—	14
ham & cheese loaf	1 oz	73	—	16
ham & cheese spread	1 oz	69	—	17
ham & cheese spread	1 tbsp	37	—	9
ham salad spread	1 tbsp	32	—	6
ham salad spread	1 oz	61	—	10
minced	1 oz	75	—	20
patties uncooked	1 (2.3 oz)	206	—	46
patties grilled	1 patty (2 oz)	203	—	43
sliced extra lean 5% fat	1 oz	37	—	13
sliced regular 11% fat	1 oz	52	—	16
steak boneless extra lean	1 oz	35	—	13
whole lean & fat roasted	3 oz	207	—	52
whole lean only roasted	3 oz	133	—	47
READY-TO-USE				
Sara Lee				
Golden Cure Smoked	2 oz	80	—	30
Honey Ham	2 oz	60	—	25

HAM DISHES

FROZEN
Weight Watchers

Handy Pocket Cheese Sauce & Ham	1 (4 oz)	200	—	5
TAKE-OUT				
croquettes	1 (3.1 oz)	217	tr	77
salad	½ cup	287	tr	237
sandwich w/ cheese	1	353	—	58

HAMBURGER

(*see also* BEEF)

FROZEN
Jimmy Dean

Burger	1 (2 oz)	220	0	40
Flamed Broiled Cheeseburger	1 (6.3 oz)	540	1	80
Mini Cheeseburger	2 (3 oz)	270	1	35
Kid Cuisine				
Beef Patty Sandwich/ Cheese	6.25 oz	430	—	35
MicroMagic				
Cheeseburger	1 pkg (4.75 oz)	450	—	80

FOOD	PORTION	CALS.	FIB.	CHOL.
MicroMagic (CONT.)				
Hamburger	1 pkg (4 oz)	350	—	55
Rudy's Farm				
Mild Burger	1 (3 oz)	360	0	65
TAKE-OUT				
double patty w/ bun	1 reg	544	—	99
double patty w/ catsup mayonnaise onion pickle tomato & bun	1 reg	649	—	94
double patty w/ catsup cheese mayonnaise mustard pickle tomato & bun	1 lg	706	—	141
double patty w/ catsup mustard mayonnaise onion pickle tomato & bun	1 lg	540	—	122
double patty w/ catsup mustard onion pickle & bun	1 reg	576	—	102
double patty w/ cheese & bun	1 reg	457	—	110
double patty w/ cheese & double bun	1 reg	461	—	80
double patty w/ cheese catsup mayonnaise onion pickle tomato & bun	1 reg	416	—	60
single patty w/ bacon catsup cheese mustard onion pickle & bun	1 lg	609	—	112
single patty w/ bun	1 lg	400	—	71
single patty w/ bun	1 reg	275	—	36
single patty w/ catsup cheese ham mayonnaise pickle tomato & bun	1 lg	745	—	122
single patty w/ catsup mustard mayonnaise onion pickle tomato & bun	1 reg	279	—	26
single patty w/ cheese & bun	1 lg	608	—	96
single patty w/ cheese & bun	1 reg	320	—	50
triple patty w/ catsup mustard pickle & bun	1 lg	693	—	142
triple patty w/ cheese & bun	1 lg	769	—	161

HAZELNUTS

Crumpy

FOOD	PORTION	CALS.	FIB.	CHOL.
Chocolate Hazelnut Spread	1 tbsp (0.5 oz)	80	0	0

HEART

FOOD	PORTION	CALS.	FIB.	CHOL.
beef simmered	3 oz	148	—	164

FOOD	PORTION	CALS.	FIB.	CHOL.
chicken simmered	1 cup (5 oz)	268	—	350
lamb braised	3 oz	158	—	212
pork, braised	1 heart (4.3 oz)	191	—	285
turkey simmered	1 cup (5 oz)	257	—	327
veal braised	3 oz	158	—	150

HEARTS OF PALM
canned	1 (1.2 oz)	9	—	0
canned	1 cup (5.1 oz)	41	—	0

HERBAL TEA
(see TEA/HERBAL TEA)

HERBS/SPICES
(see also individual names)

FOOD	PORTION	CALS.	FIB.	CHOL.
Ac'cent				
Flavor Enhancer	½ tsp	5	0	0
Herbal All Purpose Seasoning	½ tsp	0	0	0
Golden Dipt				
All Purpose Seafood	¼ tsp	2	—	0
Blackened Redfish	¼ tsp	2	—	0
Broiled Fish	¼ tsp	2	—	0
Cajun Style Shrimp & Crab	¼ tsp	2	—	0
Lemon Pepper Seafood	¼ tsp	8	—	0
Ka-Me				
Five Spice Powder	¼ tsp (1 g)	0	0	0
Lawry's				
Seasoning Blend Sloppy Joe	1 pkg	126	1	0
McIlhenny				
Crab Boil	3 oz	378	32	4
Mrs. Dash				
Extra Spicy	1 tsp (3.4 g)	12	—	0
Garlic & Herb	1 tsp (3.4 g)	12	—	0
Lemon & Herb	1 tsp (3.4 g)	12	—	0
Low Pepper Blend	1 tsp (3.4 g)	12	—	0
Original	1 tsp (3.4 g)	12	—	0
Table Blend	1 tsp (3.4 g)	12	—	0
Watkins				
Apple Bake Seasoning	¼ tsp (0.5 g)	0	0	0
Barbecue Spice	¼ tsp (0.5 g)	0	0	0
Bean Soup Seasoning	¾ tsp (2 g)	5	0	0
Beef Jerky Seasoning	2 tsp (6 g)	15	0	0
Chicken Seasoning	½ tsp (1 g)	0	0	0
Cole Slaw Seasoning	½ tsp (1.5 g)	5	0	0
Egg Sensations	1 tsp (3 g)	10	0	0

FOOD	PORTION	CALS.	FIB.	CHOL.
Watkins (CONT.)				
Fajita Seasoning	½ tsp (3 g)	10	0	0
Grill Seasoning	¼ tsp (1 g)	0	0	0
Ground Beef Seasoning	⅛ tsp (0.5 g)	0	0	0
Italian Blend	1 tsp (3 g)	1	0	0
Meat Tenderizer	⅛ tsp (0.5 g)	0	0	0
Meatloaf Seasoning	½ tsp (5 g)	15	0	0
Mexican Blend	½ tbsp (4 g)	15	0	0
Omelet & Souffle Seasoning	¾ tsp (2 g)	5	0	0
Oriental Ginger Garlic Liquid Spice Blend	1 tbsp (0.5 oz)	120	0	0
Potato Salad Seasoning	¼ tsp (1 g)	0	0	0
Pumpkin Pie Spice	¼ tsp (0.5 g)	0	0	0
Smokehouse Liquid Blend	1 tbsp (0.5 oz)	120	0	0
Soup & Vegetable Seasoning	¼ tsp (0.5 g)	0	0	0
Spanish Seasoning Blend	¼ tsp (0.5 oz)	0	0	0
curry powder	1 tsp	6	—	0
poultry seasoning	1 tsp	5	—	0
pumpkin pie spice	1 tsp	6	—	0

HERRING
FRESH

atlantic cooked	3 oz	172	—	65
atlantic cooked	1 fillet (5 oz)	290	—	110
atlantic raw	3 oz	134	—	51
pacific baked	3 oz	213	—	84
pacific fillet baked	5.1 oz	360	—	142
roe raw	3½ oz	130	—	360
READY-TO-USE				
atlantic kippered	1 fillet (1.4 oz)	87	—	33
atlantic pickled	½ oz	39	—	2

HICKORY NUTS

dried	1 oz	187	—	0

HOMINY
CANNED

Allen				
Golden	½ cup (4.5 oz)	120	4	0
Mexican	½ cup (4.5 oz)	120	3	0
White	½ cup (4.5 oz)	100	4	0
Uncle William				
Golden	½ cup (4.5 oz)	120	4	0
Mexican	½ cup (4.5 oz)	120	3	0
White	½ cup (4.5 oz)	100	4	0

FOOD	PORTION	CALS.	FIB.	CHOL.
Van Camp's				
Golden	½ cup (4.3 oz)	80	1	0
White	½ cup (4.3 oz)	80	1	0
canned	½ cup	57	—	0
HONEY				
Burleson's				
Clover	1 tbsp	60	0	0
Creamed	1 tbsp	60	0	0
Natural	1 tbsp	60	0	0
Pure	1 tbsp	60	0	0
Raw	1 tbsp	60	0	0
Rocky Mountain Clover	1 tbsp	60	0	0
Golden Blossom	1 tsp	20	—	0
Tree Of Life				
Alfalfa	1 tbsp (0.7 oz)	60	—	0
Avocado	1 tbsp (0.7 oz)	60	—	0
Buckwheat	1 tbsp (0.7 oz)	60	—	0
Clover	1 tbsp (0.7 oz)	60	—	0
Honeybear Wildflower	1 tbsp (0.7 oz)	60	—	0
Orange	1 tbsp (0.7 oz)	60	—	0
Tupelo	1 tbsp (0.7 oz)	60	—	0
Wildflower	1 tbsp (0.7 oz)	60	—	0
honey	1 tbsp (0.7 oz)	64	—	0
honey	1 cup (11.9 oz)	1031	—	0
HONEYDEW				
FRESH				
Chiquita	1 cup	70	—	0
Dole	⅒	50	1	0
cubed	1 cup	60	—	0
wedge	⅒	46	—	0
FROZEN				
Big Valley				
Balls	¾ cup (4.9 oz)	45	1	0
HORSE				
roasted	3 oz	149	—	58
HORSERADISH				
Gold's				
Hot	1 tsp	4	—	0
Red	1 tsp	4	—	0
White	1 tsp	4	—	0
Hebrew National				
White	1 tbsp	7	—	0

FOOD	PORTION	CALS.	FIB.	CHOL.
Heluva Good Cheese				
Horseradish	1 tsp (5 g)	0	—	0
Ka-Me				
Wasabi Powder	¼ tsp (1 g)	0	0	0
Kraft				
Cream Style	1 tsp (0.2 oz)	0	0	0
Horseradish Mustard	1 tsp (0.2 oz)	0	0	0
Prepared	1 tsp (0.2 oz)	0	0	0
Rosoff's				
Red	1 tbsp (0.5 oz)	8	—	0
White	1 tbsp (0.5 oz)	7	—	0
Sauceworks				
Horseradish	1 tsp (0.2 oz)	20	0	<5
Schorr's				
Red	1 tbsp (0.5 oz)	8	—	0
White	1 tbsp (0.5 oz)	7	—	0

HOT CAKES
(see PANCAKES)

HOT DOG
(see also MEAT SUBSTITUTES, SAUSAGE, SAUSAGE SUBSTITUTES)

FOOD	PORTION	CALS.	FIB.	CHOL.
CHICKEN				
Empire	1 (2 oz)	100	0	70
Health Valley				
Weiners	1	96	0	49
Wampler Longacre	1 (1.6 oz)	110	—	50
Wampler Longacre	1 (2 oz)	130	—	65
chicken	1 (1.5 oz)	116	—	45
MEAT				
Armour				
Lower Salt Jumbo	1	170	—	30
Lower Salt Jumbo Beef	1	170	—	30
Star Jumbo	1	190	—	30
Star Jumbo Beef	1	190	—	30
Chefwich				
Chili Dog	5 oz	380	—	27
Healthy Choice	1 (1.6 oz)	60	0	15
Bunsize	1 (2 oz)	70	0	20
Hebrew National				
Beef	1 (1.7 oz)	150	—	30
Cocktail Beef	6 (1.8 oz)	160	—	35
Dinner Beef	1 (4 oz)	350	—	75
Reduced Fat Beef	1 (1.7 oz)	120	—	25

FOOD	PORTION	CALS.	FIB.	CHOL.
Hormel				
Big 8	1 (2 oz)	170	0	35
Light & Lean 97	1 (1.6 oz)	45	0	15
Light & Lean 97 Beef	1 (1.6 oz)	45	—	10
Nathan's				
Natural Casing Franks	1	158	—	43
Skinless Franks	1	176	—	53
Oscar Mayer				
Beef	1 (1.6 oz)	150	0	25
Big & Juicy Deli Style Beef	1 (2.7 oz)	250	0	50
Big & Juicy Hot 'N Spicy	1 (2.7 oz)	220	0	45
Big & Juicy Original	1 (2.7 oz)	240	0	45
Big & Juicy Original Beef	1 (2.7 oz)	230	0	45
Big & Juicy Quarter Pound Beef	1 (4 oz)	350	0	65
Big & Juicy Smokie Links	1 (2.7 oz)	200	0	50
Bun-Length Beef	1 (2 oz)	180	0	35
Cheese	1 (1.6 oz)	150	0	35
Free	1 (1.8 oz)	40	—	15
Healthy Favorites Turkey & Beef	1 (2 oz)	60	0	25
Light Beef	1 (2 oz)	110	0	25
Weiners Bun-Length Pork & Turkey	1 (2 oz)	180	0	35
Weiners Little	6 (2 oz)	170	0	35
Weiners Pork & Turkey	1 (1.6 oz)	150	0	30
Weiners Light Pork Turkey Beef	1 (2 oz)	110	0	35
Russer				
Lil'Salt Deli Franks	1 (2.67 oz)	160	—	40
Shofar				
Kosher Beef	1 (1.8 oz)	150	0	20
Kosher Beef Reduced Fat Reduced Sodium	1 (1.8 oz)	120	0	25
Wrangler				
Beef	1 (2 oz)	170	0	40
Cheese	1 (2 oz)	170	0	40
Smoked	1 (2 oz)	170	0	40
beef	1 (2 oz)	180	—	35
beef	1 (1.5)	142	—	27
beef & pork	1 (1.5 oz)	144	—	22
beef & pork	1 (2 oz)	183	—	29
pork cheesefurter smokie	1 (1.5 oz)	141	—	29
TAKE-OUT				
corndog	1	460	—	79
w/ bun chili	1	297	—	51
w/ bun plain	1	242	—	44

FOOD	PORTION	CALS.	FIB.	CHOL.
TURKEY				
Empire	1 (2 oz)	90	0	35
Louis Rich	1 (1.6 oz)	90	0	40
Bun Length	1 (2 oz)	110	0	50
Turkey Cheese	1 (1.6 oz)	90	0	40
Mr. Turkey	1	110	—	40
Bun Size	1	130	—	50
Cheese	1	140	—	50
Wampler Longacre	1 (2 oz)	130	—	60
Wampler Longacre	1 (1.6 oz)	110	—	45
Weiners	1	96	0	35
turkey	1 (1.5 oz)	102	—	48
HUMMUS				
Casbah				
Mix as prep	¼ cup	120	1	0
Cedar's				
No Salt Added Hommus Tahini	2 tbsp (1 oz)	50	3	0
hummus	⅓ cup	140	—	0
hummus	1 cup	420	—	0
HYACINTH BEANS				
DRIED				
cooked	1 cup	228	—	0

ICE CREAM AND FROZEN DESSERTS

(*see also* ICES AND ICE POPS, PUDDING POPS, SHERBET, YOGURT FROZEN)

FOOD	PORTION	CALS.	FIB.	CHOL.
3 Musketeers				
Single Chocolate	1 (2 fl oz)	160	0	20
Single Vanilla	1 (2 fl oz)	160	0	15
Snack Chocolate	1 (0.72 fl oz)	60	0	5
Snack Vanilla	1 (0.72 fl oz)	60	0	5
Avari				
Creme Glace All Flavors	1 oz	10	—	0
Ben & Jerry's				
Cherry Garcia	½ cup (4 fl oz)	230	0	80
Chocolate	½ cup (4 fl oz)	230	0	55
Chocolate Chip Cookie Dough	½ cup (4 fl oz)	260	0	85
Chocolate Chip Cookie Dough	1 pop (2.5 fl oz)	240	1	45
Chocolate Fudge Brownie	½ cup (4 fl oz)	250	1	50
Chocolate Peanut Butter Chocolate Chip Cookie Dough	½ cup (4 fl oz)	280	0	55
Chunky Monkey	½ cup (4 fl oz)	270	0	70
Coffee Heath Bar Crunch	½ cup (4 fl oz)	270	0	80

FOOD	PORTION	CALS.	FIB.	CHOL.
Ben & Jerry's (CONT.)				
Heath Bar Crunch	1 pop (2.5 fl oz)	260	0	35
Heath Bar Crunch	½ cup (4 fl oz)	270	0	85
Milk Chocolate Almond	1 pop (2.5 fl oz)	250	3	35
Mint Cookie	½ cup (4 fl oz)	250	0	85
New York Super Fudge	1 pop (2.5 fl oz)	330	3	25
New York Super Fudge	½ cup (4 fl oz)	290	0	45
Pop Cherry Garcia	1 pop (3.7 fl oz)	250	2	45
Pop Heath Bar Crunch	1 pop (3.7 fl oz)	340	0	50
Pop New York Super Fudge	1 pop (3.7 fl oz)	330	3	25
Pop Rain Forest Crunch	1 pop (3.7 fl oz)	350	2	50
Rain Forest Crunch	½ cup (4 fl oz)	270	0	85
Vanilla	½ cup (4 fl oz)	215	0	95
Vanilla Chocolate Chunk	½ cup (4 fl oz)	250	0	85
Vanilla Brownie	1 bar (4 fl oz)	260	0	50
Bon Bons				
Vanilla With Milk Chocolate Coating	5 pieces	200	0	10
Vanilla With Milk Chocolate Coating	8 pieces	330	0	20
Borden				
Fat Free Strawberry	½ cup	90	—	0
Fat Free Black Cherry	½ cup	90	—	0
Fat Free Chocolate	½ cup	100	—	0
Fat Free Peach	½ cup	90	—	0
Fat Free Vanilla	½ cup	90	—	0
Bounty				
Cherry/Dark	1 (0.84 fl oz)	70	0	5
Coconut/Dark	1 (0.84 fl oz)	70	0	5
Coconut/Milk	1 (0.84 fl oz)	70	0	5
Bresler's				
All Flavors Ice Cream	3.5 oz	230	—	36
All Flavors Royale Cremes	4 oz	260	—	48
All Flavors Royale Lites	4 oz	217	—	0
Breyers				
Bar Vanilla	1 (2.7 oz)	250	tr	50
Bar Vanilla Carmel w/ Chocolate Brittle Coating	1 (2.7 oz)	260	0	45
Bar Vanilla With Chocolate Coating	1 (2.6 oz)	230	0	50
Butter Almond	½ cup	170	0	35
Butter Pecan	½ cup (2.6 oz)	180	0	35
Cherry Vanilla	½ cup	150	0	30
Chocolate	½ cup (2.6 oz)	160	1	30

FOOD	PORTION	CALS.	FIB.	CHOL.
Breyers (CONT.)				
Chocolate Chocolate Chip	½ cup (2.5 oz)	180	1	25
Chocolate Peanut Butter Twirl	½ cup (2.6 oz)	220	1	25
Chocolate Chip	½ cup (2.5 oz)	170	0	35
Chocolate Chip Cookie Dough	½ cup (2.5 oz)	190	0	40
Coffee	½ cup (2.6 oz)	150	0	35
Cookies n'Cream	½ cup (2.6 oz)	170	0	30
Deluxe Rocky Road	½ cup (2.5 oz)	190	1	25
French Vanilla	(2.5 oz)	170	0	105
Light Brownie Marble Fudge	½ cup (2.6 oz)	150	tr	30
Light Chocolate	½ cup (2.4 oz)	130	tr	30
Light Chocolate Fudge Twirl	½ cup (2.6 oz)	140	1	25
Light Heavenly Hash	½ cup (2.4 oz)	150	tr	25
Light Rocky Road Deluxe	½ cup (2.4 oz)	150	tr	25
Light Strawberry	½ cup (2.4 oz)	120	0	30
Light Toffee Fudge Parfait	½ cup (2.6 oz)	150	tr	35
Light Vanilla	½ cup (2.4 oz)	130	0	35
Light Vanilla Chocolate Strawberry	½ cup (2.4 oz)	120	0	30
Mint Chocolate Chip	½ cup (2.6 oz)	170	0	35
Mocha Almond Fudge	½ cup (2.7 oz)	190	1	30
Peach	½ cup (2.6 oz)	130	0	25
Reduced Fat Chocolate Chocolate Chip	½ cup (2.4 oz)	150	tr	25
Reduced Fat Heavenly Hash	½ cup (2.4 oz)	150	tr	25
Reduced Fat Mocha Almond Fudge	½ cup (2.5 oz)	160	tr	30
Reduced Fat Praline Almond Crunch	½ cup (2.4 oz)	140	tr	35
Reduced Fat Swiss Almond Fudge Twirl	½ cup (2.5 oz)	160	tr	30
Sandwich Vanilla	1 (2.8 oz)	250	1	25
Strawberry	½ cup (2.6 oz)	130	0	25
Toffee Bar Crunch	½ cup (2.5 oz)	180	0	40
Vanilla	½ cup (2.6 oz)	150	0	35
Vanilla Caramel Praline	½ cup (2.6 oz)	190	0	35
Vanilla Chocolate	½ cup (2.5 oz)	160	0	35
Vanilla Chocolate Strawberry	½ cup (2.5 oz)	150	0	30
Vanilla Peanut Butter Fudge Sundae	½ cup (2.5 oz)	170	0	35
Vanilla Fudge Twirl	½ cup (2.6 oz)	160	tr	35
Butterfinger	1 bar (2.5 oz)	170	0	15
Butterfinger	8 nuggets	340	0	20
Carnation				
Berry Swirl Bar Raspberry	1 bar	70	—	10

FOOD	PORTION	CALS.	FIB.	CHOL.
Carnation (CONT.)				
Berry Swirl Bar Strawberry	1 bar	70	—	9
Cheesecake Bar Original	1 bar	120	—	12
Cheesecake Bar Strawberry	1 bar	125	—	10
Chocolate Malted Bar	1 bar	70	—	19
Creamy Lites Bar Chocolate	1 bar	50	—	8
Creamy Lites Bar Strawberry	1 bar	50	—	7
Sundae Cup Strawberry	1 (3.3 oz)	200	0	30
Cool 'N Creamy				
Amarello With Chocolate Swirl	1 bar	62	—	1
Chocolate Vanilla	1 bar	54	—	1
Double Chocolate Fudge	1 bar	55	—	1
Orange Vanilla	1 bar	31	—	tr
Cool Creations				
Cookies & Cream Sandwich	1 (3.5 oz)	240	1	15
Mini Sandwich	1 (2.3 oz)	110	0	10
Cyrk				
Chocolate	3 oz	209	0	62
Maple Walnut	3 oz	299	1	62
Mint Chocolate Chip	3 oz	258	0	64
Strawberry	3 oz	208	tr	62
Vanilla	3 oz	209	0	62
DoveBar				
Almond	1 (3.67 fl oz)	335	0	35
Bite Size Almond Praline	1 (0.75 fl oz)	80	0	7
Bite Size Cherry Royale	1 (0.75 fl oz)	70	0	8
Bite Size Classic Vanilla	1 (0.75 fl oz)	70	0	8
Bite Size French Vanilla	1 (0.75 fl oz)	70	0	15
Bite Size Mint Supreme	1 (0.75 fl oz)	80	0	7
Caramel Pecan	1 (3.67 fl oz)	350	0	35
Chocolate Milk Chocolate	1 (3.8 fl oz)	340	0	40
Coffee Cashew	1 (3.67 fl oz)	335	0	35
Crunchy Cookie	1 (3.8 fl oz)	340	0	40
Peanut	1 (3.8 fl oz)	380	0	40
Single Vanilla/Dark	1 (2 fl oz)	200	0	20
Vanilla Dark Chocolate	1 (3.8 fl oz)	340	0	45
Vanilla Milk Chocolate	1 (3.8 fl oz)	340	0	40
Drumstick				
Cone Chocolate	1 (4.6 oz)	340	2	25
Cone Chocolate Dipped	1 (4.6 oz)	340	1	25
Cone Vanilla	1 (4.6 oz)	350	2	20
Cone Vanilla Caramel	1 (4.6 oz)	360	6	25
Cone Vanilla Fudge	1 (4.6 oz)	370	2	20

FOOD	PORTION	CALS.	FIB.	CHOL.
Edy's				
American Dream Rocky Road	3 oz	110	—	0
American Dream Chocolate	3 oz	90	—	0
American Dream Chocolate Chip	3 oz	100	—	0
American Dream Cookies'N'Cream	3 oz	100	—	0
American Dream Mocha Almond Fudge	3 oz	110	—	0
American Dream Strawberry	3 oz	70	—	0
American Dream Toasted Almond	3 oz	110	—	0
American Dream Vanilla	3 oz	80	—	0
American Dream Vanilla Chocolate Strawberry	3 oz	80	—	0
Light Almond Praline	4 oz	140	—	15
Light Banana-Politan	4 oz	110	—	15
Light Butter Pecan	4 oz	140	—	15
Light Cafe Au Lait	4 oz	110	—	15
Light Candy Bar	4 oz	140	—	15
Light Chocolate Chip	4 oz	120	—	15
Light Chocolate Fudge Mousse	4 oz	130	—	15
Light Cookies'N'Cream	4 oz	120	—	15
Light Dreamy Caramel Cream	4 oz	140	—	15
Light Malt Ball 'N' Fudge	4 oz	140	—	15
Light Marble Fudge	4 oz	120	—	15
Light Mocha Almond Fudge	4 oz	140	—	15
Light Peanut Butter & Chocolate	4 oz	130	—	15
Light Raspberry Truffle	4 oz	110	—	15
Light Rocky Road	4 oz	130	—	15
Light Strawberry	4 oz	110	—	15
Light Vanilla	4 oz	100	—	15
Vanilla Chocolate Strawberry	4 oz	110	—	15
Flintstones				
Cool Cream	1 (2.75 oz)	90	0	5
Push-Up	1 (2.75 oz)	100	0	5
Friendly's				
Heath English Toffee	½ cup (2.7 oz)	190	0	30
Vanilla Chocolate Strawberry	½ cup	150	tr	30
Frusen Gladje				
Butter Pecan	½ cup	280	—	60
Chocolate	½ cup	240	—	75
Chocolate Chocolate Chip	½ cup	270	—	55

FOOD	PORTION	CALS.	FIB.	CHOL.
Frusen Gladje (CONT.)				
Strawberry	½ cup	230	—	65
Swiss Chocolate Candy Almond	½ cup	270	—	55
Vanilla	½ cup	230	—	65
Vanilla Swiss Almond	½ cup	270	—	60
Good Humor				
Banana Bob	1 (3 fl oz)	155	0	5
Bar Classic Toasted Almond	1 (3.1 fl oz)	170	1	10
Bar Classic Vanilla	1 (3.1 fl oz)	190	0	15
Bar Classic Almond	1 (3.1 fl oz)	210	1	15
Bar Sidewalk Sundae	1	280	2	15
Bubble O'Bill	1 (3.6 fl oz)	170	1	15
Chip Burrrger	1 (4.7 oz)	320	1	20
Chip Sandwich	1 (4.7 oz)	320	1	20
Choco Taco	1 (4.4 fl oz)	320	1	20
Chocolate Eclair Classic	1 (3.1 fl oz)	170	1	10
Classic Candy Center Crunch Vanilla	1	280	0	15
Colonel Crunch Chocolate	1 (3.1 oz)	160	1	10
Colonel Crunch Strawberry	1 (3.1 oz)	170	0	10
Combo Cup	1 (6.2 fl oz)	200	1	35
Cone Olde Nut Sundae	1 (3.9 oz)	230	2	5
Cone Sidewalk Sundae	1 (4.2 oz)	270	1	10
Creamee Burrrger	1 (4.7 oz)	310	1	20
Crunch Classic Candy Center	1 (3.1 fl oz)	260	1	10
Far Frog	1 (3.6 fl oz)	150	1	20
Fun Box Ice Cream Sandwich	1 (3.1 fl oz)	160	1	10
King Cone	1 (5.7 fl oz)	300	2	25
King Cone Classic Vanilla	1 (4.8 oz)	300	1	20
King Cone Strawberry	1 (5.7 oz)	250	1	25
Light Chocolate Chocolate Chip	½ cup (2.4 oz)	130	tr	10
Light Chocolate Chip	½ cup (2.4 oz)	130	0	10
Light Coffee	½ cup (2.4 oz)	110	0	15
Light Cookies N'Cream	½ cup (2.4 oz)	130	0	10
Light Heavenly Hash	½ cup (2.4 oz)	140	tr	10
Light Praline Almond Crunch	½ cup (2.4 oz)	130	0	15
Light Toffee Bar Crunch	½ cup (2.4 oz)	130	0	15
Light Vanilla	½ cup (2.4 oz)	110	0	15
Light Vanilla Chocolate Strawberry	½ cup (2.4 oz)	110	0	10
Light Vanilla Fudge	½ cup (2.6 oz)	120	0	15
Magnum Almond	1 (4.2 fl oz)	270	5	30
Magnum Chocolate	1 (4.2 fl oz)	260	2	30
Number One Bar	1 (4.1 fl oz)	190	1	15

FOOD	PORTION	CALS.	FIB.	CHOL.
Good Humor (CONT.)				
Popsicle Ice Cream Sandwich	1 (3.6 fl oz)	190	1	15
Popsicle Ice Cream Bar	1 (3.1 fl oz)	160	1	15
Sandwich Giant Vanilla	1 (5.2 fl oz)	240	1	20
Sandwich Ice Cream	1	190	1	15
Sandwich Sidewalk Sundae	1 (3.1 oz)	160	1	10
Sandwich Sprinkle	1 (3.1 fl oz)	180	1	10
Sandwich Classic Chip Cookie	1 (4.1 fl oz)	300	1	18
Sandwich Giant Neapolitan	1 (5.2 fl oz)	260	1	20
Strawberry Shortcake Bar Classic	1 (3.1 fl oz)	160	1	10
Sundae Twist Cup	1	160	0	10
Toffee Taco	1 (4.4 fl oz)	300	1	15
Viennetta Chocolate	1 (4.2 fl oz)	160	1	10
Viennetta Vanilla	1 (4.2 fl oz)	160	0	20
WWF Bar	1 (3.7 fl oz)	200	1	15
X-Men Bar	1 (3 fl oz)	150	0	15
Haagen-Dazs				
Butter Pecan	4 oz	390	—	115
Chocolate	4 oz	270	—	120
Chocolate Chocolate Chip	4 oz	290	—	105
Coffee	4 oz	270	—	120
Crunch Bar Caramel Almond	1	240	—	40
Crunch Bar Peanut Butter	1	270	—	35
Crunch Bar Vanilla	1	220	—	40
Honey Vanilla	4 oz	250	—	135
Rum Raisin	4 oz	250	—	110
Strawberry	4 oz	250	—	95
Vanilla	4 oz	260	—	120
Vanilla Peanut Butter Swirl	4 oz	280	—	110
Healthy Choice				
Bordeaux Cherry Chocolate Chip	½ cup (2.5 oz)	110	tr	<5
Butter Pecan Crunch	½ cup (2.2 oz)	120	1	<5
Cappuccino Chocolate Chunk	½ cup (2.2 oz)	120	1	10
Cone Malt Caramel	½ cup (2.2 oz)	120	1	10
Cookies'N Cream	½ cup	120	tr	<5
Double Fudge Swirl	½ cup (2.2 oz)	120	1	<5
Fudge Brownie	½ cup (2.2 oz)	120	2	5
Low-Fat Black Forest	½ cup (2.5 oz)	120	1	5
Mint Chocolate Chip	½ cup (2.2 oz)	120	tr	<5
Peanut Butter Cookie Dough Fudge	½ cup (2.2 oz)	120	tr	<5
Praline & Caramel	½ cup (2.2 oz)	130	tr	<5

FOOD	PORTION	CALS.	FIB.	CHOL.
Healthy Choice (CONT.)				
Rocky Road	½ cup (2.2 oz)	140	2	<5
Vanilla	½ cup (2.2 oz)	100	1	5
Heath	1 bar (2.5 oz)	160	0	15
Heath	8 nuggets	180	0	25
Heaven				
Sundae Bars Chocolate Fudge	1 bar	150	—	7
Sundae Bars Vanilla Fudge	1 bar	150	—	7
Vanilla Caramel Nut	1 bar	225	—	9
Vanilla Nut Fudge	1 bar	222	—	9
Hood				
Bar Orange Cream	1 bar (1.8 oz)	90	0	5
Bar Vanilla	1 bar (1.6 oz)	160	0	15
Caramel Butterscotch Blast	½ cup (2.3 oz)	160	0	25
Chocolate	½ cup (2.3 oz)	140	0	30
Chocolate Chip	½ cup (2.3 oz)	160	0	30
Chocolate Eclair	1 bar (1.6 oz)	150	0	5
Christmas Tree	½ cup (2.3 oz)	140	0	30
Coffee	½ cup (2.3 oz)	140	0	30
Cookie Dough Delight	½ cup (2.3 oz)	160	0	30
Cookies N Cream	½ cup (2.3 oz)	160	0	30
Cooler Cups	1 (2.1 oz)	80	0	<5
Crispy Bar	1 (1.9 oz)	180	0	20
Egg Nog	½ cup (2.3 oz)	130	0	25
Fabulous Fudge & Peanut Butter Swirled Fudge Bars	1 bar (2.1 oz)	110	0	10
Fabulous Fudgies Assorted Bars	1 bar (2.1 oz)	100	0	10
Fat Free Raspberry Blush	½ cup (2.5 oz)	120	0	0
Fat Free Chocolate Passion	½ cup (2.5 oz)	100	0	0
Fat Free Classic Harlequin	½ cup (2.5 oz)	100	0	0
Fat Free Double Brownie Sundae	½ cup (2.5 oz)	120	0	0
Fat Free Heavenly Hash	½ cup (2.5 oz)	120	0	0
Fat Free Mississippi Mud Pie	½ cup (2.5 oz)	130	0	0
Fat Free Praline Pecan Delight	½ cup (2.5 oz)	120	0	0
Fat Free Super Strawberry Swirl	½ cup (2.5 oz)	100	0	0
Fat Free Vanilla Fudge Twist	½ cup (2.5 oz)	120	0	0
Fat Free Very Vanilla	½ cup (2.5 oz)	100	0	0
Fudge Bars	1 bar (2.7 oz)	100	0	0
Grasshopper Pie	½ cup (2.3 oz)	160	0	25
Heavenly Hash	½ cup (2.3 oz)	140	0	20
Hendrie's Cherry Chocolate Dips	1 bar (1.3 oz)	120	0	15

FOOD	PORTION	CALS.	FIB.	CHOL.

Hood (CONT.)

FOOD	PORTION	CALS.	FIB.	CHOL.
Hoodsie Cup Vanilla & Chocolate	1 (1.7 oz)	100	0	20
Light Almond Praline Delight	½ cup (2.4 oz)	110	0	15
Light Brownie Nut Sundae	½ cup (2.4 oz)	140	0	10
Light Caribbean Coffee Royale	½ cup (2.4 oz)	110	0	15
Light Chocolate Chocolate Chip Cookie Dough	½ cup (2.4 oz)	140	0	15
Light Chocolate Almond Chip Sundae	½ cup (2.4 oz)	140	0	10
Light Cookies N Cream	½ cup (2.4 oz)	130	0	15
Light Heath Toffee Chunk Swirl	½ cup (2.4 oz)	140	0	15
Light Heavenly Hash	½ cup (2.4 oz)	130	0	10
Light Maple Sugar Shack	⅓ cup (2.4 oz)	130	0	10
Light Massachusetts Mud Pie	½ cup (2.4 oz)	140	0	10
Light Raspberry Swirl	½ cup (2.4 oz)	120	0	10
Light Strawberry Supreme	½ cup (2.4 oz)	110	0	15
Light Triple Nut Cluster Sundae	½ cup (2.4 oz)	140	0	10
Light Vanilla	½ cup (2.4 oz)	110	0	15
Light Vanilla Chocolate Strawberry	½ cup (2.4 oz)	110	0	15
Low Fat No Sugar Added Caramel Swirl	½ cup (2.4 oz)	120	0	10
Low Fat No Sugar Added Chocolate Supreme	½ cup (2.4 oz)	120	0	10
Low Fat No Sugar Added Mocha Fudge	½ cup (2.4 oz)	110	0	10
Low Fat No Sugar Added Raspberry Swirl	½ cup (2.4 oz)	110	0	10
Low Fat No Sugar Added Vanilla	½ cup (2.4 oz)	100	0	10
Maple Walnut	½ cup (2.3 oz)	160	0	30
Rockets	1 (2 oz)	120	1	20
Sandwich Light	1 (2.2 oz)	160	1	10
Sandwich Vanilla	1 (2.2 oz)	180	1	20
Sports Bar	1 (2.9 oz)	250	0	25
Spumoni	½ cup (2.3 oz)	140	0	30
Strawberry	½ cup (2.3 oz)	130	0	30
Super Sortment Chocolate & Banana Fudge Bar	1 bar (2.1 oz)	100	0	10
Super Sortment Root Beer Float & Orange Cream Bar	1 bar (1.5 oz)	70	0	10
Vanilla	½ cup (2.3 oz)	140	0	30
Vanilla Chocolate Patchwork	½ cup (2.3 oz)	140	0	30

FOOD	PORTION	CALS.	FIB.	CHOL.
Hood (CONT.)				
Vanilla Chocolate Strawberry	½ cup (2.3 oz)	140	0	30
Vanilla Fudge	½ cup (2.3 oz)	140	0	25
Klondike				
Almond Bar	1 (5.2 fl oz)	310	3	25
Caramel Crunch	1 (5.2 fl oz)	300	tr	30
Chocolate Chocolate Bar	1 (5.2 fl oz)	280	tr	20
Coffee Bar	1 (5.2 fl oz)	290	0	15
Dark Chocolate Bar	1 (5.2 fl oz)	290	tr	30
Gold Bar	1 (5.2 fl oz)	340	1	34
Krispy Bar	1 (5.2 fl oz)	300	0	25
Krunch	1 (3.1 fl oz)	200	1	20
Lite Bar	1 (2.3 fl oz)	110	1	5
Lite Bar Caramel	1 (2.4 fl oz)	120	1	5
Movie Bites Chocolate	8 pieces (4.6 fl oz)	340	1	25
Movie Bites Vanilla	8 pieces (4.6 fl oz)	320	1	25
Original Bar	1 (5.2 fl oz)	290	0	15
Sandwich Chocolate	1 (5.2 fl oz)	270	2	20
Sandwich Lite	1 (2.9 fl oz)	100	1	5
Sandwich Vanilla	1 (5.2 fl oz)	250	1	20
Mars				
Almond Bar	1 (1.85 fl oz)	210	0	15
Milky Way				
Single Chocolate/Milk	1 (2 fl oz)	210	0	20
Snack Chocolate/Milk	1 (0.72 fl oz)	70	0	5
Snack Vanilla/Dark	1 (0.72 fl oz)	70	0	5
Mocha Mix				
Berry Berry Berry	½ cup	140	0	0
Dutch Chocolate	½ cup (2.3 oz)	140	0	0
Mocha Almond Fudge	½ cup (2.3 oz)	150	0	0
Neapolitan	½ cup (2.3 oz)	140	0	0
Strawberry Swirl	½ cup (2.3 oz)	140	0	0
Vanilla	½ cup (2.3 oz)	140	0	0
Nestle Crunch				
Chocolate	1 bar (3 oz)	200	0	15
Cones	1 (4.6 oz)	300	2	25
Crunch King	1 (4 oz)	270	0	20
Nuggets	8 pieces	140	0	10
Reduced Fat	1 (2.5 oz)	130	0	5
Vanilla	1 bar (3 oz)	200	0	15
Rice Dream				
Bar Chocolate	1	270	—	0
Bar Chocolate Nutty	1	330	—	0
Bar Strawberry	1	260	—	0

FOOD	PORTION	CALS.	FIB.	CHOL.
Rice Dream (CONT.)				
Bar Vanilla	1	275	—	0
Bar Vanilla Nutty	1	330	—	0
Cappuccino	½ cup	130	—	0
Carob	½ cup	130	—	0
Carob Almond	½ cup	140	—	0
Carob Chip	½ cup	140	—	0
Carob Chip Mint	½ cup	140	—	0
Cocoa Marble Fudge	½ cup	140	—	0
Dream Pie Chocolate	1	380	—	0
Dream Pie Mint	1	380	—	0
Dream Pie Mocha	1	380	—	0
Dream Pie Vanilla	1	380	—	0
Lemon	½ cup	130	—	0
Peanut Butter Fudge	½ cup	160	—	0
Strawberry	½ cup	130	—	0
Vanilla	½ cup	130	—	0
Vanilla Fudge	½ cup	140	—	0
Vanilla Swiss Almond	½ cup	140	—	0
Wildberry	½ cup	130	—	0
Sealtest				
American Glory	½ cup (2.4 oz)	130	0	25
Butter Pecan	½ cup (2.4 oz)	160	—	30
Candy Cane Crunch	½ cup (2.4 oz)	150	0	25
Chocolate	½ cup (2.4 oz)	140	tr	25
Chocolate Butter Pecan	½ cup (2.4 oz)	150	0	30
Chocolate Chip	½ cup (2.4 oz)	150	0	30
Coconut Chocolate	½ cup (2.4 oz)	160	tr	25
Coffee	½ cup (2.4 oz)	140	0	30
Cupid's Scoops	½ cup (2.5 oz)	140	0	25
Dessert Bar Free Chocolate Fudge	1	90	—	0
Dessert Bar Free Vanilla Strawberry Swirl	1	80	—	0
Dessert Bar Free Vanilla Fudge	1	80	—	0
Free Black Cherry	½ cup	100	—	0
Free Chocolate	½ cup	100	—	0
Free Peach	½ cup	100	—	0
Free Strawberry	½ cup	100	—	0
Free Vanilla	½ cup	100	—	0
Free Vanilla Strawberry Royale	½ cup	100	—	0
Free Vanilla Fudge Royale	½ cup	100	—	0
French Vanilla	½ cup (2.4 oz)	140	0	60
Fudge Royale	½ cup (2.5 oz)	150	0	25

FOOD	PORTION	CALS.	FIB.	CHOL.
Sealtest (CONT.)				
Heavenly Hash	½ cup (2.4 oz)	150	tr	25
Maple Walnut	½ cup (2.4 oz)	160	0	30
Strawberry	½ cup (2.4 oz)	130	0	25
Triple Chocolate Passion	½ cup (2.5 oz)	160	tr	25
Vanilla	½ cup (2.4 oz)	140	0	30
Vanilla Chocolate Strawberry	½ cup (2.4 oz)	140	0	25
Vanilla With Orange Sherbet	½ cup (2.7 oz)	130	0	20
Simple Pleasures				
Chocolate	4 oz	140	—	10
Chocolate Caramel Sundae Light	4 oz	90	—	15
Chocolate Light	4 oz	80	—	15
Chocolate Chip	4 oz	150	—	15
Coffee	4 oz	120	—	15
Cookies n' Cream	4 oz	150	—	10
Mint Chocolate Chip	4 oz	150	—	5
Peach	4 oz	120	—	10
Pecan Praline	4 oz	140	—	5
Rum Raisin	4 oz	130	—	15
Strawberry	4 oz	120	—	10
Toffee Crunch	4 oz	130	—	10
Vanilla	4 oz	120	—	15
Vanilla Fudge Swirl Light	4 oz	90	—	15
Snickers				
Single	1 (2 fl oz)	220	0	15
Snack	1 (1 fl oz)	110	0	5
Tofu Ice Creme				
Carob	4 fl oz	190	—	0
Vanilla	4 fl oz	190	—	0
Tofulite	4 oz	150	—	0
Tofutti				
Frutti Vanilla Apple Orchard	4 fl oz	100	—	0
Ultra Slim-Fast				
Bar Fudge	1	90	2	0
Bar Vanilla Cookie Crunch	1	90	1	0
Chocolate	4 oz	100	2	0
Chocolate Fudge	4 oz	120	2	0
Peach	4 oz	100	2	0
Pralines & Caramel	4 oz	120	2	0
Sandwich Vanilla	1	140	1	0
Sandwich Vanilla Chocolate	1	140	1	0
Sandwich Vanilla Oatmeal	1	150	3	0
Vanilla	4 oz	90	2	0

FOOD	PORTION	CALS.	FIB.	CHOL.
Ultra Slim-Fast (CONT.)				
Vanilla Fudge Cookie	4 oz	110	2	0
Weight Watchers				
Bar Chocolate Dip	1 (2 oz)	110	—	5
Bar Double Fudge	1 (1.75 oz)	60	—	5
Bar English Toffee Crunch	1 (2 oz)	120	—	5
Bar Sugar Free Chocolate Mousse	1 (1.75 oz)	35	—	5
Bar Sugar Free Chocolate Treat	1 (2.75 oz)	90	—	0
Bar Sugar Free Fat Free Orange Vanilla Treat	1 (1.75 oz)	30	—	0
Fat Free Frozen Dessert Chocolate	½ cup	80	—	5
Fat Free Frozen Dessert Chocolate Swirl	½ cup	90	—	5
Fat Free Frozen Dessert Neapolitan	½ cup	80	—	5
Fat Free Frozen Dessert Vanilla	½ cup	80	—	5
Ice Milk Chocolate Chip	½ cup	120	—	10
Ice Milk Pecan Pralines 'n Cream	½ cup	130	—	10
ONE-ders Brownies'n Creme	4 oz	130	—	10
ONE-ders Chocolate Chip	4 oz	120	—	10
ONE-ders Heavenly Hash	4 oz	130	—	10
ONE-ders Pralines'n Creme	4 oz	130	—	10
ONE-ders Strawberry	4 oz	110	—	10
chocolate	½ cup (4 fl oz)	143	—	22
dixie cup chocolate	1 (3.5 fl oz)	125	—	20
dixie cup strawberry	1 (3.5 fl oz)	112	—	17
dixie cup vanilla	1 (3.5 fl oz)	116	—	25
french vanilla soft serve	½ gal	3014	—	1226
french vanilla soft serve	½ cup (4 fl oz)	185	—	78
strawberry	½ cup (4 fl oz)	127	—	19
vanilla	½ cup (4 fl oz)	132	—	29
vanilla light	½ cup	92	—	9
vanilla rich	½ cup	178	—	45
vanilla soft serve	½ cup	111	—	10
vanilla 10% fat	½ gal	2153	—	476
vanilla 16% fat	½ gal	2805	—	256
vanilla light	½ gal	1469	—	146
vanilla light	1 cup	184	—	18
vanilla light soft serve	1 cup	223	—	13
vanilla light soft serve	½ gal	1787	—	106
TAKE-OUT				
cone vanilla light soft serve	1 (4.6 oz)	164	—	28

FOOD	PORTION	CALS.	FIB.	CHOL.
gelato chocolate hazelnut	½ cup (5.3 oz)	370	2	92
gelato vanilla	½ cup (3 oz)	211	0	151
sundae caramel	1 (5.4 oz)	303	—	25
sundae hot fudge	1 (5.4 oz)	284	—	21
sundae strawberry	1 (5.4 oz)	269	—	21

ICE CREAM CONES AND CUPS

Comet
Cups	1 (5 g)	20	tr	0
Sugar Cones	1 (12 g)	50	tr	0
Waffle Cone	1 (17 g)	70	1	0

Dutch Mill
Chocolate Covered Wafer Cups	1 (0.5 oz)	80	0	0

Keebler
Sugar Cones	1	45	—	0
Vanilla Cups	1	15	—	0

Oreo
Chocolate Cones	1 (13 g)	50	tr	0

Teddy Grahams
Cinnamon Cones	1 (0.5 oz)	60	tr	0
sugar cone	1	40	tr	0
wafer cone	1	17	tr	0

ICE CREAM TOPPINGS
(see also SYRUP)

Hershey
Chocolate Fudge	2 tbsp	100	—	5
Chocolate Shoppe Candy Bar Sprinkles York	2 tbsp (1.1 oz)	170	2	<5

Kraft
Butterscotch	2 tbsp (1.4 oz)	130	0	<5
Caramel	2 tbsp (1.4 oz)	120	0	0
Chocolate	2 tbsp (1.4 oz)	110	1	0
Hot Fudge	2 tbsp (1.4 oz)	140	tr	0
Pineapple	2 tbsp (1.4 oz)	110	0	0
Strawberry	2 tbsp (1.4 oz)	110	0	0

Marzetti
Caramel Apple	2 tbsp	60	0	5
Caramel Apple Reduced Fat	2 tbsp	30	0	5
Peanut Butter Caramel	2 tbsp	60	1	0

Smucker's
Chocolate	2 tbsp	130	—	0
Magic Shell Chocolate Fudge	2 tbsp	190	—	0
Pineapple	2 tbsp	130	—	0
Strawberry	2 tbsp	120	—	0

FOOD	PORTION	CALS.	FIB.	CHOL.
marshmallow cream	1 jar (7 oz)	615	—	0
marshmallow cream	1 oz	88	—	0
pineapple	2 tbsp (1.5 oz)	106	—	0
pineapple	1 cup (11.5 oz)	861	—	0
strawberry	1 cup (11.5 oz)	863	—	0
strawberry	2 tbsp (1.5 oz)	107	—	0
walnuts in syrup	2 tbsp (1.4 oz)	167	—	0

ICED TEA
(see TEA/HERBAL TEA)

ICES AND ICE POPS
(see also ICE CREAM AND FROZEN DESSERTS, PUDDING POPS, SHERBET, SORBET, YOGURT FROZEN)

FOOD	PORTION	CALS.	FIB.	CHOL.
Bresler's				
All Flavors Ice	3.5 oz	120	—	0
Chiquita				
Fruit & Juice Bar Cherry	1 bar (2 oz)	50	—	0
Fruit & Juice Bar Raspberry	1 bar (2 oz)	50	—	0
Fruit & Juice Bar Raspberry Banana	1 bar (2 oz)	50	—	0
Fruit & Juice Bar Strawberry	1 bar (2 oz)	50	—	0
Fruit & Juice Bar Strawberry Banana	1 bar (2 oz)	50	—	0
Cool Creations				
10 Pack	1 pop (2 oz)	60	0	0
Lion King Cone	1 (4 oz)	280	1	15
Mickey Mouse Bar	1 (4 oz)	170	0	15
Mickey Mouse Bar	1 (2.5 oz)	110	0	10
Surprise Pops	1 (2 oz)	60	0	0
Crystal Light				
Berry Blend	1 bar	13	—	0
Cherry	1 bar	13	—	0
Fruit Punch	1 bar	14	—	0
Orange	1 bar	13	—	0
Pina Colada	1 bar	14	—	0
Pineapple	1 bar	14	—	0
Pink Lemonade	1 bar	14	—	0
Raspberry	1 bar	13	—	0
Strawberry	1 bar	13	—	0
Strawberry Daiquiri	1 bar	14	—	0
Cyrk				
Ice Chocolate	4 oz	85	—	0
Ice Vanilla	4 oz	75	—	0
Sorbet Apricot	4 oz	104	1	0

FOOD	PORTION	CALS.	FIB.	CHOL.
Cyrk (CONT.)				
Sorbet Blueberry	4 oz	77	2	0
Sorbet Cherry	4 oz	98	1	0
Sorbet Lemon	4 oz	66	0	0
Sorbet Mango	4 oz	83	tr	0
Sorbet Pina Colada	4 oz	107	tr	0
Sorbet Plum	4 oz	90	1	0
Sorbet Raspberry	4 oz	88	2	0
Sorbet Strawberry	4 oz	79	1	0
Sorbet Sugar Free Apricot	4 oz	36	1	0
Sorbet Sugar Free Mango	4 oz	48	2	0
Sorbet Sugar Free Pina Colada	4 oz	66	1	0
Sorbet Sugar Free Raspberry	4 oz	35	3	0
Sorbet White Peach	4 oz	96	1	0
Dole				
Fruit 'n Juice Coconut	1 bar (4 oz)	210	0	10
Fruit 'n Juice Lemonade	1 bar (4 oz)	120	0	0
Fruit 'n Juice Lime	1 bar (4 oz)	110	0	0
Fruit 'n Juice Peach Passion	1 bar (2.5 oz)	70	0	0
Fruit 'n Juice Pineapple Coconut	1 bar (4 oz)	140	0	0
Fruit 'n Juice Pineapple Orange Banana	1 bar (2.5 oz)	70	0	0
Fruit 'n Juice Pineapple Orange Banana	1 bar (4 oz)	110	0	0
Fruit 'n Juice Raspberry	1 bar (2.5 oz)	70	0	0
Fruit 'n Juice Strawberry	1 bar (4 oz)	110	0	0
Fruit 'n Juice Strawberry	1 bar (2.5 oz)	70	0	0
Fruit Juice Grape	1 bar (1.75 oz)	45	0	0
Fruit Juice No Sugar Added Grape	1 bar (1.75 oz)	25	0	0
Fruit Juice No Sugar Added Strawberry	1 bar (1.75 oz)	25	0	0
Fruit Juice Raspberry	1 bar (1.75 oz)	45	0	0
Fruit Juice Raspberry	1 bar (1.75 oz)	25	0	0
Fruit Juice Strawberry	1 bar (1.75 oz)	45	0	0
Flintstones				
Rock Pops	1 (3.5 oz)	80	0	0
Frozfruit				
Strawberry	1 (4 oz)	80	1	0
Good Humor				
Big Stick Cherry Pineapple	1 (3.6 fl oz)	50	0	0
Big Stick Popsicle	1 (3.6 fl oz)	50	—	0
Calippo Cherry	1 (3.8 fl oz)	100	—	0

FOOD	PORTION	CALS.	FIB.	CHOL.
Good Humor (CONT.)				
Calippo Grape Lemon	1 (3.9 fl oz)	90	—	0
Calippo Orange	1 (3.9 fl oz)	90	—	0
Citrus Bites	1 (1.8 fl oz)	35	—	0
Creamsicle Orange	1 (2.8 fl oz)	110	0	10
Creamsicle Orange	1 (1.8 fl oz)	70	0	5
Creamsicle Orange Raspberry	1 (2.6 fl oz)	100	0	10
Creamsicle Sugar Free	1 (1.8 fl oz)	25	—	0
Fudgsicle Pop	1 (1.8 fl oz)	60	0	5
Fudgsicle Sugar Free	1 (1.8 fl oz)	40	1	<5
Fudgsicle Bar	1 (2.8 fl oz)	90	1	5
Fun Box Fudge Bar	1 (2.3 fl oz)	80	0	5
Fun Box Pops	1 (2 fl oz)	35	—	0
Fun Box Twin Box Cherry	1 (2.6 fl oz)	50	—	0
Fun Box Twin Pop Banana	1 (2.6 fl oz)	50	—	0
Fun Box Twin Pop Blue Raspberry	1 (2.6 fl oz)	50	—	0
Fun Box Twin Pop Cherry Lemon	1 (2.6 fl oz)	50	—	0
Fun Box Twin Pop Orange Cherry Grape	1 (2.6 oz)	50	—	0
Fun Box Twin Pop Root Beer	1 (2.6 fl oz)	50	—	0
Garfield Bar	1 (3.9 fl oz)	90	—	0
Hyperstripe	1 (2.8 fl oz)	80	—	0
Ice Stripe Cherry Orange	1 (1.5 fl oz)	35	0	0
Ice Stripe Grape Lemon	1 (1.5 fl oz)	35	0	0
Jumbo Jet Star	1 (4.7 fl oz)	80	—	0
Laser Blazer	1 (2.6 oz)	70	—	0
Popsicle All Natural	1 (1.8 fl oz)	45	—	0
Popsicle Orange Cherry Grape	1 (1.8 fl oz)	45	—	0
Popsicle Rainbow Pops	1 (1.8 fl oz)	45	—	0
Popsicle Rootbeer Banana Lime	1 (1.8 fl oz)	45	—	0
Popsicle Strawberry Raspberry Wildberry	1 (1.8 fl oz)	45	—	0
Popsicle Supersicle Traffic Signal	1	80	—	0
Popsicle Twin Pop Cherry	1 (2.6 fl oz)	70	—	0
Popsicle Twin Pop Orange Cherry Grape Lime	1 (2.6 fl oz)	70	—	0
Snow Cone	1	60	—	5
Snowfruit Coconut Bar	1 (3.75 fl oz)	150	1	10
Snowfruit Orange Bar	1	140	tr	0
Snowfruit Strawberry Bar	1	120	tr	0
Snowfruit Tropical Fruit Bar	1	110	—	0

FOOD	PORTION	CALS.	FIB.	CHOL.
Good Humor (CONT.)				
Sugar Free Pop Orange Cherry Grape	1 (1.8 fl oz)	15	—	0
Supersicle Cherry Banana	1 (4.7 fl oz)	80	—	0
Supersicle Cherry Cola	1 (4.7 fl oz)	80	—	0
Supersicle Double Fudge	1 (4.7 fl oz)	150	1	10
Supersicle Firecracker	1 (4.7 fl oz)	90	—	0
Supersicle Firecracker Jr.	1	72	—	0
Supersicle Sour Tower	1	80	—	0
Swirl Bubble Gum	1 (2.7 fl oz)	55	—	0
Swirl Cherry Banana	1 (2.7 fl oz)	55	—	0
Torpedo Cherry	1 (1.8 fl oz)	35	—	0
Twister Blue Raspberry Cherry Cherry Cola Cherry	1 (1.8 fl oz)	45	—	0
Twister Cherry Lemon Orange Lemon	1 (1.8 fl oz)	45	—	0
Vampire's Deadly Secret	1 (2.8 fl oz)	100	—	0
Watermelon Bar	1 (3.6 fl oz)	80	—	0
Hood				
Hendrie's Sizzle'N Sour Stix	1 bar (2 oz)	80	0	5
Hoodsie Pop	1 (3.3 oz)	60	—	0
Natural Blenders Pineappple	1 bar (1 oz)	60	—	0
Natural Blenders Raspberry	1 bar (1 oz)	60	—	0
Natural Blenders Strawberry	1 bar (1 oz)	60	—	0
Pop Banana	1 (3.3 oz)	60	—	0
Pop Blue Raspberry	1 (3.3 oz)	60	—	0
Pop Cherry	1 (3.3 oz)	60	—	0
Pop Grape	1 (3.3 oz)	60	—	0
Pop Orange	1 (3.3 oz)	60	—	0
Pop Root Beer	1 (3.3 oz)	60	—	0
Super Sortment Juice Bars	1 bar (1.9 oz)	40	—	0
Jell-O				
Mixed Berry	1 bar	31	—	0
Orange	1 bar	31	—	0
Orange Pineapple	1 bar	31	—	0
Raspberry	1 bar	29	—	0
Raspberry Peach	1 bar	29	—	0
Strawberry	1 bar	31	—	0
Strawberry Banana	1 bar	31	—	0
Kool-Aid				
Berry Punch	1 bar	31	—	0
Cherry	1 bar	42	—	0
Grape	1 bar	42	—	0
Mountain Berry Punch	1 bar	42	—	0

FOOD	PORTION	CALS.	FIB.	CHOL.
Lifesavers				
Ice Pops	1	35	0	0
Ice Pops Sugar Free	1	12	0	0
Tofutti				
Frutti Apricot Mango	4 fl oz	100	—	0
Frutti Three Berry	4 fl oz	100	—	0
Vitari				
Passion-Fruit	4 oz	80	—	0
Peach	4 oz	80	—	0
fruit & juice bar	1 (3 fl oz)	75	—	0
gelatin pop	1 (1.5 oz)	31	—	0
ice coconut pineapple	½ cup (4 fl oz)	109	—	0
ice fruit w/ Equal	1 bar (1.7 oz)	12	—	0
ice lime	½ cup (4 fl oz)	75	—	0
ice pop	1 (2 fl oz)	42	—	0

ICING
(*see* CAKE)

INSTANT BREAKFAST
(*see* BREAKFAST DRINKS)

JACKFRUIT

FOOD	PORTION	CALS.	FIB.	CHOL.
fresh	3½ oz	70	—	0

JALAPENO
(*see* PEPPERS)

JAM/JELLY/PRESERVES

FOOD	PORTION	CALS.	FIB.	CHOL.
BAMA				
Apple Butter	2 tsp	25	—	0
Apple Jelly	2 tsp	30	—	0
Grape Jelly	2 tsp	30	—	0
Peach Preserves	2 tsp	30	—	0
Red Plum Jam	2 tsp	30	—	0
Strawberry Preserves	2 tsp	30	—	0
Eden				
Apple Butter	1 tbsp (0.5 fl oz)	25	0	0
Estee				
Apple Reduced Calorie	1 pkg (0.5 oz)	10	—	0
Apple Slice	1 tbsp (0.5 oz)	10	—	0
Apricot	1 tbsp (0.5 oz)	5	—	0
Blackberry	1 tbsp (0.5 oz)	5	—	0
Cherry	1 tbsp (0.5 oz)	5	—	0
Grape	1 tbsp (0.5 oz)	10	—	0
Orange	1 tbsp (0.5 oz)	10	—	0

FOOD	PORTION	CALS.	FIB.	CHOL.
Estee (CONT.)				
Peach	1 tbsp (0.5 oz)	5	—	0
Red Raspberry	1 tbsp (0.5 oz)	5	—	0
Strawberry	1 tbsp (0.5 oz)	10	—	0
Strawberry	1 tbsp (0.5 oz)	10	—	0
Harvest Moon				
Apricot Fruit Spread	1 tbsp (0.6 oz)	35	—	0
Blueberry Fruit Spread	1 tbsp (0.6 oz)	35	—	0
Cherry Fruit Spread	1 tbsp (0.6 oz)	35	—	0
Grape Fruit Spread	1 tbsp (0.6 oz)	35	—	0
Peach Fruit Spread	1 tbsp (0.6 oz)	35	—	0
Raspberry Fruit Spread	1 tbsp (0.6 oz)	35	—	0
Strawberry Fruit Spread	1 tbsp (0.6 oz)	35	—	0
Home Brands				
All Flavors Jelly	2 tsp	35	—	0
All Flavors Preserves	2 tsp	35	—	0
Kraft				
Apple Jelly	1 tbsp (0.7 oz)	60	0	0
Apple Strawberry Jelly	1 tbsp (0.7 oz)	50	0	0
Apricot Preserves	1 tbsp (0.7 oz)	50	0	0
Blackberry Jelly	1 tbsp (0.7 oz)	50	0	0
Blackberry Preserves	1 tbsp (0.7 oz)	50	tr	0
Grape Jam	1 tbsp (0.7 oz)	60	0	0
Grape Jelly	1 tbsp (0.7 oz)	50	0	0
Grape Reduced Calorie	1 tbsp (0.6 oz)	20	0	0
Guava Jelly	1 tbsp (0.7 oz)	50	0	0
Orange Marmalade	1 tbsp (0.7 oz)	50	0	0
Peach Preserves	1 tbsp (0.7 oz)	50	0	0
Pineapple Preserves	1 tbsp (0.7 oz)	50	0	0
Red Currant Jelly	1 tbsp (0.7 oz)	50	0	0
Red Plum Jam	1 tbsp (0.7 oz)	60	0	0
Red Raspberry Preserves	1 tbsp (0.7 oz)	50	0	0
Strawberry Jam	1 tbsp (0.7 oz)	50	0	0
Strawberry Jelly	1 tbsp (0.7 oz)	60	0	0
Strawberry Preserves	1 tbsp (0.7 oz)	50	0	0
Strawberry Reduced Calorie	1 tbsp	20	0	0
Red Wing				
Apple Jelly	1 tbsp (0.7 oz)	50	0	0
Apple Blackberry Jelly	1 tbsp (0.7 oz)	50	0	0
Apple Cherry Jelly	1 tbsp (0.7 oz)	50	0	0
Apple Currant Jelly	1 tbsp (0.7 oz)	50	0	0
Apple Grape Jelly	1 tbsp (0.7 oz)	50	0	0
Apple Raspberry Jelly	1 tbsp (0.7 oz)	50	0	0
Apple Strawberry Jelly	1 tbsp (0.7 oz)	50	0	0

FOOD	PORTION	CALS.	FIB.	CHOL.
Red Wing (CONT.)				
Black Raspberry Jelly	1 tbsp (0.7 oz)	50	0	0
Blackberry Jelly	1 tbsp (0.7 oz)	50	0	0
Cherry Jelly	1 tbsp (0.7 oz)	50	0	0
Concord Grape Jelly	1 tbsp (0.7 oz)	50	0	0
Crabapple Jelly	1 tbsp (0.7 oz)	50	0	0
Cranberry Jelly	1 tbsp (0.7 oz)	50	0	0
Cranberry Grape Jelly	1 tbsp (0.7 oz)	50	0	0
Currant Jelly	1 tbsp (0.7 oz)	50	0	0
Damson Plum Jelly	1 tbsp (0.7 oz)	50	0	0
Elderberry Jelly	1 tbsp (0.7 oz)	50	0	0
Grape Jelly	1 tbsp (0.7 oz)	50	0	0
Mint Jelly	1 tbsp (0.7 oz)	50	0	0
Mint Apple Jelly	1 tbsp (0.7 oz)	50	0	0
Mixed Fruit Jelly	1 tbsp (0.7 oz)	50	0	0
Red Plum Jelly	1 tbsp (0.7 oz)	50	0	0
Red Raspberry Jelly	1 tbsp (0.7 oz)	50	0	0
Strawberry Jelly	1 tbsp (0.7 oz)	50	0	0
Strawberry Apple Jelly	1 tbsp (0.7 oz)	50	0	0
S&W				
Apricot Pineapple Reduced Calorie Preserves	1 tsp	4	—	0
Blueberry Reduced Calorie Jam	1 tsp	4	—	0
Concord Grape Reduced Calorie Jelly	1 tsp	4	—	0
Orange Marmalade Reduced Calorie	1 tsp	4	—	0
Red Raspberry Reduced Calorie Jam	1 tsp	4	—	0
Red Tart Cherry Reduced Calorie Preserves	1 tsp	4	—	0
Strawberry Reduced Calorie Jam	1 tsp	4	—	0
Smucker's				
All Flavors Jam	1 tsp	18	—	0
All Flavors Jelly	1 tsp	18	—	0
All Flavors Low Sugar Spread	1 tsp	8	—	0
All Flavors Preserves	1 tsp	18	—	0
All Flavors Simply Fruit	1 tsp	16	—	0
All Flavors Single Serving Jelly	½ oz	38	—	0
All Flavors Single Serving Preserves	½ oz	38	—	0
Apple Butter Autumn Harvest	1 tsp	12	—	0
Apple Butter Simply Fruit	1 tsp	12	—	0

FOOD	PORTION	CALS.	FIB.	CHOL.
Smucker's (CONT.)				
Apple Butter Natural	1 tsp	12	—	0
Apple Cider Butter	1 tsp	12	—	0
Blackberry Single Serving Imitation Jelly	1 pkg (0.4 oz)	4	—	0
Cherry Single Serving Imitation Jelly	1 pkg (0.4 oz)	4	—	0
Grape Single Serving Imitation Jelly	1 pkg (0.4 oz)	4	—	0
Orange Marmalade	1 tsp	18	—	0
Peach Butter	1 tsp	15	—	0
Pumpkin Butter Autumn Harvest	1 tsp	12	—	0
Tree Of Life				
Apricot Fruit Spread	1 tbsp (0.6 oz)	45	—	0
Blueberry Fruit Spread	1 tbsp (0.6 oz)	35	—	0
Cherry Fruit Spread	1 tbsp (0.6 oz)	40	—	0
Grape Fruit Spread	1 tbsp (0.6 oz)	35	—	0
Peach Fruit Spread	1 tbsp (0.6 oz)	45	—	0
Raspberry Fruit Spread	1 tbsp (0.6 oz)	30	—	0
Strawberry Fruit Spread	1 tbsp (0.6 oz)	35	—	0
Weight Watchers				
Grape Spread	1 tsp	8	—	0
Raspberry Spread	1 tsp	8	—	0
Strawberry Spread	1 tsp	8	—	0
White House				
Apple Butter	1 oz	50	1	0
all flavors jam	1 pkg (0.5 oz)	34	tr	0
all flavors jam	1 tbsp (0.7 oz)	48	tr	0
all flavors jelly	1 tbsp (0.7 oz)	52	tr	0
all flavors jelly	1 pkg (0.5 oz)	38	tr	0
all flavors preserve	1 tbsp (0.7 oz)	48	tr	0
apple butter	1 tbsp (0.6 oz)	33	—	0
apple butter	1 cup (9.9 oz)	519	—	0
apple jelly	3½ oz	259	—	0
apple jelly	1 tbsp (0.7 oz)	52	tr	0
apple jelly	1 pkg (0.5 oz)	38	tr	0
apricot jam	3½ oz	250	—	0
blackberry jam	3½ oz	237	—	0
cherry jam	3½ oz	250	—	0
orange jam	3½ oz	243	—	0
orange marmalade	1 pkg (0.5 oz)	34	—	0
orange marmalade	1 tbsp (0.7 oz)	49	—	0
plum jam	3½ oz	241	—	0

FOOD	PORTION	CALS.	FIB.	CHOL.
quince jam	3½ oz	236	—	0
raspberry jam	3½ oz	248	—	0
raspberry jelly	3½ oz	259	—	0
red currant jam	3½ oz	237	—	0
red currant jelly	3½ oz	265	—	0
rose hip jam	3½ oz	250	—	0
strawberry jam	3½ oz	234	—	0
strawberry jam	1 tbsp (0.7 oz)	48	tr	0
strawberry jam	1 pkg (0.5 oz)	34	tr	0
strawberry preserve	1 pkg (0.5 oz)	34	tr	0
strawberry preserve	1 tbsp (0.7 oz)	48	tr	0

JAPANESE FOOD
(see ORIENTAL FOOD)

JAVA PLUM

fresh	1 cup	82	—	0
fresh	3	5	—	0

JELLY
(see JAM/JELLY/PRESERVE)

JERUSALEM ARTICHOKE
(see ARTICHOKE)

JEW'S EAR

pepeao dried	½ cup	36	—	0
pepeao raw sliced	1 cup	25	—	0

JUJUBE

fresh	3½ oz	105	—	0

KALE
FRESH
Dole

Chopped	½ cup	17	—	0
chopped cooked	½ cup	21	—	0
raw chopped	½ cup	21	—	0
scotch chopped cooked	½ cup	18	—	0
FROZEN				
chopped cooked	½ cup	20	—	0

KETCHUP
Del Monte

	1 tbsp (0.5 oz)	15	0	0
Hain				
Natural	1 tbsp	16	—	0
Natural No Salt Added	1 tbsp	16	—	0
Healthy Choice	1 tbsp (0.5 oz)	10	0	0

FOOD	PORTION	CALS.	FIB.	CHOL.
Heinz	1 tbsp	16	—	0
Hot	1 tbsp	14	—	0
Lite	1 tbsp	8	—	0
Hunt's	1 tbsp (0.6 oz)	15	0	0
No Salt Added	1 tbsp	20	tr	0
McIlhenny	1 tbsp (0.6 oz)	23	tr	0
Spicy	1 tbsp (0.6 oz)	23	tr	tr
Red Wing				
Extra Fancy	1 tbsp (0.6 oz)	20	0	0
Smucker's	1 tsp	8	—	0
Tree Of Life	1 tbsp (0.5 oz)	10	—	0
Salsa Ketchup	1 tbsp (0.5 oz)	10	—	0
catsup	1 tbsp	16	tr	0
catsup	1 pkg (0.2 oz)	6	tr	0
low sodium	1 tbsp	16	tr	0

KIDNEY

beef simmered	3 oz	122	—	329
lamb braised	3 oz	117	—	481
pork, braised	3 oz	128	—	408
veal braised	3 oz	139	—	672

KIDNEY BEANS
CANNED

B&M				
Red Baked Beans	8 oz	250	11	5
Eden				
Organic	½ cup (4.4 oz)	100	10	0
Friends				
Red Beans	8 oz	340	—	4
Goya				
Spanish Style	7.5 oz	140	10	0
Green Giant				
Dark Red	½ cup	90	5	0
Light Red	½ cup	90	5	0
Hanover				
Dark Red	½ cup	110	—	0
Light Red In Sauce	½ cup	120	—	0
Hunt's				
Red	4 oz	100	5	0
Progresso				
Red	½ cup	100	7	0
S&W				
Dark Red Lite 50% Less Salt	½ cup	120	—	0
Dark Red Premium	½ cup	120	—	0

FOOD	PORTION	CALS.	FIB.	CHOL.
S&W (CONT.)				
Water Pack	½ cup	90	—	0
Trappey				
Dark Red	½ cup (4.5 oz)	130	8	0
Light Red	½ cup (4.5 oz)	120	8	0
Light Red New Orleans Style With Bacon	½ cup (4.5 oz)	110	6	0
Light Red With Jalapeno	½ cup (4.5 oz)	110	6	0
With Chili Gravy	½ cup (4.5 oz)	110	7	0
Van Camp's				
Dark Red	½ cup (4.6 oz)	90	6	0
Light Red	½ cup (4.6 oz)	90	6	0
kidney beans	1 cup	208	—	0
red	1 cup	216	—	0
DRIED				
Arrowhead				
Red	¼ cup (1.6 oz)	160	10	0
Hurst	1.2 oz	120	10	0
california red cooked	1 cup	219	—	0
cooked	1 cup	225	—	0
red cooked	1 cup	225	—	0
royal red cooked	1 cup	218	—	0
SPROUTS				
cooked	1 lb	152	—	0
raw	½ cup	27	—	0
KIWIS				
Dole	2	90	4	0
California Kiwifruit	2 (4.9 oz)	90	4	0
fresh	1 med	46	3	0
KNISH				
Joshua's				
Coney Island Potato	1 (4.6 oz)	280	1	0
TAKE-OUT				
potato	1 med (3.5 oz)	166	tr	36
potato	1 lg (7 oz)	332	1	72
KOHLRABI				
FRESH				
raw sliced	½ cup	19	—	0
sliced cooked	½ cup	24	—	0
KUMQUATS				
fresh	1	12	—	0

FOOD	PORTION	CALS.	FIB.	CHOL.
LAMB				
(see also LAMB DISHES)				
FRESH				
cubed lean only braised	3 oz	190	—	92
cubed lean only broiled	3 oz	158	—	77
ground broiled	3 oz	240	—	82
leg lean & fat Choice roasted	3 oz	219	—	79
loin chop w/ bone lean & fat Choice broiled	1 chop (2.3 oz)	201	—	64
loin chop w/ bone lean only Choice broiled	1 chop (1.6 oz)	100	—	44
rib chop lean & fat Choice broiled	3 oz	307	—	84
rib chop lean only Choice broiled	3 oz	200	—	78
shank lean & fat Choice braised	3 oz	206	—	90
shank lean & fat Choice roasted	3 oz	191	—	77
shoulder chop w/ bone lean & fat Choice braised	1 chop (2.5 oz)	244	—	84
shoulder chop w/ bone lean only Choice braised	1 chop (1.9 oz)	152	—	66
sirloin lean & fat Choice roasted	3 oz	248	—	82
FROZEN				
New Zealand lean & fat cooked	3 oz	259	—	93
New Zealand lean only cooked	3 oz	175	—	93
LAMB DISHES				
TAKE-OUT				
curry	¾ cup	345	—	89
stew	¾ cup	124	2	29
LAMBSQUARTERS				
chopped cooked	½ cup	29	—	0
LECITHIN				
(see SOY)				
LEEKS				
chopped cooked	¼ cup	8	—	0
cooked	1 (4.4 oz)	38	—	0
freeze dried	1 tbsp	1	—	0
raw	1 (4.4 oz)	76	—	0
raw chopped	¼ cup	16	—	0
LEMON				
FRESH				
Dole	1	18	0	0
lemon	1 med	22	—	0

FOOD	PORTION	CALS.	FIB.	CHOL.
peel	1 tbsp	0	—	0
wedge	1	5	—	0
LEMON EXTRACT				
Virginia Dare	1 tsp	22	—	0
LEMON JUICE				
Realemon	1 fl oz	6	—	0
bottled	1 tbsp	3	—	0
fresh	1 tbsp	4	—	0
frzn	1 tbsp	3	—	0
LEMONADE				
FROZEN				
Bright & Early	8 fl oz	120	—	0
Minute Maid	8 fl oz	110	—	0
Country Style	8 fl oz	120	—	0
Cranberry Lemonade	8 fl oz	80	—	0
Pink	8 fl oz	120	—	0
Raspberry	8 fl oz	120	—	0
Seneca				
as prep	8 fl oz	110	1	0
as prep w/ water	1 cup	100	—	0
not prep	1 can (6 oz)	397	—	0
MIX				
Country Time	8 fl oz	82	—	0
Pink	8 fl oz	82	—	0
Pink Sugar Free	8 fl oz	4	—	0
Sugar Free	8 fl oz	4	—	0
Crystal Light	8 fl oz	5	—	0
Kool-Aid	8 fl oz	99	—	0
Pink	8 fl oz	99	—	0
Sugar Free	8 fl oz	4	—	0
Sugar Sweetened Pink	8 fl oz	82	—	0
Wylers				
Drink Mix Unsweetened	8 oz	3	—	0
powder as prep w/ water	9 fl oz	113	—	0
powder w/ nutrasweet	1 pitcher (67 oz)	40	—	0
READY-TO-DRINK				
Crystal Geyser				
Juice Squeeze Pink	1 bottle (12 fl oz)	140	—	0
Diet Rite				
Salt/Sodium Free	8 fl oz	2	—	0
Fruitopia	8 fl oz	120	—	0
Minute Maid				
Chilled	8 fl oz	110	—	0

FOOD	PORTION	CALS.	FIB.	CHOL.
Minute Maid (CONT.)				
Cranberry Chilled	8 fl oz	120	—	0
Juices To Go	1 bottle (16 fl oz)	110	—	0
Juices To Go	1 can (11.5 fl oz)	160	—	0
Juices To Go Canberry Lemonade	1 bottle (16 fl oz)	110	—	0
Juices To Go Raspberry Lemonade	1 bottle (16 fl oz)	120	—	0
Pink Chilled	8 fl oz	110	—	0
Raspberry Chilled	8 fl oz	120	—	0
Mott's	10 fl oz	160	0	0
Nehi	8 fl oz	130	—	0
Newman's Own				
Roadside Virginia	8 fl oz	100	—	0
Ocean Spray	8 fl oz	110	0	0
With Cranberry Juice	8 fl oz	110	0	0
With Raspberry Juice	8 fl oz	110	0	0
Odwalla				
Honey	8 fl oz	70	0	0
Strawberry	8 fl oz	150	2	0
Royal Mistic				
Lemonade Limeade	16 fl oz	230	—	0
Tropical Pink	16 fl oz	230	—	0
Shasta	12 fl oz	146	—	0
Snapple	8 fl oz	110	—	0
Diet Pink	8 fl oz	13	—	0
Pink	8 fl oz	110	—	0
Strawberry	8 fl oz	110	—	0
Tropicana	1 can (11.5 oz)	160	—	0
Tropicana	8 fl oz	110	—	0
Twister Orange Cranberry	8 fl oz	130	—	0
Twister Wild Berry	8 fl oz	120	—	0
Turkey Hill	8 fl oz	110	—	0
Veryfine	8 fl oz	120	—	0
Wylers	1 can (6 fl oz)	64	—	0
Sipps	8.45 fl oz	85	—	0

LENTILS

CANNED

Health Valley

Fast Menu Hearty Lentils Garden Vegetables	7½ oz	150	16	0
Fast Menu Organic Lentils With Tofu Weiner	7½ oz	170	15	0

FOOD	PORTION	CALS.	FIB.	CHOL.
DRIED				
Hurst	1.2 oz	120	11	0
cooked	1 cup	231	—	0
MIX				
Casbah				
Pilaf as prep	1 cup	200	2	0
SPROUTS				
raw	½ cup	40	—	0
LETTUCE				
(see also SALAD)				
Dole				
Butter	1 head	21	2	0
Iceberg	⅙ med head	20	1	0
Leaf shredded	1½ cup	12	1	0
Romaine shredded	1½ cups	18	1	0
Western Express				
Heart's Of Romaine	6 leaves (3 oz)	20	1	0
bibb	1 head (6 oz)	21	2	0
boston	1 head (6 oz)	21	2	0
boston	2 leaves	2	tr	0
iceberg	1 head (19 oz)	70	5	0
iceberg	1 leaf	3	tr	0
looseleaf shredded	½ cup	5	—	0
romaine shredded	½ cup	4	tr	0
LIMA BEANS				
CANNED				
Allen				
Green	½ cup (4.5 oz)	120	8	0
Green & White	½ cup (4.5 oz)	110	9	0
Del Monte				
Green	½ cup (4.4 oz)	80	4	0
East Texas Fair				
Green	½ cup (4.5 oz)	120	8	0
S&W				
Small Fancy	½ cup	80	—	0
Seneca	½ cup	80	5	0
Trappey				
Baby Green With Bacon	½ cup (4.5 oz)	120	6	0
large	1 cup	191	—	0
lima beans	½ cup	93	—	0
DRIED				
baby cooked	1 cup	229	17	0
cooked	½ cup	104	—	0
large cooked	1 cup	217	14	0

FOOD	PORTION	CALS.	FIB.	CHOL.
FROZEN				
Birds Eye				
Baby	½ cup	130	—	0
Fordhook	½ cup	100	—	0
Green Giant				
Harvest Fresh	½ cup	80	4	0
In Butter Sauce	½ cup	100	5	5
Hanover				
Baby	½ cup	110	—	0
Fordhook	½ cup	100	—	0
cooked	½ cup	94	—	0
fordhook cooked	½ cup	85	—	0
LIME				
fresh	1	20	—	0
LIME JUICE				
Lifesavers				
Lime Punch	8 fl oz	140	—	0
Odwalla				
Summertime Lime	8 fl oz	90	0	0
Realime	1 oz	6	—	0
bottled	1 tbsp	3	—	0
fresh	1 tbsp	4	—	0
LINGCOD				
baked	3 oz	93	—	57
fillet baked	5.3 oz	164	—	101

LIQUOR/LIQUEUR

(*see also* BEER AND ALE, CHAMPAGNE, DRINK MIXERS, MALT, WINE, WINE COOLERS)

anisette	⅔ oz	74	0	0
apricot brandy	⅔ oz	64	0	0
benedictine	⅔ oz	69	0	0
bloody mary	5 oz	116	—	0
bourbon & soda	4 oz	105	—	0
coffee liqueur	1½ oz	174	—	0
cognac	3.5 oz	233	0	0
creme de menthe	1½ oz	186	—	0
curacao liqueur	⅔ oz	54	0	0
daiquiri	2 oz	111	—	0
gin	1½ oz	110	—	0
gin & tonic	7.5 oz	171	—	0
gin ricky	4 oz	150	—	0
manhattan	2 oz	128	—	0

FOOD	PORTION	CALS.	FIB.	CHOL.
martini	2½ oz	156	—	0
mint julep	10 oz	210	0	0
old-fashioned	2½ oz	127	0	0
pina colada	4½ oz	262	—	0
planter's punch	3½ oz	175	—	0
rum	1½ oz	97	—	0
screwdriver	7 oz	174	—	0
sloe gin fizz	2½ oz	132	0	0
tequila sunrise	5½ oz	189	—	0
tom collins	7½ oz	121	—	0
vodka	1½ oz	97	—	0
whiskey	1½ oz	105	—	0
whiskey sour	3 oz	123	—	0
whiskey sour mix not prep	1 pkg (0.6 oz)	64	—	0

LIVER
(see also PATE)
Dakota Lean

Beef raw	3 oz	100	—	150
beef braised	3 oz	137	—	331
beef pan-fried	3 oz	184	—	410
chicken stewed	1 cup (5 oz)	219	—	883
duck raw	1 (1.5 oz)	60	—	227
lamb braised	3 oz	187	—	426
lamb fried	3 oz	202	—	419
pork braised	3 oz	141	—	302
turkey simmered	1 cup (5 oz)	237	—	876
veal braised	3 oz	140	—	477
veal fried	3 oz	208	—	280

LOBSTER
(see also CRAYFISH)
CANNED
Progresso

Rock Lobster Sauce	½ cup	120	2	10

FRESH

northern cooked	1 cup	142	—	104
northern cooked	3 oz	83	—	61
northern raw	1 lobster (5.3 oz)	136	—	143
northern raw	3 oz	77	—	81
spiny steamed	3 oz	122	—	76
spiny steamed	1 (5.7 oz)	233	—	146

TAKE-OUT

newburg	1 cup	485	—	455

FOOD	PORTION	CALS.	FIB.	CHOL.

LOGANBERRIES
| frzn | 1 cup | 80 | — | 0 |

LONGANS
| fresh | 1 | 2 | — | 0 |

LOQUATS
| fresh | 1 | 5 | — | 0 |

LOTUS
root raw sliced	10 slices	45	—	0
root sliced cooked	10 slices	59	—	0
seeds dried	1 oz	94	—	0

LOX
(see SALMON)

LUNCHEON MEATS/COLD CUTS
(see also CHICKEN, HAM, MEAT SUBSTITUTES, TURKEY)

Carl Buddig				
Beef	1 oz	40	0	20
Corned Beef	1 oz	40	0	20
Pastrami	1 oz	40	0	20
DiLusso				
Genoa	1 oz	100	0	25
Hansel n'Gretel				
Healthy Deli Cooked Corn Beef	1 oz	35	—	11
Healthy Deli Italian Roast Beef	1 oz	31	—	16
Healthy Deli Pastrami Round	1 oz	34	—	14
Healthy Deli Regular Roast Beef	1 oz	30	—	13
Hebrew National				
Bologna Beef	2 oz	180	—	40
Bologna Beef Reduced Fat	2 oz	130	—	35
Bologna Lean Chub	2 oz	90	—	25
Bologna Midget	2 oz	180	—	40
Deli Pastrami	2 oz	80	—	30
Deli Express Corned Beef	2 oz	80	—	35
Deli Express Tongue Sliced	2 oz	120	—	50
Salami Beef	2 oz	170	—	40
Salami Beef Reduced Fat	2 oz	110	—	30
Salami Sean Chub	2 oz	90	—	30
Salami Midget	2 oz	170	—	40
Homeland				
Hard Salami	1 oz	110	0	35
Hormel				
Liverwurst Spread	4 tbsp (2 oz)	130	0	70

FOOD	PORTION	CALS.	FIB.	CHOL.
Hormel (CONT.)				
Pepperoni Chunk	1 oz	140	0	35
Pepperoni Sliced	15 slices (1 oz)	140	0	35
Pepperoni Twin	1 oz	140	0	35
Pillow Pack Genoa Salami	4 slices (1.1 oz)	120	0	30
Pillow Pack Pepperoni	1 oz	140	0	35
Pillow Pack Pepperoni	16 slices (1 oz)	140	0	35
Jones				
Liver Sausage	1 slice	80	—	43
Liver Sausage Chub	1 slice	80	—	43
Oscar Mayer				
Bologna Beef	1 slice (1 oz)	90	0	15
Bologna Garlic	1 slice (1.4 oz)	110	0	30
Bologna Light	1 slice (1 oz)	60	0	15
Bologna Light Beef	1 slice (1 oz)	60	0	10
Bologna Pork & Chicken & Beef	1 slice (1 oz)	90	0	20
Bologna Wisconsin Made Ring	2 oz	140	0	35
Braunschweiger	1 slice (1 oz)	100	0	50
Braunschweiger	2 oz	190	0	100
Braunschweiger German Brand	2 oz	200	0	90
Cotto Salami	2 slices (1.6 oz)	100	0	35
Cotto Salami Beef	2 slices (1.6 oz)	90	0	35
Free Bologna	2 slices (1.6 oz)	35	—	15
Genoa Salami	3 slices (1 oz)	100	0	25
Hard Salami	3 slices (1 oz)	100	0	25
Head Cheese	1 slice (1 oz)	50	0	25
Healthy Favorites Bologna	2 slices (1.6 oz)	45	0	15
Honey Loaf	1 slice (1 oz)	35	0	15
Liver Cheese	1 slice (1.3 oz)	120	0	80
Lunchables Bologna/American	1 pkg (4.5 oz)	450	0	85
Lunchables Deluxe Turkey/Ham	1 pkg (5.1 oz)	360	1	60
Lunchables Dessert Jello/ Honey Turkey/Cheddar	1 pkg (5.7 oz)	320	tr	50
Lunchables Fun Pack Bologna/ Wild Cherry	1 pkg (11.2 oz)	530	tr	60
Lunchables Fun Pack Ham/ Fruit Punch	1 pkg (11.2 oz)	450	tr	50
Lunchables Ham/Swiss	1 pkg (4.5 oz)	320	0	60
Lunchables Pepperoni/ American	1 pkg (4.5 oz)	480	0	95
Lunchables Salami/American	1 pkg (4.5 oz)	430	0	80
Luncheon Loaf Spiced	1 slice (1 oz)	70	0	20
New England Brand Sausage	2 slices (1.6 oz)	60	0	25
Old Fashioned Loaf	1 slice (1 oz)	60	0	15

FOOD	PORTION	CALS.	FIB.	CHOL.
Oscar Mayer (CONT.)				
Olive Loaf	1 slice (1 oz)	70	0	20
Peppered Loaf	1 slice (1 oz)	39	—	14
Pickle And Pimiento Loaf	1 slice (1 oz)	70	0	20
Salami For Beer	1 slice (1.6 oz)	110	0	30
Salami Machaich Brand Beef	2 slices (1.6 oz)	120	0	30
Sandwich Spread	2 oz	140	0	20
Summer Sausage	2 slices (1.6 oz)	140	0	40
Summer Sausage Beef	2 slices (1.6 oz)	140	0	35
Russer				
Bologna	2 oz	180	—	30
Bologna Jalapeno Pepper	2 oz	170	—	25
Bologna Wunderbar German Brand	2 oz	190	—	20
Bologna Beef	2 oz	180	—	30
Bologna Garlic	2 oz	180	—	30
Bologna Italian Brand Sweet Red Pepper	2 oz	180	—	30
Braunschweiger	2 oz	170	—	90
Cooked Salami	2 oz	120	—	50
Dutch Brand	2 oz	130	—	25
Hot Cooked Salami	2 oz	110	—	45
Italian Brand Loaf	2 oz	130	—	25
Jalapeno Loaf With Monterey Jack Cheese	2 oz	160	—	25
Kielbasa Loaf	2 oz	120	—	35
Light Bologna	2 oz	120	—	30
Light Bologna Beef	2 oz	120	—	30
Light Braunschweiger	2 oz	120	—	60
Light Old Fashioned Loaf	2 oz	90	—	30
Light P&P Loaf	2 oz	100	—	30
Light Salami Cooked	2 oz	90	—	40
Olive Loaf	2 oz	160	—	20
P&P Loaf	2 oz	160	—	25
Pepper Loaf	2 oz	90	—	30
Polish Loaf	2 oz	140	—	25
Shofar				
Salami Beef	2 oz	160	0	40
Spam				
	2 oz	170	0	40
Less Salt	2 oz	170	0	40
Lite	2 oz	110	0	45
Underwood				
Liverwurst	2.08 oz	180	—	90

FOOD	PORTION	CALS.	FIB.	CHOL.
Weight Watchers				
Bologna	2 slices (¾ oz)	35	—	15
barbecue loaf pork & beef	1 oz	49	—	11
beerwurst beef	1 slice (2¾ in x ⅟₁₆ in)	20	—	4
beerwurst beef	1 slice (4 in x ⅛ in)	75	—	13
beerwurst pork	1 slice (2¾ in x ⅟₁₆ in)	14	—	4
beerwurst pork	1 slice (4 in x ⅛ in)	55	—	13
berliner pork & beef	1 oz	65	—	13
blood sausage	1 oz	95	—	30
bologna beef	1 oz	88	—	16
bologna beef & pork	1 oz	89	—	16
bologna pork	1 oz	70	—	17
braunschweiger pork	1 slice (2½ x ¼ in)	65	—	28
braunschweiger pork	1 oz	102	—	44
corned beef loaf	1 oz	43	—	13
dutch brand loaf pork & beef	1 oz	68	—	13
headcheese pork	1 oz	60	—	23
honey loaf pork & beef	1 oz	36	—	10
honey roll sausage beef	1 oz	42	—	12
lebanon bologna beef	1 oz	60	—	20
liver cheese pork	1 oz	86	—	49
liverwurst pork	1 oz	92	—	45
luncheon meat beef	1 oz	87	—	18
luncheon meat pork & beef	1 oz	100	—	15
luncheon meat pork canned	1 oz	95	—	18
luncheon sausage pork & beef	1 oz	74	—	18
luxury loaf pork	1 oz	40	—	10
mortadella beef & pork	1 oz	88	—	16
mother's loaf pork	1 oz	80	—	13
new england sausage pork & beef	1 oz	46	—	14
olive loaf pork	1 oz	67	—	11
peppered loaf pork & beef	1 oz	42	—	13
pickle & pimiento loaf pork	1 oz	74	—	10
picnic loaf pork & beef	1 oz	66	—	11
salami cooked beef & pork	1 oz	71	—	18
salami hard pork & beef	1 pkg (4 oz)	472	—	89
salami hard pork & beef	1 slice (⅓ oz)	42	—	8
sandwich spread pork & beef	1 tbsp	35	—	6
sandwich spread pork & beef	1 oz	67	—	11
summer sausage thuringer cervelat	1 oz	98	—	19
TAKE-OUT				
Sara Lee				
Corned Beef	2 oz	70	—	40

FOOD	PORTION	CALS.	FIB.	CHOL.
Sara Lee (CONT.)				
Corned Beef Brisket	2 oz	90	—	35
Pastrami Beef	2 oz	100	1	25
Peppered Beef	2 oz	70	—	25
submarine w/ salami ham, cheese lettuce tomato onion & oil	1	456	—	35

LUPINES
dried cooked	1 cup	197	—	0

LYCHEES
Ka-Me
Whole Pitted In Syrup	15 pieces (5 oz)	130	0	0
fresh	1	6	—	0

MACADAMIA NUTS
Mauna Loa
Candy Glazed	1 oz	170	—	5
Chocolate Covered	1 oz	170	—	0
Honey Roasted	1 oz	200	—	0
Macadamia Nut Brittle	1 oz	150	—	6
Roasted & Salted	1 oz	210	—	0
dried	1 oz	199	—	0
oil roasted	1 oz	204	—	0

MACARONI
(*see* PASTA)

MACE
ground	1 tsp	8	—	0

MACKEREL
CANNED
jack	1 cup	296	—	150
jack	1 can (12.7 oz)	563	—	285
FRESH				
atlantic cooked	3 oz	223	—	64
atlantic raw	3 oz	174	—	60
jack baked	3 oz	171	—	51
jack fillet baked	6.2 oz	354	—	106
king baked	3 oz	114	—	58
king fillet baked	5.4 oz	207	—	105
pacific baked	3 oz	171	—	51
pacific fillet baked	6.2 oz	354	—	106
spanish cooked	3 oz	134	—	62
spanish cooked	1 fillet (5.1 oz)	230	—	107
spanish raw	3 oz	118	—	65

FOOD	PORTION	CALS.	FIB.	CHOL.
MALT				
Bartles & Jaymes				
Malt Cooler Black Cherry	12 fl oz	190	—	0
Malt Cooler Light Berry	12 fl oz	140	—	0
Malt Cooler Mandarin Lemon	12 fl oz	210	—	0
Malt Cooler Berry	12 fl oz	210	—	0
Malt Cooler Margarita	12 fl oz	250	—	0
Malt Cooler Original	12 fl oz	180	—	0
Malt Cooler Peach	12 fl oz	200	—	0
Malt Cooler Pina Colada	12 fl oz	270	—	0
Malt Cooler Planter's Punch	12 fl oz	220	—	0
Malt Cooler Red Sangria	12 fl oz	190	—	0
Malt Cooler Strawberry	12 fl oz	200	—	0
Malt Cooler Strawberry Daiquiri	12 fl oz	220	—	0
Malt Cooler Tropical	12 fl oz	220	—	0
Olde English	12 oz	163	—	0
Schaefer	12 oz	165	—	0
Schlitz	12 oz	177	—	0
nonalcoholic	12 fl oz	32	—	0
MALTED MILK				
Carnation				
Chocolate	3 heaping tsp (21 g)	79	—	1
Original	3 heaping tsp (21 g)	90	—	4
Kraft				
Instant Chocolate	3 tsp (0.7 oz)	80	tr	0
Instant Chocolate as prep w/ 2% milk	1 serv (9.5 oz)	200	tr	20
Instant Natural	3 tsp (0.7 oz)	90	0	5
Instant Natural as prep w/ 2% milk	1 serv (9.5 oz)	210	0	25
chocolate as prep w/ milk	1 cup	229	—	34
chocolate flavor powder	3 heaping tsp (¾ oz)	79	—	1
natural flavor as prep w/ milk	1 cup	237	—	37
natural flavor powder	3 heaping tsp (¾ oz)	87	—	4
MAMMY-APPLE				
fresh	1	431	—	0
MANGO				
fresh	1	135	—	0

FOOD	PORTION	CALS.	FIB.	CHOL.
CANNED				
Ka-Me	4 pieces (5 oz)	102	0	0
MANGO JUICE				
Kern's				
Nectar	6 fl oz	100	—	0
Libby				
Nectar	1 can (11.5 fl oz)	210	—	0
Snapple				
Diet Mango Madness	8 fl oz	13	—	0
Mango Madness Cocktail	8 fl oz	110	—	0
MARGARINE				
(see also BUTTER BLENDS, BUTTER SUBSTITUTES)				
SQUEEZE				
Parkay	1 tbsp (0.5 oz)	80	0	0
Touch of Butter	1 tbsp (0.5 oz)	80	0	0
soybean & cottonseed	1 tsp	34	—	0
STICK				
Blue Bonnet	1 tbsp	100	—	0
Chiffon	1 tbsp	100	—	0
Fleischmann's	1 tbsp	100	—	0
Light Corn Oil	1 tbsp	80	—	0
Sweet Unsalted	1 tbsp	100	—	0
Hain				
Safflower	1 tbsp	100	—	0
Safflower Unsalted	1 tbsp	100	—	0
Krona	1 tbsp	100	—	15
Land O'Lakes				
Spread	1 tbsp (0.5 oz)	90	—	0
Spread With Sweet Cream	1 tbsp (0.5 oz)	90	—	0
Spread With Sweet Cream Unsalted	1 tbsp (0.5 oz)	90	—	0
Mazola	1 tbsp (14 g)	100	—	0
Mazola	1 cup (229 g)	1650	—	0
Unsalted	1 tbsp (14 g)	100	—	0
Unsalted	1 cup (229 g)	1635	—	0
Mother's	1 tbsp	100	—	0
Unsalted	1 tbsp	100	—	0
Nucanola	1 tbsp (14 g)	90	—	0
Nucanola	1 tbsp	90	—	0
Parkay	1 tbsp (0.5 oz)	90	0	0
⅓ Less Fat	1 tbsp (0.5 oz)	70	0	0
Promise	1 tbsp	90	—	0
Touch of Butter	1 tbsp (0.5 oz)	90	0	0

FOOD	PORTION	CALS.	FIB.	CHOL.
Tree Of Life				
100% Soy	1 tbsp (0.5 oz)	100	—	0
100% Soy Salt Free	1 tbsp (0.5 oz)	100	—	0
Canola Soy	1 tbsp (0.5 oz)	100	—	0
Canola Soy Salt Free	1 tbsp (0.5 oz)	100	—	0
Weight Watchers				
Light	1 tbsp	60	—	0
corn	1 tsp	34	—	0
corn	1 stick (4 oz)	815	—	0
salted	1 stick (4 oz)	815	—	0
salted	1 tsp	39	—	0
unsalted	1 tsp	34	—	0
unsalted	1 stick (4 oz)	809	—	0
TUB				
Blue Bonnet	1 tbsp	100	—	0
Whipped	1 tbsp	80	—	0
Chiffon	1 tbsp (0.5 oz)	100	0	0
Whipped	1 tbsp (0.3 oz)	70	0	0
Fleischmann's	1 tbsp	100	—	0
Diet	1 tbsp	50	—	0
Extra Light Corn Oil Spread	1 tbsp	50	—	0
Light Corn Oil Spread	1 tbsp	80	—	0
Lightly Salted	1 tbsp	70	—	0
Sweet Unsalted	1 tbsp	100	—	0
Unsalted	1 tbsp	70	—	0
Hain				
Safflower	1 tbsp	100	—	0
Hollywood				
Safflower	1 tbsp	100	—	0
Safflower Unsalted Sweet	1 tbsp	100	—	0
Soft Spread	1 tbsp	90	0	0
I Can't Believe It's Not Butter!	1 tbsp	90	—	0
Land O'Lakes				
Spread	1 tbsp (0.5 oz)	80	—	0
Spread With Sweet Cream	1 tbsp (0.5 oz)	80	—	0
Mazola				
Diet	1 tbsp (14 g)	50	—	0
Diet	1 cup (235 g)	815	—	0
Light Corn Oil Spread	1 tbsp (14 g)	50	—	0
Mother's				
Salted	1 tbsp	100	—	0
Unsalted	1 tbsp	100	—	0
Parkay	1 tbsp (0.5 oz)	60	0	0
Light	1 tbsp (0.5 oz)	50	0	0

FOOD	PORTION	CALS.	FIB.	CHOL.
Mother's (CONT.)				
Soft	1 tbsp (0.5 oz)	100	0	0
Soft Diet	1 tbsp (0.5 oz)	50	0	0
Whipped	1 tbsp (0.3 oz)	70	0	0
Smart Beat	1 tbsp	25	—	0
Unsalted	1 tbsp	25	—	0
Tree Of Life				
Canola Soft	1 tbsp (0.5 oz)	100	—	0
Weight Watchers				
Extra Light	1 tbsp	50	—	0
Extra Light Sweet Unsalted	1 tbsp	50	—	0
corn	1 tsp	34	—	0
corn	1 cup	1626	—	0
diet	1 tsp	17	—	0
diet	1 cup	800	—	0
safflower	1 cup	1626	—	0
safflower	1 tsp	34	—	0
salted	1 tsp	34	—	0
salted	1 cup	1626	—	0
soybean salted	1 tsp	34	—	0
soybean salted	1 cup	1626	—	0
soybean unsalted	1 cup	1626	—	0
soybean unsalted	1 tsp	34	—	0
unsalted	1 cup	1626	—	0
unsalted	1 tsp	34	—	0

MARINADE
(see SAUCE)

MARJORAM
dried	1 tsp	2	—	0

MARSHMALLOW
FOOD	PORTION	CALS.	FIB.	CHOL.
Campfire				
	2 lg	40	—	0
Miniature	24	40	—	0
Joyva				
Twists Chocolate Covered	2 (1.5 oz)	190	0	0
Kraft				
Funmallows	4 (1.1 oz)	110	0	0
Funmallows Miniature	½ cup (1.1 oz)	100	0	0
Jet-Puffed	5 (1.2 oz)	110	0	0
Marshmallow Creme	2 tbsp (0.4 oz)	40	0	0
Miniature	½ cup (1.1 oz)	100	0	0
Teddy Bear Cocoa-Flavored	½ cup (1.1 oz)	100	0	0
Marshmallow Fluff	1 heaping tsp (18 g)	59	—	0
marshmallow	1 reg (0.3 oz)	23	—	0
marshmallow	1 cup (1.6 oz)	146	—	0

FOOD	PORTION	CALS.	FIB.	CHOL.

MATZO
Goodman's

FOOD	PORTION	CALS.	FIB.	CHOL.
Matzo Ball Mix 50% Less Salt	2 tbsp (0.5 oz)	50	0	0
Matzo Ball Mix as prep	2 tbsp (0.5 oz)	60	1	0
Horowitz Margareten				
Egg Milk Chocolate Coated	1 oz	97	1	8
Manischewitz				
Daily Thin Tea	1	103	tr	0
Dietetic Thins	1	91	tr	0
Egg Dark Chocolate Coated	½ matzo (1 oz)	97	1	8
Egg n' Onion	1	112	—	15
Matzo Cracker Miniatures	10	90	—	0
Matzo Farfel	1 cup	180	—	0
Matzo Meal	1 cup	514	tr	0
Passover	1	129	—	0
Passover Egg	1	132	—	25
Passover Egg Matzo Crackers	10	108	—	20
Salted Thin	1	100	tr	0
Unsalted	1	110	tr	0
Wheat Matzo Crackers	10	90	—	0
Whole Wheat w/ Bran	1	110	1	0
Streit's				
Dietetic	1 (1 oz)	100	1	0
Lightly Salted	1 (1 oz)	110	1	0
Matzoh Meal	¼ cup (1 oz)	110	1	0
Passover	1 (1 oz)	110	1	0
Unsalted	1 (0.9 oz)	100	1	0
Whole Wheat	1 (1 oz)	110	4	0
plain	1 (1 oz)	112	1	0
whole wheat	1 (1 oz)	99	3	0

MAYONNAISE
(see also MAYONNAISE TYPE SALAD DRESSING, RELISH)
Best Foods

FOOD	PORTION	CALS.	FIB.	CHOL.
Cholesterol Free Reduced Calorie	1 tbsp (15 g)	50	—	0
Cholesterol Free Reduced Calorie	1 cup (233 g)	760	—	0
Light	1 cup (233 g)	760	—	90
Light	1 tbsp (15 g)	50	—	5
Real	1 cup	1570	—	95
Real	1 tbsp	100	—	5
Hain				
Canola	1 tbsp	100	—	5

FOOD	PORTION	CALS.	FIB.	CHOL.
Hain (CONT.)				
Canola	1 tbsp	60	—	0
Cold Processed	1 tbsp	110	—	5
Eggless No Salt Added	1 tbsp	110	—	0
Light Low Sodium	1 tbsp	60	—	10
Real No Salt Added	1 tbsp	110	—	5
Safflower	1 tbsp	110	—	5
Hellman's	1 tbsp	100	—	5
Hellman's	1 cup (220 g)	1570	—	95
Cholesterol Free Reduced Calorie	1 tbsp (15 g)	50	—	0
Cholesterol Free Reduced Calorie	1 cup (233 g)	760	—	0
Light Reduced Calorie	1 cup (233 g)	760	—	90
Light Reduced Calorie	1 tbsp (15 g)	50	—	5
Hollywood	1 tbsp	110	—	5
Canola	1 tbsp	100	—	5
Safflower	1 tbsp	100	—	5
Kraft				
Free	1 tbsp (0.6 oz)	10	0	0
Light	1 tbsp (0.5 oz)	50	0	0
Real	1 tbsp (0.5 oz)	100	0	10
McIlhenny				
Spicy	1 tbsp (0.5 oz)	108	tr	8
Mother's	1 tbsp	100	—	10
Red Wing				
"H" Style	1 tbsp (0.5 oz)	110	—	10
Smart Beat				
Canola Oil	1 tbsp	40	—	0
Weight Watchers				
Fat Free	1 tbsp	12	—	0
Light	1 tbsp	50	—	5
Low Sodium	1 tbsp	50	—	5
mayonnaise	1 cup	1577	—	130
mayonnaise	1 tbsp	99	—	8
reduced calorie	1 cup	556	—	58
reduced calorie	1 tbsp	34	—	4
sandwich spread	1 tbsp	60	—	12

MAYONNAISE TYPE SALAD DRESSING

(*see also* MAYONNAISE, RELISH)

Bright Day	1 tbsp	60	—	0
Miracle Whip	1 tbsp (0.5 oz)	70	0	5
Free	1 tbsp (0.6 oz)	15	0	0

FOOD	PORTION	CALS.	FIB.	CHOL.
Miracle Whip (cont.)				
Light	1 tbsp (0.5 oz)	40	0	0
Smart Beat	1 tbsp (15 g)	12	—	0
Spin Blend	1 tbsp	60	—	10
Cholesterol Free	1 tbsp	40	—	0
Weight Watchers				
Fat Free Whipped Dressing	1 tbsp	16	—	0
mayonnaise type salad dressing	1 cup	916	—	60
mayonnaise type salad dressing	1 tbsp	57	—	4
reduced calorie w/o cholesterol	1 cup	1084	—	0
reduced calorie w/o cholesterol	1 tbsp	68	—	0
MEAT STICKS				
Tombstone				
Beef Jerky	1 stick (0.5 oz)	35	0	15
Beef Sticks	1 (0.8 oz)	110	0	20
Snappy Sticks	1 (0.8 oz)	110	0	20
jerky beef	1 lg piece (0.7 oz)	67	—	22
jerky beef	1 oz	96	—	32
smoked	1 (0.7)	109	—	26
smoked	1 oz	156	—	38
MEAT SUBSTITUTES				
(*see also* BACON SUBSTITUTES, CHICKEN SUBSTITUTES, SAUSAGE				
SUBSTITUTES, TURKEY SUBSTITUTES)				
Green Giant				
Harvest Burgers Original	1 (3 oz)	140	5	0
Harvest Direct				
TVP Beef Chunks	3.5 oz	280	18	0
TVP Beef Chunks Flavored	3.5 oz	250	17	0
TVP Beef Strips	3.5 oz	280	18	0
TVP Ground Beef	3.5 oz	280	18	0
TVP Ground Beef Flavored	3.5 oz	250	17	0
Jaclyn's				
Salisbury Steak Style Dinner	11 oz	260	—	0
Sirloin Strips Style Dinner	12 oz	290	—	0
Ken & Robert's				
Veggie Burger	1 (62 g)	110	—	0
LaLoma				
Corn Dogs	1 (71 g)	190	—	0
Dinner Cuts	2 pieces (99 g)	110	—	0
Griddle Steaks	1 piece (54 g)	140	—	0
Nuteena	½ in slice (65 g)	160	—	0
Patty Mix	¼ cup (16 g)	50	—	0
Redi-Burger	½ in slice (68 g)	130	—	0

FOOD	PORTION	CALS.	FIB.	CHOL.
LaLoma (CONT.)				
Savory Dinner Loaf Mix not prep	¼ cup (16 g)	50	—	0
Savory Meatballs	7 (70 g)	190	—	0
Sizzle Burger	1 patty (71 g)	220	—	0
Sozzle Franks	2 (68 g)	170	—	0
Swiss Steak	1 piece (92 g)	170	—	0
Tender Bits	4 pieces (57 g)	80	—	0
Tender Rounds	6 pieces (73 g)	120	—	0
Vege-Burger	½ cup (108 g)	110	—	0
Vita-Burger Chunk	¼ cup (21 g)	70	—	0
Vita-Burger Granules	3 tbsp (21 g)	70	—	0
Lightlife				
American Grill	2.75 oz	110	—	0
Barbecue Grill	2.75 oz	130	—	0
Smart Deli Slices	2 slices (1.5 oz)	44	—	0
Smart Dogs	1 (1.5 oz)	40	—	0
Smart Dogs To Go	1 (5 oz)	115	—	0
Tofu Pups	1 (1.5 oz)	92	—	0
Vegetarian Sloppy Joe	4.3 oz	130	—	0
Midland Harvest				
Burger n' Loaf Chili w/o Beans	0.8 oz	90	2	0
Burger n' Loaf Herbs & Spice	3.2 oz	140	4	0
Burger n' Loaf Italian	3.2 oz	140	4	0
Burger n' Loaf Original	3.2 oz	140	4	0
Burger n' Loaf Sloppy Joe w/o Sauce	0.8 oz	80	1	0
Burger n' Loaf Taco	2.7 oz	90	1	0
Sovex				
Better Than Burger?	½ cup (1.9 oz)	165	9	0
Spring Creek				
Soysage	1 patty (1.6 oz)	63	—	0
White Wave				
Meatless Healthy Franks	1 (1.5 oz)	90	0	0
Meatless Jumbo Franks	1 (3 oz)	170	0	0
Meatless Sandwich Slices Beef	2 slices (1.6 oz)	90	1	0
Meatless Sandwich Slices Bologna	2 slices (1.6 oz)	120	1	0
Meatless Sandwich Slices Pastrami	2 slices (1.6 oz)	90	1	0
Meatless Healthy Franks	1 (1.5 oz)	90	—	0
Veggie Burger	1 patty (2.5 oz)	110	2	0
Zoglo's				
Crispy Vegetarian Cutlets	1 (3.5 oz)	200	2	0

FOOD	PORTION	CALS.	FIB.	CHOL.
Zoglo's (CONT.)				
Savory Vegetarian Kebabs	1 serv (2.8 oz)	135	2	0
Tender Vegetarian Burgers	1 (2.6 oz)	150	2	0
Vegetable Patties	1 (2.6 oz)	130	2	0
Vegetarian Franks	1 (2.6 oz)	125	2	0

MELON
(*see also individual names*)
FRESH
Chiquita

Cantalene	1 cup	60	—	0
Honey Mist	1 cup	80	—	0

FROZEN
Big Valley

Mixed	¾ cup (4.9 oz)	40	1	0
melon balls	1 cup	55	—	0

MEXICAN FOOD
(*see also* SALSA, SAUCE, TORTILLA)

MILK
(*see also* CHOCOLATE, COCOA, MILK DRINKS)
CANNED
Carnation

Evaporated	2 tbsp	40	—	10
Evaporated Lowfat	2 tbsp	25	—	5
Lite Evaporated Skimmed	½ cup (4 fl oz)	100	—	5
Sweetened Condensed	2 tbsp	130	—	10
Pet				
Evaporated	½ cup	170	—	36
Evaporated Filled	½ cup	150	—	5
Evaporated Light Skimmed	½ cup	100	—	10
condensed sweetened	1 oz	123	—	13
condensed sweetened	1 cup	982	—	104
evaporated	½ cup	169	—	37
evaporated skim	½ cup	99	—	5

DRIED
Carnation

Nonfat	⅓ cup dry	80	—	<5
Sanalac				
as prep	8 oz	80	0	4
buttermilk	1 tbsp	25	—	5
nonfat instantized	1 pkg (3.2 oz)	244	—	12

FRESH
BodyWise

Nonfat	8 fl oz	100	0	5

FOOD	PORTION	CALS.	FIB.	CHOL.
CalciMilk	8 fl oz	102	0	10
Farmland				
1%	8 fl oz	100	0	10
2%	8 fl oz	130	0	20
Cholesterol Reduced	8 oz	150	—	10
Easylac 1%	8 fl oz	100	—	10
Easylac Nonfat	8 fl oz	90	—	5
Skim	8 fl oz	80	0	<5
Skim Plus	8 fl oz	100	—	5
Friendship				
Buttermilk	8 fl oz	120	0	15
Lactaid				
1%	8 fl oz	102	0	10
Nonfat	8 fl oz	86	0	4
1%	1 cup	102	—	10
1%	1 qt	409	—	39
1% protein fortified	1 qt	477	—	39
1% protein fortified	1 cup	119	—	10
2%	1 qt	485	—	73
2%	1 cup	121	—	18
buttermilk	1 qt	396	—	34
buttermilk	1 cup	99	—	9
goat	1 qt	672	—	111
goat	1 cup	168	—	28
human	1 cup	171	—	34
indian buffalo	1 cup	236	—	46
low sodium	1 cup	149	—	33
skim	1 qt	342	—	18
skim	1 cup	86	—	4
skim protein fortified	1 qt	400	—	20
skim protein fortified	1 cup	100	—	5
whole	1 cup	150	—	33
SHELF-STABLE				
Parmalat				
1%	1 cup (8 oz)	110	0	15
2%	1 cup (8 oz)	130	0	20
Skim	1 cup (8 oz)	90	0	5
Whole	1 cup (8 oz)	160	0	35

MILK DRINKS

(*see also* BREAKFAST DRINKS, CHOCOLATE, COCOA)

FOOD	PORTION	CALS.	FIB.	CHOL.
Body Wise				
Chocolate Nonfat Milk	1 cup (8 fl oz)	180	1	5

FOOD	PORTION	CALS.	FIB.	CHOL.
Hershey				
Chocolate Milk 2%	1 cup	190	—	20
Hood				
Chocolate Lowfat	1 cup (8 oz)	150	0	10
Lactaid				
Chocolate Milk 1%	8 fl oz	158	tr	7
Parmalat				
Chocolate 2%	1 box (8 oz)	180	1	20
chocolate milk	1 cup	208	—	30
chocolate milk	1 qt	833	—	122
chocolate milk 1%	1 cup	158	—	7
chocolate milk 1%	1 qt	630	—	29
chocolate milk 2%	1 cup	179	—	17
strawberry flavor mix as prep w/ whole milk	9 oz	234	—	33

MILK SUBSTITUTES

(*see also* COFFEE WHITENERS)

FOOD	PORTION	CALS.	FIB.	CHOL.
Better Than Milk				
Carob	8 fl oz	130	—	0
Chocolate	8 fl oz	125	—	0
Light	8 fl oz	80	—	0
Natural	8 fl oz	90	—	0
Eden				
Original	1 pkg (8.8 oz)	135	0	0
Original	8 fl oz	130	0	0
EdenBlend				
Original	8 fl oz	120	0	0
EdenRice				
Original	8 fl oz	110	0	0
Edensoy				
Carob	8 fl oz	150	0	0
Extra Original	1 pkg (8.8 oz)	140	0	0
Extra Original	8 fl oz	130	0	0
Extra Vanilla	1 pkg (8.8 fl oz)	150	0	0
Extra Vanilla	8 fl oz	140	0	0
Vanilla	8 fl oz	150	0	0
Vanilla	1 pkg (8.8 fl oz)	150	0	0
Health Valley				
Soo Moo	1 cup	120	0	0
Rice Dream				
Carob Lite	8 fl oz	150	—	0
Chocolate	8 fl oz	190	—	0
Chocolate	8 fl oz	190	—	0
Lite Organic Original	8 fl oz	130	—	0

FOOD	PORTION	CALS.	FIB.	CHOL.
Rice Dream (CONT.)				
Lite Vanilla	8 fl oz	130	—	0
Spring Creek				
!Honey Vanilla	1 oz	23	—	0
Original	1 oz	21	—	0
Plain	1 oz	15	—	0
Vegelicious	8 fl oz	100	—	0
Vitamite	8 fl oz	100	—	0
Vitasoy				
Carob Supreme	8 fl oz	150	—	0
Cocoa Light	8 fl oz	140	—	0
Cocoa Rich	8 fl oz	160	—	0
Original Creamy	8 fl oz	100	—	0
Original Light	8 fl oz	90	—	0
Vanilla Delite	8 fl oz	150	—	0
Vanilla Light	8 fl oz	110	—	0
Westsoy				
Cocoa Lite	8 fl oz	140	—	0
Plain Lite	8 fl oz	100	—	0
Vanilla Lite	8 fl oz	110	—	0
First Alternative	8 fl oz	80	—	0
imitation milk	1 cup	150	—	tr
imitation milk	1 qt	600	—	2

MILKFISH

baked	3 oz	162	—	57

MILKSHAKE

Hood				
Shake Up Chocolate	1 cup (8 oz)	240	0	20
Shake Up Strawberry	1 cup (8 oz)	220	0	20
Shake Up Vanilla	1 cup (8 oz)	220	0	20
MicroMagic				
Chocolate	1 (10.5 oz)	290	—	40
Milky Way				
Shake	1 (10 fl oz)	390	0	60
Parmalat				
Shake A Shake Chocolate	1 box (6 oz)	180	1	15
Shake A Shake Orange Vanilla	1 box (6 oz)	110	0	10
Shake A Shake Vanilla	1 box (6 oz)	170	0	15
chocolate	10 oz	360	—	37
strawberry	10 oz	319	—	31
thick shake chocolate	10.6 oz	356	—	32
thick shake vanilla	11 oz	350	—	37
vanilla	10 oz	314	—	32

FOOD	PORTION	CALS.	FIB.	CHOL.
MILLET				
cooked	½ cup	143	—	0
MINERAL/BOTTLED WATER				
Artesia				
Almund	7 oz	0	—	0
Cranberi	7 oz	0	—	0
Lemin	7 oz	0	—	0
Orange	7 oz	0	—	0
Canada Dry				
Sparkling Water	8 fl oz	0	0	0
Crystal Geyser				
Sparking Natural Wild Cherry	1 bottle (12 fl oz)	0	—	0
Sparkling Lemon	1 bottle (12 fl oz)	0	—	0
Sparkling Mineral	1 bottle (12 fl oz)	0	—	0
Sparkling Natural Cola Berry	1 bottle (12 fl oz)	0	—	0
Sparkling Orange	1 bottle (12 fl oz)	0	—	0
Diamond Spring	1 qt	0	—	0
Evian	1 liter	0	0	0
Glennpatrick				
Irish Spring Pure	8 oz	0	—	0
LaCroix				
Sparkling Berry	12 fl oz	0	—	0
Sparkling Lemon	12 fl oz	0	—	0
Sparkling Lime	12 fl oz	0	—	0
Sparkling Orange	12 fl oz	0	—	0
Sparkling Regular	12 fl oz	0	—	0
Mountain Valley	1 qt	0	—	0
San Pellegrino	1 liter (33.8 oz)	0	—	0
Saratoga				
Sparkling	1 liter	0	—	0
MISO				
Eden				
Genmai Miso Organic	1 tbsp (0.5 oz)	25	tr	0
Hacho Miso Organic	1 tbsp (0.5 oz)	35	1	0
Kome Miso Organic	1 tbsp (0.6 oz)	25	tr	0
Mugi Miso Organic	1 tbsp (0.6 oz)	25	1	0
Shiro Miso Organic	1 tbsp (0.6 oz)	35	1	0
miso	½ cup	284	7	0
MOLASSES				
Brer Rabbit				
Dark	2 tbsp	110	—	0
Light	2 tbsp	110	—	0

FOOD	PORTION	CALS.	FIB.	CHOL.
McIlhenny	1 tbsp (0.7 oz)	66	tr	0
Tree Of Life				
Blackstrap	1 tbsp (0.5 oz)	45	—	0
blackstrap	1 tbsp (0.7 oz)	47	—	0
blackstrap	1 cup (11.5 oz)	771	—	0
molasses	1 cup (11.5 oz)	873	—	0
molasses	1 tbsp (0.7 oz)	53	—	0

MONKFISH
baked	3 oz	82	—	27

MOOSE
roasted	3 oz	114	—	66

MOTH BEANS
dried cooked	1 cup	207	—	0

MOUSSE
FROZEN
Pepperidge Farm				
San Francisco Chocolate Mousse	1	490	—	150
Sara Lee				
Chocolate	1 slice (2.7 oz)	260	—	20
Chocolate Light	1 (3 oz)	170	—	10
Weight Watchers				
Chocolate	1 (2.5 oz)	160	—	5
Praline Pecan	1 (2.71 oz)	180	—	5
HOME RECIPE				
chocolate	½ cup (7.1 oz)	447	—	299
crab	¼ cup	364	—	136
orange	½ cup	87	—	1
MIX				
Jell-O				
Rich & Luscious Chocolate	½ cup	145	—	9
Rich & Luscious Chocolate Fudge	½ cup	143	—	9
Knorr				
Dark Chocolate as prep	½ cup	90	—	5
Milk Chocolate as prep	½ cup	90	—	5
White Chocolate as prep	½ cup	80	—	5
Royal				
Chocolate Mousse No-Bake	⅛ pie	130	—	0
TAKE-OUT				
chocolate	½ cup (7.1 oz)	447	—	299

FOOD	PORTION	CALS.	FIB.	CHOL.
MUFFIN				
FROZEN				
Health Valley				
Almond & Date Oat Bran Fancy Fruit	1	180	8	0
Fat Free Apple Spice	1	140	5	0
Fat Free Banana	1	130	5	0
Fat Free Raisin Spice	1	140	5	0
Oat Bran Fancy Fruit Blueberry	1	140	8	0
Oat Bran Fancy Fruit Raisin	1	180	8	0
Rice Bran Fancy Fruit Raisin	1	210	6	0
Pepperidge Farm				
Banana Nut	1	170	—	30
Blueberry	1	170	1	25
Cholesterol Free Multi Grain Muesli	1	200	—	0
Cholesterol Free Oatbran With Apple	1	190	—	0
Cholesterol Free Raisin Bran	1	170	—	0
Cinnamon Swirl	1	190	1	35
Corn	1	180	—	30
Sara Lee				
Apple Oat Bran	1	190	—	0
Apple Spice	1	220	—	0
Blueberry	1	200	—	0
Blueberry Free & Light	1	120	—	0
Golden Corn	1	240	—	0
Oat Bran	1	210	—	0
Raisin Bran	1	220	—	0
HOME RECIPE				
blueberry as prep w/ 2% milk	1 (2 oz)	163	—	21
blueberry as prep w/ whole milk	1 (2 oz)	165	—	23
corn as prep w/ 2% milk	1 (2 oz)	180	—	24
corn as prep w/ whole milk	1 (2 oz)	183	—	25
plain as prep w/ 2% milk	1 (2 oz)	169	—	22
plain as prep w/ whole milk	1 (2 oz)	172	—	24
wheat bran as prep w/ 2% milk	1 (2 oz)	161	—	19
wheat bran as prep w/ whole milk	1 (2 oz)	164	—	20
MIX				
Arrowhead				
Bran	⅓ cup (1.4 oz)	150	7	0
Oat Bran Wheat Free	⅓ cup (1.5 oz)	160	7	0
Betty Crocker				
Apple Cinnamon	1	120	—	25

FOOD	PORTION	CALS.	FIB.	CHOL.
Betty Crocker (CONT.)				
Apple Cinnamon No Cholesterol Recipe	1	110	—	0
Banana Nut	1	120	—	25
Banana Nut No Cholesterol Recipe	1	110	—	0
Cinnamon Streusel	1	200	—	30
Oat Bran	1	190	—	35
Oat Bran No Cholesterol Recipe	1	180	—	0
Twice The Blueberries	1	120	—	20
Twice The Blueberries No Cholesterol Recipe	1	110	—	0
Wild Blueberry	1	120	—	25
Wild Blueberry Light	1	70	—	20
Wild Blueberry Light No Cholesterol Recipe	1	70	—	0
Wild Blueberry No Cholesterol Recipe	1	110	—	0
Flako				
Corn	⅓ cup (1.4 oz)	160	1	0
Hain				
Oat Bran Apple Cinnamon	1	140	5	0
Oat Bran Banana Nut	1	140	4	0
Oat Bran Raspberry Spice	1	140	4	0
Jiffy				
Apple Cinnamon as prep	1	190	1	33
Banana Nut as prep	1	180	1	27
Blueberry as prep	1	190	1	36
Bran Date	1	110	—	10
Bran With Dates as prep	1	170	3	36
Corn as prep	1	180	1	0
Honey Date as prep	1	170	1	30
Oatmeal as prep	1	180	2	27
Wanda's				
Blue Corn	¼ cup mix per serv (1.2 oz)	130	1	0
blueberry	1 (1¾ oz)	149	—	23
corn	1 (1.75 oz)	160	—	31
wheat bran as prep	1 (1¾ oz)	138	—	34
READY-TO-EAT				
Arnold				
Bran'nola	1 (2.3 oz)	160	2	0
Raisin	1 (2.3 oz)	160	2	0
Dutch Mill				
Apple Oat Bran	1 (2 oz)	180	1	0

FOOD	PORTION	CALS.	FIB.	CHOL.
Dutch Mill (CONT.)				
Banana Walnut	1 (2 oz)	220	1	5
Carrot	1 (2 oz)	190	1	30
Corn	1 (2 oz)	190	1	40
Cranberry Orange	1 (2 oz)	170	1	55
Raisin Bran	1 (2 oz)	230	3	30
Freihofer's				
Corn Toasters	1 (1.3 oz)	130	0	15
Hostess				
Mini Apple Cinnamon	5 (2 oz)	260	3	45
Mini Banana Nut	5 (2 oz)	260	tr	40
Mini Blueberry	5 (2 oz)	240	tr	40
Mini Chocolate Chip	5 (2 oz)	260	1	35
Muffin Loaf Blueberry	1 (3.8 oz)	440	2	80
Oat Bran	1 (1.5 oz)	160	tr	0
Oat Bran Banana Nut	1 (1.5 oz)	150	1	0
Weight Watchers				
Apple Cinnamon	1 (2.5 oz)	200	1	0
Lemon Poppy Seed	1 (2.5 oz)	200	1	0
blueberry	1 (2 oz)	158	2	17
oat bran wheat free	1 (2 oz)	154	4	0
MULBERRIES				
fresh	1 cup	61	—	0
MULLET				
striped cooked	3 oz	127	—	54
striped raw	3 oz	99	—	42
MUNG BEANS				
DRIED				
cooked	1 cup	213	—	0
SPROUTS				
canned	½ cup	8	—	0
cooked	½ cup	13	—	0
raw	½ cup	16	—	0
stir fried	½ cup	31	—	0
MUNGO BEANS				
dried cooked	1 cup	190	—	1
MUSHROOMS				
CANNED				
B In B				
With Garlic	¼ cup	12	1	0
	¼ cup	12	1	0
Empress				
Button	2 oz	14	—	0

FOOD	PORTION	CALS.	FIB.	CHOL.
Empress (CONT.)				
Button Sliced	2 oz	14	—	0
Pieces & Stems	2 oz	14	—	0
Straw Broken	2 oz	10	—	0
Green Giant				
Oriental Straw	¼ cup	12	1	0
Pieces And Stems	¼ cup	12	1	0
Sliced	¼ cup	12	1	0
Whole	¼ cup	12	1	0
Ka-Me				
Stir Fry	½ cup (4.5 oz)	20	2	0
Straw Whole Peeled	½ cup (4.5 oz)	20	2	0
Seneca	½ cup	25	2	0
chanterelle	3½ oz	12	6	0
pieces	½ cup	19	—	0
whole	1 (0.4 oz)	3	—	0
DRIED				
chanterelle	3½ oz	89	60	0
shitake	4 (½ oz)	44	—	0
FRESH				
chanterelle	3½ oz	11	6	0
enoki raw	1 (4 in)	2	—	0
morel	3½ oz	9	7	0
raw	1 (½ oz)	5	tr	0
raw sliced	½ cup	9	tr	0
shitake cooked	4 (2.5 oz)	40	—	0
sliced cooked	½ cup	21	1	0
whole cooked	1 (0.4 oz)	3	—	0
FROZEN				
Empire				
Breaded	7 (2.8 oz)	90	1	0

MUSSELS

blue raw	3 oz	73	—	24
blue raw	1 cup	129	—	42
fresh blue cooked	3 oz	147	—	48

MUSTARD

Blanchard & Blanchard				
Mustard	1 tsp (5 g)	0	0	0
Eden				
Hot Organic	1 tsp (5 g)	0	0	0
Grey Poupon				
Country Dijon	1 tsp	6	0	0
Dijon	1 tsp	6	0	0

FOOD	PORTION	CALS.	FIB.	CHOL.
Grey Poupon (CONT.)				
Parisian	1 tsp	6	0	0
Hain				
Stone Ground	1 tbsp	14	—	0
Stone Ground No Salt Added	1 tbsp	14	—	0
Heinz				
Mild Yellow	1 tbsp	8	—	0
Spicy Brown	1 tbsp	14	—	0
Ka-Me				
Hot Mustard Powder Chinese Style	¼ tsp (1 g)	5	1	0
Kosciuszko				
Spicy Brown	1 tsp	5	—	0
Kraft	1 tsp (0.2 oz)	0	0	0
McIlhenny				
Coarse Ground	1 tsp (0.2 oz)	4	tr	0
Spicy	1 tsp (0.2 oz)	6	1	0
Plochman				
Dijon	1 tsp (5 g)	7	—	0
Spoonable Salad	1 tsp (5 g)	4	—	0
Squeeze Salad	1 tsp (5 g)	4	—	0
Stone Ground	1 tsp (5 g)	6	—	0
Tree Of Life				
Dijon	1 tsp (5 g)	0	—	0
Dijon Imported	1 tsp (5 g)	5	—	0
Low Sodium	1 tsp (5 g)	3	—	0
Stone Ground	1 tsp (5 g)	0	—	0
Yellow	1 tsp (5 g)	0	—	0
dry mustard seed yellow	1 tsp	15	—	0
yellow ready-to-use	1 tsp	5	—	0
MUSTARD GREENS				
CANNED				
Allen	½ cup (4.1 oz)	30	3	0
Sunshine	½ cup (4.1 oz)	25	2	0
FRESH				
chopped cooked	½ cup	11	—	0
raw chopped	½ cup	7	—	0
FROZEN				
chopped cooked	½ cup	14	—	0
NATTO				
natto	½ cup	187	—	0
NAVY BEANS				
CANNED				
Allen	½ cup (4.5 oz)	110	6	0

FOOD	PORTION	CALS.	FIB.	CHOL.
Eden				
Organic	½ cup (4.3 oz)	100	7	0
Hanover	½ cup	100	—	0
Trappey				
With Bacon	½ cup (4.5 oz)	110	7	0
With Bacon & Jalapeno	½ cup (4.5 oz)	110	7	0
navy	1 cup	296	—	0
DRIED				
cooked	1 cup	259	—	0
SPROUTS				
cooked	3½ oz	78	—	0
raw	½ cup	35	—	0
NECTARINE				
Dole	1	70	3	0
fresh	1	67	2	0
NEUFCHATEL				
Philadelphia	1 oz	70	0	20
Spreadery				
Classic Ranch	2 tbsp (1 oz)	60	0	20
Garden Vegetable	2 tbsp (1 oz)	70	0	20
Garlic & Herb	2 tbsp (1 oz)	80	0	20
With Strawberry	1 oz	70	—	15
WisPride				
Garden Vegetable Cup	2 tbsp (1.1 oz)	60	0	15
Garlic & Herb Cup	2 tbsp (1.1 oz)	60	0	15
neufchatel	1 oz	74	—	22
neufchatel	1 pkg (3 oz)	221	—	65

NON-DAIRY CREAMERS
(*see* COFFEE WHITENERS)

NON-DAIRY WHIPPED TOPPINGS
(*see* WHIPPED TOPPINGS)

NOODLES
(*see also* PASTA DINNERS)

CANNED				
Dinty Moore				
Noodles & Chicken	1 can (7.5 oz)	180	1	30
Micro Cup Meals				
Noodles & Chicken	1 cup (7.5 oz)	180	1	30
Noodles & Chicken	1 cup (10.4 oz)	250	2	45
Van Camp's				
Noodlee Weenee	1 can (8 oz)	230	1	20
DRY				
Creamette				
Egg	2 oz	221	—	70

FOOD	PORTION	CALS.	FIB.	CHOL.
Golden Grain				
Egg	2 oz	210	2	65
Hodgson Mill				
Veggie Egg not prep	2 oz	200	2	35
Whole Wheat Spinach Egg not prep	2 oz	190	5	30
Whole Wheat Egg not prep	2 oz	190	4	30
Ka-Me				
Chinese Egg	½ cup (2 oz)	210	2	53
Chinese Plain	½ cup (2 oz)	200	1	0
Chuka Soba Curly Noodles	2 oz	200	1	0
Lo Mein Wide Chinese	½ cup (2 oz)	200	1	0
Py Mai Fun Rice Sticks	2 oz	193	0	0
Sai Fun Bean Thread	1 cup (2 oz)	190	1	0
Soba Shin Shu Japanese Buckwheat	2 oz	200	2	0
Tomoshiraga Somen Noodles	2 oz	190	1	0
Udon Japanese Thick	2 oz	190	1	0
La Choy				
Chow Mein Narrow	½ cup	150	tr	0
Chow Mein Wide	½ cup	150	tr	0
Rice	½ cup	130	tr	0
Mueller's				
Egg	2 oz (57 g)	220	—	55
Noodle Trio	2 oz (57 g)	220	—	55
Noodles By Leonardo				
Egg Fine not prep	1 cup (2 oz)	210	2	80
Egg Medium not prep	1 cup (2 oz)	210	2	80
Egg Wide not prep	1 cup (2 oz)	210	2	80
San Giorgio				
Egg	2 oz	210	—	70
Shofar				
No Yolks	2 oz	210	3	0
cellophane	1 cup	492	—	0
chow mein	1 cup	237	—	0
egg	1 cup (38 g)	145	—	36
egg cooked	1 cup	212	—	53
japanese soba	2 oz	192	—	0
japanese soba cooked	½ cup	56	—	0
japanese somen	2 oz	203	—	0
japanese somen cooked	½ cup	115	—	0
spinach/egg	1 cup	145	—	36
spinach/egg cooked	1 cup	211	—	52

FOOD	PORTION	CALS.	FIB.	CHOL.
DRY MIX				
Kraft				
Chicken Egg Noodle	1 cup	330	1	60
La Choy				
Ramen Noodles Chicken as prep	1 cup	200	4	0
Raman Noodles Beef as prep	1 cup	200	4	0
Lipton				
Noodles & Sauce Romanoff	½ cup	136	—	31
Minute				
Microwave Chicken Flavored	½ cup	157	—	36
Microwave Parmesan	½ cup	178	—	47
Noodles By Leonardo				
Macaroni & Cheese as prep	1 cup (2.5 oz)	250	2	0
FRESH				
Herb's				
Egg Fine	2 oz	220	2	60
Egg Medium	2 oz	220	2	60
Kluski Medium	2 oz	220	2	60
Kluski Wide	2 oz	220	2	60
FROZEN				
Luigino's				
Stroganoff	1 cup (7.5 oz)	290	2	50
Stroganoff	1 pkg (8 oz)	310	2	55
TAKE-OUT				
noodle pudding	½ cup	132	—	27
NOPALES				
cooked	1 cup (5.2 oz)	23	—	0
raw sliced	½ cup (1.5 oz)	7	—	0
raw sliced	1 cup (3 oz)	14	—	0
NUTMEG				
Watkins				
	¼ tsp (0.5 g)	0	0	0
ground	1 tsp	12	—	0

NUTRITIONAL SUPPLEMENTS

(*see also* BREAKFAST BAR, BREAKFAST DRINKS)

FOOD	PORTION	CALS.	FIB.	CHOL.
DIET				
Sego				
Lite Chocolate	10 fl oz	150	—	5
Lite Dutch Chocolate	10 fl oz	150	—	5
Lite French Vanilla	10 fl oz	150	—	5
Lite Strawberry	10 fl oz	150	—	5
Lite Vanilla	10 fl oz	150	—	5

FOOD	PORTION	CALS.	FIB.	CHOL.
Sego (CONT.)				
Very Chocolate	10 fl oz	225	—	5
Very Chocolate Malt	10 fl oz	225	—	5
Very Strawberry	10 fl oz	225	—	5
Very Vanilla	10 fl oz	225	—	5
Slim-Fast				
Powder Chocolate as prep w/ skim milk	8 oz	190	2	9
Powder Chocolate Malt as prep w/ skim milk	8 oz	190	2	9
Powder Strawberry as prep w/ skim milk	8 oz	190	2	9
Powder Vanilla as prep w/ skim milk	8 oz	190	2	6
Sweet Success				
Chewy Bar Chocolate Brownie	1 (1.6 oz)	120	3	<5
Chewy Bar Chocolate Peanut Butter	1 (1.6 oz)	120	3	<5
Chewy Bar Chocolate Raspberry	1 (1.6 oz)	120	3	<5
Chewy Bar Chocolate Chip	1 (1.6 oz)	120	3	<5
Chewy Bar Oatmeal Raisin	1 (1.6 oz)	120	3	<5
Chocolate Raspberry Truffle	1 can (10 fl oz)	200	6	5
Chocolate Raspberry as prep w/ skim milk	9 fl oz	180	6	6
Chocolate Mocha Supreme	1 can (10 fl oz)	200	6	5
Chocolate Mocha Supreme as prep w/ skim milk	9 fl oz	180	6	6
Classic Chocolate Chip as prep w/ skim milk	9 fl oz	180	6	6
Creamy Milk Chocolate	1 can (10 fl oz)	200	6	5
Creamy Milk Chocolate	1 carton (12 fl oz)	220	6	<5
Creamy Milk Chocolate as prep w/ skim milk	9 fl oz	180	6	6
Creamy Vanilla Delight as prep w/ skim milk	9 fl oz	180	6	6
Dark Chocolate Fudge	1 can (10 fl oz)	200	6	5
Dark Chocolate Fudge	1 carton (12 fl oz)	220	6	<5
Dark Chocolate Fudge as prep w/ skim milk	9 fl oz	180	6	6
Rich Chocolate Almond	1 can (10 fl oz)	200	6	5
Rich Chocolate Almond	1 carton (12 fl oz)	220	6	<5
Rich Chocolate Almond as prep w/ skim milk	9 fl oz	180	6	6

FOOD	PORTION	CALS.	FIB.	CHOL.
Sweet Success (CONT.)				
Smooth Vanilla Creme	1 can (10 fl oz)	200	6	5
Ultra Slim-Fast				
Cafe Mocha as prep w/ skim milk	8 oz	200	6	8
Chocolate Royale as prep w/ skim milk	8 oz	200	5	8
Crunch Bar Cocoa Almond	1	110	3	0
Crunch Bar Cocoa Raspberry	1	100	3	0
Crunch Bar Vanilla Almond	1	110	3	0
Dutch Chocolate as prep w/ water	8 oz	220	4	8
French Vanilla as prep w/ skim milk	8 oz	190	4	8
French Vanilla as prep w/ water	8 oz	220	4	8
Fruit Juice Mix as prep w/ fruit juice	8 oz	200	6	12
Nutrition Bar Peanut Butter	1	140	7	5
Nutrition Bar Dutch Chocolate	1	130	6	5
Pina Colada as prep w/ skim milk	8 oz	180	6	8
Ready-To-Drink Chocolate Royale	12 oz	250	5	5
Ready-To-Drink French Vanilla	12 oz	220	5	5
Ready-To-Drink Strawberry Supreme	12 oz	220	5	5
Strawberry Supreme as prep w/ water	8 oz	220	4	8
Strawberry as prep w/ skim milk	8 oz	190	4	8
REGULAR				
BeneFit				
Nutrition Bar	1 (2 oz)	240	tr	0
EggPro	4 oz	200	—	18
Fi-Bar				
Apple	1 (1 oz)	90	5	0
Cocoa Almond	1	130	4	0
Cocoa Peanut	1	130	4	0
Cranberry & Wild Berries	1 (1 oz)	100	4	0
Lemon	1 (1 oz)	90	4	0
Mandarin Orange	1 (1 oz)	99	5	0
Nuggets Almond Cappuccino Crunch	1 pkg	136	—	0
Nuggets Almond Butter Crunch	1 pkg	163	—	0

FOOD	PORTION	CALS.	FIB.	CHOL.
Fi-Bar (CONT.)				
Nuggets Coconut Almond Crunch	1 pkg	136	—	0
Nuggets Peanut Butter Crunch	1 pkg	160	—	0
Raspberry	1 (1 oz)	100	4	0
Strawberry	1 (1 oz)	100	4	0
Treat Yourself Right Almond	1	152	5	0
Treat Yourself Right Peanutty Butter	1	152	5	0
Vanilla Almond	1	130	4	0
Vanilla Peanut	1	130	4	0
Gookinaid				
Lemonade	1 cup (8 fl oz)	45	—	0
Malsovit				
Mealwafers	2	152	—	0
Meal On The Go				
Apple	1 bar (3 oz)	294	5	0
Banana w/ Pecans	1 bar (3 oz)	289	8	0
Original	1 bar (3 oz)	286	7	0
Nutra/Balance				
Frozen Pudding Butterscotch	4 oz	225	—	0
Frozen Pudding Chocolate	4 oz	225	—	0
Frozen Pudding Tapioca	4 oz	225	—	0
Frozen Pudding Vanilla	4 oz	225	—	0
NutraShake				
With Fiber Vanilla	6 oz	300	—	0
With Fiber Strawberry	6 oz	300	—	0
NutriShake				
Chocolate	4 oz	200	—	18
Strawberry	4 oz	200	—	18
Vanilla	4 oz	200	—	18
Vita-J				
Apple Juice	11.5 fl oz	8	—	0
Fruit Punch	11.5 fl oz	8	—	0
Grapefruit Cocktail w/ Raspberry	11.5 fl oz	8	—	0
Orange Juice	11.5 fl oz	8	—	0

NUTS MIXED
(see also INDIVIDUAL NAMES)

FOOD	PORTION	CALS.	FIB.	CHOL.
Eagle				
Cashews & Peanuts Honey Roasted	1 oz	170	—	0
Mixed	1 oz	180	—	0

FOOD	PORTION	CALS.	FIB.	CHOL.
Eagle (CONT.)				
Mixed Deluxe	1 oz	180	—	0
Fisher				
Mixed Deluxe Lightly Salted	1 oz	180	—	0
Mixed Deluxe Salted	1 oz	180	—	0
Mixed Oil Roasted 25% More Cashews Lightly Salted	1 oz	180	—	0
Mixed Oil Roasted 25% More Cashews Salted	1 oz	180	—	0
Nut & Fruit Pina Colada	1 oz	150	—	0
Nut & Fruit Raisin Cranberry	1 oz	150	—	0
Nut & Fruit Tropical Fruit	1 oz	140	—	0
Nut Toppings Oil Roasted With Peanuts	1 oz	190	—	0
Peanuts Cashews	1 oz	170	—	0
Guy's				
Mixed With Peanuts	1 oz	180	—	0
Tasty Mix	1 oz	130	—	0
Planters				
Cashews & Peanuts Honey Roasted	1 oz	170	—	0
Mixed Lightly Salted	1 oz	170	—	0
Peanuts & Cashews Honey Roasted	1 oz	170	—	0
dry roasted w/ peanuts	1 oz	169	—	0
dry roasted w/ peanuts salted	1 oz	169	—	0
oil roasted w/ peanuts	1 oz	175	—	0
oil roasted w/ peanuts salted	1 oz	175	—	0
oil roasted w/o peanuts	1 oz	175	—	0
oil roasted w/o peanuts salted	1 oz	175	—	0

OCTOPUS

fresh steamed	3 oz	140	—	82

OHELOBERRIES

fresh	1 cup	39	—	0

OIL

(see also FAT)

Arrowhead				
Hazelnut	1 tbsp (0.5 fl oz)	120	0	0
Bertolli				
Classico	1 tbsp	120	—	0
Extra Light	1 tbsp	120	—	0
Extra Virgin	1 tbsp	120	—	0

FOOD	PORTION	CALS.	FIB.	CHOL.
Bertolli (CONT.)				
Crisco	1 tbsp (0.5 fl oz)	120	—	0
Corn Canola	1 tbsp (0.5 fl oz)	120	—	0
Puritan Canola	1 tbsp (0.5 fl oz)	120	0	0
Eden				
Hot Pepper Sesame	1 tbsp (0.5 oz)	130	0	0
Toasted Sesame	1 tbsp (0.5 oz)	130	0	0
Hain				
All Blend	1 tbsp	120	—	0
Almond	1 tbsp	120	—	0
Apricot Kernel	1 tbsp	120	—	0
Avocado	1 tbsp	120	—	0
Canola	1 tbsp	120	—	0
Canola Organic	1 tbsp	120	—	0
Coconut	1 tbsp	120	—	0
Corn	1 tbsp	120	—	0
Garlic & Oil	1 tbsp	120	—	0
Olive	1 tbsp	120	—	0
Peanut	1 tbsp	120	—	0
Rice Bran	1 tbsp	120	—	0
Safflower	1 tbsp	120	—	0
Safflower Hi-Oleic	1 tbsp	120	—	0
Safflower Organic	1 tbsp	120	—	0
Sesame	1 tbsp	120	—	0
Soy	1 tbsp	120	—	0
Sunflower	1 tbsp	120	—	0
Sunflower Organic	1 tbsp	120	—	0
Walnut	1 tbsp	120	—	0
Hollywood				
Canola	1 tbsp	120	—	0
Peanut	1 tbsp	120	—	0
Safflower	1 tbsp	120	—	0
Soy	1 tbsp	120	—	0
Sunflower	1 tbsp	120	—	0
House Of Tsang				
Hot Chili Sesame	1 tsp (5 g)	45	0	0
Mongolian Fire	1 tsp (5 g)	45	0	0
Pure Sesame	1 tsp (5 g)	45	0	0
Singapore Curry	1 tsp (5 g)	45	0	0
Wok Oil	1 tbsp (0.5 oz)	130	0	0
Italica	1 tbsp	120	—	0
Ka-Me				
Chili Hot	1 tbsp (0.5 fl oz)	130	0	0
Sesame	1 tbsp (0.5 fl oz)	130	0	0

FOOD	PORTION	CALS.	FIB.	CHOL.
Ka-Me (CONT.)				
Sesame Tempura	1 tbsp (0.5 fl oz)	130	0	0
Mazola	1 cup (221 g)	1955	—	0
Mazola	1 tbsp (14 g)	120	—	0
No Stick	2.5 sec spray (0.2 g)	2	—	0
Orville Redenbacher's	1 tbsp	120	0	0
Pam	1 sec spray (0.266 g)	2	—	0
Butter	1 sec spray (0.266 g)	2	—	0
Olive Oil	1 sec spray (0.266 g)	2	—	0
Pump	1 spray (0.43 g)	4	—	0
Planters				
Peanut	1 tbsp	120	—	0
Popcorn	1 tbsp	120	—	0
Pompeian	1 tbsp	130	—	0
Progresso				
Olive	1 tbsp	119	0	0
Olive Extra Light	1 tbsp	119	0	0
Olive Extra Virgin	1 tbsp	119	0	0
Smart Beat				
Canola	1 tbsp (14 g)	120	—	0
Smart Beat	1 tbsp	120	—	0
Tree Of Life				
Almond	1 tbsp (0.5 g)	130	—	0
Apricot Kernal	1 tbsp (0.5 g)	130	—	0
Avocado	1 tbsp (0.5 g)	130	—	0
Macadamia Nut	1 tbsp (0.5 g)	130	—	0
Olive Extra Virgin Organic	1 tbsp (0.5 g)	130	—	0
Sesame	1 tbsp (0.5 g)	130	—	0
Toasted Sesame	1 tbsp (0.5 g)	130	0	0
Weight Watchers				
Butter Spray	1 sec spray	2	—	0
Cooking Spray	1 sec spray	2	—	0
Wesson				
Canola	1 tbsp	120	0	0
Cooking Spray Lite	0.5 sec spray	0	0	0
Corn	1 tbsp	120	0	0
Olive	1 tbsp	120	0	0
Sunflower	1 tbsp	120	0	0
Vegetable	1 tbsp	120	0	0
almond	1 tbsp	120	—	0

FOOD	PORTION	CALS.	FIB.	CHOL.
almond	1 cup	1927	—	0
apricot kernel	1 cup	1927	—	0
apricot kernel	1 tbsp	120	—	0
avocado	1 tbsp	124	—	0
avocado	1 cup	1927	—	0
babassu palm	1 tbsp	120	—	0
butter oil	1 cup	1795	—	524
butter oil	1 tbsp	112	—	33
canola	1 cup	1927	—	0
canola	1 tbsp	124	—	0
coconut	1 tbsp	117	—	0
corn	1 cup	1927	—	0
corn	1 tbsp	120	—	0
cottonseed	1 tbsp	120	—	0
cottonseed	1 cup	1927	—	0
cupu assu	1 tbsp	120	—	0
grapeseed	1 tbsp	120	—	0
hazelnut	1 cup	1927	—	0
hazelnut	1 tbsp	120	—	0
mustard	1 cup	1927	—	0
mustard	1 tbsp	124	—	0
oat	1 tbsp	120	—	0
olive	1 cup	1909	—	0
olive	1 tbsp	119	—	0
palm	1 tbsp	120	—	0
palm	1 cup	1927	—	0
palm kernel	1 tbsp	117	—	0
palm kernel	1 cup	1879	—	0
peanut	1 cup	1909	—	0
peanut	1 tbsp	119	—	0
poppyseed	3.5 fl oz	900	—	0
poppyseed	1 tbsp	120	—	0
rice bran	1 tbsp	120	—	0
safflower	1 tbsp	120	—	0
safflower	1 cup	1927	—	0
sesame	1 tbsp	120	—	0
sheanut	1 tbsp	120	—	0
soybean	1 cup	1927	—	0
soybean	1 tbsp	120	—	0
sunflower	1 cup	1927	—	0
sunflower	1 tbsp	120	—	0
teaseed	1 tbsp	120	—	0
tomatoseed	1 tbsp	120	—	0
vegetable soybean & cottonseed	1 cup	1927	—	0

FOOD	PORTION	CALS.	FIB.	CHOL.
vegetable soybean & cottonseed	1 tbsp	120	—	0
walnut	1 cup	1927	1	0
walnut	1 tbsp	120	—	0
wheat germ	1 tbsp	120	—	0
FISH OIL				
Hain				
Cod Liver	1 tbsp	120	—	85
Cod Liver Cherry	1 tbsp	120	—	75
Cod Liver Mint	1 tbsp	120	—	85
cod liver	1 tbsp	123	—	78
herring	1 tbsp	123	—	104
menhaden	1 tbsp	123	—	71
salmon	1 tbsp	123	—	66
sardine	1 tbsp	123	—	97
OKRA				
CANNED				
Allen				
Cut	½ cup (4.4 oz)	25	3	0
McIlhenny				
Pickled	2 pieces (1 oz)	7	1	0
Trappey				
Cocktail Hot	2 pieces (1 oz)	8	1	0
Cocktail Mild	1 pieces (1 oz)	9	1	0
Creole Gumbo	½ cup (4.2 oz)	35	3	0
Cut	½ cup (4.4 oz)	25	3	0
FRESH				
raw	8 pods	36	—	0
raw sliced	½ cup	19	—	0
sliced cooked	½ cup	25	—	0
sliced cooked	8 pods	27	—	0
FROZEN				
Hanover				
Cut	½ cup	25	—	0
Whole	½ cup	35	—	0
sliced cooked	1 pkg (10 oz)	94	—	0
sliced cooked	½ cup	34	—	0
OLIVES				
Progresso				
Olive Appetizer	½ cup	180	—	0
Olive Condite	½ cup	130	—	0
Salad Olives	½ cup	120	—	0
S&W				
Ripe Extra Large	3.5 oz	163	—	0

FOOD	PORTION	CALS.	FIB.	CHOL.
S&W (CONT.)				
Ripe Pitted Large	3.5 oz	163	—	0
Tee Pee				
Spanish Green	2 oz	98	—	0
green	4 med	15	tr	0
green	3 extra lg	15	tr	0
ripe	1 jumbo	7	—	0
ripe	1 lg	5	tr	0
ripe	1 sm	4	tr	0
ripe	1 colossal	12	—	0
ONION				
CANNED				
S&W				
Whole Small	½ cup	35	—	0
Vlasic				
Lightly Spiced Cocktail Onions	1 oz	4	—	0
Watkins				
Liquid Spice	1 tbsp (0.5 oz)	120	0	0
chopped	½ cup	21	—	0
whole	1 (2.2 oz)	12	—	0
DRIED				
Watkins				
Flakes	¼ tsp (1 g)	0	0	0
flakes	1 tbsp	16	—	0
powder	1 tsp	7	—	0
FRESH				
Antioch Farms				
Vidalia	1 med	60	3	0
Dole				
Green chopped	1 tbsp	2	tr	0
chopped cooked	½ cup	47	—	0
raw chopped	½ cup	30	—	0
raw chopped	1 tbsp	4	tr	0
scallions raw chopped	1 tbsp	2	tr	0
scallions raw sliced	½ cup	16	1	0
welsh raw	3½ oz	34	—	0
FROZEN				
Birds Eye				
Polybag Whole Small	½ cup	30	2	0
Small With Cream Sauce	½ cup	100	1	10
Kineret				
Rings	6 (3 oz)	200	0	0
Ore Ida				
Chopped	¾ cup (3 oz)	25	1	0

FOOD	PORTION	CALS.	FIB.	CHOL.
Ore Ida (CONT.)				
Onion Ringers	6 pieces (3 oz)	240	2	0
Southland				
Chopped	2 oz	15	—	0
chopped cooked	½ cup	30	—	0
chopped cooked	1 tbsp	4	—	0
rings	7 (2.5 oz)	285	—	0
rings cooked	2 (0.7 oz)	81	—	0
whole cooked	3½ oz	28	—	0
TAKE-OUT				
rings breaded & fried	8 to 9	275	—	14

ORANGE
CANNED
Del Monte				
Mandarin In Heavy Syrup	½ cup (4.4 oz)	80	tr	0
Dole				
Mandarin Segments	½ cup	70	—	0
Pineapple Mandarin Segments	½ cup	80	—	0
Empress				
Mandarin	5.5 oz	100	—	0
Mandarin From Japan	5.5 oz	35	—	0
S&W				
Mandarin Natural Style	½ cup	60	—	0
Mandarin Selected Sections in Heavy Syrup	½ cup	76	—	0
Mandarin Unsweetened	½ cup	28	—	0
FRESH				
Dole	1	50	6	0
california valencia	1	59	3	0
california navel	1	65	3	0
florida	1	69	4	0
peel	1 tbsp	6	—	0
sections	1 cup	85	4	0

ORANGE EXTRACT
Virginia Dare	1 tsp	22	—	0

ORANGE JUICE
BAMA	8.45 fl oz	120	—	0
Bright & Early				
Chilled	8 fl oz	120	—	0
Frozen	8 fl oz	120	—	0
Del Monte	8 fl oz	110	tr	0
Hawaiian Punch	6 oz	100	—	0

FOOD	PORTION	CALS.	FIB.	CHOL.
Hi-C	1 can (11.5 fl oz)	180	—	0
Box	8.45 fl oz	130	—	0
Hood				
From Concentrate	1 cup (8 oz)	120	—	0
Select	1 cup (8 oz)	120	—	0
With Calcium	1 cup (8 oz)	120	—	0
Juice Works	6 oz	90	—	0
Kool-Aid	8 oz	98	—	0
Sugar Sweetened	8 oz	79	—	0
Libby	6 fl oz	80	—	0
Minute Maid				
Box	8.45 fl oz	120	—	0
Calcium Rich Chilled	8 fl oz	120	—	0
Calcium Rich frzn	8 fl oz	120	—	0
Chilled	8 fl oz	110	—	0
Country Style Chilled	8 fl oz	110	—	0
Country Style frzn	8 fl oz	110	—	0
Juices To Go	1 can (11.5 fl oz)	160	—	0
Juices To Go	1 bottle (16 fl oz)	110	—	0
Juices To Go	1 bottle (10 fl oz)	140	—	0
Orange Punch Box	8.45 fl oz	130	—	0
Premium Choice Chilled	8 fl oz	110	—	0
Pulp Free Chilled	8 fl oz	110	—	0
Pulp Free frzn	8 fl oz	110	—	0
Reduced Acid frzn	8 fl oz	110	—	0
Mott's				
From Concentrate	10 fl oz	130	0	0
Ocean Spray	8 fl oz	120	0	0
S&W				
100% Unsweetened	6 oz	83	—	0
Sippin' Pak				
100% Pure	8.45 fl oz	110	—	0
Sipps	8.45 oz	130	—	0
Snapple				
Juice	10 fl oz	130	—	0
Orangeade	8 fl oz	120	—	0
Tang				
Breakfast Crystals Sugar Free as prep	6 oz	5	—	0
Breakfast Crystals as prep	6 oz	86	—	0
Fruit Box	8.45 oz	127	—	0
Tropical Orange	8.45 fl oz	146	—	0
Tree Of Life	8 fl oz	110	0	0
Tree Top	6 oz	90	—	0

FOOD	PORTION	CALS.	FIB.	CHOL.
Tropicana	1 container (10 fl oz)	130	—	0
Frozen as prep	6 fl oz	110	—	0
Season's Best	1 bottle (7 fl oz)	90	—	0
Season's Best	1 can (11.5 fl oz)	140	—	0
Season's Best	8 fl oz	110	—	0
Season's Best	1 bottle (10 fl oz)	130	—	0
Season's Best Calcium	8 fl oz	110	—	0
Season's Best Homestyle	8 fl oz	110	—	0
Season's Best Vitamin	8 fl oz	110	—	0
Veryfine				
100%	8 oz	121	—	0
Orange Drink	8 oz	140	—	0
canned	1 cup	104	—	0
chilled	1 cup	110	—	0
fresh	1 cup	111	—	0
frzn as prep	1 cup	112	1	0
frzn not prep	6 oz	339	2	0
orange drink	6 oz	94	—	0

OREGANO

Watkins

Liquid Spice	1 tbsp (0.5 oz)	120	0	0
ground	1 tsp	5	—	0

ORGAN MEATS

(*see* BRAINS, GIBLETS, GIZZARD, HEART, KIDNEY, LIVER, SWEETBREADS)

ORIENTAL FOOD

(*see also* DINNER, NOODLES, RICE)

CANNED

Chun King

Divider Pak Beef Chow Mein	8 oz	110	—	20
Divider Pak Beef Chow Mein	7 oz	100	—	15
Divider Pak Beef Pepper Oriental	7 oz	110	—	15
Divider Pak Chicken Chow Mein	8 oz	120	—	10
Divider Pak Pork Chow Mein	7 oz	120	—	25
Divider Pak Shrimp Chow Mein	7 oz	100	—	30
Stir Fry Entree Chow Mein w/ Beef	6 oz	290	—	50
Stir Fry Entree Chow Mein w/ Chicken	6 oz	220	—	45
Stir Fry Entree Egg Foo Young	5 oz	140	—	140
Stir Fry Entree Sukiyaki	6 oz	290	—	50

FOOD	PORTION	CALS.	FIB.	CHOL.
Chun King (CONT.)				
Stir Fry Entree Pepper Steak	6 oz	250	—	50
La Choy				
Bi-Pack Beef Pepper	¾ cup	80	2	17
Bi-Pack Chow Mein Chicken	¾ cup	80	1	18
Bi-Pack Chow Mein Pork	¾ cup	80	2	14
Bi-Pack Chow Mein Shrimp	¾ cup	70	1	19
Bi-Pack Sweet & Sour Chicken	¾ cup	120	2	13
Bi-Pack Teriyaki Chicken	¾ cup	85	1	20
Dinner Chow Mein Chicken	¾ pkg	300	2	16
Entree Beef Pepper Oriental	¾ cup	100	2	36
Entree Chow Mein Beef	¾ cup	40	2	16
Entree Chow Mein Chicken	¾ cup	70	4	16
Entree Chow Mein Meatless	¾ cup	25	2	0
Entree Chow Mein Shrimp	¾ cup	35	2	50
Entree Sweet & Sour Chicken	¾ cup	240	1	19
Entree Sweet & Sour Pork	¾ cup	250	1	18
chow mein chicken	1 cup	95	—	8
FRESH				
egg roll wrapper	1	83	—	3
wonton wrappers	1	23	—	1
FROZEN				
Birds Eye				
Easy Recipe Chicken Teriyaki not prep	½ pkg	160	4	0
Easy Recipe Oriental Beef not prep	½ pkg	100	8	0
Internationals Chinese Stir Fry not prep	3.3 oz	35	2	0
Japanese Stir Fry International not prep	3.3 oz	30	2	0
Chun King				
Beef Pepper Oriental	13 oz	319	—	40
Chow Mein Chicken	13 oz	370	—	85
Crunchy Walnut Chicken	13 oz	310	—	45
Egg Rolls Chicken	1 (3.6 oz)	220	—	20
Egg Rolls Meat & Shrimp	1 (3.6 oz)	220	—	20
Egg Rolls Shrimp	1 (3.6 oz)	200	—	20
Fried Rice w/ Chicken	8 oz	260	—	75
Fried Rice w/ Pork	8 oz	270	—	55
Imperial Chicken	13 oz	300	—	30
Restaurant Style Egg Rolls Pork	1 (3 oz)	180	—	25
Sweet & Sour Pork	13 oz	400	—	25
Dining Light				
Chicken Chow Mein	9 oz	180	—	30

FOOD	PORTION	CALS.	FIB.	CHOL.
Empire				
Large Egg Rolls	1 (3 oz)	190	2	2
Miniature Egg Rolls	6 (4.8 oz)	280	4	0
La Choy				
Restaurant Style Egg Roll Almond Chicken	1 (3 oz)	120	—	5
Restaurant Style Egg Roll Pork	1 (3 oz)	150	—	7
Restaurant Style Egg Roll Shrimp	1 (3 oz)	130	—	5
Restaurant Style Egg Roll Sweet & Sour Chicken	1 (3 oz)	150	—	5
Snack Egg Roll Chicken	1 (1.45 oz)	90	—	4
Snack Egg Roll Lobster	1 (1.45 oz)	75	—	4
Snack Egg Roll Meat & Shrimp	1 (1.45 oz)	80	—	4
Snack Egg Roll Shrimp	1 (1.45 oz)	75	—	4
Lean Cuisine				
Chicken Chow Mein With Rice	1 pkg (9 oz)	210	2	35
Luigino's				
Chicken & Almonds With Rice	1 pkg (8 oz)	250	3	20
Chop Suey Pork With Rice	1 pkg (8.5 oz)	210	2	15
Egg Rolls Chicken	1 pkg (6 oz)	360	2	25
Egg Rolls Pork & Shrimp	1 pkg (6 oz)	340	3	25
Egg Rolls Shrimp	1 pkg (6 oz)	350	4	20
Egg Rolls Sweet & Sour Chicken	1 pkg (6 oz)	400	4	25
Egg Rolls Sweet & Sour Pork	1 pkg (6 oz)	360	4	15
Egg Rolls Szechwan Vegetable	1 pkg (6 oz)	350	3	10
Lo Mein Chicken	1 pkg (8 oz)	320	3	15
Lo Mein Shrimp	1 pkg (8 oz)	190	4	15
Oriental Beef & Peppers With Rice	1 pkg (8 oz)	230	2	10
Stouffer's				
Chicken Chow Mein With Rice	1 pkg (10.6 oz)	260	3	30
Chicken Oriental	1 pkg (9.75 oz)	320	2	40
Stir-Fry Teriyaki	1 pkg (9 oz)	260	4	30
Tyson				
Stir Fry Kit With Yoshida Oriental Sauce	10.6 oz	330	—	80
MIX				
La Choy				
Dinner Classics Pepper Steak	¾ cup	180	1	60
Dinner Classics Egg Foo Young	2 patties + 3 oz sauce	170	1	275
Dinner Classics Sweet & Sour	¾ cup	310	tr	50

FOOD	PORTION	CALS.	FIB.	CHOL.
TAKE-OUT				
chicken teriyaki	¾ cup	399	—	92
chop suey w/ beef & pork	1 cup	300	—	68
chop suey w/ pork	1 cup	375	2	62
chow mein chicken	1 cup	255	—	75
chow mein pork	1 cup	425	3	89
chow mein shrimp	1 cup	221	3	55
wonton fried	½ cup (1 oz)	111	1	31
wonton soup	1 cup	205	1	89
OYSTERS				
CANNED				
Bumble Bee				
Whole	½ cup (3.5 oz)	100	0	55
eastern	3 oz	58	—	46
eastern	1 cup	170	—	136
FRESH				
eastern cooked	3 oz	117	—	93
eastern cooked	6 med	58	—	46
eastern raw	6 med	58	—	46
eastern raw	1 cup	170	—	136
TAKE-OUT				
battered & fried	6 (4.9 oz)	368	—	109
breaded & fried	6 (4.9 oz)	368	—	109
eastern breaded & fried	3 oz	167	—	69
eastern breaded & fried	6 med (88 g)	173	—	72
oysters rockefeller	3 oysters	66	—	38
stew	1 cup	278	tr	100
PANCAKE/WAFFLE SYRUP				
(see also SYRUP)				
Alaga				
Breakfast	2 tbsp	108	—	0
Butter Lite	2 tbsp	54	—	0
Honey Flavored	2 tbsp	124	—	0
Lite	2 tbsp	54	—	0
Aunt Jemima				
Butter Rich	¼ cup (2.8 oz)	210	—	0
Butterlite	¼ cup (2.8 oz)	210	—	0
Butterlite	¼ cup (2.5 oz)	100	—	0
Lite	¼ cup (2.5 oz)	100	—	0
Brer Rabbit				
Dark	2 tbsp	120	—	0
Light	2 tbsp	120	—	0
Estee				
Lite Maple	¼ cup (2.4 oz)	80	—	0

FOOD	PORTION	CALS.	FIB.	CHOL.
Golden Griddle	1 cup (321 g)	885	—	0
Golden Griddle	1 tbsp (20 g)	50	—	0
Karo	1 tbsp (21 g)	60	—	0
Log Cabin				
Country Kitchen	1 oz	103	—	0
Lite	1 oz	49	—	0
Mrs. Richardson's				
Lite	¼ cup (2.5 oz)	100	—	0
Original Recipe	¼ cup (2.8 oz)	210	—	0
Red Wing	¼ cup (2 oz)	210	0	0
Lite	¼ cup (2 oz)	100	0	0
Tastee				
Maple	2 tbsp	113	—	0
Tastee	2 tbsp	121	—	0
Tree Of Life				
Maple	¼ cup (2.1 oz)	200	—	0
Weight Watchers	1 tbsp	25	—	0
Whitfield				
White Label	2 tbsp	121	—	0
Yellow Label	2 tbsp	125	—	0
Yellow Label Butter Flavor	2 tbsp	117	—	0
Yellow Label Maple Flavor	2 tbsp	117	—	0
low calorie	1 tbsp	12	0	0
maple	2 tbsp	122	—	0
maple	1 cup (11.1 oz)	824	—	0
maple	1 tbsp (0.8 oz)	52	—	0
pancake syrup	1 tbsp (0.7 oz)	57	—	0
pancake syrup	1 cup (11 oz)	903	—	0
pancake syrup light	1 oz	46	—	0
pancake syrup w/ butter	1 cup (11 oz)	933	—	14
pancake syrup w/ butter	1 tbsp (0.7 oz)	59	—	1

PANCAKES

FROZEN

Aunt Jemima				
Blueberry	3 (3.4 oz)	210	2	15
Buttermilk	3 (3 oz)	180	2	15
Lowfat	3 (3.4 oz)	130	8	0
Original	3 (3.4 oz)	200	2	15
Healthy Starts				
Pancakes w/ LeanLinks	6 oz	360	—	0
Jimmy Dean				
Flapstick	1 (2.5 oz)	240	1	20
Flapstick Blueberry	1 (2.5 oz)	260	1	15

FOOD	PORTION	CALS.	FIB.	CHOL.
Quaker				
Lite Pancakes & Lite Links	1 pkg (6 oz)	310	—	48
Lite Pancakes & Lite Syrup	1 pkg (6 oz)	260	—	32
Pancakes & Sausages	1 pkg (6 oz)	420	—	62
Weight Watchers				
Buttermilk	2 (2.5 oz)	140	—	10
buttermilk	1 (4 in diam) (1.3 oz)	83	—	3
plain	1 (4 in diam) (1.3 oz)	83	—	3
HOME RECIPE				
blueberry	1 (4 in diam)	84	—	21
plain	1 (4 in diam)	86	—	23
MIX				
Arrowhead				
Multigrain Pancake & Waffle Mix	¼ cup (1.2 oz)	120	3	0
Aunt Jemima				
Buckwheat Pancake & Waffle Mix	¼ cup (1.4 oz)	120	4	0
Buttermilk Pancake & Waffle Mix	⅓ cup (1.9 oz)	190	2	10
Original Pancake & Waffle Mix	⅓ cup (1.6 oz)	150	1	0
Pancake & Waffle Mix Regular	⅓ cup (1.9 oz)	190	1	15
Pancake & Waffle Mix Whole Wheat	¼ cup (1.4 oz)	130	3	0
Bisquick				
Apple Cinnamon Shake 'N Pour	3 (4 in diam)	240	—	0
Blueberry Shake 'N Pour	3 (4 in diam)	270	—	0
Buttermilk Shake 'N Pour	3 (4 in diam)	250	—	0
Original Shake 'N Pour	3 (4 in diam)	250	—	0
Estee				
Pancake Mix Fat Free as prep	4 (4 in diam)	180	1	0
Fast Shake				
Blueberry	1 serving (2.5 oz)	251	—	2
Buttermilk	1 serving (2.5 oz)	258	—	2
Original	1 serving (2.5 oz)	266	—	tr
Health Valley				
Pancake Mix not prep	1 oz	100	3	0
Hodgson Mill				
Buckwheat	⅓ cup (1.8 oz)	160	1	0
Stone-Buhr				
Buckwheat	¼ cup (1.4 oz)	130	3	0
Oat Bran	¼ cup (1.4 oz)	130	2	0

FOOD	PORTION	CALS.	FIB.	CHOL.
Stone-Buhr (CONT.)				
Whole Wheat	¼ cup (1.4 oz)	120	3	0
Wanda's				
Blue Corn	⅓ cup mix per serv (1.7 oz)	170	2	0
buckwheat	1 (4 in diam)	62	—	20
sugar free low sodium	1 (3 in diam)	44	—	0
whole wheat	1 (4 in diam)	92	—	27
TAKE-OUT				
buckwheat	1 (4 in diam)	55	—	20
potato	1 (4 in diam)	78	tr	60
w/ butter & syrup	3	519	—	57

PANCREAS
(see SWEETBREADS)

PAPAYA
CANNED
Ka-Me				
	¾ cup	120	1	0
FRESH				
Produce Marketing Assoc				
Papaya	½	80	—	0
cubed	1 cup	54	—	0
papaya	1	117	—	0

PAPAYA JUICE
Goya				
Nectar	6 oz	110	—	0
Kern's				
Nectar	6 fl oz	110	—	0
Libby				
Nectar	1 can (11.5 fl oz)	210	—	0
nectar	1 cup	142	—	0

PAPRIKA
Watkins				
	¼ tsp (0.5 oz)	0	0	0
paprika	1 tsp	6	—	0

PARSLEY
Dole				
Chopped	1 tbsp	10	tr	0
dry	1 tbsp	1	—	0
dry	1 tsp	1	—	0
fresh chopped	½ cup	11	—	0

PARSNIPS
| fresh cooked | 1 (5.6 oz) | 130 | — | 0 |

FOOD	PORTION	CALS.	FIB.	CHOL.
fresh sliced cooked	½ cup	63	—	0
raw sliced	½ cup	50	—	0

PASSION FRUIT
purple fresh	1	18	—	0

PASSION FRUIT JUICE
Snapple
Passion Supreme	10 fl oz	160	—	0
purple	1 cup	126	—	0
yellow	1 cup	149	—	0

PASTA
(*see also* NOODLES, PASTA DINNERS, PASTA SALAD)
DRY
Anthony
Pasta	2 oz	210	tr	0

Bella Via
Angel Hair	2 oz	200	—	0
Artichoke Angel Hair as prep	⅝ cup	200	—	0
Artichoke Spaghetti as prep	⅝ cup	200	—	0
Elbows	2 oz	200	—	0
Fettucini as prep	⅝ cup	200	—	0
Linguini	2 oz	200	—	0
Penne as prep	⅝ cup	200	—	0
Rotelli	2 oz	200	—	0
Shells	2 oz	200	—	0
Spaghetti	2 oz	200	—	0
Ziti	2 oz	200	—	0

Classico
Gnocchi Di Toscana	1 cup (2 oz)	210	2	0

Creamette
Linguini Egg	2 oz	221	—	70
Rotelle	2 oz	210	—	0
Rotini Rainbow	2 oz	210	—	0
Spaghetti Egg	2 oz	221	—	70
Spaghetti Thin	2 oz	210	—	0
Ziti	2 oz	210	—	0

DeFino
Lasagna No Boil	1 oz	102	—	0
Ribbons No Boil	2 oz	204	—	0

Delverde
Spaghetti Whole Wheat	2 oz	206	5	0

Eden
Elbows Whole Wheat Organic	2 oz	210	6	0

FOOD	PORTION	CALS.	FIB.	CHOL.
Eden (CONT.)				
Elbows Whole Wheat Vegetable Organic	2 oz	210	6	0
Kudzu And Sweet Potato Pasta	2 oz	190	0	0
Kudzu Kiri Pasta	2 oz	190	0	0
Mung Bean Pasta Harusame	2 oz	190	0	0
Ribbons Durum Wheat Curry Organic	2 oz	220	3	0
Ribbons Durum Wheat Organic	2 oz	220	3	0
Ribbons Durum Wheat Paella Organic	2 oz	220	3	0
Ribbons Durum Wheat Parsley Garlic Organic	2 oz	220	3	0
Ribbons Durum Wheat Pesto Organic	2 oz	220	3	0
Ribbons Whole Wheat Spinach Organic	2 oz	200	7	0
Rice Pasta Bifun	2 oz	200	0	0
Shells Durum Wheat Vegetable Organic	2 oz	210	2	0
Soba 100% Buckwheat	2 oz	200	3	0
Soba 40% Buckwheat	2 oz	190	3	0
Soba Lotus Root	2 oz	190	4	0
Soba Mugwort	2 oz	190	2	0
Soba Wild Yam Jinenjo	2 oz	190	2	0
Spaghetti Durum Wheat Organic	2 oz	210	2	0
Spaghetti Kamut Organic	2 oz	210	6	0
Spaghetti Pasley Garlic Organic	2 oz	210	2	0
Spaghetti Whole Wheat Organic	2 oz	210	6	0
Spirals Durum Wheat Vegetable Organic	2 oz	210	2	0
Spirals Kamut Organic	2 oz	210	6	0
Spirals Sesame Rice Organic	2 oz	200	6	0
Spirals Whole Wheat Vegetable Organic	2 oz	210	6	0
Udon	2 oz	190	3	0
Udon Brown Rice	2 oz	190	2	0
Gioia				
Pasta	2 oz	210	tr	0
Golden Grain				
Pasta	2 oz	203	0	0
Hanover				
Spaghetti Wheels	½ cup	90	—	0

FOOD	PORTION	CALS.	FIB.	CHOL.
Health Valley				
Lasagna Whole Wheat	2 oz	170	7	0
Lasagna Spinach Whole Wheat	2 oz	170	7	0
Spaghetti Amaranth	2 oz	170	9	0
Spaghetti Oat Bran	2 oz	120	4	0
Spaghetti Spinach Whole Wheat	2 oz	170	7	0
Spaghetti Whole Wheat	2 oz	170	7	0
Hodgson Mill				
Spaghetti Whole Wheat Spinach not prep	2 oz	190	5	0
Veggie Bows not prep	2 oz	200	1	0
Veggie Rotini not prep	2 oz	200	1	0
Veggie Wagon Wheels not prep	2 oz	200	1	0
Whole Wheat Spirals not prep	2 oz	190	6	0
La Molisana				
Radiatori	2 oz	230	—	0
Lupini				
Elbow uncooked	½ cup (2 oz)	190	5	0
Spaghetti Light uncooked	½ cup (2 oz)	190	5	0
Spaghetti With Triticale	½ pkg (2 oz)	190	6	0
Luxury				
Pasta	2 oz	210	tr	0
Merlino's				
Pasta	2 oz	210	tr	0
Mueller's				
Dinosaurs	2 oz (57 g)	210	—	0
Jungle Animals	2 oz (57 g)	210	—	0
Lasagne	2 oz (57 g)	210	—	0
Monsters	2 oz (57 g)	210	—	0
Outer Space	2 oz	210	—	0
Spaghetti	2 oz (57 g)	210	—	0
Teddy Bears	2 oz (57 g)	210	—	0
Twists Tri Color	2 oz (57 g)	210	—	0
Noodles By Leonardo				
Capellini not prep	½ cup (2 oz)	200	2	0
Elbows not prep	½ cup (2 oz)	200	2	0
Fettucini not prep	½ cup (2 oz)	200	2	0
Linguine not prep	½ cup (2 oz)	200	2	0
Rigatoni not prep	½ cup (2 oz)	200	2	0
Rotini not prep	½ cup (2 oz)	200	2	0
Shells not prep	½ cup (2 oz)	200	2	0
Spaghetti not prep	½ cup (2 oz)	200	2	0
Spaghettini not prep	½ cup (2 oz)	200	2	0

FOOD	PORTION	CALS.	FIB.	CHOL.
Noodles By Leonardo (CONT.)				
Vermicelli not prep	½ cup (2 oz)	200	2	0
Penn Dutch				
Pasta	2 oz	210	tr	0
Pomi				
Capellini	2 oz	210	—	0
Prince				
Egg	2 oz	221	1	70
Pasta	2 oz	210	tr	0
Rainbow	2 oz	210	1	0
Spinach Egg	2 oz	220	1	70
Pritikin				
Spaghetti Whole Wheat	⅛ box (2 oz)	190	—	0
Spiral	⅔ cup (2 oz)	190	—	0
Red Cross				
Pasta	2 oz	210	tr	0
Ronco				
Pasta	2 oz	210	tr	0
Ronzoni				
Elbows	¾ cup (2 oz)	210	—	0
Fettucini	¾ cup (2 oz)	210	—	0
Fusilli	¾ cup (2 oz)	210	—	0
Lasagne	¾ cup (2 oz)	210	—	0
Manicotti	¾ cup (2 oz)	210	—	0
Mostaccioli	¾ cup (2 oz)	210	—	0
Rigatoni	¾ cup (2 oz)	210	—	0
Rotelle uncooked	¾ cup (2 oz)	210	—	0
Rotini uncooked	¾ cup (2 oz)	210	—	0
Shells uncooked	¾ cup (2 oz)	210	—	0
Shells Jumbo	¾ cup (2 oz)	210	—	0
Spaghetti not prep	¾ cup (2 oz)	210	—	0
Tubettini	¾ cup (2 oz)	210	—	0
San Giorgio				
Bowties Egg	2 oz	210	—	70
Capellini	2 oz	210	2	0
Elbow Macaroni	2 oz	210	2	0
Fettuccine Egg	2 oz	210	—	70
Fettuccini Florentine	2 oz	210	—	70
Lasagne	2 oz	210	2	0
Linguini	2 oz	210	2	0
Manicotti	2 oz	210	2	0
Mostaccioli Rigati	2 oz	210	—	0
Rigatoni	2 oz	210	2	0
Rotini	2 oz	210	2	0

FOOD	PORTION	CALS.	FIB.	CHOL.
San Giorgio (CONT.)				
Shells	2 oz	210	2	0
Spaghetti	2 oz	210	2	0
Spaghetti Thin	2 oz	210	2	0
Vermicelli	2 oz	210	2	0
Ziti Cut	2 oz	210	2	0
Tree Of Life				
Cajun as prep	⅝ cup (4.9 oz)	200	1	0
Confetti as prep	⅝ cup (4.9 oz)	200	1	0
Garlic & Parsley as prep	⅝ cup (4.9 oz)	200	1	0
Jamaican Spice as prep	⅝ cup (4.9 oz)	200	1	0
Lemon Pepper as prep	⅝ cup (4.9 oz)	200	1	0
Spinach as prep	⅝ cup (4.9 oz)	200	1	0
Tex Mex as prep	⅝ cup (4.9 oz)	200	1	0
Thai as prep	⅝ cup (4.9 oz)	200	1	0
Tomato Basil as prep	⅝ cup (4.9 oz)	200	1	0
Vimco				
Pasta	2 oz	210	tr	0
corn cooked	1 cup	176	—	0
elbows	1 cup	389	—	0
elbows cooked	1 cup	197	—	0
protein-fortified cooked	1 cup	188	—	0
shells	1 cup	389	—	0
shells cooked	1 cup	197	—	0
spaghetti	2 oz	211	—	0
spaghetti cooked	1 cup	197	—	0
spaghetti protein-fortified cooked	1 cup	229	—	0
spinach spaghetti	2 oz	212	—	0
spinach spaghetti cooked	1 cup	183	—	0
spirals	1 cup	389	—	0
spirals cooked	1 cup	197	—	0
vegetable	1 cup	308	—	0
vegetable cooked	1 cup	171	—	0
whole wheat	1 cup	365	—	0
whole wheat cooked	1 cup (4.9 oz)	174	—	0
whole wheat spaghetti	2 oz	198	—	0
whole wheat spaghetti cooked	1 cup	174	—	0
FRESH				
Contadina				
Angel's Hair	1¼ cup (2.8 oz)	240	2	90
Fettuccine	1¼ cup (2.9 oz)	250	2	85
Fettuccine Cholesterol Free	1 cup (2.9 oz)	240	2	0
Light Ravioli Cheese	1 cup (3.1 oz)	240	2	60
Light Ravioli Garden Vegetable	1¼ cup (3.8 oz)	290	3	65

FOOD	PORTION	CALS.	FIB.	CHOL.
Contadina (CONT.)				
Light Tortellini Garlic & Cheese	1 cup (3.6 oz)	280	3	55
Linguine	1¼ cup (3 oz)	260	2	95
Linguine Cholesterol Free	1¼ cup (3.1 oz)	250	2	0
Ravioli Beef And Garlic	1¼ cup (4 oz)	350	3	110
Ravioli Cheese	1 cup (3.1 oz)	280	2	85
Ravioli Chicken And Rosemary	1¼ cup (4 oz)	330	3	85
Tagliatelli Spinach	1¼ cup (3.1 oz)	270	4	105
Tortellini Spinach Three Cheese	¾ cup (3.1 oz)	280	3	55
Tortelloni Cheese	¾ cup (3 oz)	260	3	45
Tortelloni Cheese And Basil	1 cup (4 oz)	360	3	65
Tortelloni Chicken And Prosciutto	1 cup (3.8 oz)	360	3	75
Tortelloni Chicken And Vegetable	¾ cup (2.9 oz)	260	2	45
Tortelloni Spicy Italian Sausage And Bell Pepper	1 cup (3.6 oz)	330	3	90
Di Giorno				
Angel's Hair	2 oz	160	1	0
Fettuccine	2.5 oz	190	2	0
Fettuccine Spinach	2.5 oz	190	2	0
Linguine	2.5 oz	190	2	0
Linguine Herb	2.5 oz	190	2	0
Ravioli Italian Herb Cheese	1 cup (3.8 oz)	350	2	45
Ravioli Light Cheese & Garlic	1 cup (3.7 oz)	270	1	5
Ravioli Light Tomato & Cheese	1 cup (3.7 oz)	280	2	10
Ravioli With Italian Sausage	¾ cup (3.6 oz)	340	2	50
Tortellini Cheese	¾ cup (2.8 oz)	260	1	30
Tortellini Mozzarella Garlic	1 cup (3.5 oz)	300	1	45
Tortellini Mushroom	1 cup (3.4 oz)	290	2	30
Tortellini Red Hot Pepper Cheese	1 cup (3.4 oz)	310	3	40
Tortellini With Chicken And Herbs	1 cup (3.2 oz)	260	1	35
Tortellini With Meat	¾ cup (3.1 oz)	290	1	40
Herb's				
Fettucine Bell Pepper Basil	2 oz	220	2	60
Fettucine Parsley Garlic	2 oz	220	2	60
Fettucine Spinach	2 oz	220	2	60
Ribbons Vegetable	2 oz	220	2	60
Ribbons Whole Wheat	2 oz	200	7	0
Rotini Mixed Vegetable	2 oz	210	2	0
Shells Mixed Vegetable	2 oz	210	2	0

FOOD	PORTION	CALS.	FIB.	CHOL.
Trios				
Ravioli Cracked Pepper Garlic Cheese	1 cup (4.3 oz)	340	0	50
plain made w/ egg cooked	2 oz	75	—	19
spinach made w/ egg cooked	2 oz	74	—	19
HOME RECIPE				
made w/ egg cooked	2 oz	74	—	23
made w/o egg cooked	2 oz	71	—	0
PASTA DINNERS				
(*see also* DINNER, PASTA SALAD)				
CANNED				
Chef Boyardee				
ABC's & 1,2,3's In Cheese Flavor Sauce	7.5 oz	180	—	3
ABC's & 1,2,3's w/ Mini Meatballs	7.5 oz	260	2	17
Beef Ravioli	7.5 oz	190	2	11
Beefaroni	7.5 oz	220	2	18
Cheese Ravioli In Meat Sauce	7.5 oz	200	—	10
Dinosaurs In Cheese Flavor Sauce	7.5 oz	180	—	3
Dinosaurs w/ Meatballs	7.5 oz	240	4	17
Elbows In Beef Sauce	7.5 oz	210	—	15
Lasagna	7.5 oz	230	—	18
Lasagna In Garden Vegetable Sauce	7.5 oz	170	—	3
Macaroni & Cheese	7.5 oz	180	1	20
Microwave Main Meal Beans & Pasta	10.5 oz	200	10	10
Microwave Main Meal Beef Ravioli Suprema	10.5 oz	290	5	10
Microwave Main Meal Cheese Ravioli Suprema	10.5 oz	290	5	10
Microwave Main Meal Fettuccine	10.5 oz	290	6	25
Microwave Main Meal Lasagna	10.5 oz	290	5	20
Microwave Main Meal Meat Tortellini	10.5 oz	220	6	30
Microwave Main Meal Noodles w/ Chicken	10.5 oz	170	3	20
Microwave Main Meal Peas & Pasta	10.5 oz	190	6	0
Microwave Main Meal Spaghetti Suprema	10.5 oz	200	7	20

FOOD	PORTION	CALS.	FIB.	CHOL.
Chef Boyardee (CONT.)				
Microwave Main Meal Zesty Macaroni	10.5 oz	290	5	25
Microwave Main Meal Ziti In Sauce	10.5 oz	210	7	0
Pasta Rings & Meatballs	7.5 oz	220	4	25
Rigatoni	7.5 oz	210	—	17
Rings & Franks	7.5 oz	190	3	20
Shells In Mushroom Sauce	7.5 oz	170	—	2
Shells In Meat Sauce	7.5 oz	210	—	15
Spaghetti & Meat Balls	7.5 oz	230	—	20
Tic Tac Toes In Cheese Flavor Sauce	7.5 oz	170	3	2
Tic Tac Toes w/ Mini Meatballs	7.5 oz	250	3	16
Turtles In Sauce	7.5 oz	160	2	3
Turtles w/ Meatballs	7.5 oz	210	2	20
Dinty Moore				
American Classics Lasagna With Meat & Sauce	1 bowl (10 oz)	260	3	15
Hormel				
Lasagna	1 can (7.5 oz)	250	1	25
Spaghetti & Meatballs	1 can (7.5 oz)	210	2	20
Kid's Kitchen				
Cheezy Mac & Beef	1 cup (7.5 oz)	250	0	30
Microwave Meals Beefy Macaroni	1 cup (7.5 oz)	190	2	30
Microwave Meals Macaroni & Cheese	1 cup (7.5 oz)	260	1	35
Microwave Meals Mini Ravioli	1 cup (7.5 oz)	240	3	20
Microwave Meals Spaghetti Ring & Meatballs	1 cup (7.5 oz)	250	3	20
Noodle Rings & Chicken	1 cup (7.5 oz)	150	1	20
Spaghetti Rings & Franks	1 cup (7.5 oz)	230	3	15
Micro Cup Meals				
Lasagna	1 cup (7.5 oz)	230	2	35
Lasagna & Beef Tomato Sauce	1 cup	359	3	34
Macaroni & Cheese	1 cup (7.5 oz)	260	1	35
Macaroni & Beef With Vegetables	1 cup	285	6	26
Ravioli Tomato Sauce	1 cup (7.5 oz)	260	3	20
Spaghetti & Meat Sauce	1 cup (7.5 oz)	220	4	30
Top Shelf				
Italian Lasagna	1 bowl (10 oz)	350	3	50
Spaghetti With Meat Sauce	1 bowl (10 oz)	240	3	20

FOOD	PORTION	CALS.	FIB.	CHOL.
Van Camp's				
Spaghetti Weenee	1 can (8 oz)	230	1	20
DRY MIX				
Casbah				
Pasta Fasul	1 pkg (1.6 oz)	150	2	0
Hain				
Pasta & Sauce Creamy Parmesan	¼ pkg	150	—	10
Pasta & Sauce Primavera	¼ pkg	140	—	10
Pasta & Sauce Tangy Cheddar	¼ pkg	180	—	3
Kraft				
Cheddar Cheese Egg Noodle	1 cup (8 oz)	430	1	70
Macaroni & Cheese Deluxe Original	1 cup (6.1 oz)	320	1	25
Macaroni & Cheese Dinosaurs	1 cup (6.8 oz)	390	1	10
Macaroni & Cheese Flintstones	1 cup (6.8 oz)	390	1	10
Macaroni & Cheese Milk White Cheddar	1 cup (6.8 oz)	390	1	10
Macaroni & Cheese Original	1 cup (6.9 oz)	390	1	10
Macaroni & Cheese Santa Mac	1 cup	390	1	10
Macaroni & Cheese Spirals	1 cup (6.8 oz)	390	1	10
Macaroni & Cheese Super Mario Bros	1 cup (6.8 oz)	390	1	10
Macaroni & Cheese Teddy Bears	1 cup (6.8 oz)	390	1	10
Macaroni & Cheese Thick 'N Creamy	1 cup (6.1 oz)	320	2	25
Spaghetti Mild American	1 cup (8.1 oz)	270	3	<5
Spaghetti Tangy Italain	1 cup (7.9 oz)	270	3	<5
Spaghetti With Meat Sauce	1 cup (8.2 oz)	330	3	15
Minute				
Microwave Cheddar Cheese Broccoli And Pasta as prep	½ cup	160	—	11
Nile Spice				
Pasta'n Sauce Mediterranean	1 pkg	210	2	10
Pasta'n Sauce Parmesan	1 pkg	200	1	10
Pasta'n Sauce Primavera	1 pkg	200	2	10
Uncle Ben				
Country Inn Pasta & Sauce Angel Hair Parmesan	1 serv (2.2 oz)	245	3	13
Country Inn Pasta & Sauce Broccoli & White Cheddar	1 serv (2.2 oz)	240	2	8
Country Inn Pasta & Sauce Butter & Herb	1 serv (2 oz)	230	1	10

FOOD	PORTION	CALS.	FIB.	CHOL.
Uncle Ben (CONT.)				
Country Inn Pasta & Sauce Creamy Garlic	1 serv (2.4 oz)	261	2	8
Country Inn Pasta & Sauce Fettuccine Alfredo	1 serv (2.2 oz)	310	2	12
Country Inn Pasta & Sauce Herb Linguine	1 serv (2.2 oz)	240	2	5
Country Inn Pasta & Sauce Mushroom Fettuccine	1 serv (2.2 oz)	250	2	12
Country Inn Pasta & Sauce Vegetable Alfredo	1 serv (2.2 oz)	240	2	11
Velveeta				
Rotini & Cheese Broccoli	1 cup (7.2 oz)	400	2	45
Shells & Cheese Bacon	1 cup (6.8 oz)	360	1	40
Shells & Cheese Original	1 cup (6.6 oz)	360	1	40
Shells & Cheese Salsa	1 cup (7.5 oz)	380	2	40
FROZEN				
Banquet				
Macaroni & Cheese	9 oz	240	—	10
Noodles & Chicken	10 oz	170	—	40
Spaghetti & Meat Sauce	8.75 oz	160	—	10
Birds Eye				
Easy Recipe Chicken Primavera not prep	½ pkg	80	7	0
Easy Recipe Chicken Alfredo not prep	½ pkg	160	3	0
Budget Gourmet				
Cheese Ravioli	1 pkg (9.5 oz)	290	—	30
Lasagna Italian Sausage	1 pkg (10 oz)	430	—	45
Lasagna Vegetable	1 pkg (10.5 oz)	390	—	15
Lasagna Three Cheese	1 pkg (10 oz)	390	—	70
Lasagna With Meat Sauce	1 pkg (9.4 oz)	290	—	30
Linguini With Shrimp & Clams	1 pkg (9.5 oz)	280	—	45
Linguini With Shrimp And Clams	1 pkg (10 oz)	270	—	50
Macaroni & Cheese With Cheddar & Parmesan	1 pkg (10.5 oz)	330	—	30
Macaroni And Cheese	1 pkg (5.75 oz)	230	—	35
Manicotti Cheese	1 pkg (10 oz)	440	—	75
Pasta Alfredo With Broccoli	1 pkg (5.5 oz)	210	—	30
Penne Pasta With Chunky Tomato Sauce & Italian Sausage	1 pkg (10 oz)	320	—	5
Rigatoni In Cream Sauce With Broccoli & Chicken	1 pkg (10.8 oz)	290	—	30

FOOD	PORTION	CALS.	FIB.	CHOL.
Budget Gourmet (CONT.)				
Spaghetti With Chunky Tomato & Meat Sauce	1 pkg (10 oz)	300	—	35
Tortellini Cheese	1 pkg (5.5 oz)	200	—	20
Ziti In Marinara Sauce	1 pkg (6.25 oz)	200	—	10
Dining Light				
Cheese Cannelloni	9 oz	310	—	70
Cheese Lasagna	9 oz	260	—	30
Fettucini	9 oz	290	—	35
Lasagna	9 oz	240	—	25
Spaghetti	9 oz	220	—	20
Formagg				
Penne Pasta Alfredo	⅔ cup (5 oz)	190	0	0
Penne Pasta Primavera	⅔ cup (5 oz)	190	0	0
Vegetable Pasta & Ceasar Italian Garden	⅔ cup (5 oz)	190	0	0
Green Giant				
Garden Gourmet Creamy Mushroom	1 pkg	220	3	25
Garden Gourmet Pasta Dijon	1 pkg	260	4	55
Garden Gourmet Pasta Florentine	1 pkg	230	4	25
Garden Gourmet Rotini Cheddar	1 pkg	230	5	20
One Serve Cheese Tortellini	1 pkg	260	—	25
One Serve Macaroni & Cheese	1 pkg	230	—	25
One Serve Pasta Marinara	1 pkg	180	—	0
One Serve Pasta Parmesan With Green Peas	1 pkg	170	—	10
Pasta Accents Creamy Cheddar	½ cup	100	—	5
Pasta Accents Garden Herb	½ cup	80	—	5
Pasta Accents Garlic Seasoning	½ cup	110	—	5
Pasta Accents Pasta Primavera	½ cup	110	—	5
Healthy Choice				
Beef Macaroni Casserole	1 meal (8.5 oz)	200	5	15
Cheese Ravioli Parmigiana	1 meal (9 oz)	250	6	20
Chicken Fettucini Alfredo	1 meal (8.5 oz)	250	3	30
Classics Pasta Shells Marinara	1 meal (12 oz)	360	5	25
Classics Turkey Fettuccine Alla Crema	1 meal (12.5 oz)	350	5	30
Fettucini Alfredo	1 meal (8 oz)	240	3	10
Lasagna Roma	1 meal (13.5 oz)	390	9	15
Macaroni & Cheese	1 meal (9 oz)	290	4	15
Spaghetti Bolognese	1 meal (10 oz)	260	5	15

FOOD	PORTION	CALS.	FIB.	CHOL.
Healthy Choice (CONT.)				
Three Cheese Manicotti	1 meal (11 oz)	310	7	20
Vegetable Pasta Italiano	1 meal (10 oz)	220	6	0
Zucchini Lasagna	1 meal (14 oz)	330	11	10
Kid Cuisine				
Macaroni & Cheese w/ Mini Franks	9 oz	360	—	35
Mini-Cheese Ravioli	8.75 oz	290	—	15
Spaghetti w/ Meat Sauce	9.25 oz	310	—	30
Le Menu				
Entree LightStyle Garden Vegetables Lasagna	10½ oz	260	—	25
Entree LightStyle Lasagna With Meat Sauce	10 oz	290	—	30
Entree LightStyle Meat Sauce & Cheese Tortellini	8 oz	250	—	15
Entree LightStyle Spaghetti With Beef Sauce And Mushrooms	9 oz	280	—	15
LightStyle 3-Cheese Stuffed Shells	10 oz	280	—	25
LightStyle Cheese Tortellini	10 oz	230	—	15
Lean Cuisine				
Cannelloni Cheese	1 pkg (9.1 oz)	270	3	30
Cheddar Bake With Pasta	1 pkg (9 oz)	220	3	20
Chicken Fettucini	1 pkg (9 oz)	270	2	45
Fettucini Alfredo	1 pkg (9 oz)	270	2	15
Fettucini Primavera	1 pkg (10 oz)	260	4	35
Lasagna Classic Cheese	1 pkg (11.5 oz)	290	5	30
Lasagna Tuna	1 pkg (9.75 oz)	230	3	20
Lasagna Zucchini	1 pkg (11 oz)	240	4	15
Lasagna With Meat Sauce	1 pkg (10.25 oz)	270	5	25
Macaroni & Cheese	1 pkg (9 oz)	270	2	20
Macaroni & Beef	1 pkg (10 oz)	280	3	25
Marinara Twist	1 pkg (10 oz)	240	4	5
Ravioli Cheese	1 pkg (8.5 oz)	250	4	55
Rigatoni	1 pkg (9 oz)	180	4	20
Spaghetti With Meat Sauce	1 pkg (11.5 oz)	290	4	20
Spaghetti & Meatballs	1 pkg (9.5 oz)	290	4	30
Luigino's				
& Pomodora Sauce With Meatballs	1 pkg (9 oz)	320	2	15
& Pomodoro Sauce With Meatballs	1 cup (6.3 oz)	270	2	10

FOOD	PORTION	CALS.	FIB.	CHOL.
Luigino's (CONT.)				
Cheese Tortellini & Alfredo Sauce With Broccoli	1 pkg (8 oz)	390	2	65
Cheese Ravioli & Alfredo With Broccoli Sauce	1 pkg (8.5 oz)	420	2	70
Fettuccine Alfredo	1 cup (7.5 oz)	330	3	20
Fettuccine Alfredo	1 pkg (9.4 oz)	390	4	30
Fettuccine Alfredo With Broccoli	1 pkg (9.2 oz)	360	4	25
Fettuccine Carbonara	1 pkg (9 oz)	360	3	35
Lasagna Alfredo	1 pkg (9 oz)	360	2	30
Lasagna Alfredo	1 cup (6.3 oz)	300	2	25
Lasagna Pollo	1 pkg (9 oz)	320	3	30
Lasagna With Meat Sauce	1 cup (7.2 oz)	240	2	15
Lasagna With Meat Sauce	1 pkg (9 oz)	290	2	20
Lasagna With Vegetables	1 pkg (9 oz)	290	2	20
Linguini With Red Sauce & Clams	1 pkg (9 oz)	260	3	0
Linguini With Clams & Sauce	1 pkg (9 oz)	270	2	10
Linguini With Seafood	1 pkg (9 oz)	290	4	0
Macaroni & Cheese	1 cup (7.2 oz)	310	2	15
Macaroni & Cheese	1 pkg (9 oz)	370	3	20
Marinara Sauce Penne Pasta Italian Sausage & Peppers	1 cup (7.4 oz)	290	2	30
Marinara Sauce Penne Pasta Italian Sausage & Peppers	1 pkg (9 oz)	350	2	35
Meat Ravioli & Pomodoro Sauce	1 pkg (8.5 oz)	320	3	50
Minestrone With Penne Pasta	1 cup (6.3 oz)	180	1	5
Penne Pollo	1 pkg (9 oz)	330	3	20
Penne Primavera	1 pkg (9 oz)	350	3	25
Rigatoni Pomodoro Italiano	1 pkg (9 oz)	290	4	0
Shells & Cheese With Jalapenos	1 pkg (8.5 oz)	360	2	30
Spaghetti Bolognese	1 pkg (9 oz)	270	4	20
Spaghetti Marinara	1 pkg (10 oz)	250	3	0
Spinach Ravioli & Primavera Sauce	1 pkg (8.5 oz)	360	2	45
Morton				
Spaghetti & Meat Sauce	8.5 oz	170	—	10
Mrs. Paul's				
Entrees Light Seafood Lasagne	9½ oz	290	—	57
Entrees Light Seafood Rotini	9 oz	240	—	25
Seafood Totini	9 oz	240	—	25

FOOD	PORTION	CALS.	FIB.	CHOL.
Palmazone				
Macaroni 'n Cheese	½ pkg (6 oz)	260	—	20
Senor Felix's				
Lasagna Southwestern	1 serv (6 oz)	160	2	15
Stouffer's				
Beef Ravioli	1 pkg (9.5 oz)	370	5	80
Cheese Tortellini With Alfredo Sauce	1 pkg (8.9 oz)	550	5	160
Cheese Tortellini With Tomato Sauce	1 pkg (9.25 oz)	290	4	105
Cheese Manicotti	1 pkg (9 oz)	340	7	50
Cheese Ravioli With Tomato Sauce	1 pkg (9.5 oz)	360	4	85
Cheese Shells With Tomato Sauce	1 pkg (9.25 oz)	340	5	50
Fettucini Alfredo	1 pkg (10 oz)	480	3	100
Four Cheese Lasagna	1 pkg (10.75 oz)	410	3	55
Homestyle Chicken Fettucini	1 pkg (10.5 oz)	380	3	65
Lasagna With Meat Sauce	1 cup (7 oz)	260	4	35
Lasagna With Meat Sauce	1 pkg (10.5 oz)	360	5	50
Lunch Express Fettucini Primavera	1 pkg (10.25 oz)	420	4	95
Lunch Express Lasagna With Meat Sauce	1 pkg (10 oz)	350	4	40
Lunch Express Swedish Meatballs With Pasta	1 pkg (10.25 oz)	530	3	65
Lunch Express Cheese Lasagna Casserole	1 pkg (9.5 oz)	270	5	15
Lunch Express Cheese Ravioli	1 pkg (8.5 oz)	310	2	60
Lunch Express Chicken Fettucini	1 pkg (10.25 oz)	250	4	35
Lunch Express Chicken Alfredo	1 pkg (9.6 oz)	360	3	60
Lunch Express Macaroni & Cheese & Broccoli	1 pkg (9.5 oz)	240	5	20
Lunch Express Macaroni & Cheese With Broccoli	1 pkg (10.4 oz)	360	3	30
Lunch Express Pasta & Chicken Marinara	1 pkg (9.1 oz)	270	4	20
Lunch Express Pasta & Tuna Casserole	1 pkg (9.6 oz)	280	4	20
Lunch Express Pasta & Turkey Dijon	1 pkg (9.9 oz)	270	6	30
Lunch Express Rigatoni With Meat Sauce	1 pkg (10.75 oz)	340	3	30

FOOD	PORTION	CALS.	FIB.	CHOL.
Stouffer's (CONT.)				
Lunch Express Spaghetti With Meat Sauce	1 pkg (9.6 oz)	320	5	30
Macaroni & Cheese	1 cup (6 oz)	330	2	30
Macaroni & Beef	1 pkg (11.5 oz)	340	4	50
Noodles Romanoff	1 pkg (12 oz)	460	4	60
Spaghetti With Meat Sauce	1 pkg (12.9 oz)	430	6	40
Spaghetti With Meatballs	1 pkg (12.6 oz)	420	5	45
Tuna Noodle Casserole	1 pkg (10 oz)	330	3	40
Turkey Tettrazini	1 pkg (10 oz)	360	2	40
Vegetable Lasagna	1 cup (8 oz)	280	2	25
Vegetable Lasagna	1 pkg (10.5 oz)	370	3	35
Tabatchnick				
Macaroni & Cheese	7.5 oz	280	2	26
Tyson				
Parmigiana	1 pkg (11.25 oz)	380	—	36
Ultra Slim-Fast				
Pasta Primavera	12 oz	340	5	25
Spaghetti With Beef & Mushroom Sauce	12 oz	370	0	25
Weight Watchers				
Angel Hair Pasta	10 oz	200	—	10
Baked Cheese Ravioli	9 oz	240	—	30
Cheese Tortellini	9 oz	310	—	15
Cheese Manicotti	9.25 oz	260	—	25
Chicken Fettucini	8.25 oz	280	—	40
Fettucini Alfredo	8 oz	230	—	25
Garden Lasagne	11 oz	260	—	15
Italian Cheese Lasagne	11 oz	290	—	20
Lasagne	10.25 oz	240	—	5
Spaghetti With Meat Sauce	10 oz	240	—	5
HOME RECIPE				
macaroni & cheese	1 cup	430	—	44
spaghetti w/ meatballs & tomato sauce	1 cup	330	—	89
SHELF-STABLE				
Lunch Bucket				
Lasagna With Meatsauce	1 pkg (7.5 oz)	220	—	30
Light'n Healthy Italian Style Pasta	1 pkg (7.5 oz)	130	—	10
Light'n Healthy Pasta In Wine Sauce	1 pkg (7.5 oz)	130	—	10
Light'n Healthy Pasta'n Garden Vegetables	1 pkg (7.5 oz)	150	—	0

FOOD	PORTION	CALS.	FIB.	CHOL.
Lunch Bucket (CONT.)				
Pasta'n Chicken	1 pkg (7.5 oz)	180	—	45
Spaghetti'n Meatsauce	1 pkg (7.5 oz)	240	—	30
My Own Meal				
Cheese Tortellini	1 pkg (10 oz)	340	6	15
TAKE-OUT				
lasagna	1 piece (2.5 in x 2.5 in)	374	2	107
macaroni & cheese	1 cup	230	—	24
manicotti	¾ cup (6.4 oz)	273	2	77
rigatoni w/ sausage sauce	¾ cup	260	3	59
spaghetti w/ meatballs & cheese	1 cup	407	—	104

PASTA MACHINE MIX

Wanda's

Dried Tomato	⅓ cup mix per serv (1.9 oz)	202	1	0
Durum & Semolina	⅓ cup mix per serv (1.9 oz)	199	1	0
Semolina Blend	⅓ cup mix per serv (1.9 oz)	202	1	0
Spinach	⅓ cup mix per serv (1.9 oz)	202	1	0
Whole Wheat & Semolina	⅓ cup mix per serv (1.9 oz)	198	4	0

PASTA SALAD

MIX

Kraft

Pasta Salad Classic Ranch With Bacon	¾ cup (4.7 oz)	360	2	15
Pasta Salad Creamy Ceasar	¾ cup (4.8 oz)	350	2	15
Pasta Salad Garden Primavera	¾ cup (5 oz)	280	2	<5
Pasta Salad Light Italian	¾ cup (5 oz)	190	2	<5
Pasta Salad Parmesan Peppercorn	¾ cup (4.9 oz)	360	2	20
TAKE-OUT				
elbow macaroni salad	3.5 oz	160	—	0
italian style pasta salad	3.5 oz	140	—	0
mustard macaroni salad	3.5 oz	190	—	0
pasta salad w/ vegetables	3.5 oz	140	—	0

PASTRY

(*see* BROWNIE, CAKE, DANISH PASTRY)

PATE

CANNED

Sells

Liver	2.08 oz	190	—	90

FOOD	PORTION	CALS.	FIB.	CHOL.
goose liver smoked	1 tbsp (13 g)	60	—	20
goose liver smoked	1 oz	131	—	43

PEACH
CANNED
Del Monte

Halves Cling In Heavy Syrup	½ cup (4.5 oz)	100	1	0
Halves Cling Lite	½ cup (4.4 oz)	60	1	0
Halves Cling Melba In Heavy Syrup	½ cup (4.5 oz)	100	1	0
Halves Freestone In Heavy Syrup	½ cup (4.5 oz)	100	1	0
Sliced Cling Fruit Naturals	½ cup (4.4 oz)	60	1	0
Sliced Cling In Heavy Syrup	½ cup (4.5 oz)	100	1	0
Sliced Cling Lite	½ cup (4.4 oz)	60	1	0
Sliced Freestone In Heavy Syrup	½ cup (4.5 oz)	100	1	0
Sliced Freestone Lite	½ cup (4.4 oz)	60	1	0
Snack Cups Diced Fruit Naturals	1 serv (4.5 oz)	60	1	0
Snack Cups Diced Fruit Naturals EZ-Open Lid	1 serv (4.2 oz)	60	1	0
Snack Cups Diced In Heavy Syrup	1 serv (4.5 oz)	100	1	0
Snack Cups Diced In Heavy Syrup EZ-Open Lid	1 serv (4.2 oz)	90	1	0
Snack Cups Diced Lite	1 serv (4.5 oz)	60	1	0
Snack Cups Diced Lite EZ-Open Lid	1 serv (4.2 oz)	60	1	0
Whole Cling In Heavy Syrup	½ cup (4.2 oz)	100	tr	0
Hunt's				
Halves	4 oz	90	tr	0
Slices	4 oz	90	tr	0
Libby				
Halves Yellow Cling Lite	½ cup (4.4 oz)	60	1	0
Sliced Yellow Cling Lite	½ cup (4.4 oz)	60	1	0
S&W				
Halves Clingstone	½ cup	100	—	0
Halves Clingstone Diet	½ cup	30	—	0
Halves Clingstone Unsweetened	½ cup	30	—	0
Halves Freestone Diet	½ cup	30	—	0
Halves Freestone In Heavy Syrup	½ cup	100	—	0
Sliced Clingstone Diet	½ cup	30	—	0

FOOD	PORTION	CALS.	FIB.	CHOL.
S&W (CONT.)				
Sliced Clingstone Unsweetened	½ cup	30	—	0
Sliced Freestone In Heavy Syrup	½ cup	100	—	0
Sliced Yellow Cling Natural Style	½ cup	90	—	0
Sliced Yellow Cling Premium In Heavy Syrup	½ cup	100	—	0
Slices Freestone Diet	½ cup	30	—	0
Whole Yellow Cling Spiced In Heavy Syrup	½ cup	90	—	0
Yellow Cling Natural Lite	½ cup	50	—	0
halves in heavy syrup	1 half	60	—	0
halves in light syrup	1 half	44	—	0
halves juice pack	1 half	34	—	0
halves water pack	1 half	18	—	0
spiced in heavy syrup	1 cup	180	—	0
spiced in heavy syrup	1 fruit	66	—	0
DRIED				
Del Monte				
Sun Dried	⅓ cup (1.4 oz)	90	5	0
Mariani	¼ cup	140	—	0
halves	10	311	11	0
halves	1 cup	383	13	0
halves cooked w/ sugar	½ cup	139	—	0
halves cooked w/o sugar	½ cup	99	—	0
FRESH				
Dole	2	70	1	0
peach	1	37	1	0
sliced	1 cup	73	—	0
FROZEN				
Big Valley				
Freestone	⅔ cup (4.9 oz)	50	1	0
slices sweetened	1 cup	235	—	0
PEACH JUICE				
Goya				
Nectar	6 oz	110	—	0
Kern's				
Nectar	6 fl oz	110	—	0
Libby				
Nectar	1 can (11.5 fl oz)	210	—	0
Mott's				
Fruit Basket Orchard Peach Juice Cocktail as prep	8 fl oz	130	0	0

FOOD	PORTION	CALS.	FIB.	CHOL.
Smucker's	8 oz	120	—	0
Snapple				
Dixie Peach	10 fl oz	140	—	0
nectar	1 cup	134	—	0
PEANUT BUTTER				
Arrowhead				
Creamy	2 tbsp (1.1 oz)	200	1	0
Crunchy	2 tbsp (1.1 oz)	200	1	0
BAMA				
Creamy	2 tbsp	200	—	0
Crunchy	2 tbsp	200	—	0
Jelly & Peanut Butter	2 tbsp	150	—	0
Crazy Richard's				
Natural Creamy	2 tbsp (1.1 oz)	190	—	0
Erewhon				
Chunky	2 tbsp (32 g)	190	—	0
Chunky Unsalted	2 tbsp (32 g)	190	—	0
Creamy	2 tbsp (32 g)	190	—	0
Creamy Unsalted	2 tbsp (32 g)	190	—	0
Estee				
Chunky Sodium Free	2 tbsp (1 oz)	190	2	0
Chunky Sodium Free Sorbitol Sweetened	2 tbsp (1 oz)	190	2	0
Creamy Sodium Free	2 tbsp (1 oz)	190	2	0
Creamy Sodium Free Sorbitol Sweetened	2 tbsp (1 oz)	190	2	0
Health Valley				
Chunky No Salt	2 tbsp	170	2	0
Creamy No Salt	2 tbsp	170	3	0
Hollywood				
Creamy	1 tbsp	35	1	0
Crunchy	1 tbsp	35	1	0
Unsalted	1 tbsp	35	1	0
Home Brand	2 tbsp	210	—	0
Natural Lightly Salted	2 tbsp	210	—	0
Natural Unsalted	2 tbsp	210	—	0
No-Sugar Added	2 tbsp	180	—	0
Jif				
Creamy	2 tbsp (1.1 ox)	190	2	0
Extra Crunchy	2 tbsp (1.1 oz)	190	2	0
Peter Pan				
Creamy	2 tbsp	190	2	0
Creamy Salt Free	2 tbsp	190	2	0

FOOD	PORTION	CALS.	FIB.	CHOL.
Peter Pan (CONT.)				
Crunchy	2 tbsp	190	2	0
Crunchy Salt Free	2 tbsp	190	2	0
Red Wing				
Creamy	2 tbsp (1.1 oz)	200	2	0
Crunchy	2 tbsp (1.1 oz)	200	2	0
Reese's				
Peanut Butter Chips	¼ cup (1.5 oz)	230	—	5
Simply Jif				
Creamy	2 tbsp (1.1 oz)	180	2	0
Extra Crunchy	2 tbsp (1.1 oz)	180	2	0
Skippy				
Creamy	1 cup (263 g)	1540	—	0
Creamy w/ 2 slices white bread	1 sandwich	340	—	0
Reduced Fat Creamy	2 tbsp	190	1	0
Super Chunk	2 tbsp (32 g)	190	—	0
Super Chunk	1 cup (260 g)	1540	—	0
Super Chunk w/ slices white bread	1 sandwich	340	—	0
Smucker's				
Goober Grape	2 tbsp	180	—	0
Honey Sweetened	2 tbsp	200	—	0
Natural	2 tbsp	200	—	0
Natural No-Salt Added	2 tbsp	200	—	0
Tree Of Life				
Creamy	2 tbsp (1 oz)	190	1	0
Creamy No Salt	2 tbsp (1 oz)	190	1	0
Creamy Organic	2 tbsp (1 oz)	190	1	0
Creamy Organic No Salt	2 tbsp (1 oz)	190	1	0
Crunchy	2 tbsp (1 oz)	190	1	0
Crunchy No Salt	2 tbsp (1 oz)	190	1	0
Crunchy Organic	2 tbsp (1 oz)	190	1	0
Crunchy Organic No Salt	2 tbsp (1 oz)	190	1	0
Peanut Wonder 78% Less Fat	2 tbsp (1 oz)	100	1	0
chunky	1 cup	1520	17	0
chunky	2 tbsp	188	2	0
chunky w/o salt	2 tbsp	188	2	0
chunky w/o salt	1 cup	1520	17	0
smooth	1 cup	1517	15	0
smooth	2 tbsp	188	2	0
smooth w/o salt	2 tbsp	188	2	0
smooth w/o salt	1 cup	1517	15	0

FOOD	PORTION	CALS.	FIB.	CHOL.
PEANUTS				
Beer Nuts				
Peanuts	1 pkg (1 oz)	180	—	0
Eagle				
Honey Roasted	1 oz	170	—	0
Honey Roasted Cinnamon	1 oz	170	—	0
Honey Roasted Maple	1 oz	170	—	0
Low Salt	1 oz	170	—	0
Virginia Fancy	1 oz	90	—	0
Fisher				
Party Peanuts	1 oz	160	—	0
Salted-In-Shell shelled	1 oz	170	—	0
Spanish Roasted	1 oz	180	—	0
Frito Lay				
Dry Roasted	1.2 oz	190	—	0
Salted	1 oz	170	—	0
Guy's				
Dry Roasted	1 oz	170	—	0
Spanish Salted	1 oz	170	—	0
Lance				
Honey Toasted	1 pkg (39 g)	230	—	0
Roasted w/ Shell	1 pkg (50 g)	190	—	0
Salted	1 pkg (32 g)	190	—	0
Salted Tube	1 pkg (42 g)	240	—	0
Little Debbie				
Salted	1 pkg (1.2 oz)	230	2	0
Planters				
	1 bag (0.5 oz)	80	—	0
Cocktail Lightly Salted	1 oz	170	2	0
Cocktail Unsalted	1 oz	170	—	0
Dry Roasted Lightly Salted	1 oz	160	3	0
Dry Roasted Unsalted	1 oz	170	—	0
Fresh Roast Lightly Salted	1 oz	160	2	0
Fresh Roast Salted	1 oz	170	2	0
Honey Roasted	1 oz	170	—	0
Honey Roasted Dry Roasted	1 oz	160	—	0
Spanish	1 oz	170	—	0
Spanish Raw	1 oz	160	—	0
Weight Watchers				
Honey Roasted	0.7 oz	100	—	0
chocolate coated	1 cup (5.2 oz)	773	—	13
chocolate coated	10 (1.4 oz)	208	—	4
cooked	½ cup	102	—	0
dry roasted	1 cup	855	12	0

FOOD	PORTION	CALS.	FIB.	CHOL.
dry roasted	1 oz	164	2	0
oil roasted	1 oz	163	2	0
oil roasted	1 cup	837	13	0
oil roasted w/o salt	1 oz	163	2	0
oil roasted w/o salt	1 cup	837	13	0
spanish oil roasted	1 oz	162	2	0
spanish oil roasted w/o salt	1 oz	162	2	0
unroasted	1 oz	159	—	0
valencia oil roasted	1 cup	848	9	0
valencia oil roasted	1 oz	165	2	0
valencia oil roasted w/o salt	1 oz	165	2	0
valencia oil roasted w/o salt	1 cup	848	9	0
virginia oil roasted	1 oz	161	—	0
virginia oil roasted	1 cup	826	—	0

PEAR
CANNED
Del Monte

FOOD	PORTION	CALS.	FIB.	CHOL.
Halves Fruit Naturals	½ cup (4.4 oz)	60	1	0
Halves In Heavy Syrup	½ cup (4.5 oz)	100	1	0
Halves Lite	½ cup (4.4 oz)	60	1	0
Sliced In Heavy Syrup	½ cup (4.5 oz)	100	1	0
Sliced Lite	½ cup (4.4 oz)	60	1	0
Snack Cups Diced In Heavy Syrup	1 serv (4.5 oz)	100	1	0
Snack Cups Diced In Heavy Syrup EZ-Open Lid	1 serv (4.2 oz)	90	1	0
Snack Cups Diced Lite	1 serv (4.5 oz)	60	1	0
Snack Cups Diced Lite EZ-Open Lid	1 serv (4.2 oz)	60	1	0
Hunt's				
Halves	4 oz	90	tr	0
Libby				
Halves Lite	½ cup (4.3 oz)	60	1	0
Sliced Lite	½ cup (4.3 oz)	60	1	0
S&W				
Halves Bartlett In Heavy Syrup	½ cup	100	—	0
Halves Bartlett Peeled Unsweetened	½ cup	35	—	0
Halves Peeled Diet	½ cup	35	—	0
Quartered Peeled Diet	½ cup	35	—	0
Sliced Natural Light Bartlett	½ cup	60	—	0
Sliced Natural Style	½ cup	80	—	0
halves in heavy syrup	1 cup	188	—	0

FOOD	PORTION	CALS.	FIB.	CHOL.
halves in heavy syrup	1 half	68	—	0
halves in light syrup	1 half	45	—	0
halves juice pack	1 cup	123	—	0
halves water pack	1 half	22	—	0
DRIED				
Mariani	¼ cup	150	—	0
halves	1 cup	472	—	0
halves	10	459	—	0
halves cooked w/ sugar	½ cup	196	—	0
halves cooked w/o sugar	½ cup	163	—	0
FRESH				
Dole	1	100	4	0
asian	1 (4.3 oz)	51	—	0
pear	1	98	4	0
sliced w/ skin	1 cup	97	4	0

PEAR JUICE

FOOD	PORTION	CALS.	FIB.	CHOL.
Goya				
Nectar	6 oz	120	—	0
Kern's				
Nectar	6 fl oz	120	—	0
Libby				
Nectar	1 can (11.5 fl oz)	220	3	0
nectar	1 cup	149	—	0

PEAS

FOOD	PORTION	CALS.	FIB.	CHOL.
CANNED				
Allen				
Crowder	½ cup (4.5 oz)	110	8	0
Purple Hull	½ cup (4.4 oz)	120	6	0
Crest Top				
Early June	½ cup (4.5 oz)	100	6	0
Del Monte				
Sweet	½ cup (4.4 oz)	60	4	0
Sweet 50% Less Salt	½ cup (4.4 oz)	60	4	0
Sweet No Salt Added	½ cup (4.4 oz)	60	4	0
Sweet Very Young	½ cup (4.4 oz)	60	4	0
East Texas Fair				
Cream Peas	½ cup (4.4 oz)	120	5	0
Crowder	½ cup (4.5 oz)	110	8	0
Lady Peas With Snaps	½ cup (4.3 oz)	100	4	0
Peas 'n Pork	½ cup (4.5 oz)	110	5	0
Pepper Peas	½ cup (4.5 oz)	120	6	0
Purple Hull	½ cup (4.4 oz)	120	6	0
White Acre	½ cup (4.3 oz)	100	5	0

FOOD	PORTION	CALS.	FIB.	CHOL.
Friends				
Small Pea Beans	8 oz	360	—	6
Green Giant				
Sweet	½ cup	50	4	0
Homefolks				
Crowder	½ cup (4.5 oz)	110	8	0
Purple Hull	½ cup (4.4 oz)	120	6	0
Owatonna				
Early June or Sweet	½ cup	70	—	0
S&W				
Petit Pois	½ cup	70	—	0
Sweet	½ cup	70	—	0
Sweet Water Pack	½ cup	40	—	0
Veri-Green Sweet	½ cup	70	—	0
Seneca	½ cup	50	5	0
Natural Pack	½ cup	60	4	0
Sunshine				
Field Peas	½ cup (4.4 oz)	120	6	0
Lady Peas	½ cup (4.3 oz)	100	5	0
Trappey				
Field Peas With Bacon	½ cup (4.5 oz)	90	5	0
Field Peas With Snaps And Bacon	½ cup (4.5 oz)	110	4	0
Van De Kamp's				
Baked Pea Beans	8 oz	270	11	5
green	½ cup	59	—	0
green low sodium	½ cup	59	—	0
DRIED				
split cooked	1 cup	231	—	0
FRESH				
Dole				
Sugar Peas	½ cup	30	2	0
edible-pod cooked	½ cup	34	2	0
edible-pod raw	½ cup	30	2	0
green cooked	½ cup	67	—	0
green raw	½ cup	58	—	0
FROZEN				
Birds Eye				
Green	½ cup	80	4	0
In Butter Sauce	½ cup	80	3	5
Polybag Deluxe Tender Tiny	½ cup	60	4	0
Polybag Green	½ cup	70	2	0
Sugar Snap Deluxe	½ cup	45	4	0
Tender Tiny Deluxe	½ cup	60	4	0

FOOD	PORTION	CALS.	FIB.	CHOL.
Chun King				
Chinese Pea Pods	1.5 oz	20	—	0
Green Giant				
Harvest Fresh Early June	½ cup	60	3	0
Harvest Fresh Sugar Snap	½ cup	30	2	0
Harvest Fresh Sweet	½ cup	50	3	0
In Butter Sauce	½ cup	80	4	5
One Serve In Butter Sauce	1 pkg	90	5	5
Sugar Snap Sweet Select	½ cup	30	2	0
Sweet	½ cup	50	4	0
Hanover				
Petite	½ cup	70	—	0
Snow Peas	½ cup	35	—	0
Sweet	½ cup	70	—	0
La Choy				
Snow Pea Pods	½ pkg (3 oz)	35	—	0
Le Seur				
Early Select	½ cup	60	4	0
Le Suer Early In Butter Sauce	½ cup	80	3	5
Tree Of Life	⅔ cup (3.1 oz)	70	4	0
edible-pod cooked	1 pkg (10 oz)	132	—	0
edible-pod cooked	½ cup	42	—	0
green cooked	½ cup	63	—	0
SHELF-STABLE				
Green Giant				
Mini Sweet	½ cup	60	4	0
SPROUTS				
raw	½ cup	77	—	0
PECANS				
Eagle				
Honey Roasted	1 oz	200	—	0
Planters				
Halves	1 oz	190	—	0
Pieces	1 oz	190	—	0
dried	1 oz	190	2	0
dry roasted	1 oz	187	—	0
dry roasted salted	1 oz	187	—	0
halves dried	1 cup	721	7	0
oil roasted	1 oz	195	—	0
oil roasted salted	1 oz	195	—	0
PECTIN				
Certo	1 tbsp	2	—	0
Slim Set	1 tbsp	3	tr	0

FOOD	PORTION	CALS.	FIB.	CHOL.
Slim Set	1 pkg	208	14	0
Sure-Jell	¼ pkg	38	—	0
Light	¼ pkg	33	—	0
powder	1 pkg (1.75 oz)	163	—	0
powder	¼ pkg (0.4 oz)	39	—	0
PEPPER				
Ac'cent				
Lemon	½ tsp	0	0	0
Seasoned	½ tsp	0	0	0
Lawry's				
Lemon	1 tsp	6	tr	0
Watkins				
Black	¼ tbsp (0.5 g)	0	0	0
Cajun	¼ tbsp (0.5 g)	0	0	0
Cracked Black	¼ tbsp (0.5 g)	0	0	0
Dijon	¼ tbsp (0.5 g)	0	0	0
Garlic Peppercorn Blend	¼ tbsp (1 g)	0	0	0
Herb	¼ tbsp (0.5 g)	0	0	0
Italian	¼ tbsp (0.5 g)	0	0	0
Lemon	¼ tbsp (1 g)	0	0	0
Mexican	¼ tbsp (0.5 g)	0	0	0
Red Pepper Flakes	¼ tsp (0.5 oz)	0	0	0
Royal Pepper Blend	¼ tbsp (0.5 g)	0	0	0
black	1 tsp	5	—	0
cayenne	1 tsp	6	—	0
red	1 tsp	6	—	0
white	1 tsp	7	—	0
PEPPERS				
CANNED				
Chi-Chi's				
Chilies Diced Green	2 tbsp (1.2 oz)	10	0	0
Chilies Green Whole	¾ pepper (1 oz)	10	0	0
Jalapenos Green Wheels	1 oz	10	0	0
Jalapenos Green Whole	1 oz	10	0	0
Jalapenos Red Wheels	1 oz	10	0	0
Jalapenos Red Whole	1 oz	15	0	0
Del Monte				
Chilpotie In Spice Sauce	2 tbsp (1.1 oz)	20	1	0
Hot Chili	4 (1 oz)	10	tr	0
Jalapeno Pickled Sliced	2 tbsp (1.1 oz)	5	tr	0
Jalapeno Pickled Whole	2 tbsp (1.1 oz)	5	tr	0
Jalapeno Whole	1 (0.7 oz)	3	tr	0
Jalapeno Nacho Pickled Sliced	2 tbsp (1 oz)	5	tr	0

FOOD	PORTION	CALS.	FIB.	CHOL.
Hebrew National				
Filet	¼ pepper (1 oz)	9	—	0
Hot Cherry	⅓ pepper (1 oz)	11	—	0
Red Filet	¼ pepper (1 oz)	9	—	0
McIlhenny				
Jalapeno Nacho Slices	12 slices (1.1 oz)	7	1	0
Old El Paso				
Green Chilies Chopped	2 tbsp	5	1	0
Green Chilies Whole	1	10	1	0
Jalapenos Peeled	3	10	1	0
Jalapenos Slices	2 tbsp	15	1	0
Progresso				
Hot Cherry	½ cup	190	—	0
Hot Cherry Pickled	½ cup	130	—	0
Piccalilli	½ cup	190	—	0
Roasted	½ cup	20	2	0
Sweet Fried	½ jar	37	1	0
Tuscan	½ cup	20	—	0
Rosoff's				
Sweet	¼ pepper (1 oz)	9	—	0
Schorr's				
Filet Peppers	1 oz	9	—	0
Trappey				
Banana Mild	3 peppers (1 oz)	6	1	0
Banana Sliced Rings	21 slices (1 oz)	6	1	0
Cherry Hot	2 peppers (1 oz)	7	1	0
Cherry Mild	2 peppers (1 oz)	10	1	0
Dulcito Italian Pepperoncini	4 peppers (1 oz)	8	1	0
In Vinegar Hot	15 peppers (1 oz)	9	tr	0
Jalapeno Hot Sliced	21 slices (1 oz)	4	1	tr
Jalapeno Whole	2 peppers (1 oz)	11	1	tr
Serano	7 peppers (1 oz)	7	tr	0
Tempero Golden Greek Pepperoncini	4 peppers (1 oz)	7	1	0
Torrido Santa Fe Grande	3 peppers (1 oz)	10	tr	0
Vlasic				
Hot Banana Pepper Rings	1 oz	4	—	0
Hot Cherry	1 oz	10	—	0
Jalapeno Mexican Hot	1 oz	8	—	0
Mexican Tiny Hot	1 oz	6	—	0
Mild Cherry	1 oz	8	—	0
Mild Greek Pepperoncini Salad Peppers	1 oz	4	—	0
chili green hot	1 (2.6 oz)	18	—	0

FOOD	PORTION	CALS.	FIB.	CHOL.
chili green hot chopped	½ cup	17	—	0
chili red hot	1 (2.6 oz)	18	—	0
chili red hot chopped	½ cup	17	—	0
green halves	½ cup	13	—	0
jalapeno chopped	½ cup	17	—	0
red halves	½ cup	13	—	0
DRIED				
green	1 tbsp	1	—	0
red	1 tbsp	1	—	0
FRESH				
Dole				
Bell	1 med	25	2	0
chili green hot raw	1	18	—	0
chili green hot raw chopped	½ cup	30	—	0
chili red hot raw	1 (1.6 oz)	18	—	0
chili red raw chopped	½ cup	30	—	0
green chopped cooked	½ cup	19	—	0
green cooked	1 (2.6 oz)	20	—	0
green raw	1 (2.6 oz)	20	1	0
green raw chopped	½ cup	13	1	0
red chopped cooked	½ cup	19	—	0
red cooked	1 (2.6 oz)	20	—	0
red raw	1 (2.6 oz)	20	1	0
red raw chopped	½ cup	13	1	0
yellow raw	1 (6.5 oz)	50	—	0
yellow raw	10 strips	14	—	0
FROZEN				
Old El Paso				
Jalapenos Pickled	2	5	—	0
Southland				
Green Diced	2 oz	10	—	0
Sweet Red & Green Cut	2 oz	15	—	0
green chopped not prep	1 oz	6	—	0
red chopped	1 oz	6	—	0

PERCH
FRESH				
cooked	1 fillet (1.6 oz)	54	—	53
cooked	3 oz	99	—	98
ocean perch atlantic cooked	1 fillet (1.8 oz)	60	—	27
ocean perch atlantic cooked	3 oz	103	—	46
ocean perch atlantic raw	3 oz	80	—	36
raw	3 oz	77	—	76

FOOD	PORTION	CALS.	FIB.	CHOL.
FROZEN				
Van De Kamp's				
Battered	2 pieces	310	—	30
Ocean Perch Light Fillets	1 piece	280	—	25
Ocean Perch Natural Fillets	4 oz	130	—	40
PERSIMMONS				
dried japanese	1	93	—	0
fresh	1	32	—	0
fresh japanese	1	118	—	0
PHYLLO DOUGH				
Ekizian				
phyllo dough	½ lb	865	—	123
	1 oz	85	—	0
sheet	1	57	—	0
PICKLES				
Claussen				
Bread 'N Butter Slices	1 slice	7	—	0
Dill Spears	1 spear	4	—	0
Kosher Halves	1 half	9	—	0
Kosher Slices	1 slice	1	—	0
Kosher Whole	1	9	—	0
No Garlic Dills	1	17	—	0
Del Monte				
Dill Halves	¼ pickle (1 oz)	5	tr	0
Dill Hamburger Chips	5 pieces (1 oz)	5	0	0
Dill Sweet Chips	5 pieces (1 oz)	40	tr	0
Dill Sweet Gherkin	2 pickles (1 oz)	40	tr	0
Dill Sweet Midgets	3 pickles (1 oz)	40	tr	0
Dill Sweet Whole	2 pickles (1 oz)	40	tr	0
Dill Tiny Kosher	1½ pickle (1 oz)	5	tr	0
Dill Whole Pickles	1½ pickle (1 oz)	5	tr	0
Hebrew National				
Half Sour	½ pickle (1 oz)	4	—	0
Kosher	⅓ pickle (1 oz)	4	—	0
Kosher Barrel Cured Dill	1 pkg	23	—	0
Kosher Barrel Cured Hot Dill	1 pkg	23	—	0
Kosher Chips	3 slices (1 oz)	4	—	0
Kosher Halves	⅓ pickle (1 oz)	4	—	0
Kosher Large	⅙ pickle (1 oz)	4	—	0
Kosher Spears	½ spear (1 oz)	4	—	0
Sour Garlic	⅓ pickle (1 oz)	3	—	0
McIlhenny				
Hot N' Sweet	4 (1 oz)	42	tr	0

FOOD	PORTION	CALS.	FIB.	CHOL.
Rosoff's				
Half Sour	⅓ pickle (1 oz)	4	—	0
Half Sour Spears	½ spear (1 oz)	4	—	0
Kosher	⅓ pickle (1 oz)	4	—	0
Kosher Halves	⅓ pickle (1 oz)	4	—	0
Schorr's				
Garlic	⅓ pickle (1 oz)	3	—	0
Half Sour	½ spear (1 oz)	4	—	0
Half Sour	⅓ pickle (1 oz)	4	—	0
Kosher Deli	½ pickle (1 oz)	4	—	0
Kosher Halves	⅓ pickle (1 oz)	4	—	0
Kosher Spears	½ spear (1 oz)	4	—	0
Kosher Whole	⅓ pickle (1 oz)	4	—	0
Vlasic				
Bread & Butter Chips	1 oz	30	—	0
Bread & Butter Chunks	1 oz	25	—	0
Bread & Butter Stixs	1 oz	18	—	0
Deli Bread & Butter	1 oz	25	—	0
Deli Dill Halves	1 oz	4	—	0
Half-The-Salt Hamburger Dill Chips	1 oz	2	—	0
Half-The-Salt Kosher Crunchy Dills	1 oz	4	—	0
Half-The-Salt Kosher Dill Spears	1 oz	4	—	0
Half-The-Salt Sweet Butter Chips	1 oz	30	—	0
Hot & Spicy Garden Mix	1 oz	4	—	0
Kosher Baby Dills	1 oz	4	—	0
Kosher Crunchy Dills	1 oz	4	—	0
Kosher Dill Gherkins	1 oz	4	—	0
Kosher Dill Spears	1 oz	4	—	0
Kosher Snack Chunks	1 oz	4	—	0
No Garlic Dill Spears	1 oz	4	—	0
Original Dills	1 oz	2	—	0
Polish Snack Chunk Dills	1 oz	4	—	0
Zesty Crunchy Dills	1 oz	4	—	0
Zesty Dill Snack Chunks	1 oz	4	—	0
Zesty Dill Spears	1 oz	4	—	0
dill	1 (2.3 oz)	12	—	0
dill low sodium	1 (2.3 oz)	12	1	0
dill low sodium sliced	1 slice	1	tr	0
dill sliced	1 slice	1	tr	0
gherkins	3½ oz	21	—	0

FOOD	PORTION	CALS.	FIB.	CHOL.
kosher dill	1 (2.3 oz)	12	1	0
polish dill	1 (2.3 oz)	12	1	0
quick sour	1 (1.2 oz)	4	—	0
quick sour low sodium	1 (1.2 oz)	4	—	0
quick sour sliced	1 slice	1	—	0
sweet	1 (1.2 oz)	41	tr	0
sweet gherkin	1 sm (½ oz)	20	—	0
sweet low sodium	1 (1.2 oz)	41	tr	0
sweet sliced	1 slice	7	tr	0
PIE				
(*see also* PIE CRUST)				
CANNED FILLING				
Libby				
Pumpkin Pie Mix	½ cup	100	2	0
apple	1 can (21 oz)	599	6	0
apple	⅛ can (2.6 oz)	74	1	0
cherry	⅛ can (2.6 oz)	85	—	0
cherry	1 can (21 oz)	683	—	0
pumpkin pie mix	1 cup	282	—	0
FROZEN				
Kineret				
Apple Homestyle	⅙ pie (4 oz)	313	1	0
Mrs. Smith's				
Apple	⅛ of 9 in pie (4.6 oz)	370	2	0
Apple	⅙ of 8 in pie (4.3 oz)	270	1	0
Apple	⅒ of 10 in pie (4.6 oz)	280	1	0
Apple SmartStyle	⅕ of 8 in pie (4 oz)	220	2	0
Apple Cranberry	⅙ of 8 in pie (4.3 oz)	280	1	0
Apple Lattice Ready To Serve	⅕ of 8 in pie (4.6 oz)	310	2	0
Banana Cream	¼ of 8 in pie (3.4 oz)	250	1	0
Berry	⅙ of 8 in pie (4.3 oz)	280	0	0
Blackberry	⅙ of 8 in pie (4.3 oz)	280	1	0
Blueberry	⅙ of 8 in pie	260	1	0
Blueberry Cheese Yogurt SmartStyle	¼ of 7 in pie (4.2 oz)	270	1	10

FOOD	PORTION	CALS.	FIB.	CHOL.
Mrs. Smith's (CONT.)				
Boston Cream	1/8 of 8 in pie (2.4 oz)	170	0	25
Cherry	1/8 of 9 in pie (4.6 oz)	320	1	0
Cherry	1/10 of 10 in pie (4.6 oz)	410	—	10
Cherry	1/6 of 8 in pie	270	1	0
Cherry SmartStyle	1/5 of 8 in pie (4 oz)	230	1	0
Cherry Lattice Ready To Serve	1/5 of 8 in pie (4.6 oz)	320	1	0
Chocolate Cream	1/4 of 8 in pie (3.4 oz)	290	1	0
Coconut Cream	1/4 of 8 in pie (3.4 oz)	280	0	0
Coconut Custard	1/5 of 8 in pie (5 oz)	280	0	75
Dutch Apple	1/8 of 9 in pie (4.5 oz)	300	2	0
Dutch Apple	1/6 of 8 in pie	310	1	0
Dutch Apple	1/10 of 10 in pie (4.6 oz)	320	1	0
French Silk Cream	1/6 of 8 in pie (4.8 oz)	410	1	5
Hearty Pumpkin	1/5 of 8 in pie (5.2 oz)	280	2	60
Lemon Cream	1/4 of 8 in pie (3.4 oz)	270	0	0
Lemon Meringue	1/5 of 8 in pie (4.8 oz)	300	0	65
Mince	1/6 of 8 in pie (4.3 oz)	300	2	0
Peach	1/6 of 8 in pie	260	1	0
Peach	1/8 of 9 in pie (4.6 oz)	310	1	0
Peach Cheese Yogurt SmartStyle	1/4 of 7 in pie (4.2 oz)	270	1	10
Pecan	1/8 of 10 in pie (4.5 oz)	500	1	60
Pumpkin	1/5 of 8 in pie (5.2 oz)	270	1	45
Pumpkin	1/9 of 10 in pie (5.1 oz)	250	1	50
Red Raspberry	1/6 of 8 in pie (4.3 oz)	280	0	0

FOOD	PORTION	CALS.	FIB.	CHOL.
Mrs. Smith's (CONT.)				
Strawberry Banana Yogurt SmartStyle	¼ of 7 in pie (4.2 oz)	240	1	0
Strawberry Rhubarb	⅙ of 8 in pie (4.3 oz)	280	0	0
Strawberry Rhubarb	⅕ of 8 in pie (4.8 oz)	520	1	70
Strawberry SmartStyle	⅕ of 8 in pie (4 oz)	210	2	0
Pepperidge Farm				
Hyannis Boston Cream Pie	1	230	2	70
Mississippi Mud	1	310	—	60
Sara Lee				
Apple Homestyle	1 slice (4 oz)	280	—	0
Apple Homestyle High	1 slice (4.9 oz)	400	—	0
Apple Streusel Free & Light	1 slice (2.9 oz)	170	—	0
Blueberry Homestyle	1 slice (4 oz)	300	—	0
Cherry Homestyle	1 slice (4 oz)	270	—	0
Cherry Streusel Free & Light	1 slice (3.6 oz)	160	—	0
Dutch Apple Homestyle	1 slice (4 oz)	300	—	0
Mince Homestyle	1 slice (4 oz)	300	—	0
Peach Homestyle	1 slice (3.4 oz)	280	—	0
Pecan Homestyle	1 slice (3.4 oz)	400	—	55
Pumpkin Homestyle	1 slice (4 oz)	240	—	40
Raspberry Homestyle	1 slice (4 oz)	280	—	0
Weight Watchers				
Apple	1 slice (3.5 oz)	165	—	0
Chocolate Mocha	1 (2.75 oz)	180	—	5
apple	⅛ of 9 in pie (4.4 oz)	297	2	0
blueberry	⅛ of 9 in pie (4.4 oz)	289	—	0
cherry	⅛ of 9 in pie (4.4 oz)	325	1	0
chocolate creme	⅙ of 8 in pie (4 oz)	344	—	6
coconut creme	⅙ of 7 in pie (2.2 oz)	191	1	0
lemon meringue	⅙ of 8 in pie (4.5 oz)	303	1	51
peach	⅙ of 8 in pie (4.1 oz)	261	—	0
HOME RECIPE				
apple	⅛ of 9 in pie (5.4 oz)	411	3	0

FOOD	PORTION	CALS.	FIB.	CHOL.
banana cream	⅛ of 9 in pie (5.2 oz)	398	—	75
blueberry	⅛ of 9 in pie (5.2 oz)	360	—	0
butterscotch	⅛ of 9 in pie (4.5 oz)	355	—	78
cherry	⅛ of 9 in pie (6.3 oz)	486	—	0
coconut creme	⅛ of 9 in pie (4.7 oz)	396	—	77
custard	⅛ of 9 in pie (4.5 oz)	262	2	87
lemon meringue	⅛ of 9 in pie (4.5 oz)	362	2	68
mince	⅛ of 9 in pie (5.8 oz)	477	—	0
pecan	⅛ of 9 in pie (4.3 oz)	502	4	106
pumpkin	⅛ of 9 in pie (5.4 oz)	316	4	65
vanilla cream	⅛ of 9 in pie (4.4 oz)	350	—	78
MIX				
Jell-O				
Banana Cream as prep w/ whole milk	⅙ pie 8 in	103	—	11
Chocolate Cream Pie No Bake Dessert	⅛ pie	260	—	29
Chocolate Mousse	⅛ pie	259	—	29
Coconut Cream	⅛ pie	258	—	29
Coconut Cream as prep w/ whole milk	⅙ pie 8 in	111	—	11
Lemon	⅙ pie 8 in	175	—	92
Pumpkin	⅛ pie	253	—	31
Royal				
Key Lime Pie Filling	mix for 1 serving	50	—	0
Lemon Pie Filling	mix for 1 serving	50	0	0
chocolate mousse no-bake	⅛ of 9 in pie (3.3 oz)	247	—	0
READY-TO-EAT				
coconut custard	⅙ of 8 in pie (3.6 oz)	271	—	36
custard	⅙ pie 9 in	330	—	169
pecan	⅙ of 8 in pie (4 oz)	452	4	36

FOOD	PORTION	CALS.	FIB.	CHOL.
pumpkin	⅛ of 8 in pie (3.8 oz)	229	3	22
SNACK				
Drake's				
Apple	1 (2 oz)	210	—	0
Blueberry	1 (2 oz)	210	—	0
Cherry	1 (2 oz)	220	—	0
Lemon	1 (2 oz)	210	—	0
Lance				
Pecan	1 (38 g)	350	—	40
Little Debbie				
Marshmallow Banana	1 pkg (1.4 oz)	160	0	0
Marshmallow Banana	1 pkg (2 oz)	240	0	0
Marshmallow Banana	1 pkg (2.7 oz)	320	0	0
Marshmallow Chocolate	1 pkg (1.4 oz)	160	1	0
Marshmallow Chocolate	1 pkg (2.7 oz)	320	1	0
Marshmallow Chocolate	1 pkg (2 oz)	240	1	0
Oatmeal Creme	1 pkg (1.3 oz)	170	1	0
Oatmeal Creme	1 pkg (3 oz)	360	2	0
Oatmeal Creme	1 pkg (2.5 oz)	300	1	0
Raisin Creme	1 pkg (1.2 oz)	140	1	0
Raisin Creme	1 pkg (2.5 oz)	290	0	0
Tastykake				
Apple	1 pkg (113 g)	300	2	0
Banana Creme	1 pkg (120 g)	380	2	25
Blueberry	1 pkg (113 g)	310	2	0
Cherry	1 pkg (113 g)	300	2	0
Coconut Creme	1 pkg (113 g)	380	2	65
French Apple	1 pkg (120 g)	350	2	0
Lemon	1 pkg (113 g)	320	2	40
Lemon Lime	1 pkg (113 g)	320	1	45
Peach	1 pkg (113 g)	300	—	0
Pineapple Cheese	1 pkg (120 g)	340	2	20
Pumpkin	1 pkg (4 oz)	320	2	30
Strawberry	1 pkg (113 g)	340	1	0
Tasty Klair	1 pkg (113 g)	400	2	55
apple	1 (3 oz)	266	—	13
cherry	1 (3 oz)	266	—	13
lemon	1 (3 oz)	266	—	13
PIE CRUST				
(see also PIE)				
FROZEN				
Pet-Ritz				
Deep Dish	⅙ pie (1 oz)	130	—	7

FOOD	PORTION	CALS.	FIB.	CHOL.
Pet-Ritz (CONT.)				
Graham Cracker	⅙ pie (0.83 oz)	110	—	7
Regular	⅙ pie (0.83 oz)	110	—	7
Tart Shells	1	150	—	7
puff pastry baked	1 shell (1.4 oz)	223	—	0
HOME RECIPE				
9-inch crust	1	900	—	0
baked	9 in shell (6.3 oz)	949	—	0
baked	⅛ 9 in crust (0.8 oz)	119	—	0
MIX				
Betty Crocker	1/16 pkg	120	—	0
Sticks	1/16 pkg	120	—	0
Flako	¼ cup (0.9 oz)	130	1	5
Jiffy				
as prep	⅐ crust	180	tr	5
as prep	⅛ of 9 in pie (0.7 oz)	100	—	0
as prep	9 in crust (5.6 oz)	801	—	0
READY-TO-EAT				
Generic Label				
Graham	⅛ pie (0.7 oz)	110	1	0
Honey Maid				
Graham	⅙ crust (1 oz)	140	tr	0
Nabisco				
Nilla	⅙ crust (1 oz)	140	0	<5
Oreo	⅙ crust (1 oz)	140	tr	0
Ready Crust				
Chocolate	1 (3 in diam)	110	—	0
Chocolate	⅛ pie 9 in	100	—	0
Graham	⅛ pie 9 in	100	—	0
Graham	1 (3 in diam)	110	—	0
chocolate cookie crumb baked	9 in crust (7.7 oz)	1130	—	3
chocolate cookie crumb baked	⅛ of 9 in pie (1 oz)	139	—	0
chocolate cookie crumb chilled	⅛ of 9 in pie (1 oz)	142	—	0
chocolate cookie crumb chilled	9 in crust (7.8 oz)	1127	—	3
graham cracker baked	⅛ of 9 in pie (1 oz)	148	—	0
graham cracker baked	9 in crust (8.4 oz)	1181	—	0
graham cracker chilled	9 in crust (8.6 oz)	1182	—	0
graham cracker chilled	⅛ of 9 in pie (1 oz)	150	—	0
vanilla wafer cracker crumbs baked	⅛ of 9 in pie (0.8 oz)	119	—	9
vanilla wafer cracker crumbs baked	9 in crust (6.1 oz)	937	—	69

FOOD	PORTION	CALS.	FIB.	CHOL.
vanilla wafer cracker crumbs chilled	⅛ of 9 in pie (0.8 oz)	117	—	9
vanilla wafer cracker crumbs chilled	9 in crust (6.2 oz)	934	—	69
REFRIGERATED				
Pillsbury				
All Ready	⅛ of 2 crust pie	240	—	15
PIEROGI				
FROZEN				
Empire				
Potato Cheese	3 (4.6 oz)	260	5	5
Potato Onion	3 (4.6 oz)	250	4	0
Golden				
Potato Cheese	3 (4 oz)	250	—	35
Mrs. T's				
Potato And Cheddar Cheese	1 (1.3 oz)	60	—	<2
Potato And Onion	1 (1.3 oz)	50	—	<2
Sauerkraut	1	60	—	2
TAKE-OUT				
pierogi	¾ cup (4.4 oz)	307	—	49
PIG'S EARS AND FEET				
Hormel				
Pickled Feet	2 oz	80	0	45
Pickled Hocks	2 oz	110	0	45
ears, frzn, simmered	1 ear (3.7 oz)	183	—	99
feet pickled	1 oz	58	—	26
feet pickled	1 lb	923	—	419
feet, simmered	2.5 oz	138	—	71
PIGEON				
w/ skin & bone	3.5 oz	169	—	110
PIGEON PEAS				
dried cooked	½ cup	102	—	0
dried cooked	1 cup	204	—	0
PIGNOLIA				
(*see* PINE NUTS)				
PIKE				
northern cooked	½ fillet (5.4 oz)	176	—	78
northern cooked	3 oz	96	—	43
northern raw	3 oz	75	—	33
roe raw	3½ oz	130	—	360

FOOD	PORTION	CALS.	FIB.	CHOL.
walleye baked	3 oz	101	—	94
walleye fillet baked	4.4 oz	147	—	137

PILLNUTS

pillnuts- canarytree dried	1 oz	204	—	0

PIMIENTOS

Dromedary	1 oz	10	—	0
canned	1 tbsp	3	—	0
canned	1 slice	0	—	0

PINE NUTS

pignolia dried	1 oz	146	—	0
pignolia dried	1 tbsp	51	—	0
pinyon dried	1 oz	161	—	0

PINEAPPLE
CANNED

Del Monte				
Chunks In Heavy Syrup	½ cup (4.3 oz)	90	1	0
Chunks In Its Own Juice	½ cup (4.4 oz)	70	1	0
Crushed In Heavy Syrup	½ cup (4.4 oz)	90	1	0
Crushed In Its Own Juice	½ cup (4.3 oz)	70	1	0
Sliced In Heavy Syrup	½ cup (4.1 oz)	90	1	0
Sliced In Its Own Juice	½ cup (4 oz)	60	1	0
Snack Cups Tidbits In Juice	1 serv (4.5 oz)	70	1	0
Snack Cups Tidbits In Juice EZ-Open Lid	1 serv (4.2 oz)	60	1	0
Spears In Its Own Juice	½ cup (4.3 oz)	70	1	0
Tidbits In Its Own Juice	½ cup (4.3 oz)	70	1	0
Wedges In Its Own Juice	½ cup (4.3 oz)	70	1	0
Dole				
All Cuts Juice Pack	½ cup	70	—	0
All Cuts Syrup Pack	½ cup	90	—	0
Empress				
Chunk	4 oz	70	—	0
Crushed	4 oz	70	—	0
Sliced	4 oz	70	—	0
Libby				
Crushed	1 cup with juice	140	—	0
Sliced In Unsweetened Juice	1 cup with juice	140	—	0
S&W				
Hawaiian Slice In Heavy Syrup	½ cup	90	—	0
Hawaiian Slice Juice Pack	½ cup	70	—	0
Sliced Unsweetened	½ cup	60	—	0
chunks in heavy syrup	1 cup	199	—	0

FOOD	PORTION	CALS.	FIB.	CHOL.
chunks juice pack	1 cup	150	—	0
crushed in heavy syrup	1 cup	199	—	0
slices in heavy syrup	1 slice	45	—	0
slices in light syrup	1 slice	30	—	0
slices juice pack	1 slice	35	—	0
slices water pack	1 slice	19	—	0
tidbits in heavy syrup	1 cup	199	—	0
tidbits in juice	1 cup	150	—	0
tidbits in water	1 cup	79	—	0
FRESH				
Chiquita	1 cup	90	—	0
Dole	2 slices	90	2	0
diced	1 cup	77	2	0
slice	1 slice	42	1	0
FROZEN				
chunks sweetened	½ cup	104	—	0

PINEAPPLE JUICE

Bright & Early				
Frozen	8 fl oz	120	—	0
Del Monte	6 fl oz	80	0	0
Del Monte	8 fl oz	110	0	0
Del Monte	1 serv (11.5 oz)	190	1	0
Dole				
100% frzn as prep	8 fl oz	130	0	0
Chilled	6 fl oz	90	—	0
Minute Maid				
Box	8.45 fl oz	130	—	0
Frozen	8 fl oz	130	—	0
Frozen	8 fl oz	110	—	0
S&W				
Unsweetened	6 oz	100	—	0
Tree Top	6 oz	100	—	0
Veryfine				
100%	8 oz	125	—	0
canned	1 cup	139	—	0
frzn as prep	1 cup	129	—	0
frzn not prep	6 oz	387	—	0

PINK BEANS
CANNED
Goya				
Spanish Style	7.5 oz	140	10	0
DRIED				
cooked	1 cup	252	—	0

FOOD	PORTION	CALS.	FIB.	CHOL.
PINTO BEANS				
CANNED				
Allen	½ cup (4.5 oz)	110	7	0
Brown Beauty	½ cup (4.5 oz)	110	7	0
East Texas Fair	½ cup (4.5 oz)	110	7	0
Eden				
Organic	½ cup (4.4 oz)	90	6	0
Gebhardt	4 oz	100	5	0
Goya				
Spanish Style	7.5 oz	140	10	0
Green Giant	½ cup	90	5	0
Picante	½ cup	100	6	0
Old El Paso	½ cup	100	8	0
Progresso	½ cup	110	7	0
Trappey				
Jalapinto With Bacon	½ cup (4.5 oz)	120	8	0
With Bacon	½ cup (4.5 oz)	120	7	0
pinto	1 cup	186	—	0
DRIED				
Arrowhead	¼ cup (1.5 oz)	150	8	0
Bean Cuisine	½ cup	115	5	0
Hurst	1.2 oz	120	10	0
With Spanish Seasoning	1.3 oz	120	6	0
cooked	1 cup	235	—	0
FROZEN				
cooked	3 oz	152	—	0
SPROUTS				
cooked	3½ oz	22	—	0
raw	3½ oz	62	—	0
PINYON				
(*see* PINE NUTS)				
PISTACHIOS				
Dole				
Shelled	1 oz	163	—	0
Shells On	1 oz	90	—	0
Fisher				
Red Tint	1 oz	170	—	0
Lance	1 pkg (32 g)	100	—	0
Planters				
Dry Roasted	1 oz	170	—	0
Red Salted	1 oz	170	—	0
dried	1 cup	739	14	0
dried	1 oz	164	3	0

FOOD	PORTION	CALS.	FIB.	CHOL.
dry roasted	1 oz	172	—	0
dry roasted salted	1 oz	172	—	0
dry roasted salted	1 cup	776	—	0
PITANGA				
fresh	1 cup	57	—	0
fresh	1	2	—	0
PIZZA				
DOUGH				
Boboli				
Shell + Sauce	⅛ lg shell (2.6 oz)	170	1	5
Shell + Sauce	⅛ sm shell (2.6 oz)	170	1	5
House of Pasta				
Frozen	⅛ of 14 in pie (1.9 oz)	140	1	0
Jiffy				
as prep	¼ crust	180	2	0
Sassafras				
Cornmeal Pizza Crust	1 slice (1.4 oz)	140	1	0
Italian Pizza Crust Mix	1 slice (1.4 oz)	140	1	0
Wanda's				
Crust Mix Oregano & Basil	⅒ pie (1.4 oz)	149	1	0
Crust Mix Oregano & Basil Whole Wheat	⅒ pie (1.4 oz)	141	5	0
Watkins				
Crust Mix	⅛ pkg (1.8 oz)	180	2	0
FROZEN				
Celeste				
Italian Bread Deluxe	1 (5.1 oz)	290	3	15
Italian Bread Garlic & Herb Zesty Chicken	1 (5 oz)	260	3	20
Italian Bread Pepperoni	1 (5 oz)	320	3	20
Italian Bread Zesty Four Cheese	1 (4.6 oz)	300	3	25
Large Cheese	¼ pie (4.4 oz)	320	3	25
Large Deluxe	¼ pie (5.5 oz)	350	4	20
Large Pepperoni	¼ pie (4.7 oz)	350	3	20
Large Suprema With Meat	⅕ pie (4.6 oz)	290	3	15
Large Zesty Four Cheese	¼ pie (4.4 oz)	330	3	30
Small Cheese	1 (7.5 oz)	540	4	45
Small Deluxe	1 (8.2 oz)	540	6	25
Small Hot & Zesty Four Cheese	1 (7 oz)	530	4	50
Small Original Four Cheese	1 (7 oz)	540	4	50
Small Pepperoni	1 (6.7 oz)	520	4	25

FOOD	PORTION	CALS.	FIB.	CHOL.
Celeste (CONT.)				
Small Sausage	1 (7.5 oz)	530	5	25
Small Suprema Vegetable	1 (7.5 oz)	480	5	5
Small Suprema With Meat	1 (9 oz)	580	7	30
Small Zesty Four Cheese	1 (7 oz)	530	4	50
Empire	½ pie (5 oz)	340	2	30
3 Pack	1 (3 oz)	210	7	20
Bagel	1 (2 oz)	150	0	15
English Muffin	1 (2 oz)	130	1	15
Healthy Choice				
French Bread Cheese	1 (5.6 oz)	310	6	10
French Bread Pepperoni	1 (6 oz)	360	5	25
French Bread Sausage	1 (6 oz)	330	6	20
French Bread Supreme	1 (6.35 oz)	340	5	25
Kid Cuisine				
Cheese	1 (6.85 oz)	380	—	25
Hamburger	1 (6.85 oz)	330	—	15
Kineret	1 slice (4.9 oz)	490	2	20
Bagel Pizza	2 (4 oz)	300	1	30
Lean Cuisine				
French Bread Cheese	1 pkg (6 oz)	350	4	20
French Bread Deluxe	1 pkg (6.1 oz)	350	5	30
French Bread Pepperoni	1 pkg (5.25 oz)	330	4	25
MicroMagic				
Deep Dish Combination	1 (6.5 oz)	605	—	28
Deep Dish Pepperoni	1 (6.5 oz)	615	—	42
Deep Dish Sausage	1 (6.5 oz)	590	—	18
Old El Paso				
Pizza Burrito Cheese	1	320	0	20
Pizza Burrito Pepperoni	1	260	0	20
Pizza Burrito Sausage	1	260	0	15
Small World				
Four Cheese	1 (4 oz)	240	1	13
Special Delivery				
Organic	⅓ pizza (5.3 oz)	320	1	20
Organic Soy Kaas	⅓ pizza (5.3 oz)	320	1	0
Stouffer's				
French Bread Bacon Cheddar	1 piece (5.8 oz)	440	4	30
French Bread Cheese	1 piece (5.2 oz)	350	3	15
French Bread Cheeseburger	1 piece (6 oz)	440	5	55
French Bread Deluxe	1 piece (6.2 oz)	440	5	35
French Bread Double Cheese	1 piece (5.9 oz)	420	5	30
French Bread Garden Vegetable	1 piece (5.8 oz)	340	4	15
French Bread Pepperoni	1 piece (5.6 oz)	420	3	35

FOOD	PORTION	CALS.	FIB.	CHOL.
Stouffer's (CONT.)				
French Bread Pepperoni & Mushroom	1 piece (6.1 oz)	430	3	30
French Bread Sausage	1 piece (6 oz)	420	4	35
French Bread Sausage & Pepperoni	1 piece (6.25 oz)	460	4	40
French Bread Vegetable Deluxe	1 piece (6.4 oz)	380	5	25
French Bread White Pizza	1 piece (5.1 oz)	460	5	25
Lunch Express Deluxe	1 pkg (6.6 oz)	460	4	45
Lunch Express Double Cheese	1 pkg (5.9 oz)	420	3	35
Lunch Express Pepperoni	1 pkg (5.75 oz)	440	4	40
Lunch Express Sausage	1 pkg (6.5 oz)	460	3	40
Lunch Express Sausage & Pepperoni	1 pkg (6.4 oz)	500	4	60
Tombstone				
12 in Canadian Bacon	⅕ pie (5.5 oz)	360	2	40
12 in Cheese & Hamburger	⅕ pie (4.4 oz)	320	2	30
12 in Cheese & Pepperoni	⅕ pie (4.4 oz)	340	2	35
12 in Cheese & Sausage	⅕ pie (4.4 oz)	320	2	30
12 in Cheese Sausage & Mushroom	⅕ pie (4.5 oz)	320	2	30
12 in Deluxe	⅕ pie (4.7 oz)	320	2	30
12 in Extra Cheese	⅕ pie (5.1 oz)	370	2	30
12 in Sausage & Pepperoni	⅕ pie (4.4 oz)	340	2	35
12 in Special Order Four Cheese	⅕ pie (5.2 oz)	400	2	40
12 in Special Order Four Meat	⅙ pie (4.7 oz)	350	2	40
12 in Special Order Pepperoni	⅙ pie (4.5 oz)	360	2	40
12 in Special Order Super Supreme	⅙ pie (4.8 oz)	350	2	40
12 in Special Order Three Sausage	⅙ pie (4.6 oz)	340	2	35
12 in Supreme	⅕ pie (4.6 oz)	330	2	35
12 in ThinCrust Italian Style Three Cheese	¼ pie (4.8 oz)	380	2	45
9 in Cheese & Hamburger	⅓ pie (4.1 oz)	310	2	30
9 in Cheese & Pepperoni	⅓ pie (4.1 oz)	340	2	30
9 in Cheese & Sausage	⅓ pie (4.1 oz)	310	2	30
9 in Deluxe	⅓ pie (4.5 oz)	320	2	30
9 in Extra Cheese	⅓ pie (5.6 oz)	420	3	30
9 in Pepperoni & Sausage	⅓ pie (4.4 oz)	360	2	35
9 in Special Order Four Meat	⅓ pie (5.3 oz)	400	2	45
9 in Special Order Pepperoni	⅓ pie (5.1 oz)	400	2	45

FOOD	PORTION	CALS,	FIB.	CHOL.
Tombstone (CONT.)				
9 in Special Order Super Supreme	⅓ pie (5.5 oz)	400	2	45
9 in Special Order Three Sausage	⅓ pie (5.2 oz)	390	2	40
Double Top Pepperoni With Double Cheese	⅙ pie (4.5 oz)	350	2	45
Double Top Sausage & Pepperoni With Double Cheese	⅙ pie (4.7 oz)	360	2	45
Double Top Sausage With Double Cheese	⅙ pie (4.7 oz)	350	2	40
For One ½ Less Fat Cheese	1 pie (6.5 oz)	360	3	15
For One ½ Less Fat Pepperoni	1 pie (6.7 oz)	400	4	35
For One ½ Less Fat Supreme	1 pie (7.7 oz)	400	4	35
For One ½ Less Fat Vegetable	1 pie (7.2 oz)	360	5	15
For One Cheese & Pepperoni	1 pie (7 oz)	580	3	50
For One Extra Cheese	1 pie (7 oz)	540	3	45
For One Italian Sausage	1 pie (7 oz)	560	2	55
For One Sausage & Pepperoni	1 pie (7 oz)	590	3	55
For One Supreme	1 pie (7.5 oz)	570	3	50
Light Supreme	⅕ pie (4.8 oz)	270	3	20
Light Vegetable	⅕ pie (4.6 oz)	240	3	10
ThinCrust Italian Style Four Meat Combo	¼ pie (5.1 oz)	410	2	50
ThinCrust Italian Style Pepperoni	¼ pie (5 oz)	420	2	55
ThinCrust Italian Style Sausage	¼ pie (5.1 oz)	400	2	50
ThinCrust Italian Style Supreme	¼ pie (5.3 oz)	400	2	45
ThinCrust Mexican Style Supreme Taco	¼ pie (5.1 oz)	380	2	50
Weight Watchers				
Cheese	1 (6.03 oz)	300	—	10
Deluxe Combination	1 (7.32 oz)	320	—	10
Deluxe French Bread	1 (5.94 oz)	260	—	10
Pepperoni	1 (6.08 oz)	320	—	15
Sausage	1 (6.43 oz)	340	—	10
SAUCE				
Boboli	1 pkg (1.2 oz)	20	1	0
Boboli	¼ cup (2.5 oz)	40	1	0
Eden				
Pizza Pasta Sauce	½ cup (4.4 oz)	80	3	0
Ragu				
Quick Traditional	3 tbsp (1.7 oz)	35	—	0
Tree Of Life	¼ cup (1.9 oz)	30	—	0

FOOD	PORTION	CALS.	FIB.	CHOL.
TAKE-OUT				
Cheese Deep Dish Individual	1 (5.5 oz)	460	2	20
cheese	⅛ pie 12 in	140	—	9
cheese	12 in pie	1121	—	74
cheese meat & vegetables	⅛ pie 12 in	184	—	21
cheese meat & vegetables	12 in pie	1472	—	165
pepperoni	12 in pie	1445	—	115
pepperoni	⅛ pie 12 in	181	—	14
PLANTAINS				
Top Banana				
All Natural Plantain Chips	1 oz	150	—	0
FRESH				
sliced cooked	½ cup	89	—	0
uncooked	1 (6.3 oz)	218	—	0
PLUMS				
CANNED				
S&W				
Halves Purple Fancy Unpeeled In Extra Heavy Syrup	½ cup	135	—	0
Whole Purple Fancy Unpeeled In Extra Heavy Syrup	½ cup	135	—	0
Whole Unpeeled Diet	½ cup	52	—	0
purple in heavy syrup	3	119	—	0
purple in heavy syrup	1 cup	320	—	0
purple in light syrup	3	83	—	0
purple in light syrup	1 cup	158	—	0
purple juice pack	3	55	—	0
purple juice pack	1 cup	146	—	0
purple water pack	3	39	—	0
purple water pack	1 cup	102	—	0
FRESH				
Dole	2	70	1	0
plum	1	36	—	0
sliced	1 cup	91	—	0
POI				
poi	½ cup	134	—	0
POKEBERRY SHOOTS				
Allen	½ cup (4.1 oz)	35	3	0
FRESH				
cooked	½ cup	16	—	0
raw	½ cup	18	—	0

FOOD	PORTION	CALS.	FIB.	CHOL.
POLENTA				
(see CORNMEAL)				
POLLACK				
atlantic fillet baked	5.3 oz	178	—	137
atlantic baked	3 oz	100	—	77
POMEGRANATES				
pomegranate	1	104	—	0
POMPANO				
florida cooked	3 oz	179	—	54
florida raw	3 oz	140	—	43
POPCORN				
(see also CHIPS, POPCORN CAKES, PRETZELS, SNACKS)				
Barrel O' Fun				
Baked Curl	1 oz	150	0	0
Caramel Corn	1 oz	115	1	0
Corn Pop	1 oz	190	0	0
White Cheddar Pops	1 oz	170	0	0
Cape Cod	½ oz	80	—	0
Light	½ oz	60	—	0
Cheetos				
Cheddar Cheese	0.5 oz	80	—	0
Chesters	0.5 oz	70	—	0
Cheddar Cheese	0.5 oz	80	—	0
Microwave	3 cups	110	—	0
Microwave Butter	3 cups	120	—	0
Microwave Cheese	3 cups	110	—	0
Eagle	½ oz	80	—	0
Estee				
No Sugar Added Caramel	1 cup (1 oz)	120	1	0
Greenfield				
Caramel	1 cup (1 oz)	120	—	0
Jiffy Pop				
Bag Butter	3 cups	90	2	0
Bag Lite	3 cups	70	2	0
Bag Regular	3 cups	100	2	0
Glazed Popcorn Clusters	1 oz	120	1	5
Microwave Butter	4 cup	140	3	0
Microwave Regular	4 cup	140	3	0
Pan Butter	4 cup	130	2	0
Pan Regular	4 cup	130	2	0
Lance				
Cheese	1 pkg (25 g)	130	—	5

FOOD	PORTION	CALS.	FIB.	CHOL.
in blade chop lean & fat braised	1 chop (2.4 oz)	275	—	72
in blade chop lean & fat panfried	1 chop (3.1 oz)	368	—	85
in blade chop lean only braised	1 chop (1.8 oz)	156	—	57
in blade chop lean only broiled	1 chop (2.1 oz)	177	—	59
in blade chop lean only panfried	1 chop (2.2 oz)	175	—	60
in blade chop lean only roasted	1 chop (2.5 oz)	198	—	63
loin blade lean & fat, braised	3 oz	348	—	92
loin blade lean & fat, broiled	3 oz	334	—	83
loin blade lean & fat, panfried	3 oz	352	—	81
loin blade lean & fat, roasted	3 oz	310	—	76
loin blade lean only, broiled	3 oz	255	—	85
loin blade lean only, panfried	3 oz	240	—	82
loin blade lean only, roasted	3 oz	238	—	76
loin chop lean & fat braised	1 chop (2.5 oz)	261	—	73
loin chop lean & fat roasted	1 chop (2.9 oz)	262	—	74
loin chop lean & fat, braised	1 chop (2.3 oz)	267	—	67
loin chop lean & fat, broiled	1 chop (2.7 oz)	295	—	76
loin chop lean & fat, panfried	1 chop (2.9 oz)	337	—	72
loin chop lean & fat, roasted	1 chop (2.8 oz)	274	—	68
loin chop lean only, braised	1 chop (1.8 oz)	147	—	51
loin chop lean only, broiled	1 chop (2.1 oz)	165	—	60
loin chop lean only, panfried	1 chop (2 oz)	157	—	49
loin chop lean only, roasted	1 chop (2.3 oz)	167	—	54
loin lean & fat, braised	3 oz	312	—	87
loin lean & fat, broiled	3 oz	294	—	80
loin lean only, braised	3 oz	232	—	90
loin lean only, broiled	3 oz	218	—	81
loin lean only, roasted	3 oz	204	—	77
loin w/ fat, roasted	3 oz	271	—	77
lungs braised	3 oz	84	—	329
pancreas braised	3 oz	186	—	268
rib chop lean only, braised	1 chop (1.8 oz)	147	—	51
rib chop lean only, broiled	1 chop (2.1 oz)	162	—	69
rib chop lean only, panfried	1 chop (2oz)	160	—	60
rib chop lean only, roasted	1 chop (2.2 oz)	162	—	52
rib chop lean & fat, braised	1 chop (2.2 oz)	246	—	64
rib chop lean & fat, broiled	1 chop (2.6 oz)	264	—	72
rib chop lean & fat, panfried	1 chop (2.9 oz)	343	—	74
rib chop lean & fat, roasted	1 chop (2.6 oz)	252	—	64
shoulder arm picnic cured lean & fat roasted	3 oz	238	—	49
shoulder arm picnic cured lean only roasted	3 oz	145	—	41
shoulder arm picnic lean only, braised	3 oz	211	—	97

FOOD	PORTION	CALS.	FIB.	CHOL.
Lance (CONT.)				
Plain	1 pkg (25 g)	140	—	0
White Cheddar Cheese	1 pkg (25 g)	140	—	5
Louise's				
Fat-Free Apple Cinnamon	1 oz	100	1	0
Fat-Free Buttery Toffee	1 oz	100	1	0
Fat-Free Caramel	1 oz	100	1	0
Newman's Own				
Oldstyle Picture Show	3½ cups	80	—	0
Oldstyle Picture Show Microwave Natural Butter	3 cups	150	4	0
Oldstyle Picture Show Microwave No Salt	3 cups	150	4	0
Oldstyle Picture Show Microwave Light Butter	3 cups	90	4	0
Oldstyle Picture Show Microwave Light Natural	3 cups	90	4	0
Orville Redenbacher's				
Gourmet Hot Air	3 cups	40	3	0
Gourmet Original	3 cups	80	3	0
Gourmet White	3 cups	80	3	0
Microwave Gourmet	3 cups	100	3	0
Microwave Gourmet Butter Toffee	2½ cups	210	2	tr
Microwave Gourmet Caramel	2½ cups	240	2	tr
Microwave Gourmet Cheddar Cheese	3 cups	130	3	2
Microwave Gourmet Salt Free	3 cups	100	3	0
Microwave Gourmet Salt Free Butter	3 cups	100	3	0
Microwave Gourmet Sour Cream 'n Onion	3 cups	160	3	0
Microwave Gourmet Butter	3 cups	100	3	0
Microwave Gourmet Frozen	3 cups	100	3	0
Microwave Gourmet Frozen Butter	3 cups	100	3	0
Microwave Gourmet Light	3 cups	70	3	0
Microwave Gourmet Light Butter	3 cups	70	3	0
Pop Secret				
Butter Flavor	3 cups	100	2	1
Butter Flavor Singles	6 cups	250	4	0
Light Butter Flavor	3 cups	70	2	0
Light Butter Flavor Singles	6 cups	140	4	0

FOOD	PORTION	CALS.	FIB.	CHOL.
Pop Secret (CONT.)				
Light Natural Flavor	3 cups	70	2	0
Light Natural Flavor Singles	6 cups	150	4	0
Natural Flavor	3 cups	100	2	0
Natural Flavor Salt Free	3 cups	100	2	0
Pop Chips	1½ cups (1 oz)	130	1	0
Pop Qwiz Butter Flavor	3 cups	100	2	0
Pop Qwiz Natural Flavor	3 cups	100	2	0
Smartfood				
Cheddar Cheese	0.5 oz	80	—	6
Light Butter	0.5 oz	70	—	8
Snyder's				
Butter	1 oz	140	3	0
Ultra Slim-Fast				
Lite N' Tasty	½ oz	60	2	0
Weight Watchers				
Microwave	1 oz	100	—	0
air-popped	1 cup (0.3 oz)	31	2	0
air-popped	1 oz	108	4	0
carmel coated w/ peanuts	⅔ cup (1 oz)	114	1	0
cheese	1 cup (0.4 oz)	58	1	1
cheese	1 oz	149	3	3
oil popped	1 oz	142	3	0
oil popped	1 cup (0.4 oz)	55	1	0

POPCORN CAKES

Mother's				
Butter Flavor	1 (0.3 oz)	35	0	0
Unsalted	1 (0.3 oz)	35	0	0
Quaker				
Butter	1 (0.3 oz)	35	—	0
Caramel	1 (0.5 oz)	50	—	0
Nacho	1 (0.4 oz)	40	—	0
White Cheddar	1 (0.4 oz)	40	—	0
popcorn cake	1 (0.3 oz)	38	—	0

POPOVER

home recipe as prep w/ 2% milk	1 (1.4 oz)	87		46
home recipe as prep w/ whole milk	1 (1.4 oz)	90		47

POPPY SEEDS

poppy seeds	1 tsp	15		0

PORK

(*see also* BACON, BACON SUBSTITUTES, CANADIAN BACON, HAM, LUNCHEON MEAT/COLD CUTS, SAUSAGE)

FOOD	PORTION	CALS.		

The values for cooked pork may differ slightly from va raw pork. When meat is cooked some moisture and fat changing the nutritive value slightly. As a rule of thumb, assumed that a 4 oz raw portion will equal a 3 oz cooked of meat.

FOOD	PORTION	CALS.		CHOL.
CANNED				
Hormel				
Pickled Tidbits	2 oz	100		
FRESH				
Oscar Mayer				
Sweet Morsel Smoked Boneless Pork Shoulder	3 oz	180	0	
blade chop, roasted	1 (3.1 oz)	321	—	
center loin chop, broiled	1 (3.1 oz)	275	—	
center loin chop lean & fat braised	1 chop (2.6 oz)	266	—	
center loin chop lean & fat broiled	1 chop (3.1 oz)	275	—	
center loin chop lean & fat panfried	1 chop (3.1 oz)	333	—	92
center loin chop lean & fat roasted	1 chop (3.1 oz)	268	—	80
center loin chop lean only braised	1 chop (2.1 oz)	166	—	68
center loin chop lean only broiled	1 chop (2.5 oz)	166	—	71
center loin chop lean only panfried	1 chop (2.4 oz)	178	—	71
center loin chop lean only roasted	1 chop (2.4 oz)	180	—	68
center loin lean & fat, braised	3 oz	301	—	91
center loin lean & fat, panfried	3 oz	318	—	87
center loin lean only, broiled	3 oz	196	—	83
center loin lean only, panfried	3 oz	226	—	91
center loin lean only, roasted	3 oz	204	—	78
center loin, roasted	3 oz	259	—	78
ham fresh rump half lean & fat, roasted	3 oz	233	—	81
ham fresh rump half lean only, roasted	3 oz	187	—	81
ham fresh shank half lean & fat, roasted	3 oz	258	—	78
ham fresh shank half lean only, roasted	3 oz	183	—	78
ham fresh whole lean & fat, roasted	3 oz	250	—	79
ham fresh whole lean only, roasted	3 oz	187	—	80
leg loin & shoulder lean only, roasted	3 oz	198	—	79
loin blade chop lean & fat braised	1 chop (3.1 oz)	321	—	70

FOOD	PORTION	CALS.	FIB.	CHOL.
shoulder arm picnic lean only, roasted	3 oz	194	—	81
shoulder arm picnic lean & fat, braised	3 oz	293	—	93
shoulder arm picnic lean & fat, roasted	3 oz	281	—	80
shoulder blade boston steak lean & fat braised	1 steak (5.6 oz)	594	—	178
shoulder blade boston steak lean & fat broiled	1 steak (6.5 oz)	647	—	190
shoulder blade boston steak lean & fat roasted	1 steak (6.5 oz)	594	—	179
shoulder blade boston steak lean only braised	1 steak (4.6 oz)	382	—	151
shoulder blade boston steak lean only broiled	1 steak (5.3 oz)	413	—	159
shoulder blade boston steak lean only roasted	1 steak (5.5 oz)	404	—	155
shoulder blade roll cured lean & fat	3 oz	304	—	60
shoulder boston blade lean & fat, braised	3 oz	316	—	95
shoulder boston blade lean & fat, broiled	3 oz	297	—	87
shoulder boston blade lean & fat, roasted	3 oz	273	—	82
shoulder boston blade lean only, braised	3 oz	250	—	99
shoulder boston blade lean only, broiled	3 oz	233	—	89
shoulder boston blade lean only, roasted	3 oz	218	—	83
shoulder whole lean only, roasted	3 oz	207	—	82
shoulder whole, roasted	3 oz	277	—	81
sirloin chop lean & fat, braised	1 chop (2.4 oz)	250	—	75
sirloin chop lean & fat, broiled	1 chop (2.8 oz)	278	—	81
sirloin chop lean & fat, roasted	1 chop (2.8 oz)	244	—	76
sirloin chop lean only, braised	1 chop (1.9 oz)	149	—	63
sirloin chop lean only, broiled	1 chop (2.3 oz)	165	—	67
sirloin chop lean only, roasted	1 chop (2.5 oz)	175	—	67
spareribs, braised	3 oz	338	—	103
spleen braised	3 oz	127	—	428
tail simmered	3 oz	336	—	110
tenderloin lean only, roasted	3 oz	141	—	79

FOOD	PORTION	CALS.	FIB.	CHOL.
TAKE-OUT				
Sara Lee				
Pork Roast	2 oz	70	—	40

PORK DISHES
FROZEN
Jimmy Dean

BBQ Pork Rib Sandwich	1 (5.4 oz)	440	1	55

POSOLE
(see HOMINY)

POT PIE
FROZEN
Banquet

Vegetable Pie w/ Beef	7 oz	510	—	25
Vegetable Pie w/ Chicken	7 oz	550	—	35
Vegetable Pie w/ Turkey	7 oz	510	—	40
Empire				
Chicken	1 (8.1 oz)	440	11	30
Turkey	1 (8.1 oz)	470	11	25
Morton				
Beef	7 oz	430	—	29
Vegetable Pie w/ Beef	7 oz	430	—	30
Vegetable Pie w/ Chicken	7 oz	420	—	35
Vegetable Pie w/ Turkey	7 oz	420	—	40
Stouffer's				
Beef Pie	1 pkg (10 oz)	450	3	65
Chicken Pie	1 pkg (10 oz)	520	3	70
Chicken Pie	½ pkg (8 oz)	460	3	65
Turkey	1 cup (8 oz)	500	3	55
Turkey	1 pkg (10 oz)	530	3	65
TAKE-OUT				
beef	⅓ pie 9 in (7.4 oz)	515	—	42
chicken	⅓ pie 9 in (8.1 oz)	545	—	56

POTATO
(see also CHIPS, KNISH)
CANNED
Allen

Refried Potatoes	½ cup (4.5 oz)	150	11	0
Butterfield				
Diced	⅔ cup (5.7 oz)	100	3	0
Sliced	½ cup (5.7 oz)	100	4	0
Whole	2½ pieces (5.6 oz)	90	2	0

FOOD	PORTION	CALS.	FIB.	CHOL.
Del Monte				
New Sliced	⅔ cup (5.4 oz)	60	2	0
New Whole	⅔ cup (5.5 oz)	60	2	0
Hormel				
Au Gratin & Bacon	1 can (7.5 oz)	250	2	25
Scalloped & Ham	1 can (7.5 oz)	260	1	35
Hunt's				
Whole New	4 oz	70	tr	0
Micro Cup Meals				
Scalloped Potatoes & Ham	1 cup (10.4 oz)	360	3	40
Scalloped Potatoes With Ham	1 cup (7.5 oz)	260	2	35
S&W				
New Potatoes Extra Small	½ cup	45	—	0
Seneca				
Whole	½ cup	80	2	0
Sunshine				
Whole	2½ pieces (5.6 oz)	90	2	0
potatoes	½ cup	54	—	0
FRESH				
Yukon Gold	1 (5.3 oz)	110	—	0
baked skin only	1 skin (2 oz)	115	2	0
baked w/ skin	1 (6½ oz)	220	—	0
baked w/o skin	1 (5 oz)	145	2	0
baked w/o skin	½ cup	57	1	0
boiled	½ cup	68	1	0
microwaved	1 (7 oz)	212	—	0
microwaved w/o skin	½ cup	78	—	0
raw w/o skin	1 (3.9 oz)	88	—	0
FROZEN				
Budget Gourmet				
Baked With Broccoli And Cheese	1 pkg (10.5 oz)	300	—	30
Cheddared Potatoes	1 pkg (5.5 oz)	260	—	35
Cheddared Potatoes With Broccoli	1 pkg (5 oz)	150	—	20
Three Cheese Potatoes	1 pkg (5.75 oz)	220	—	30
Empire				
Crinkle Cut French Fries	½ cup (3 oz)	90	7	0
Latkes Potato Pancakes	1 (2 oz)	80	8	0
Latkes Mini Potato Pancakes	2 (2 oz)	90	6	0
Golden				
Potato Pancakes	1 (1.33 oz)	71	—	4
Green Giant				
One Serve Au Gratin	1 pkg	200	—	20
One Serve Potatoes & Broccoli	1 pkg	130	—	5

FOOD	PORTION	CALS.	FIB.	CHOL.
Green Giant (CONT.)				
In Cheese Sauce				
Healthy Choice				
Cheddar Broccoli Potatoes	1 meal (10.5 oz)	310	8	10
Garden Potato Casserole	1 meal (9.25 oz)	200	6	10
Kineret				
Crinkle Cut	18 pieces (3 oz)	120	2	0
Kugel	1 piece (2.5 oz)	150	1	30
Latkes	1 (1.5 oz)	90	2	0
Latkes Mini	10 (3 oz)	160	2	0
Lean Cuisine				
Deluxe Cheddar	1 pkg (10.4 oz)	270	3	30
Oh Boy!				
Stuffed With Cheddar Cheese	1 (6 oz)	130	4	0
Stuffed With Real Bacon	1 (6 oz)	120	4	5
Ore Ida				
Cheddar Browns	1 patty (3 oz)	90	1	<5
Cottage Fries	14 pieces (3 oz)	130	1	0
Crispers!	17 pieces (3 oz)	220	2	0
Crispers! Nacho	10 pieces (3 oz)	170	2	0
Crispers! Texas	3 oz	170	2	0
Crispy Crowns!	12 pieces (3 oz)	100	2	0
Crispy Crunchies	12 pieces (3 oz)	160	2	0
Deep Fries Crinkle Cuts	18 pieces (3 oz)	160	2	0
Deep Fries French Fries	22 pieces (3 oz)	160	2	0
Dinner Fries Country Style	8 pieces (3 oz)	110	1	0
Fast Fries	23 pieces (3 oz)	140	2	0
Fast Fries Ranch	22 pieces (3 oz)	150	1	0
Golden Crinkles	16 pieces (3 oz)	120	2	0
Golden Fries	16 pieces (3 oz)	120	1	0
Golden Patties	1 (2.5 oz)	140	2	0
Golden Twirls	28 pieces (3 oz)	160	2	0
Hash Browns Country Style	1 cup (2.6 oz)	60	1	0
Hash Browns Shredded	1 patty (3 oz)	70	1	0
Hash Browns Southern Style	¾ cup (3 oz)	70	2	0
Hot Tots	9 pieces (3 oz)	150	2	0
Mashed Natural Butter	½ cup (2.1 oz)	80	tr	<5
Microwave Crinkle Cuts	1 pkg (3.5 oz)	180	2	0
Microwave Hash Browns	1 patty (2 oz)	110	tr	0
Microwave Tater Tots	1 pkg (3.75 oz)	190	2	0
O'Brien Potatoes	¾ cup (3 oz)	60	2	0
Pixie Crinkles	33 pieces (3 oz)	140	3	0
Shoestrings	38 pieces (3 oz)	150	2	0
Snackin' Fries	1 pkg (5 oz)	180	3	0

FOOD	PORTION	CALS.	FIB.	CHOL.
Ore Ida (CONT.)				
Snackin' Fries Extra Zesty	1 pkg (5 oz)	180	4	0
Tater ABC's	10 pieces (3 oz)	190	2	0
Tater Tots	9 pieces (3 oz)	160	2	0
Tater Tots Bacon	9 pieces (3 oz)	150	1	0
Tater Tots Onion	9 pieces (3 oz)	150	2	0
Toaster Hash Browns	2 patties (3.5 oz)	190	1	0
Topped Broccoli & Cheese	½ (6 oz)	150	4	10
Topped Salsa & Cheese	½ (5.5 oz)	160	3	10
Topped Vegetable Primavera	1 (6.13 oz)	160	—	<5
Twice Baked Butter	1 (5 oz)	200	4	0
Twice Baked Cheddar Cheese	1 (5 oz)	190	3	0
Twice Baked Ranch	1 (5 oz)	180	3	0
Twice Baked Sour Cream & Chives	1 (5 oz)	180	3	0
Waffle Fries	15 pieces (3 oz)	140	2	0
Wedges With Skin	9 pieces (3 oz)	110	2	0
Zesties!	12 pieces (3 oz)	160	1	0
Stouffer's				
Au Gratin	½ cup (2.25 oz)	130	1	15
Baked Broccoli & Cheese	1 pkg (10.1 oz)	320	4	25
Baked Cheddar Cheese & Bacon	1 pkg (9.4 oz)	380	5	40
Lunch Express Baked Broccoli & Cheese	1 pkg (10.25 oz)	250	6	25
Scalloped	½ cup (2.25 oz)	130	2	5
Weight Watchers				
Baked Broccoli & Cheese	10.5 oz	270	—	5
Baked Broccoli & Ham	11.5 oz	280	—	100
Baked Chicken Divan	11.25 oz	280	—	30
Baked Homestyle Turkey	11.75 oz	250	—	60
french fries	10 strips	111	2	0
french fries thick cut	10 strips	109	—	0
potato puffs	½ cup	138	—	0
potato puffs as prep	1	16	—	0
HOME RECIPE				
au gratin	½ cup	160	—	29
mashed	½ cup	111	—	2
scalloped	½ cup	105	—	14
MIX				
Country Store				
Mashed not prep	⅓ cup	70	—	0
Kraft				
Potatoes & Cheese Au Gratin	½ cup	130	—	40

FOOD	PORTION	CALS.	FIB.	CHOL.
Kraft (CONT.)				
Potatoes & Cheese Broccoli Au Gratin	½ cup	120	—	40
Potatoes & Cheese Scalloped	½ cup	140	—	25
Potatoes & Cheese Scalloped With Ham	½ cup	150	—	15
instant mashed flakes as prep w/ whole milk & butter	½ cup	118	—	15
instant mashed flakes not prep	½ cup	78	—	0
instant mashed granules as prep w/ whole milk & butter	½ cup	114	—	15
instant mashed granules not prep	½ cup	372	—	0
REFRIGERATED				
Simply Potatoes				
Au Gratin	¼ pkg (3 oz)	130	—	21
Hash Browns	⅕ pkg (4 oz)	100	—	0
Hash Browns Onion	⅕ pkg (4 oz)	120	—	0
Hash Browns Southwest Style	⅕ pkg (4 oz)	100	—	0
Mashed	⅕ pkg (4 oz)	90	—	0
Scalloped	¼ pkg (3 oz)	100	—	17
SHELF-STABLE				
Lunch Bucket				
Scalloped	1 pkg (7.5 oz)	160	—	35
Pantry Express				
Augratin	½ cup	120	2	5
TAKE-OUT				
au gratin w/ cheese	½ cup	178	—	18
baked topped w/ cheese sauce	1	475	—	19
baked topped w/ cheese sauce & bacon	1	451	—	30
baked topped w/ cheese sauce & broccoli	1	402	—	20
baked topped w/ cheese sauce & chili	1	481	—	31
baked topped w/ sour cream & chives	1	394	—	23
french fried in beef tallow	1 lg	358	—	20
french fried in beef tallow	1 reg	237	—	13
french fried in vegetable oil	1 reg	235	—	0
french fried in vegetable oil	1 lg	355	—	0
hash brown	½ cup	151	—	9
mashed w/ whole milk & margarine	⅓ cup	66	—	2
mustard potato salad	3.5 oz	120	—	0

FOOD	PORTION	CALS.	FIB.	CHOL.
o'brien	1 cup	157	—	7
potato pancakes	1 (1.3 oz)	101	—	35
potato salad	½ cup	179	—	86
potato salad	⅓ cup	108	—	57
potato salad w/ vegetables	3.5 oz	120	—	0
scalloped	½ cup	127	—	7

POTATO STARCH
Manischewitz	1 cup	570	—	0
potato starch	3½ oz	335	—	0

POUT
ocean baked	3 oz	86	—	57
ocean fillet baked	4.8 oz	139	—	91

PRESERVE
(see JAM/JELLY/PRESERVE)

PRETZELS
(see also CHIPS, POPCORN, SNACKS)

A & Eagle	1 oz	110	—	0
Beer	1 oz	110	—	0
Barrel O' Fun				
Mini	1 oz	110	1	0
Sticks	1 oz	110	1	0
Twists	1 oz	110	1	0
Estee				
Dutch Unsalted	2 (1.1 oz)	130	1	0
Nuggets Ranch Reduced Sodium	23 (1 oz)	130	tr	0
Nuggets Reduced Sodium	30 (1 oz)	120	1	0
Unsalted	23 (1 oz)	120	1	0
Formagg				
Pretzel Nuts	1 oz	120	tr	0
J&J				
Soft	1 (2.25 oz)	170	—	0
Soft Bites	5 bites	110	—	0
Lance				
Twist	1 pkg (42 g)	150	—	0
Manischewitz				
Bagel Pretzels Original	4 (1 oz)	110	1	0
Mister Salty				
Dutch	2 (1.1 oz)	120	1	0
Mini	22 (1 oz)	110	1	0
Sticks Fat Free	47 (1 oz)	110	1	0
Twist Fat Free	9 (1 oz)	110	1	0

FOOD	PORTION	CALS.	FIB.	CHOL.
Mr. Phipps				
Chipps Original	16 (1 oz)	120	tr	0
Chips Lower Sodium	16 (1 oz)	120	tr	0
Chips Original Fat Free	16 (1 oz)	100	tr	0
Quinlan				
Beers	1 oz	110	1	0
Hard Sourdough	1 oz	110	1	0
Logs	1 oz	110	1	0
Nuggets	1 oz	110	1	0
Rods	1 oz	110	1	0
Sticks	1 oz	110	1	0
Thins	1 oz	110	1	0
Rold Gold				
Bavarian	3 pieces (1 oz)	120	—	0
Pretzel Chips	1 oz	110	—	0
Pretzel Chips Cheese	1 oz	120	—	0
Rods	3 pieces (1 oz)	110	—	0
Sour Dough	1½ pieces (1 oz)	110	—	0
Snack Mix	½ cup (1 oz)	140	—	0
Sticks	50 pieces (1 oz)	110	—	0
Thin Twist	10 pieces (1 oz)	110	—	0
Tiny Twist	15 pieces (1 oz)	110	—	0
Snyder's				
Logs	1 oz	310	—	0
Minis	1 oz	310	—	0
Minis Unsalted	1 oz	310	—	0
Nibblers	1 oz	310	—	0
Oat Bran	1 oz	120	—	0
Old Fashioned Hard	1 oz	111	—	0
Old Fashioned Hard Unsalted	1 oz	100	—	0
Old Tyme	1 oz	310	—	0
Old Tyme Unsalted	1 oz	110	—	0
Rods	1 oz	310	—	0
Sourdough Hard Buttermilk Ranch	1 oz	130	0	0
Sourdough Hard Cheddar Cheese	1 oz	160	0	0
Sourdough Hard Honey Mustard & Onion	1 oz	130	0	0
Stix	1 oz	310	—	0
Very Thins	1 oz	310	—	0
Sunshine				
California Pretzels	1 oz	110	1	0

FOOD	PORTION	CALS.	FIB.	CHOL.
Ultra Slim-Fast				
Lite N' Tasty	1 oz	100	4	0
Wege				
Sourdough	1 oz	102	—	0
Unsalted	1 oz	102	—	0
Whole Wheat	1 oz	109	—	0
dutch twist	4 (2.1 oz)	229	2	0
pretzels	1 oz	108	1	0
rods	4 (2 oz)	229	2	0
sticks	10	10	—	tr
sticks	120 (2 oz)	229	2	0
twist	1 (½ oz)	65	—	tr
twists	10 (2.1 oz)	229	2	0
whole wheat	2 med (2 oz)	205	—	0
whole wheat	2 sm (1 oz)	103	—	0

PRICKLYPEAR

fresh	1	42	—	0

PRUNE JUICE

Del Monte	8 fl oz	170	1	0
S&W				
Unsweetened	6 oz	120	—	0
canned	1 cup	181	3	0

PRUNES

CANNED
in heavy syrup	5	90	—	0
in heavy syrup	1 cup	245	—	0

DRIED
Del Monte				
Pitted	¼ cup (1.4 oz)	120	3	0
Unpitted	⅓ cup (1.4 oz)	110	1	0
Mariani				
Pitted	¼ cup	140	—	0
Whole	¼ cup	140	—	0
Sunsweet				
Orange Essence Pitted Prunes	6 (1.4 oz)	100	3	0
cooked w/ sugar	½ cup	147	7	0
cooked w/o sugar	½ cup	113	6	0
dried	10	201	6	0
dried	1 cup	385	12	0

PUDDING

(*see also* CUSTARD, PUDDING POPS)
HOME RECIPE
bread pudding	1 recipe 6 serv (26.4 oz)	1266	—	434

FOOD	PORTION	CALS.	FIB.	CHOL.
bread pudding	½ cup (4.4 oz)	212	—	83
bread w/ raisins	½ cup	180	—	77
chocolate as prep w/ 2% milk	½ cup (5.5 oz)	206	—	9
chocolate as prep w/ whole milk	½ cup (5.5 oz)	221	—	17
corn	⅔ cup	181	—	122
rice	½ cup (5.3 oz)	217	—	17
MIX				
Knorr				
Creme Caramel Flan & Sauce as prep	½ cup + 1 tbsp sauce	190	—	20
My*T*Fine				
Butterscotch	mix for 1 serving	90	—	0
Chocolate	mix for 1 serving	100	0	0
Chocolate Almond	mix for 1 serving	100	—	0
Chocolate Fudge	mix for 1 serving	100	1	0
Lemon	mix for 1 serving	90	—	0
Vanilla	mix for 1 serving	90	0	0
Vanilla Tapioca	mix for 1 serving	80	—	0
Royal				
Banana Cream	mix for 1 serving	80	0	0
Banana Cream Instant	mix for 1 serving	90	—	0
Butterscotch	mix for 1 serving	90	0	0
Butterscotch Instant	mix for 1 serving	90	—	0
Cherry Vanilla Instant	mix for 1 serving	90	0	0
Chocolate	mix for 1 serving	90	0	0
Chocolate Chocolate Chip Instant	mix for 1 serving	110	0	0
Chocolate Instant	mix for 1 serving	110	0	0
Chocolate Peanut Butter Instant	mix for 1 serving	110	0	0
Dark 'n Sweet Chocolate	mix for 1 serving	90	1	0
Dark'N-Sweet Instant	mix for 1 serving	110	0	0
Lemon Instant	mix for 1 serving	90	—	0
Pistachio Instant	mix for 1 serving	90	0	0
Strawberry Instant	mix for 1 serving	100	—	0
Vanilla	mix for 1 serving	80	0	0
Vanilla Chocolate Chip Instant	mix for 1 serving	90	0	0
Vanilla Instant	mix for 1 serving	90	—	0
lemon	½ cup (5.1 oz)	163	—	77
MIX WITH 2% MILK				
Jell-O				
Banana Instant Sugar Free	½ cup	84	—	9
Chocolate Instant Sugar Free	½ cup	92	—	9
Chocolate Sugar Free	½ cup	91	—	9
Pistachio Instant Sugar Free	½ cup	94	—	9

FOOD	PORTION	CALS.	FIB.	CHOL.
Jell-O (CONT.)				
Vanilla Instant Sugar Free	½ cup	82	—	9
banana	½ cup (4.9 oz)	142	—	9
banana instant	½ cup (5.2 oz)	152	—	9
chocolate	½ cup (5 oz)	150	—	9
chocolate instant	½ cup (5.2 oz)	149	—	9
coconut cream	½ cup (4.9 oz)	148	—	9
coconut cream instant	½ cup (5.2 oz)	157	—	0
lemon instant	½ cup (5.2 oz)	155	—	9
rice	½ cup (5.1 oz)	161	—	9
tapioca	½ cup (5 oz)	147	—	9
vanilla	½ cup (4.9 oz)	141	—	9
vanilla instant	½ cup (5 oz)	147	—	9
MIX WITH SKIM MILK				
D-Zerta				
Butterscotch	½ cup	68	—	2
Chocolate	½ cup	65	—	2
Vanilla	½ cup	69	—	2
Emes				
Dietetic	½ cup (4 fl oz)	71	—	0
MIX WITH WHOLE MILK				
Jell-O				
Banana Cream Instant	½ cup	165	—	17
Butter Pecan Instant	½ cup	170	—	17
Butterscotch	½ cup	169	—	17
Butterscotch Instant	½ cup	164	—	17
Chocolate Instant	½ cup	176	—	17
Chocolate Tapioca Americana	½ cup	169	—	17
Chocolate Fudge Instant	½ cup	175	—	17
Coconut Cream Instant	½ cup	178	—	17
French Vanilla	½ cup	169	—	17
French Vanilla Instant	½ cup	165	—	17
Golden Egg Custard Americana	½ cup	167	—	85
Lemon Instant	½ cup	168	—	17
Milk Chocolate Instant	½ cup	179	—	17
Pineapple Cream Instant	½ cup	165	—	17
Pistachio Instant	½ cup	170	—	17
Rice Americana	½ cup	175	—	17
Vanilla	½ cup	156	—	17
Vanilla Instant	½ cup	168	—	17
Vanilla Tapioca Americana	½ cup	160	—	17
banana	½ cup (4.9 oz)	157	—	17
banana instant	½ cup (5.2 oz)	167	—	17
chocolate	½ cup (5 oz)	158	—	17

FOOD	PORTION	CALS.	FIB.	CHOL.
chocolate instant	½ cup (5.2 oz)	164	—	17
coconut cream	½ cup (4.9 oz)	160	—	17
coconut cream instant	½ cup (5.2 oz)	172	—	17
lemon instant	½ cup (5.2 oz)	169	—	17
rice	½ cup (5.1 oz)	175	—	17
tapioca	½ cup (5 oz)	161	—	17
vanilla	½ cup (4.9 oz)	155	—	17
vanilla instant	½ cup (5 oz)	181	—	16
READY-TO-USE				
Del Monte				
Sanck Cups Banana	1 serv (4 oz)	140	0	0
Snack Cups Butterscotch	1 serv (4 oz)	140	0	0
Snack Cups Chocolate	1 serv (4 oz)	160	0	0
Snack Cups Chocolate Peanut Butter	1 serv (4 oz)	160	0	0
Snack Cups Chocolate Fudge	1 serv (4 oz)	150	0	0
Snack Cups Lite Chocolate	1 serv (4 oz)	100	0	0
Snack Cups Lite Vanilla	1 serv (4 oz)	90	0	0
Snack Cups Tapioca	1 serv (4 oz)	140	0	0
Snack Cups Vanilla	1 serv (4 oz)	150	0	0
Imagine Foods				
Lemon Dream	1 (4 oz)	120	—	0
Jell-O				
Chocolate	1 (4 oz)	171	—	1
Chocolate Caramel Swirl	1 (4 oz)	175	—	2
Chocolate Vanilla Swirl	1 (4 oz)	175	—	2
Chocolate Vanilla Swirl	1 (5.5 oz)	240	—	2
Chocolate Fudge	1 (4 oz)	171	—	1
Chocolate Fudge Milk Chocolate Swirl	1 (4 oz)	171	—	2
Light Chocolate	1 (4 oz)	104	—	5
Light Chocolate Vanilla	1 (4 oz)	104	—	5
Light Chocolate Fudge	1 (4 oz)	101	—	3
Light Vanilla	1 (4 oz)	104	—	6
Milk Chocolate	1 (4 oz)	173	—	2
Tapicoa	1 (5.5 oz)	229	—	2
Tapioca	1 (4 oz)	167	—	2
Vanilla	1 (4 oz)	182	—	2
Vanilla	1 (5.5 oz)	250	—	2
Vanilla Chocolate Swirl	1 (4 oz)	178	—	2
Snack Pack				
Banana	4.25 oz	145	0	1
Butterscotch	4.25 oz	170	0	1
Chocolate	4.25 oz	170	0	1

FOOD	PORTION	CALS.	FIB.	CHOL.
Snack Pack (CONT.)				
Chocolate Marshmallow	4.25 oz	165	0	1
Chocolate Fudge	4.25 oz	165	0	1
Lemon	4.25 oz	150	tr	0
Light Chocolate	4.25 oz	100	0	1
Light Tapioca	4.25 oz	100	0	1
Tapioca	4.25 oz	150	0	1
Vanilla	4.25 oz	170	0	1
Swiss Miss				
Butterscotch	4 oz	180	0	5
Chocolate	4 oz	180	0	5
Chocolate Fudge	4 oz	220	0	5
Chocolate Sundae	4 oz	220	0	5
Light Chocolate	4 oz	100	0	0
Light Chocolate Fudge	4 oz	100	0	0
Light Vanilla	4 oz	100	0	0
Light Vanilla Chocolate Parfait	4 oz	100	0	0
Tapicoa	4 oz	160	0	5
Vanilla	4 oz	190	0	5
Vanilla Parfait	4 oz	180	0	1
Vanilla Sundae	4 oz	200	0	5
Ultra Slim-Fast				
Butterscotch	4 oz	100	2	0
Chocolate	4 oz	100	2	0
Vanilla	4 oz	100	2	0
chocolate	1 pkg (5 oz)	189	—	5
lemon	1 pkg (5 oz)	177	—	0
vanilla	1 pkg (4 oz)	146	—	8
TAKE-OUT				
bread pudding	½ cup (4.4 oz)	212	—	83
rice w/ raisins	½ cup	246	4	136
tapicoa	½ cup	169	—	111
tapioca	½ cup (5.3 oz)	189	—	124
vanilla	½ cup (4.3 oz)	130	—	17

PUDDING POPS

(*see also* ICE CREAM AND FROZEN DESSERTS, PUDDING)

Jell-O				
Chocolate	1 pop	79	—	1
Chocolate Caramel Swirl	1 pop	74	—	1
Chocolate Vanilla Swirl	1 pop	78	—	1
Chocolate Fudge	1 pop	79	—	1
Chocolate Peanut Butter Swirl	1 bar	78	—	1
Chocolate Swirl	1 pop	80	—	1

FOOD	PORTION	CALS.	FIB.	CHOL.
Jell-O (CONT.)				
Deluxe Chocolate Covered	1 pop	201	—	2
Deluxe Peanuts And Chocolate	1 bar	185	—	2
Milk Chocolate	1 pop	80	—	1
Vanilla	1 pop	77	—	1
chocolate	1 (1.6 oz)	72	—	1
vanilla	1 (1.6 oz)	75	—	1
PUMMELO				
fresh	1	228	—	0
sections	1 cup	71	—	0
PUMPKIN				
CANNED				
Libby				
Solid Pack	½ cup	60	4	0
Owatonna	½ cup	40	—	0
pumpkin	½ cup	41	—	0
FRESH				
cooked mashed	½ cup	24	—	0
flowers cooked	½ cup	10	—	0
flowers raw	1	0	—	0
leaves cooked	½ cup	7	—	0
leaves raw	½ cup	4	—	0
raw cubed	½ cup	15	—	0
SEEDS				
dried	1 oz	154	—	0
roasted	1 cup	1184	—	0
roasted	1 oz	148	—	0
salted & roasted	1 cup	1184	—	0
salted & roasted	1 oz	148	—	0
whole roasted	1 oz	127	—	0
whole roasted	1 cup	285	—	0
whole salted roasted	1 cup	285	—	0
whole salted roasted	1 oz	127	—	0
PURSLANE				
cooked	1 cup	21	—	0
raw	1 cup	7	—	0
QUAHOGS				
(*see* CLAMS)				
QUICHE				
HOME RECIPE				
lorraine	⅛ pie 8 in	600	—	285

FOOD	PORTION	CALS.	FIB.	CHOL.
QUINCE				
fresh	1	53	—	0
QUINOA				
Arrowhead	¼ cup (1.4 oz)	140	4	0
Eden				
not prep	¼ cup (1.6 oz)	170	3	0
quinoa	½ cup	318	—	0
RABBIT				
domestic w/o bone roasted	3 oz	167	—	70
wild w/o bone stewed	3 oz	147	—	104
RADICCHIO				
raw shredded	½ cup	5	—	0
RADISHES				
DRIED				
chinese	½ cup	157	—	0
daikon	½ cup	157	—	0
FRESH				
Dole	7	20	0	0
chinese raw	1 (12 oz)	62	—	0
chinese raw sliced	½ cup	8	—	0
chinese sliced cooked	½ cup	13	—	0
daikon raw	1 (12 oz)	62	—	0
daikon raw sliced	½ cup	8	—	0
daikon sliced cooked	½ cup	13	—	0
red raw	10	7	—	0
red sliced	½ cup	10	—	0
white icicle raw	1 (½ oz)	2	—	0
white icicle raw sliced	½ cup	7	—	0
SPROUTS				
raw	½ cup	8	—	0
RAISINS				
Cinderella				
Seedless	½ cup	250	—	0
Del Monte	1 box (1.5 oz)	140	3	0
Del Monte	1 box (1 oz)	90	2	0
Del Monte	¼ cup (1.4 oz)	130	2	0
Del Monte	1 box (0.5 oz)	45	tr	0
Golden	¼ cup (1.4 oz)	130	2	0
Yogurt Raisins Strawberry	1 pkg (0.9 oz)	110	tr	0
Yogurt Raisins Vanilla	1 pkg (1 oz)	120	tr	0
Yogurt Raisins Vanilla	1 pkg (0.9 oz)	110	tr	0

FOOD	PORTION	CALS.	FIB.	CHOL.
Del Monte (CONT.)				
Yogurt Raisins Vanilla	3 tbsp (1 oz)	130	1	0
Dole				
Golden	½ cup	250	—	0
Seedless	½ cup	250	—	0
Tree Of Life				
Organic	¼ cup (1.4 oz)	130	2	0
chocolate coated	10 (0.4 oz)	39	—	0
chocolate coated	1 cup (6.7 oz)	741	—	5
golden seedless	1 cup	437	8	0
seedless	1 tbsp	27	—	0
seedless	1 cup	434	8	0

RASPBERRIES
CANNED
in heavy syrup	½ cup	117	—	0
FRESH				
Dole				
	1 cup	45	9	0
raspberries	1 cup	61	—	0
raspberries	1 pint	154	—	0
FROZEN				
Big Valley				
Raspberries	⅔ cup (4.9 oz)	80	3	0
Birds Eye				
Whole In Lite Syrup	½ cup	100	4	0
sweetened	1 cup	256	—	0
sweetened	1 pkg (10 oz)	291	—	0

RASPBERRY JUICE
Crystal Geyser				
Juice Squeeze Mountain Raspberry	1 bottle (12 fl oz)	135	—	0
Kool-Aid				
Sugar Free	8 oz	2	—	0
Smucker's	8 oz	120	—	0

RED BEANS
CANNED
Allen	½ cup (4.5 oz)	160	9	0
B&M				
Small Baked	8 oz	223	11	5
Green Giant	½ cup	90	5	0
Hunt's				
Small	4 oz	90	6	0
Van Camp's	½ cup (4.6 oz)	90	5	0

FOOD	PORTION	CÁLS.	FIB.	CHOL.
DRIED				
Bean Cuisine	½ cup	115	5	0
MIX				
Bean Cuisine				
Pasta & Beans Barcelona Red With Radiatore	½ cup	170	—	tr
Mahatma				
Red Beans & Rice	1 cup	190	7	0
RELISH				
Claussen				
Pickle Relish	1 tbsp	14	—	0
Del Monte				
Hamburger	1 tbsp (0.5 oz)	20	tr	0
Hot Dog	1 tbsp (0.5 oz)	15	tr	0
Sweet Pickle	1 tbsp (0.5 oz)	20	0	0
Hellman's				
Sandwich Spread	1 tbsp (15 g)	55	—	5
Old El Paso				
Jalapeno	2 tbsp	5	—	0
Vlasic				
Dill	1 oz	2	—	0
Hamburger	1 oz	40	—	0
Hot Piccalilli	1 oz	35	—	0
India	1 oz	30	—	0
Sweet	1 oz	30	—	0
cranberry orange	½ cup	246	—	0
hamburger	½ cup	158	—	0
hamburger	1 tbsp	19	—	0
hot dog	½ cup	111	—	0
hot dog	1 tbsp	14	—	0
sweet	1 tbsp	19	—	0
sweet	½ cup	159	—	0
RHUBARB				
fresh	½ cup	13	—	0
frzn	½ cup	60	—	0
frzn as prep w/ sugar	½ cup	139	—	0
RICE				
(*see also* BRAN, CEREAL, FLOUR, RICE CAKES, WILD RICE)				
BROWN				
Arrowhead				
Basmati	¼ cup (1.5 oz)	150	2	0
Quick Regular	⅓ cup (1.5 oz)	150	2	0

FOOD	PORTION	CALS.	FIB.	CHOL.
Arrowhead (CONT.)				
Quick Spanish Style	¼ pkg (1.4 oz)	150	2	0
Quick Vegetable Herb	¼ pkg (1.4 oz)	150	3	0
Quick Wild Rice & Herb	¼ pkg (1.3 oz)	140	3	0
Minute				
Precooked as prep	½ cup	121	1	0
Near East				
Pilaf as prep	1 cup	220	2	0
S&W				
Quick Natural Long Grain	3.5 oz	110	—	0
Quick Natural Long Grain cooked	3.5 oz	119	—	0
Uncle Ben	1 serv (1.6 oz)	158	1	0
long-grain cooked	½ cup	109	2	0
medium-grain cooked	½ cup	109	—	0
CANNED				
Van Camp's				
Spanish	1 cup (9 oz)	180	3	0
DRY MIX				
Casbah				
Jambalaya	1 pkg (1.4 oz)	130	1	0
La Fiesta	1 pkg (1.59 oz)	170	0	0
Nutted Pilaf as prep	1 cup	220	1	0
Pilaf as prep	1 cup	200	tr	0
Spanish Pilaf as prep	1 cup	200	1	0
Thai Yum	1 pkg (1.7 oz)	180	1	0
Chun King				
Stir Fry Entree	.25 oz	20	—	0
Goodman's				
Rice & Vermicelli For Beef	¾ cup	160	0	5
Rice & Vermicelli For Chicken	¾ cup	160	1	0
Hain				
Rice Almondine	½ cup	130	—	0
La Choy				
Chinese Fried Rice	¾ cup	190	tr	0
Lipton				
Rice & Sauce Chicken Broccoli	½ cup	129	—	2
Rice & Sauce Long Grain & Wild Rice Original	½ cup	121	0	0
Rice & Sauce Skillet Style Spanish	½ cup	104	—	0
Mahatma				
Broccoli & Cheese	1 cup	200	2	5
Jambalaya	1 cup (2 oz)	190	tr	0

FOOD	PORTION	CALS.	FIB.	CHOL.
Mahatma (CONT.)				
Long Grain & Wild	1 cup (2 oz)	190	2	0
Pilaf	1 cup (2 oz)	190	tr	0
Spanish	1 cup (2 oz)	180	2	0
Yellow Rice Mix	1 cup	190	tr	0
Minute				
Microwave Broccoli Almondin	½ cup	143	—	8
Microwave Cheddar Cheese Broccoli	½ cup	164	—	11
Microwave French Pilaf	½ cup	133	—	8
Microwave Long Grain Brown And Wild	½ cup	140	—	8
Microwave Rice With Savory Cheese Sauce as prep	½ cup	162	—	11
Minute Rice				
Drunstick With Vermicelli as prep	½ cup	153	—	10
Rib Roast With Vermicelli as prep	½ cup	151	—	10
Near East				
Barley Pilaf as prep	1 cup	220	5	0
Beef Pilaf as prep	1 cup	220	1	0
Curry Rice as prep	1 cup	220	1	0
Lentil Pilaf as prep	1 cup	210	0	0
Long Grain & Wild as prep	1 cup	220	2	0
Pilaf Chicken as prep	1 cup	220	1	0
Pilaf Kosher as prep	1 cup	220	1	0
Spanish Pilaf as prep	1 cup	230	1	0
Old El Paso				
Mexican	½ cup	140	—	0
Pritikin				
Mexican	⅓ cup (2 oz)	200	—	0
Oriental	⅓ cup (2 oz)	190	—	0
Success				
Beef Oriental	½ cup	190	2	0
Broccoli & Cheese	½ cup	200	2	10
Brown & Wild	½ cup	190	3	0
Classic Chicken	½ cup	150	1	0
Long Grain & Wild	½ cup	190	1	0
Pilaf	½ cup	200	2	0
Spanish	½ cup	190	1	0
Uncle Ben				
Brown & Wild Fast Cooking	1 serv (1.3 oz)	120	1	tr
Country Inn Broccoli Almondine	1 serv (1.2 oz)	124	1	tr

FOOD	PORTION	CALS.	FIB.	CHOL.
Uncle Ben (CONT.)				
Country Inn Broccoli & White Cheddar	1 serv (1.2 oz)	131	1	3
Country Inn Broccoli Au Gratin	1 serv (1.1 oz)	116	1	2
Country Inn Chicken With Wild Rice	1 serv (1.1 oz)	108	1	1
Country Inn Creamy Chicken & Mushroom	1 serv (1.3 oz)	138	1	2
Country Inn Creamy Chicken & Wild Rice	1 serv (1.3 oz)	135	1	4
Country Inn Green Bean Almondine	1 serv (1.2 oz)	128	1	2
Country Inn Herbed Au Gratin	1 serv (1.2 oz)	119	1	3
Country Inn Homestyle Chicken & Vegetables	1 serv (1.3 oz)	139	1	7
Country Inn Rice Florentine	1 serv (1.2 oz)	212	1	3
Country Inn Vegetable Pilaf	1 serv (1.2 oz)	115	1	1
Country inn Chicken Stock	1 serv (1.2 oz)	123	1	3
Long Grain & Wild Chicken Stock Sauce	1 serv (1.3 oz)	133	1	5
Long Grain & Wild Fast Cooking	1 serv (1 oz)	101	1	1
Long Grain & Wild Garden Vegetable Blend	1 serv (1.3 oz)	128	1	1
Long Grain & Wild Original	1 serv (1 oz)	96	1	tr
FROZEN				
Birds Eye				
Rice & Broccoli Au Gratin	½ pkg	150	1	10
Budget Gourmet				
Oriental Rice With Vegetables	1 pkg (5.75 oz)	230	—	20
Rice Pilaf With Green Beans	1 pkg (5.5 oz)	230	—	10
Green Giant				
Garden Gourmet Asparagus Pilaf	1 pkg	190	3	10
Garden Gourmet Sherry Wild Rice	1 pkg	210	3	10
One Serve Rice 'N Broccoli In Cheese Sauce	1 pkg	180	—	5
One Serve Rice Peas 'N Mushrooms With Sauce	1 pkg	130	—	5
Rice Originals Italian Rice 'N Spinach In Cheese Sauce	½ cup	140	—	10
Rice Originals Pilaf	½ cup	110	—	2
Rice Originals Rice 'N Broccoli In Cheese Sauce	½ cup	120	—	5

FOOD	PORTION	CALS.	FIB.	CHOL.
Green Giant (CONT.)				
Rice Originals Rice Medley	½ cup	100	—	5
Rice Originals White & Wild	½ cup	130	—	0
Luigino's				
Fried Rice Chicken	1 pkg (8 oz)	250	2	55
Fried Rice Pork	1 pkg (8 oz)	250	2	60
Fried Rice Pork & Shrimp	1 pkg (8 oz)	250	2	55
Fried Rice Shrimp	1 pkg (8 oz)	220	2	60
Risotto Parmesano	1 pkg (8 oz)	360	2	50
TAKE-OUT				
pilaf	½ cup	84	3	22
spanish	¾ cup	363	—	35
WHITE				
Arrowhead				
Basmati	¼ cup (1.5 oz)	150	tr	0
Minute				
Boil In Bag Long Grain as prep	½ cup	94	—	0
Long Grain as prep	⅔ cup	150	1	8
Minute Rice				
Long Grain & Wild as prep	½ cup	149	—	10
Minute Rice				
as prep	⅔ cup	141	1	5
S&W				
Long Grain cooked	3.5 oz	106	—	0
Superfino				
Arborio Rice	½ cup	100	—	0
Uncle Ben				
Boil-In-Bag	1 serv (0.9 oz)	94	tr	0
Converted	1 serv (1.2 oz)	123	tr	0
In An Instant	1 serv (1.1 oz)	111	tr	0
glutinous cooked	½ cup	116	—	0
long-grain cooked	½ cup	131	tr	0
long-grain instant cooked	½ cup	80	tr	0
long-grain parboiled cooked	½ cup	100	tr	0
medium-grain cooked	½ cup	132	—	0
short-grain cooked	½ cup	133	—	0
starch	3½ oz	343	—	0

RICE CAKES
(*see also* POPCORN CAKES)

Hain				
Mini Apple Cinnamon	½ oz	60	0	0
Mini Barbeque	½ oz	70	0	0
Mini Cheese	½ oz	60	0	<5

FOOD	PORTION	CALS.	FIB.	CHOL.
Hain (CONT.)				
Mini Honey Nut	½ oz	60	0	0
Mini Nacho Cheese	½ oz	70	0	<5
Mini Plain	½ oz	60	0	0
Mini Plain No Salt Added	½ oz	60	0	0
Mini Ranch	½ oz	70	—	0
Mini Teriyaki	½ oz	50	0	0
Ka-Me				
Cheese	16 pieces (1 oz)	120	0	0
Onion	16 pieces (1 oz)	120	0	0
Plain	16 pieces (1 oz)	120	0	0
Seaweed	16 pieces (1 oz)	120	0	0
Sesame	16 pieces (1 oz)	120	0	0
Unsalted	16 pieces (1 oz)	120	0	0
Mother's				
Mini Apple	5 (0.5 oz)	50	0	0
Mini Caramel	5 (0.5 oz)	50	0	0
Mini Cinnamon	5 (0.5 oz)	50	0	0
Mini Plain Unsalted	7 (0.5 oz)	60	0	0
Multigrain Lightly Salted	1 (0.3 oz)	35	0	0
Rye Unsalted	1 (0.3 oz)	35	1	0
Wheat Unsalted	1 (0.3 oz)	35	1	0
Pritikin				
Mini Apple Crisp	5 (0.5 oz)	50	—	0
Multigrain	1 (0.3 oz)	35	—	0
Multigrain Unsalted	1 (0.3 oz)	35	—	0
Plain	1 (0.3 oz)	35	—	0
Plain Unsalted	1 (0.3 oz)	35	—	0
Sesame Low Sodium	1 (0.3 oz)	35	—	0
Sesame Unsalted	1 (0.3 oz)	35	—	0
Quaker				
Apple Cinnamon	1 (0.4 oz)	40	—	0
Banana Crunch	1 (0.5 oz)	50	—	0
Cinnamon Crunch	1 (0.5 oz)	50	—	0
Mini Apple Cinnamon	6 (0.5 oz)	50	—	0
Mini Banana Crunch	6 (0.5 oz)	50	—	0
Mini Butter Popped Corn	6 (0.5 oz)	50	—	0
Mini Caramel Corn	6 (0.5 oz)	50	—	0
Mini Cinnamon Crunch	6 (0.5 oz)	50	—	0
Mini Honey Nut	6 (0.5 oz)	50	—	0
Mini White Cheddar	6 (0.5 oz)	50	—	0
Salt-Free	1 (0.3 oz)	35	—	0
Salted	1 (0.3 oz)	35	—	0

FOOD	PORTION	CALS.	FIB.	CHOL.
Tree Of Life				
Fat Free Mini Apple Cinnamon	15	60	0	0
Fat Free Mini Caramel	15	60	0	0
Fat Free Mini Honey Nut	15	60	0	0
Fat Free Mini Jalapeno	15	60	0	0
Fat Free Mini Plain	15	50	0	0
brown rice	1 (0.3 oz)	35	tr	0
brown rice & buckwheat	1 (0.3 oz)	34	tr	0
brown rice & buckwheat unsalted	1 (0.3 oz)	34	tr	0
brown rice & corn	1 (0.3 oz)	35	—	0
brown rice & rye	1 (0.3 oz)	35	tr	0
brown rice & sesame seed	1 (0.3 oz)	35	—	0
brown rice multigrain	1 (0.3 oz)	35	—	0
brown rice multigrain unsalted	1 (0.3 oz)	35	—	0
brown rice unsalted	1 (0.3 oz)	35	tr	0

ROCKFISH

pacific cooked	1 fillet (5.2 oz)	180	—	66
pacific cooked	3 oz	103	—	38
pacific raw	3 oz	80	—	29

ROE

(see individual fish names)

fish	3.5 oz	39	—	105
fresh baked	1 oz	58	—	136
fresh baked	3 oz	173	—	408

ROLL

(see also BISCUIT, CROISSANT, ENGLISH MUFFIN, MUFFIN, POPOVER, SCONE)

FROZEN

Weight Watchers				
Cinnamon Rolls	1 (2.1 oz)	180	—	5
HOME RECIPE				
dinner as prep w/ 2% milk	1 (2½ in)	111	—	12
dinner as prep w/ whole milk	1 (2½ in)	112	—	13
raisin & nut	1 (2 oz)	196	—	13
MIX				
Natural Ovens				
German Hard	1 (2.1 oz)	138	1	0
Gourmet Dinner	1 (1 oz)	50	2	0
Hearty Sandwich	1 (1.8 oz)	110	2	0
READY-TO-EAT				
Alvarado St. Bakery				
Burger Buns	1 (2.2 oz)	140	3	0

FOOD	PORTION	CALS.	FIB.	CHOL.
Alvarado St. Bakery (CONT.)				
Hot Dog Buns	1 (2.2 oz)	140	3	0
Arnold				
Augusto Pan Cubano	1	230	2	0
Bakery Light	1 (1.5 oz)	80	4	0
Bran'nola Buns	1 (1.5 oz)	100	3	0
Dinner Plain	1 (0.7 oz)	50	1	tr
Dinner Sesame	1 (0.7 oz)	50	1	tr
Dutch Egg	1	130	2	0
Hamburger	1	120	2	0
Hot Dog	1 (1.5 oz)	110	2	0
Hot Dog Bran'nola	1 (1.5 oz)	110	1	0
Hot Dog New England Style	1	110	1	0
Italian 8-inch Savoni	1	210	3	0
Onion Premium	1 (2.6 oz)	180	2	0
Onion Soft	1	140	2	0
Potato	1	140	2	0
Sandwich Soft Sesame	1	130	2	0
August Bros.				
Kaiser	1	170	2	0
Onion	1	160	2	0
Sesame Cubano	1	170	2	0
Bread Du Jour				
Bavarian Cracked Wheat	1 (1.2 oz)	90	1	0
Crusty Italian	1 (1.2 oz)	80	tr	0
French Petite	1 (3.5 oz)	230	2	0
Rye	1 (1.2 oz)	90	1	0
Sourdough	1 (2.2 oz)	140	2	0
Country Kitchen				
Frankfurt	1	120	—	0
Dicarlo's				
Extra Sourdough	1 (1.6 oz)	100	1	0
French	1 (1 oz)	70	tr	0
Hollywood				
Dark Bread	1	40	—	0
Dinner Light Pan Special Formula	1	60	—	0
Sliced Light Special Formula	1	80	—	0
Home Pride				
Dinner Wheat	1 (1.9 oz)	160	2	0
Hamburger Potato Bun	1 (1.9 oz)	130	2	0
Hot Dog Potato Bun	1 (1.9 oz)	130	2	0
Sandwich Roll Wheat	1 (1.9 oz)	160	2	0
White	2 (1.6 oz)	130	1	0

FOOD	PORTION	CALS.	FIB.	CHOL.
Martin's				
Big Marty Poppy	1	170	3	0
Big Marty Sesame	1	170	3	0
Hoagie	1	240	3	0
Hoagie Sesame	1	240	4	0
Potato Dinner	1	100	1	0
Potato Long	1	140	2	0
Potato Party	1	50	1	0
Potato Sandwich	1	140	2	0
Sandwich Whole Wheat 100% Stoneground	1	160	5	0
Matthew's				
Salad Roll	1	110	2	0
Sandwich	1	110	2	0
Pepperidge Farm				
Brown 'N Serve Club	1	100	1	0
Brown 'N Serve French	½ roll	180	1	0
Brown 'N Serve Hearth	1	50	tr	0
Dinner	1	60	tr	<5
Dinner Country Style Classic	1	50	0	0
Finger Poppy Seed	1	50	tr	<5
Finger Sesame Seed	1	60	tr	<5
Frankfurter Dijon	1	160	2	0
Frankfurter Side Sliced	1	140	1	0
Frankfurter w/ Poppy Seeds	1	130	1	0
Frankfurter Top Sliced	1	140	1	0
French Style	1	100	1	0
Hamburger	1	130	1	0
Hamburger	1	130	1	0
Heat & Serve Butter Crescent	1	110	tr	15
Heat & Serve Golden Twist	1	110	tr	5
Hoagie Soft	1	210	1	0
Old Fashioned	1	50	tr	5
Parker House	1	60	tr	5
Party	1	30	tr	0
Potato Sandwich	1	160	1	0
Sandwich Onion w/ Poppy Seeds	1	150	1	0
Sandwich Salad	1	110	—	10
Sandwich w/ Sesame Seeds	1	140	1	0
Soft Family	1	100	1	0
Sourdough French	1	100	1	0
Roman Meal				
Brown & Serve	2 (2 oz)	140	2	0

FOOD	PORTION	CALS.	FIB.	CHOL.
Roman Meal (CONT.)				
Dinner	2 (2 oz)	136	2	0
Hamburger	1 (1.6 oz)	111	2	0
Hotdog	1 (1.5 oz)	103	2	0
Sandwich	1 (2.7 oz)	181	3	0
Sandwich	1 (2.7 oz)	181	3	0
San Francisco				
Sourdough	1 (1.8 oz)	180	3	0
The Baker				
Honey Cinnamon Raisin	1 (2 oz)	150	4	0
Wonder				
Brown 'N Serve Wheat	1 (1 oz)	70	tr	0
Brown 'N Serve White	1 (1 oz)	70	tr	0
Brown 'N Serve Buttermilk	1 (1 oz)	70	tr	0
Dinner White Light	1 (1 oz)	60	4	0
Hamburger	1 (1.5 oz)	110	tr	0
Hamburger Light	1 (1.5 oz)	80	5	0
Hamburger Wheat	1 (2.2 oz)	170	1	0
Hot Dog	1 (1.5 oz)	110	tr	0
Hot Dog Light	1 (1.5 oz)	80	5	0
Tea Dinner Rolls	1 (1.5 oz)	80	5	0
brown & serve	1 (1 oz)	85	—	0
cinnamon raisin	1 (2¾ in)	223	1	40
dinner	1 (1 oz)	85	—	0
french	1 (1.3 oz)	105	—	0
hamburger multi-grain	1 (1½ oz)	113	2	0
hamburger reduced calorie	1 (1½ oz)	84	3	0
hard	1 (3½ in)	167	—	0
hotdog multi-grain	1 (1½ oz)	113	2	0
hotdog reduced calorie	1 (1½ oz)	84	3	0
kaiser	1 (3½ in)	167	—	0
oat bran	1 (1.2 oz)	78	1	0
rye	1 (1 oz)	81	—	0
submarine	1 (4.7 oz)	155	—	tr
wheat	1 (1 oz)	77	—	0
whole wheat	1 (1 oz)	75	—	0
REFRIGERATED				
Pillsbury				
Best Quick Cinnamon Rolls w/ Icing	1	110		0
Butterflake	1	140		0
Crescent	1	100		0
crescent	1 (1 oz)	98	—	0

FOOD	PORTION	CALS.	FIB.	CHOL.
ROSE APPLE				
fresh	3½ oz	32	—	0
ROSE HIP				
fresh	3½ oz	91	—	0
ROSELLE				
fresh	1 cup	28	—	0
ROSEMARY				
dried	1 tsp	4	—	0
ROUGHY				
orange baked	3 oz	75	—	22
RUTABAGA				
CANNED				
Sunshine				
Diced	½ cup (4.2 oz)	30	3	0
FRESH				
cooked mashed	½ cup	41	—	0
raw cubed	½ cup	25	—	0
SABLEFISH				
baked	3 oz	213	—	53
fillet baked	5.3 oz	378	—	95
smoked	1 oz	72	—	18
smoked	3 oz	218	—	55
SAFFLOWER				
seeds dried	1 oz	147	—	0
SAFFRON				
saffron	1 tsp	2	—	0
SAGE				
Watkins				
ground	¼ tsp (0.5 g)	0	0	0
ground	1 tsp	2	—	0
SALAD				
(see also LETTUCE, PASTA SALAD)				
MIX				
Dole				
Caesar Salad	⅓ pkg (3.5 oz)	170	1	5
Classic Blend	3.5 oz	25	1	0
Coleslaw Blend	3.5 oz	30	2	0
French Blend	3.5 oz	25	1	0
Italian Blend	3.5 oz	25	1	0
Salad-In-A- Minute Oriental	3.5 oz	110	2	0

FOOD	PORTION	CALS.	FIB.	CHOL.
Dole (CONT.)				
Salad-In-A- Minute Spinach	3.5 oz	180	3	0
Fresh Express				
American Salad	1½ cups (3 oz)	20	1	0
Caesar Salad	1½ cups (3 oz)	140	1	10
European Salad	1½ cups (3 oz)	20	1	0
Garden Salad	1½ cups (3 oz)	20	1	0
Italian Salad	1½ cups (3 oz)	20	1	0
Oriental Salad	1½ cups (3 oz)	120	1	0
Rivera Salad	1½ cups (3 oz)	10	1	0
Spinach Salad	1½ cups (3 oz)	130	3	0
TAKE-OUT				
chef w/o dressing	1½ cups	386	—	244
tossed w/o dressing	1½ cups	32	—	0
tossed w/o dressing	¾ cup	16	—	0
tossed w/o dressing w/ cheese & egg	1½ cups	102	—	98
tossed w/o dressing w/ chicken	1½ cups	105	—	72
tossed w/o dressing w/ pasta & seafood	1½ cups (14.6 oz)	380	—	50
tossed w/o dressing w/ shrimp	1½ cups	107	—	180
waldorf	½ cup	79	1	8

SALAD DRESSING
HOME RECIPE

vinegar & oil	1 tbsp	72	—	0
MIX				
Good Seasons				
Blue Cheese & Herbs as prep	1 tbsp	72	—	tr
Buttermilk Farm as prep	1 tbsp	58	—	5
Cheese Garlic as prep	1 tbsp	72	—	tr
Cheese Italian as prep	1 tbsp	72	—	tr
Classic Dill	1 pkg	28	—	0
Italian as prep	1 tbsp	71	—	0
Italian Lite as prep	1 tbsp	27	—	0
Italian No Oil as prep	1 tbsp	7	—	0
Lemon & Herbs as prep	1 tbsp	71	—	0
Lite Cheese Italian as prep	1 tbsp	27	—	tr
Lite Ranch as prep	1 tbsp	29	—	3
Mild Italian as prep	1 tbsp	73	—	0
Ranch as prep	1 tbsp	57	—	5
Zesty Italian as prep	1 tbsp	71	—	0
Hain				
No Oil 1000 Island	1 tbsp	12	—	tr

FOOD	PORTION	CALS.	FIB.	CHOL.
Hain (CONT.)				
No Oil Bleu Cheese	1 tbsp	14	—	<5
No Oil Buttermilk	1 tbsp	11	—	0
No Oil Caesar	1 tbsp	6	—	0
No Oil French	1 tbsp	12	—	0
No Oil Garlic & Cheese	1 tbsp	6	—	0
No Oil Herb	1 tbsp	2	—	0
No Oil Italian	1 tbsp	2	—	0
READY-TO-USE				
Estee				
Creamy French Fat Free	1 pkg (0.5 oz)	5	—	0
Creamy Garlic Fat Free	1 pkg (0.5 oz)	5	—	0
Fat Free Thousand Island	1 pkg (0.5 oz)	5	—	0
Hain				
1000 Island	1 tbsp	50	—	0
Canola Garden Tomato	1 tbsp	60	—	0
Canola Italian	1 tbsp	50	—	0
Canola Spicy French Mustard	1 tbsp	50	—	5
Canola Tangy Citrus	1 tbsp	50	—	0
Creamy Ceasar	1 tbsp	60	—	<5
Creamy Ceasar Low Salt	1 tbsp	60	—	<5
Creamy French	1 tbsp	60	—	0
Creamy Italian	1 tbsp	80	—	0
Creamy Italian No Salt Added	1 tbsp	80	—	0
Cucumber Dill	1 tbsp	80	—	5
Dijon Vinaigrette	1 tbsp	50	—	<5
Garlic & Sour Cream	1 tbsp	70	—	0
Honey & Sesame	1 tbsp	60	—	0
Italian Cheese Vinaigrette	1 tbsp	55	—	<5
Old Fashioned Buttermilk	1 tbsp	70	—	0
Poppyseed Rancher's	1 tbsp	60	—	<5
Savory Herb No Salt Added	1 tbsp	90	—	0
Swiss Cheese Vinaigrette	1 tbsp	60	—	<5
Traditional Italian No Salt Added	1 tbsp	60	—	0
Traditional Italian	1 tbsp	80	—	0
Healthy Sensation				
Blue Cheese	1 tbsp	19	—	1
French	1 tbsp	21	—	0
Honey Dijon	1 tbsp	26	—	0
Italian	1 tbsp	7	—	0
Ranch	1 tbsp	15	—	0
Thousand Island	1 tbsp	20	—	0

FOOD	PORTION	CALS.	FIB.	CHOL.
Hollywood				
Ceasar	1 tbsp	70	0	0
Creamy French	1 tbsp	70	0	0
Creamy Italian	1 tbsp	90	0	0
Dijon Vinaigrette	1 tbsp	60	0	0
Italian Cheese	1 tbsp	80	0	0
Italian	1 tbsp	90	0	0
Old Fashion Buttermilk	1 tbsp	75	0	0
Poppy Seed Rancher's	1 tbsp	75	0	0
Thousand Island	1 tbsp	60	0	5
Kraft				
Bacon & Tomato	2 tbsp (1.1 oz)	140	0	<5
Buttermilk Ranch	2 tbsp (1 oz)	150	0	<5
Caesar Ranch	2 tbsp (1 oz)	140	0	10
Catalina With Honey	2 tbsp (1.2 oz)	140	0	0
Catalina French	2 tbsp (1.2 oz)	140	0	0
Ceasar	2 tbsp (1.1 oz)	130	0	<5
Chunky Blue Cheese	2 tbsp (1.2 oz)	90	0	10
Coleslaw	2 tbsp (1.2 oz)	150	0	25
Creamy Ceasar	2 tbsp (1 oz)	140	0	10
Creamy Garlic	2 tbsp (1.1 oz)	110	0	0
Creamy Italian	2 tbsp (1.1 oz)	110	0	0
Cucumber Ranch	2 tbsp (1.1 oz)	150	0	0
Deliciously Right Bacon & Tomato	2 tbsp (1.1 oz)	60	0	<5
Deliciously Right Caesar	2 tbsp (1.1 oz)	50	0	<5
Deliciously Right Catalina French	2 tbsp (1.2 oz)	80	0	0
Deliciously Right Creamy Italian	2 tbsp (1.1 oz)	50	0	0
Deliciously Right Cucumber Ranch	2 tbsp (1.1 oz)	60	0	0
Deliciously Right French	2 tbsp (1.2 oz)	50	0	0
Deliciously Right Italian	2 tbsp (1.1 oz)	70	0	0
Deliciously Right Ranch	2 tbsp (1.1 oz)	110	0	10
Deliciously Right Thousand Island	2 tbsp (1.2 oz)	70	0	5
Free Blue Cheese	2 tbsp (1.2 oz)	50	0	0
Free Catalina	2 tbsp (1.2 oz)	45	tr	0
Free French	2 tbsp (1.2 oz)	50	tr	0
Free Honey Dijon	2 tbsp (1.2 oz)	50	1	0
Free Italian	2 tbsp (1.1 oz)	10	0	0
Free Peppercorn Ranch	2 tbsp (1.2 oz)	50	1	0
Free Ranch	1 tbsp (1.2 oz)	50	tr	0
Free Red Wine Vinegar	2 tbsp (1.1 oz)	15	0	0

FOOD	PORTION	CALS.	FIB.	CHOL.
Kraft (CONT.)				
Free Thousand Island	2 tbsp (1.2 oz)	45	1	0
French	2 tbsp (1.1 oz)	120	0	0
Honey Dijon	2 tbsp (1.1 oz)	150	0	0
House Italian	2 tbsp (1.1 oz)	120	0	<5
Oil-Free Italian	2 tbsp (1.1 oz)	5	0	0
Peppercorn Ranch	2 tbsp (1 oz)	170	0	10
Pesto Italian	2 tbsp (1.1 oz)	140	0	0
Ranch	2 tbsp (1 oz)	170	0	5
Roka Blue Cheese	2 tbsp (1.2 oz)	90	0	10
Russian	2 tbsp (1.2 oz)	130	0	0
Salsa Ranch	2 tbsp (1 oz)	130	0	10
Salsa Zesty Garden	2 tbsp (1.1 oz)	70	tr	0
Sour Cream & Onion Ranch	2 tbsp (1 oz)	170	0	10
Thousand Island	2 tbsp (1.1 oz)	110	0	10
Thousand Island With Bacon	2 tbsp (1 oz)	120	0	0
Zesty Italian	2 tbsp (1.1 oz)	110	0	0
Marzetti				
Bacon Spinach Salad	2 tbsp	80	15	1
Blue Cheese	2 tbsp	160	0	20
Buttermilk Parmesan Pepper	2 tbsp	170	0	10
Buttermilk Parmesan Ranch	2 tbsp	160	0	10
Buttermilk Veggie Dip	2 tbsp	170	0	3
Buttermilk & Herb	2 tbsp	180	0	3
Buttermilk Bacon Ranch	2 tbsp	180	0	10
Buttermilk Blue Cheese	2 tbsp	160	0	10
Buttermilk Ranch	2 tbsp	180	0	4
Caesar	2 tbsp	150	0	0
Caesar Ranch	2 tbsp	190	0	5
California French	2 tbsp	160	0	0
Celery Seed	2 tbsp	160	0	0
Chunky Blue Cheese	2 tbsp	150	0	25
Classic Caesar Ranch	2 tbsp	190	0	5
Country French	2 tbsp	150	0	10
Cracked Peppercorn	2 tbsp	140	0	30
Creamy Garlic Italian	2 tbsp	160	0	15
Creamy Italian	2 tbsp	150	0	15
Crispy Celery Seed	2 tbsp	160	0	0
Dijon Honey Mustard	2 tbsp	140	0	20
Dijon Ranch	2 tbsp	170	0	25
Dutch Sweet 'N Sour	2 tbsp	160	0	0
Fat Free California French	2 tbsp	45	0	0
Fat Free Honey Dijon	2 tbsp	60	1	0
Fat Free Honey French	2 tbsp	45	0	0

FOOD	PORTION	CALS.	FIB.	CHOL.
Marzetti (CONT.)				
Fat Free Italian	2 tbsp	15	0	0
Fat Free Peppercorn Ranch	2 tbsp	30	1	0
Fat Free Ranch	2 tbsp	30	1	0
Fat Free Raspberry	2 tbsp	70	0	0
Fat Free Slaw	2 tbsp	45	0	15
Fat Free Sweet & Sour	2 tbsp	45	0	0
Fat Free Thousand Island	2 tbsp	35	0	0
Garden Ranch	2 tbsp	180	0	3
Gusto Italian	2 tbsp	120	0	0
Honey Dijon	2 tbsp	140	0	15
Honey Dijon Ranch	2 tbsp	150	0	25
Honey French	2 tbsp	160	0	0
Honey French Blue Cheese	2 tbsp	160	0	0
House Caesar	2 tbsp	150	0	5
Italian With Olive Oil	2 tbsp	120	0	0
Light Slaw	2 tbsp	60	0	30
Light Blue Cheese	2 tbsp	60	0	15
Light Buttermilk Ranch	2 tbsp	90	0	10
Light California French	2 tbsp	80	0	0
Light Chunky Blue Cheese	2 tbsp	80	0	15
Light French	2 tbsp	40	0	0
Light French	2 tbsp	40	0	0
Light Honey French	2 tbsp	80	0	0
Light Italian	2 tbsp	60	0	0
Light Ranch	2 tbsp	90	0	5
Light Red Wine Vinegar & Oil	2 tbsp	20	0	0
Light Sweet & Sour	2 tbsp	100	0	0
Light Thousand Island	2 tbsp	70	0	20
Old Fashioned Poppyseed	2 tbsp	140	0	10
Olde Venice Italian	2 tbsp	130	0	0
Olde World Caesar	2 tbsp	150	0	5
Parmesan Pepper	2 tbsp	160	0	10
Peppercorn Ranch	2 tbsp	180	0	10
Poppyseed	2 tbsp	160	0	15
Potato Salad Dressing	2 tbsp	120	0	15
Ranch	2 tbsp	180	0	3
Red Wine Vinegar & Oil	2 tbsp	130	0	0
Romano Cheese Caesar	2 tbsp	150	0	15
Romano Italian	2 tbsp	160	0	0
Savory Italian	2 tbsp	110	0	0
Slaw	2 tbsp	170	0	30
Southern Slaw	2 tbsp	100	0	20
Sweet & Saucy	2 tbsp	140	0	0

FOOD	PORTION	CALS.	FIB.	CHOL.
Marzetti (CONT.)				
Sweet & Sour	2 tbsp	160	0	0
Thousand Island	2 tbsp	150	0	25
Vintage Champagne	2 tbsp	150	0	0
Wilde Raspberry	2 tbsp	150	0	0
Newman's Own				
Italian Light	1 tbsp (0.5 fl oz)	10	—	0
Olive Oil & Vinegar	1 tbsp (0.5 fl oz)	80	—	0
Ranch	1 tbsp (0.5 fl oz)	90	—	5
Pfeiffer				
1000 Island	2 tbsp	140	0	20
California French	2 tbsp	140	0	0
French	2 tbsp	150	0	10
Honey Dijon	2 tbsp	140	0	15
Lite Italian	2 tbsp	50	0	0
Ranch	2 tbsp	180	0	3
Savory Italian	2 tbsp	110	0	0
Pritikin				
Dijon Balsamic Vinaigrette	2 tbsp (1 oz)	3	—	0
French	2 tbsp (1 oz)	35	—	0
Honey Dijon	2 tbsp (1 oz)	45	—	0
Honey French	2 tbsp (1 oz)	40	—	0
Italian	2 tbsp (1 oz)	20	—	0
Raspberry Vinaigrette	2 tbsp (1 oz)	45	—	0
Red Wing				
"K" Dressing	1 tbsp (0.5 oz)	70	0	5
Chunky Blue Cheese	2 tbsp (1 oz)	130	0	0
Creamy Ranch	2 tbsp (1 oz)	150	0	15
French Traditional	2 tbsp (1 oz)	130	0	0
Italian Traditional	2 tbsp (1 oz)	100	0	0
Spicy Sweet French	2 tbsp (1 oz)	130	0	0
Thousand Island Thick & Rich	2 tbsp (1 oz)	110	0	15
S&W				
French Low Calorie	1 tbsp	18	—	0
Italian No-Oil	1 tbsp	2	—	0
Russian Low Calorie	1 tbsp	25	—	0
Seven Seas				
Creamy Italian	2 tbsp (1.1 oz)	110	0	0
Free Italian	2 tbsp (1.1 oz)	10	0	0
Free Ranch	2 tbsp (1.2 oz)	50	1	0
Free Red Wine Vinegar	2 tbsp (1.1 oz)	15	0	0
Green Goddess	2 tbsp (1 oz)	120	0	0
Herbs & Spices	2 tbsp (1.1 oz)	120	0	0
Ranch	2 tbsp (1 oz)	150	0	5

FOOD	PORTION	CALS.	FIB.	CHOL.
Seven Seas (CONT.)				
Red Wine Vinegar & Oil	2 tbsp (1.1 oz)	110	0	0
Reduced Calorie Creamy Italian	2 tbsp (1.1 oz)	60	0	0
Reduced Calorie Italian With Olive Oil	2 tbsp (1.1 oz)	50	0	0
Reduced Calorie Ranch	2 tbsp (1.1 oz)	100	0	0
Reduced Calorie Red Wine Vinegar & Oil	2 tbsp (1.1 oz)	60	0	0
Two Cheese Italian	2 tbsp (1.1 oz)	70	0	0
Viva Buttermilk	2 tbsp (1.1)	150	0	0
Viva Caesar	2 tbsp (1.1 oz)	120	0	0
Viva Italian	2 tbsp (1.1 oz)	110	0	0
Viva Reduced Calorie Italian	2 tbsp (1.1 oz)	45	0	0
Tree Of Life				
Cafe Venice	2 tbsp (1 oz)	100	0	0
Fat Free Honey French	2 tbsp (1 oz)	35	—	0
Fat Free Italian Garlic	2 tbsp (1 oz)	20	—	0
Fat Free Oriental Ginger	2 tbsp (1 oz)	15	—	0
Frisco's Raspberry	2 tbsp (1 oz)	120	0	0
Maison Caesar	2 tbsp (1 oz)	70	0	5
Shanghai Palace	2 tbsp (1 oz)	80	0	0
Ultra Slim-Fast				
French	1 tbsp	20	0	0
Italian	1 tbsp	6	0	0
W.J. Clark				
Ginger Orange Vinaigrette	1 tbsp	73	0	0
Herbs & Romano	1 tbsp	67	0	0
Lemon Peppercorn	1 tbsp	72	0	0
Lime Cilantro Vinaigrette	1 tbsp	73	0	0
Poppy Seed	1 tbsp	75	0	0
Sweet Pepper Basil	1 tbsp	69	0	0
Tarragon Honey Mustard	1 tbsp	66	0	0
Walden Farms				
Bleu Cheese Fat Free	2 tbsp (1 oz)	25	0	8
Creamy Italian With Parmesan Fat Free	1 tbsp (1 oz)	25	0	0
Fat Free Balsamic Vinaigrette	2 tbsp (1 oz)	15	0	0
Fat Free Caesar	2 tbsp (1 oz)	25	0	0
Fat Free Italian	2 tbsp (1 oz)	10	0	0
Fat Free Raspberry Vinaigrette	2 tbsp (1 oz)	20	0	0
Fat Free Russian	2 tbsp (1 oz)	30	0	5
French Style Fat Free	2 tbsp (1 oz)	25	0	0
Honey Dijon Fat Free	2 tbsp (1 oz)	25	0	0
Italian Sodium Free Fat Free	2 tbsp (1 oz)	10	0	0

FOOD	PORTION	CALS.	FIB.	CHOL.
Walden Farms (CONT.)				
Italian Sugar Free Fat Free	2 tbsp (1 oz)	0	0	0
Italian With Sun Dried Tomato	2 tbsp (1 oz)	15	0	0
Ranch Fat Free	2 tbsp (1 oz)	25	0	0
Ranch With Sun Dried Tomato	2 tbsp (1 oz)	25	0	0
Thousand Island Fat Free	2 tbsp (1 oz)	35	0	5
Weight Watchers				
Russian	1 tbsp	50	—	5
Thousand Island	1 tbsp	50	—	5
Wishbone				
Blue Chees Chunky Lite	1 tbsp	40	0	1
Blue Cheese Chunky	1 tbsp	73	—	1
Classic Olive Oil Italian	1 tbsp	33	—	0
Classic Lite Dijon Vinaigrette	1 tbsp	30	—	0
Classic Lite Olive Oil Italian	1 tbsp	20	—	0
Creamy Italian	1 tbsp	54	—	tr
Deluxe French	1 tbsp	57	0	0
Dijon Vinaigrette Classic	1 tbsp	57	0	0
French Fat Free	1 tbsp	6	—	0
French Lite	1 tbsp	30	0	0
French Sweet 'N Spicy Lite	1 tbsp	17	—	0
French Red	1 tbsp	64	—	0
French Sweet 'N Spicy	1 tbsp	61	—	0
Italian	1 tbsp	45	—	0
Italian Lite	1 tbsp	6	—	0
Italian Cream Lite	1 tbsp	26	—	tr
Lite Caesar With Olive Oil	1 tbsp	28	—	1
Lite French Red	1 tbsp	17	—	0
Lite Olive Oil Vinaigrette	1 tbsp	16	—	0
Lite Red Wine Vinaigrette Olive Oil	1 tbsp	20	—	0
Olive Oil Vinaigrette	1 tbsp	30	—	0
Ranch	1 tbsp	76	—	6
Ranch Lite	1 tbsp	42	0	5
Red Wine Olive Oil Vinaigrette	1 tbsp	34	—	0
Robusto Italian	1 tbsp	46	0	0
Russian	1 tbsp	54	tr	0
Russian Lite	1 tbsp	21	—	0
Thousand Island	1 tbsp	66	—	7
Thousand Island Lite	1 tbsp	22	—	1
french reduced calorie	1 tbsp	22	—	1
italian reduced calorie	1 tbsp	16	—	1
russian reduced calorie	1 tbsp	23	—	1
sesame seed	1 tbsp	68	—	0
thousand island reduced calorie	1 tbsp	24	—	2

FOOD	PORTION	CALS.	FIB.	CHOL.

SALMON
CANNED
Bumble Bee

FOOD	PORTION	CALS.	FIB.	CHOL.
Keta	3.5 oz	160	—	60
Pink	3.5 oz	160	—	50
Pink Skinless & Boneless	3.25 oz	120	—	25
Red	3.5 oz	180	—	60
Red Skinless & Boneless	3.25 oz	130	—	30
Deming's				
Alaska Pink	½ cup	140	—	65
Alaska Red Sockeye	½ cup	170	—	65
Double Q				
Alaska Pink	½ cup	140	—	65
chum w/ bone	3 oz	120	—	33
chum w/ bone	1 can (13.9 oz)	521	—	144
sockeye w/ bone	1 can (12.9 oz)	566	—	161
sockeye w/ bone	3 oz	130	—	37
FRESH				
atlantic baked	3 oz	155	—	60
chinook baked	3 oz	196	—	72
chum baked	3 oz	131	—	81
coho cooked	3 oz	157	—	42
coho cooked	½ fillet (5.4 oz)	286	—	76
coho raw	3 oz	124	—	33
pink baked	3 oz	127	—	57
sockeye cooked	3 oz	183	—	74
sockeye cooked	½ fillet (5.4 oz)	334	—	135
sockeye raw	3 oz	143	—	53
SMOKED				
chinook	1 oz	33	—	7
chinook	3 oz	99	—	20
TAKE-OUT				
salmon cake	1 (3 oz)	241	—	104

SALSA
(see also KETCHUP, MEXICAN FOOD, SAUCE)
Chi-Chi's

FOOD	PORTION	CALS.	FIB.	CHOL.
Hot	2 tbsp (1 oz)	10	0	0
Medium	1 tbsp (1 oz)	10	0	0
Mild	2 tbsp (1 oz)	10	0	0
Verde Medium	2 tbsp (1.2 oz)	15	0	0
Verde Mild	2 tbsp (1.2 oz)	15	0	0
Del Monte				
Mexicana	2 tbsp (1.1 oz)	5	1	0

FOOD	PORTION	CALS.	FIB.	CHOL.
Del Monte (CONT.)				
Taquera	2 tbsp (1.1 oz)	5	1	0
Verde	2 tbsp (1.1 oz)	10	tr	0
Frito Lay				
Hot	1 oz	12	—	0
Medium	1 oz	12	—	0
Mild	1 oz	12	—	0
Hain				
Hot	¼ cup	22	—	0
Heluva Good Cheese				
Cheese & Salsa	2 tbsp (1.1 oz)	80	0	10
Thick & Chunky Hot	2 tbsp (1.2 oz)	10	0	0
Thick & Chunky Mild	2 tbsp (1.2 oz)	10	0	0
Hot Cha Cha				
Medium	2 tbsp (1 oz)	5	—	0
Louise's				
Fat Free BBQ Black Bean	1 oz	10	0	0
Fat Free Black Bean	1 oz	10	0	0
Fat Free Medium	1 oz	10	1	0
Fat Free Mild	1 oz	10	1	0
Fat Free Nacho Queso	1 oz	15	0	0
Newman's Own				
Bandito Hot	1 tbsp (0.7 oz)	6	—	0
Bandito Medium	1 tbsp (0.7 oz)	6	—	0
Bandito Mild	1 tbsp (0.7 oz)	6	—	0
Old El Paso				
Homestyle Chunky Mild	2 tbsp	5	—	0
Medium	2 tbsp	5	—	0
Picante Salsa Hot	2 tbsp	10	—	0
Picante Salsa Medium	2 tbsp	10	—	0
Picante Salsa Mild	2 tbsp	10	—	0
Thick'n Chunky Green Chili	2 tbsp	3	—	0
Thick'n Chunky Hot	2 tbsp	10	—	0
Thick'n Chunky Medium	2 tbsp	10	—	0
Thick'n Chunky Mild	2 tbsp	10	—	0
Thick'n Chunky Salsa Verde	2 tbsp	10	1	0
Ortega				
Hot Green Chili	1 tbsp	6	—	0
Medium Green Chili	1 tbsp	6	—	0
Mild Green Chili	1 tbsp	8	—	0
Pace				
Thick & Chunky	2 tbsp (1 fl oz)	12	1	0
Roserita				
Chunky Hot	3 tbsp (1.5 oz)	25	tr	0

FOOD	PORTION	CALS.	FIB.	CHOL.
Roserita (CONT.)				
Chunky Medium	3 tbsp (1.5 oz)	25	tr	0
Chunky Mild	3 tbsp (1.5 oz)	25	tr	0
Taco Salsa Chunky Medium	3 tbsp (1.5 oz)	25	tr	0
Taco Salsa Chunky Mild	3 tbsp (1.5 oz)	25	tr	0
Tree Of Life				
Hot	2 tbsp (1 oz)	10	—	0
Medium	2 tbsp (1 oz)	10	—	0
Mild	2 tbsp (1 oz)	10	—	0
No Salt	2 tbsp (1 oz)	10	—	0
Watkins				
Salsa Seasoning Blend	⅛ tsp (0.5 g)	0	0	0
Tropical	2 tbsp (1 oz)	60	0	0
SALSIFY				
fresh sliced cooked	½ cup	46	—	0
raw sliced	½ cup	55	—	0
SALT SUBSTITUTES				
Morton	1 tsp	2	—	0
Papa Dash				
Lite Lite Lite Salt	¼ tsp (0.5 g)	1	—	0
Salt Lover's Blend	¼ tsp (0.7 g)	tr	—	0
SALT/SEASONED SALT				
(see also SALT SUBSTITUTE)				
Hain				
Sea Salt	1 tsp	0	—	0
Sea Salt Iodized	1 tsp	0	—	0
Morton				
Garlic	1 tsp	3	—	0
Iodized	1 tsp	tr	—	0
Kosher	1 tsp	0	—	0
Lite	1 tsp	tr	—	0
Nature's Season Seasoning Blend	1 tsp	3	—	0
Non-Iodized	1 tsp	0	—	0
Seasoned	1 tsp	4	—	0
Watkins				
Bacon Cheese Salt	¼ tbsp (1 g)	0	0	0
Butter Salt	¼ tbsp (1 g)	0	0	0
Cheese Salt	¼ tbsp (1 g)	0	0	0
Garlic Salt	¼ tsp (1 g)	0	0	0
Salt & Vinegar Seasoning	¼ tsp (1 g)	0	0	0
Seasoning Salt	¼ tsp (1 g)	0	0	0

FOOD	PORTION	CALS.	FIB.	CHOL.
Watkins (CONT.)				
Sour Cream & Onion Salt	¼ tbsp (1 g)	0	0	0
salt	1 tsp (6 g)	0	—	0
salt	1 tbsp (18 g)	0	—	0
SAPODILLA				
fresh	1	140	—	0
fresh cut up	1 cup	199	—	0
SAPOTES				
fresh	1	301	—	0
SARDINES				
CANNED				
Del Monte				
In Tomato Sauce	1 fish (1.4 oz)	50	tr	25
Port Clyde				
In Louisiana Hot Sauce	1 can (3.75 oz)	170	0	105
In Mustard Sauce	1 can (3.75 oz)	150	1	110
In Mustard Sauce	1 can (3.75 oz)	150	1	110
In Soybean Oil Select Small	1 can (3.3 oz)	220	0	115
In Soybean Oil With Hot Chilies	1 can (3.3 oz)	155	0	80
In Soybean Oil drained	1 can (3.3 oz)	220	0	115
In Soybean Oil drained	1 can (3.3 oz)	220	0	115
In Spring Water	1 can (3.3 oz)	170	0	140
In Tomato Sauce	1 can (3.75 oz)	150	0	100
atlantic in oil w/ bone	1 can (3.2 oz)	192	—	131
atlantic in oil w/ bone	2	50	—	34
pacific in tomato sauce w/ bone	1	68	—	23
pacific in tomato sauce w/ bone	1 can (13 oz)	658	—	225
SAUCE				
(*see also* BARBECUE SAUCE, GRAVY, PIZZA, SALSA, SPAGHETTI SAUCE TOMATO)				
DRY				
Chun King				
Sweet 'n Sour Entree Mix	3.8 oz	370	—	0
Kikkoman				
Marinade For Meat	1 oz pkg	64	—	0
Sweet & Sour	2⅛ oz pkg	228	—	0
Teriyaki	1½ oz pkg	125	—	0
bearnaise as prep w/ milk & butter	1 cup	701	—	189
cheese as prep w/ milk	1 cup	307	—	53
curry as prep w/ milk	1 cup	270	—	35
mushroom as prep w/ milk	1 cup	228	—	34
sourcream as prep w/ milk	1 cup	509	—	91

FOOD	PORTION	CALS.	FIB.	CHOL.
stroganoff as prep	1 cup	271	—	38
sweet & sour as prep	1 cup	294	—	0
teriyaki as prep	1 cup	131	—	0
white as prep w/ milk	1 cup	241	—	34
JARRED				
Armour				
Chili Hot Dog	¼ cup (2.2 oz)	120	—	20
Meatless Sloppy Joe Sauce	¼ cup (2.2 oz)	30	—	0
Best Foods				
Tartar	1 tbsp (14 g)	70	—	5
Bright Day				
Tartar	1 tbsp	50	—	0
Chi-Chi's				
Taco Thick & Chunky	1 tbsp (0.5 oz)	10	0	0
Del Monte				
Cocktail	¼ cup (2.7 oz)	100	0	0
Sloppy Joe Hickory Flavor	¼ cup (2.4 oz)	70	0	0
Sloppy Joe Italian Style	¼ cup (2.4 oz)	70	0	0
Sloppy Joe Original	¼ cup (2.4 oz)	70	0	0
El Molino				
Taco Red Mild	2 tbsp	10	—	0
Gebhardt				
Enchilada Sauce	3 tbsp (1.5 oz)	25	tr	tr
Hot Dog Chili Sauce	2 tbsp	30	tr	3
Hot Sauce	½ tsp	tr	tr	0
Gold's				
Rib	1 oz	60	—	0
Golden Dipt				
Cajun Style	1 oz	90	—	0
Creole	1 oz	20	—	0
Dijonaisse	1 oz	52	—	0
French White	1 oz	55	—	0
Ginger Teriyaki Marinade	1 oz	120	—	0
Lemon Butter Dill	1 oz	100	—	0
Lemon Herb Marinade	1 oz	130	—	0
Seafood Cocktail	1 tbsp	20	—	0
Seafood Cocktail Extra Hot	1 tbsp	20	—	0
Tartar	1 tbsp	70	—	10
Tartar Lite	1 tbsp	50	—	5
Guiltless Gourmet				
Picante Hot	1 oz	6	tr	0
Picante Medium	1 oz	6	tr	0
Heinz				
Worcestershire	1 tbsp	6	—	0

FOOD	PORTION	CALS.	FIB.	CHOL.
Hellman's				
Tartar	1 tbsp (14 g)	70	—	5
Heluva Good Cheese				
Cocktail	¼ cup (1.6 oz)	40	—	0
Hormel				
Not-So-Sloppy-Joe Sauce	¼ cup (2.2 oz)	70	1	0
House Of Tsang				
Bangkok Padang	1 tbsp (0.6 oz)	45	0	0
Hoisin	1 tsp (6 g)	15	0	0
Mandarin Marinade	1 tbsp (0.6 oz)	25	0	0
Saigon Sizzle	1 tbsp (0.6 oz)	40	0	0
Spicy Brown Bean	1 tsp (6 g)	15	0	0
Stir Fry Sweet & Sour	1 tbsp (0.6 oz)	35	0	0
Stir Fry Szechuan Spicy	1 tbsp (0.6 oz)	20	0	0
Stir Fry Classic	1 tbsp (0.6 oz)	25	0	0
Sweet & Sour Concentrate	1 tsp (6 g)	10	0	0
Teriyaki Korean	1 tbsp (0.6 oz)	30	0	0
Just Rite				
Hot Dog	2 oz	60	tr	7
Ka-Me				
Black Bean Sauce	1 tbsp (0.5 oz)	10	1	0
Chili Sauce Hot Garlic	1 tbsp (0.5 oz)	15	1	0
Duck Sauce	2 tbsp (1 oz)	80	0	0
Fish Sauce	1 tbsp (0.5 fl oz)	10	0	0
Hoisin Sauce	2 tbsp (1 oz)	45	1	0
Hot Sauce	1 tsp (5 g)	0	0	0
Lemon Sauce	1 tbsp (0.5 oz)	45	0	0
Mandarin Orange Sauce	2 tbsp (1 oz)	80	0	0
Oyster Sauce	1 tbsp (0.5 fl oz)	10	0	0
Plum	2 tbsp (1 fl oz)	80	0	0
Stir Fry Sauce	1 tbsp	10	0	0
Sweet & Sour	2 tbsp (1 fl oz)	50	0	0
Szechuan	1 tbsp (0.5 oz)	20	2	0
Tamari	1 tbsp (0.5 fl oz)	10	0	0
Tempura Sauce	2 tbsp (1 fl oz)	15	0	0
Teriyaki Sauce	1 tbsp (0.5 fl oz)	10	0	0
Kikkoman				
Stir-Fry	1 tbsp	16	1	1
Sweet & Sour	1 tbsp	19	tr	tr
Teriyaki	1 tbsp	15	0	0
Kraft				
Sandwich Spread & Burger Sauce	1 tbsp (0.5 oz)	50	0	<5
Sweet'n Sour	2 tbsp (1.3 oz)	80	0	0

FOOD	PORTION	CALS.	FIB.	CHOL.
Kraft (CONT.)				
Tartar Sauce Nonfat	2 tbsp (1.1 oz)	25	tr	0
La Choy				
Duck Sauce Sweet & Sour	1 tbsp	25	tr	0
Sweet & Sour	1 tbsp	25	tr	0
Lawry's				
Teriyaki Marinade	2 tbsp	72	tr	0
Lea & Perrins				
Worcestershire	1 tsp	5	—	0
Worcestershire White Wine	1 tsp	4	—	0
Manwich				
Mexican	2.5 oz	35	1	0
Sloppy Joe	2.5 oz	40	1	0
Marzetti				
Teriyaki Stir-Fry	2 tbsp (1.1 oz)	48	tr	tr
	2 tbsp	80	0	0
McIlhenny				
7 Spice Chili	2 tbsp (1.1 oz)	48	tr	tr
Tabasco	2 tbsp (1.1 fl oz)	16	1	tr
	1 tsp	1	tr	tr
Mrs. Dash				
Steak	1 tbsp	17	—	0
Newman's Own				
Bandito Diavalo Spicy	4 oz	70	—	0
Old El Paso				
Enchilada Green	2 tbsp	11	—	0
Enchilada Hot	¼ cup	30	—	0
Enchilada Mild	¼ cup	25	—	0
Picante Thick'n Chunky Hot	2 tbsp	10	—	0
Picante Thick'n Chunky Medium	2 tbsp	10	—	0
Picante Thick'n Chunky Mild	2 tbsp	10	—	0
Taco Hot	1 tbsp	5	—	0
Taco Medium	1 tbsp	5	—	0
Taco Mild	1 tbsp	5	—	0
Tomatoes & Jalapenos	¼ cup	11	1	0
Tomatoes & Green Chilies	¼ cup	10	—	0
Ortega				
Taco Thick & Smooth Hot	1 tbsp	8	0	0
Taco Thick & Smooth Mild	1 tbsp	8	0	0
Taco Western Style	1 oz	8	—	0
Pace				
Picante	2 tbsp (1 fl oz)	7	tr	0
Progresso				
Alfredo	½ cup	340	—	95
Primavera Creamy	½ cup	190	1	54

FOOD	PORTION	CALS.	FIB.	CHOL.
Red Wing				
Chili Sauce	1 tbsp (0.6 oz)	20	0	0
Seafood Cocktail	¼ cup (2 oz)	90	0	0
Sauce Arturo	¼ cup (2.2 fl oz)	50	0	0
Sauceworks				
Cocktail	¼ cup (2.3 oz)	60	tr	0
Sweet'n Sour	2 tbsp (1.2 oz)	60	0	0
Tartar	2 tbsp (1.1 oz)	100	0	10
Tartar Natural Lemon & Herb	2 tbsp (1 oz)	150	0	15
Simmer Chef				
Golden Honey Mustard	½ cup (4 fl oz)	150	1	0
Hearty Onion & Mushroom	½ cup (4 fl oz)	50	1	0
Tabasco				
Picante	2 tbsp (1.5 oz)	17	1	0
Trappey				
Indi-Pep West Indian Style Pepper Sauce	1 tsp (0.1 oz)	1	tr	0
Mexi Pep Louisiana Hot Sauce	1 tsp (0.1 oz)	tr	tr	0
Pepper Sauce	1 tsp (0.2 oz)	1	tr	0
Red Devil Buffalo Style Hot Sauce	1 tsp (0.1 oz)	1	tr	0
Red Devil Cayenne Pepper Sauce	1 tsp (0.1 oz)	1	tr	0
Worcestershire Chef Magic	1 tsp (0.1 oz)	3	tr	0
Watkins				
Beef Marinade	¼ tbsp (2 g)	5	0	0
Calypso Hot Pepper Sauce	1 tsp (5 g)	10	0	0
Carribean Red Pepper Sauce	1 tsp (5 g)	10	0	0
Chicken & Pork Marinade	¼ tbsp (2 g)	5	0	0
Fish & Seafood Marinade	¼ tbsp (2 g)	10	0	0
Inferno Hot Pepper Sauce	2 tbsp (1 oz)	35	1	0
Weight Watchers				
Tartar	1 tbsp	35	—	5
Wise				
Picante	2 tbsp	12	—	0
teriyaki	1 tbsp	15	—	0
teriyaki	1 oz	30	—	0
SHELF-STABLE				
Cheez Whiz				
Cheese Sauce With Mild Salsa Zap-A-Pack	2 tbsp (1.2 oz)	90	0	20
Zap-A-Pack	2 tbsp (1.2 oz)	90	0	20

SAUERKRAUT
CANNED

Claussen	½ cup	17	—	0

FOOD	PORTION	CALS.	FIB.	CHOL.
Del Monte	½ cup (4.2 oz)	15	2	0
Eden				
Organic	½ cup (3.9 oz)	25	3	0
Hebrew National				
Gallon Kraut	½ cup	25	—	0
S&W	½ cup	25	—	0
Seneca	2 tbsp	5	1	0
SnowFloss				
Kraut	4 oz	28	1	0
Kraut Bavarian Style	4 oz	64	1	0
Vlasic				
Old Fashioned	1 oz	4	—	0
canned	½ cup	22	—	0

SAUERKRAUT JUICE

| *S&W* | 4 oz | 14 | — | 0 |

SAUSAGE

(see also HOT DOG, SAUSAGE SUBSTITUTES)

Aidells				
Andouille Cajun Cooked	1 (3.5 oz)	220	—	40
Burmese Curry Cooked	1 (3.5 oz)	220	—	20
Chicken & Apple Fresh	1 (1.9 oz)	110	—	20
Chicken & Apple Smoked	1 (3.5 oz)	220	0	30
Chicken & Turkey New Mexico Smoked	1 (3.5 oz)	220	—	40
Chicken & Turkey Thai Fresh	1 (3.5 oz)	200	—	35
Chicken & Turkey Thai Smoked	1 (3.5 oz)	220	—	30
Chicken & Turkey With Sun-Dried Tomatoes & Basil Fresh	1 (3.5 oz)	200	—	35
Chicken & Turkey With Sun-Dried Tomatoes & Basil Smoked	1 (3.5 oz)	200	—	30
Creole Hot Cooked	1 (3.5 oz)	220	—	30
Duck & Turkey Smoked	1 (3.5 oz)	220	—	60
Hunter's Cooked	1 (3.5 oz)	240	—	35
Italain Mild Fresh	1 (3.5 oz)	230	—	40
Italian Hot Fresh	1 (3.5 oz)	230	—	40
Lamb & Beef With Rosemary Fresh	1 (3.5 oz)	220	—	35
Lemon Chicken Cooked	1 (3.5 oz)	220	—	35
Mexican Chorizo Beef Fresh	1 (3.5 oz)	400	—	70
Whiskey Fennel Cooked	1 (3.5 oz)	230	—	65

FOOD	PORTION	CALS.	FIB.	CHOL.
Armour				
Vienna Sausage 25% Less Fat	3 (1.9 oz)	130	—	50
Vienna Sausage In BBQ Sauce	3 (2.1 oz)	160	—	45
Vienna Sausage In Beef Stock	3 (1.9 oz)	170	—	50
Vienna Sausage In Hot Sauce	3 (2.1 oz)	170	—	50
Vienna Sausage Smoked	3 (1.9 oz)	170	—	50
Banner				
Sausage Tripe	2 oz	90	—	85
Bilinski's				
Chicken Italian With Peppers & Onions	1 (3 oz)	120	—	80
Golden Brown				
Beef	1	80	—	18
Mild	1	100	—	18
Spicy	1	100	—	18
Hebrew National				
Beef Knocks	1 (3 oz)	260	—	55
Polish Beef	1 link	240	—	50
Hormel				
Light & Lean 97 Dinner Smoked	2 oz	60	0	20
Pickled Hot	6 (2 oz)	140	0	40
Pickled Smoked	6 (2 oz)	140	0	40
Vienna	2 oz	140	0	45
Vienna Chicken	2 oz	90	0	55
Jimmy Dean				
Brick Sausage	2.5 oz	270	0	55
Bulk	2.5 oz	300	0	55
Hickory Smoked Dinner Sausage	2 oz	170	0	35
Pattie Pre-Cooked	1 (1.9 oz)	230	0	45
Polska Kielbasa	2 oz	170	0	35
Sage Pattie	1 (2 oz)	200	0	45
Sausage Pattie Raw	1 (2 oz)	200	0	40
Skinless Link	2 (2 oz)	200	0	45
Skinless Link	4 (2 oz)	200	0	45
Jones				
Brown & Serve Bacon	1	90	—	19
Brown & Serve Beef	1	90	—	18
Brown & Serve Light	1	60	—	16
Brown & Serve Regular	1	100	—	19
Cello Beef	1 slice (1 oz)	130	—	25

FOOD	PORTION	CALS.	FIB.	CHOL.
Jones (CONT.)				
Cello Hot Country	1 slice (1 oz)	110	—	24
Cello Original	1 slice (1 oz)	100	—	24
Dinner Link	1	280	—	48
Golden Brown Light Links	1	60	—	16
Golden Brown Mild Pattie	1	150	—	29
Italian	1	160	—	44
Light Link	1	70	—	21
Little Link	1	140	—	24
Patties	1	150	—	36
Scrapple	1 slice (1½ oz)	90	—	24
Scrapple	1 slice	90	—	24
Little Sizzlers				
Brown & Serve	2 patties (1.4 oz)	190	0	40
Brown & Serve	3 links (2.1 oz)	190	0	45
Cooked	3 links (1.4 oz)	210	0	45
Cooked	2 patties (2 oz)	250	0	50
Heat & Serve Pork cooked	3 links (1.4 oz)	210	0	45
Louis Rich				
Polska Kielbasa	2 oz	80	0	35
Turkey	2.5 oz	110	0	50
Turkey & Cheese Smoked	2 oz	90	0	35
Turkey Links	2 (2 oz)	90	0	45
Turkey Smoked	2 oz	90	0	35
Mr. Turkey				
Breakfast	2.5 oz	130	—	65
Hearty Blend Polish Kielbasa	1 oz	70	—	23
Hearty Blend Smoked	1 oz	70	—	23
Hot Smoked	1 oz	45	—	15
Italian Smoked	1 oz	45	—	15
Polish Kielbasa	1 oz	45	—	15
Smoked	1 oz	45	—	15
Old Smokehouse				
Summer Sausage	1 oz	110	0	30
Oscar Mayer				
Pork cooked	2 links (1.7 oz)	170	0	40
Smokies Beef	1 (1.5 oz)	120	0	25
Smokies Cheese	1 (1.5 oz)	130	0	30
Smokies Links	1 (1.5 oz)	130	0	25
Smokies Little	6 (2 oz)	170	0	35
Perdue				
Breakfast Links Turkey cooked	1 (1.3 oz)	40	—	19
Breakfast Patties Turkey cooked	1 (1.3 oz)	61	—	27
Hot Italian Turkey cooked	1 (2 oz)	94	—	43

FOOD	PORTION	CALS.	FIB.	CHOL.
Perdue (CONT.)				
Sweet Italian Turkey cooked	1 (2 oz)	94	—	43
Rudy's Farm				
Italian Mild	2.5 oz	240	0	50
Italian Hot	2.5 oz	240	0	50
Italian Mild Natural Casing	1 (2 oz)	190	0	40
Morning Right Link	3 (2.9 oz)	150	0	40
Morning Right Pattie	2 (2.9 oz)	150	0	40
Pattie Pre-Cooked	1 (1.4 oz)	100	1	35
Smoked	4 (2.1 oz)	200	0	40
Sweet Link	1 (3.9 oz)	380	0	80
Shofar				
Knockwurst Beef	1 (3 oz)	260	0	50
Tyson				
Country Pork	3.5 oz	320	—	49
Wampler Longacre				
Turkey	1 link (1 oz)	60	—	30
Turkey	1 pattie (2 oz)	120	—	60
bratwurst pork, cooked	1 link (3 oz)	256	—	51
bratwurst pork	1 oz	92	—	18
bratwurst pork & beef	1 link (2.5 oz)	226	—	44
country-style pork, cooked	1 link (½ oz)	48	—	11
country-style pork, cooked	1 patty (1 oz)	100	—	22
italian pork, cooked	1 (2.4 oz)	216	—	52
italian pork, cooked	1 (3 oz)	268	—	65
kielbasa pork	1 oz	88	—	19
knockwurst pork & beef	1 oz	87	—	16
knockwurst pork & beef	1 (2.4 oz)	209	—	39
polish pork	1 oz	92	—	20
polish pork	1 (8 oz)	739	—	158
pork, cooked	1 patty (1 oz)	100	—	22
pork, cooked	1 link (½ oz)	48	—	11
smoked beef cooked	1 sausage (1.4 oz)	134	—	29
smoked pork	1 sm link (½ oz)	62	—	11
smoked pork	1 link (2.4 oz)	265	—	46
smoked pork & beef	1 link (2.4 oz)	229	—	48
smoked pork & beef	1 sm link (½ oz)	54	—	11
vienna canned	1 (½ oz)	45	—	8
vienna canned	7 (4 oz)	315	—	59
TAKE-OUT				
pork	1 link (.5 oz)	48	—	11
pork	1 patty (1 oz)	100	—	22

FOOD	PORTION	CALS.	FIB.	CHOL.
SAUSAGE DISHES				
Jimmy Dean				
Italian Sausage & Mozzarella Sandwich	1 (4.5 oz)	380	2	40
SAUSAGE SUBSTITUTES				
LaLoma				
Linketts	2 (71 g)	140	—	0
Little Links	2 (46 g)	90	—	0
Lightlife				
Lean Links Breakfast	1.25 oz	69	—	0
Lean Links Italian	1.5 oz	83	—	0
White Wave				
Meatless Healthy Links	2 (1.6 oz)	140	3	0
SAVORY				
ground	1 tsp	4	—	0
SCALLOP				
FRESH				
raw	3 oz	75	—	28
FROZEN				
Mrs. Paul's				
Fried	2 oz	160	—	10
HOME RECIPE				
breaded & fried	2 lg	67	—	19
TAKE-OUT				
breaded & fried	6 (5 oz)	386	—	107
SCONE				
Finnegan's				
Irish Raisin	1 (2.7 oz)	90	1	0
HOME RECIPE				
apricot scone	1	232	—	34
SCROD				
FROZEN				
Gorton's				
Microwave Entree Baked	1 pkg	320	—	80
SEA BASS				
(*see* BASS)				
SEATROUT				
(*see* TROUT)				
SEAWEED				
Eden				
Agar Agar Bars	1 tbsp (2.5 oz)	10	2	0

FOOD	PORTION	CALS.	FIB.	CHOL.
Eden (CONT.)				
Agar Agar Flakes	1 tbsp (2.5 oz)	10	2	0
Arame	½ cup (0.3 oz)	30	7	0
Hiziki	½ cup (0.3 oz)	30	6	0
Kombu	3.5 in piece (3.3 g)	10	1	0
Nori	1 sheet (2.5 g)	10	1	0
Sushi Nori	1 sheet (2.5 g)	10	1	0
Wakame	½ cup (0.3 oz)	25	4	0
Wakame Flakes	½ cup (0.3 oz)	25	4	0
Maine Coast				
Alaria	⅓ cup (7 g)	18	2	0
Dulse	⅓ cup (7 g)	18	2	0
Kelp	⅓ cup (7 g)	17	3	0
Kelp Crunch	1 bar (1 oz)	129	2	0
Kelp Crunch Peanut-Raisin	1 bar (1 oz)	129	2	0
Laver	⅓ cup (7 g)	22	3	0
Sea Seasoning Dulse	1 g	3	—	0
Sea Seasoning Dulse With Celery	1 g	3	—	0
Sea Seasoning Dulse With Garlic	1 g	3	—	0
Sea Seasoning Dulse With Sesame	1 g	3	—	0
Sea Seasoning Kelp	1 g	3	—	0
Sea Seasoning Kelp With Cayenne	1 g	3	—	0
Sea Seasoning Nori	1 g	3	—	0
Sea Seasoning Nori With Ginger	1 g	3	—	0
agar dried	1 oz	87	—	0
agar fresh	1 oz	tr	—	0
irishmoss fresh	1 oz	14	—	0
kelp fresh	1 oz	12	—	0
kombu fresh	1 oz	12	—	0
laver fresh	1 oz	10	—	0
nori fresh	1 oz	10	—	0
spirulina dried	1 oz	83	—	0
spirulina fresh	1 oz	7	—	0
tangle fresh	1 oz	12	—	0
wakame fresh	1 oz	13	—	0

SEITAN
(*see* WHEAT)

SEMOLINA
dry	½ cup	303	3	0

FOOD	PORTION	CALS.	FIB.	CHOL.
SESAME				
Arrowhead				
Sesame Tahini	1 oz	170	—	0
Casbah				
Tahini Sauce Mix as prep	¼ cup	160	tr	0
Eden				
Sesame Shake	½ tsp (1.5 g)	10	tr	0
Sesame Shake Garlic	½ tsp (1.5 g)	10	tr	0
Sesame Shake Organic Seaweed	½ tsp (1.5 g)	10	tr	0
Erewhon				
Sesame Butter	2 tbsp (32 g)	190	—	0
Sesame Tahini	2 tbsp (32 g)	200	—	0
Joyva				
Tahini	2 tbsp (1 oz)	200	1	0
Stone-Buhr				
Seeds Raw	4 tsp (1 oz)	180	1	0
seeds	1 tsp	16	—	0
seeds dried	1 tbsp	52	—	0
seeds dried	1 cup	825	—	0
seeds roasted & toasted	1 oz	161	—	0
sesame butter	1 tbsp	95	—	0
sesame crunch candy	20 pieces (1.2 oz)	181	—	0
sesame crunch candy	1 oz	146	—	0
sesame sticks	1 oz	153	—	0
sesame sticks unsalted	1 oz	153	—	0
tahini from roasted & toasted kernels	1 tbsp	89	—	0
tahini from stone ground kernels	1 tbsp	86	—	0
tahini from unroasted kernels	1 tbsp	85	—	0
SESBANIA				
flower	1	1	—	0
flowers	1 cup	5	—	0
flowers cooked	1 cup	23	—	0
SHAD				
roe raw	3½ oz	130	—	360
SHALLOTS				
dried	1 tbsp	3	—	0
raw chopped	1 tbsp	7	—	0
SHARK				
batter-dipped & fried	3 oz	194	—	50
raw	3 oz	111	—	43

FOOD	PORTION	CALS.	FIB.	CHOL.

SHELLFISH
(see individual names, SHELLFISH SUBSTITUTES)

SHELLFISH SUBSTITUTES
Louis Kemp

Crab Delights Chunk Style	2 oz	54	—	10
Lobster Delights	2 oz	60	—	10
Maryland Style Cakes	2.5 oz	154	—	26
Ocean Magic				
Imitation King Crab	3 oz	80	—	15
crab imitation	3 oz	87	—	17
scallop imitation	3 oz	84	—	18
shrimp imitation	3 oz	86	—	31
surimi	1 oz	28	—	8
surimi	3 oz	84	—	25

SHELLIE BEANS
CANNED

shellie beans	½ cup	37	—	0

SHERBET
(see also ICES AND ICE POPS)

Bresler's				
All Flavors	3.5 oz	140	—	6
Hood				
Lime Orange Lemon	½ cup (3.1 oz)	120	0	<5
Orange	½ cup (3.1 oz)	120	0	<5
Rainbow Swirl	½ cup (3.1 oz)	120	0	<5
Raspberry Orange Lime	½ cup (3.1 oz)	120	0	<5
Sealtest				
Lime	½ cup (3 oz)	130	0	5
Orange	½ cup (3 oz)	130	0	5
Rainbow Orange Red Raspberry Lime	½ cup (3 oz)	130	0	5
Red Raspberry	½ cup (3 oz)	130	0	5
orange	½ cup (4 fl oz)	132	—	5
orange	½ gal	2158	—	113
orange	1 bar (2.75 fl oz)	91	—	3
orange home recipe	½ cup	120	—	9

SHRIMP
CANNED

canned	3 oz	102	—	147
canned	1 cup	154	—	222
FRESH				
cooked	3 oz	84	—	166

FOOD	PORTION	CALS.	FIB.	CHOL.
cooked	4 large	22	—	43
raw	4 large	30	—	43
raw	3 oz	90	—	130
FROZEN				
Gorton's				
Microwave Crunchy Shrimp	5 oz	380	—	65
Mrs. Paul's				
Entrees Light Seafood & Clams With Linguini	10 oz	240	—	40
READY-TO-USE				
American Original Foods				
Fried	4 oz	253	—	27
TAKE-OUT				
breaded & fried	4 large	73	—	53
breaded & fried	3 oz	206	—	150
breaded & fried	6 to 8 (6 oz)	454	—	201
jambalaya	¾ cup	188	8	50
SMELT				
rainbow cooked	3 oz	106	—	76
rainbow raw	3 oz	83	—	60
SNACKS				
(*see also* CHIPS, FRUIT SNACKS, NUTS MIXED, POPCORN, PRETZELS)				
Bakem-ets	21 pieces (1 oz)	160	—	25
Hot'N Spicy	21 pieces (1 oz)	150	—	25
Cheetos				
Cheddar Valley	26 pieces (1 oz)	160	1	0
Crunchy	26 pieces (1 oz)	150	1	0
Curls	15 pieces (1 oz)	150	1	0
Flamin' Hot	26 pieces (1 oz)	150	1	0
Light	38 pieces (1 oz)	140	1	0
Paws	16 pieces (1 oz)	160	1	0
Puffed Ball	38 pieces (1 oz)	160	1	0
Puffs	33 pieces (1 oz)	160	1	0
Chex				
Snack Mix Barbeque	½ cup (1.1 oz)	130	1	0
Snack Mix Cool Sour Cream And Onion	½ cup (1 oz)	130	2	0
Snack Mix Golden Cheddar	½ cup (1 oz)	130	1	0
Snack Mix Traditional	⅔ cup (1.2 oz)	150	2	0
Combos				
Cheddar	1 pkg (1.7 oz)	250	1	5
Cheddar Cheese Cracker	1 oz	140	0	5
Cheddar Cheese Pretzel	1 pkg (1.8 oz)	240	1	5

FOOD	PORTION	CALS.	FIB.	CHOL.
Combos (CONT.)				
Cheddar Cheese Pretzel	1 oz	130	0	0
Chili Cheese With Corn Shell	1 oz	140	1	0
Chili Cheese w/ Corn Shell	1 pkg (1.7 oz)	230	2	5
Mustard Pretzel	1 pkg (1.8 oz)	230	1	0
Mustard Pretzel	1 oz	130	1	0
Nacho	1 pkg (1.8 oz)	230	1	0
Nacho Cheese Pretzel	1 oz	130	1	0
Nacho Cheese With Tortilla Shell	1 oz	140	1	0
Nacho Cheese w/ Tortilla Shell	1 pkg (1.7 oz)	230	1	0
Pepperoni & Cheese Pizza	1 oz	140	0	5
Pepperoni & Cheese Pizza	1 pkg (1.7 oz)	240	1	5
Pizzeria Pretzel	1 pkg (1.8 oz)	230	1	0
Pizzeria Pretzel	1 oz	130	1	0
Tortilla Ranch	1 oz	140	1	5
Tortilla Ranch	1 bag (1.7 oz)	240	1	5
Cornnuts				
Barbecue	1 oz	120	2	0
Nacho Cheese	1 oz	120	2	0
Original	1 oz	120	2	0
Original	1 pkg (2 oz)	260	4	0
Picante	1 oz	120	2	0
Ranch	1 oz	120	2	0
Doo Dads	1 oz	130	—	0
Eagle				
Cheese Crunch	1 oz	160	—	0
Energy Food Factory				
Poprice Cheddar Cheese	½ oz	60	—	0
Poprice Herb & Garlic	½ oz	50	—	0
Poprice Lite	½ oz	50	—	0
Poprice Original No Salt	½ oz	45	—	0
Estee				
Snack Crisps Apple Cinnamon	27 crisps (1 oz)	130	1	0
Snack Crisps Apple Cinnamon	1 pkg (0.66 oz)	90	tr	0
Snack Crisps Chocolate	30 crisps (1 oz)	130	2	0
Snack Crisps Chocolate	1 pkg (0.66 oz)	90	1	0
Snack Crisps Lemon	30 (1 oz)	130	tr	5
Snack Crisps Lemon	1 pkg (0.66 oz)	90	tr	0
Snack Crisps Ranch	30 (1 oz)	130	tr	5
Snack Crisps Ranch	1 pkg (0.6 oz)	90	0	5
Snack Crisps White Cheddar	1 pkg (0.6 oz)	90	tr	5
Snack Crisps With Cheddar	27 crisps (1 oz)	130	tr	5

FOOD	PORTION	CALS.	FIB.	CHOL.
Frito Lay				
Corn Nuggets Toasted	1.38 oz	170	—	0
Funyums				
Onion Rings	11 pieces (1 oz)	140	1	0
Handi-Snacks				
Peanut Butter'n Crackers	1 pkg (1.1 oz)	180	1	0
Peanut Butter'n Grahamsticks	1 pkg (1.1 oz)	170	1	0
Health Valley				
Cheddar Lites	0.75 oz	40	tr	tr
Cheddar Lites With Green Onion	0.75 oz	40	tr	0
Lance				
Cheese Balls	1 pkg (32 g)	190	—	5
Crunchy Cheese Twists	1 pkg (42 g)	260	—	0
Gold-N-Chees	1 pkg (39 g)	180	—	5
Pork Skins	1 pkg (14 g)	80	—	20
Pork Skins BBQ	1 pkg (14 g)	80	—	20
Munchos				
	16 pieces (1 oz)	160	—	0
Snyder's				
Cheddar Cheese Twists	1 oz	150	—	0
Kruncheez	1 oz	160	—	0
Onion Toasters	1 oz	150	3	0
Snack Mix	1 oz	170	tr	0
Sopaipillas Apple & Cinnamon	1 oz	150	1	0
Ultra Slim-Fast				
Lite N' Tasty Cheese Curls	1 oz	110	3	0
Weight Watchers				
Cheese Curls	½ oz	70	—	0
oriental mix	1 oz	155	—	0
pork skins	½ oz	77	—	14
pork skins	1 oz	154	—	27
pork skins barbecue	½ oz	76	—	16
pork skins barbecue	1 oz	152	—	33
trail mix	1 cup (5.3 oz)	693	—	0
trail mix	1 oz	131	—	0
trail mix tropical	1 oz	115	—	0

SNAIL

cooked	3 oz	233	—	110
raw	3 oz	117	—	55

SNAP BEANS
CANNED

green	½ cup	13	1	0
green low sodium	½ cup	13	1	0

FOOD	PORTION	CALS.	FIB.	CHOL.
italian	½ cup	13	1	0
italian low sodium	½ cup	13	1	0
yellow	½ cup	13	1	0
yellow low sodium	½ cup	13	1	0
FRESH				
green cooked	½ cup	22	—	0
green raw	½ cup	17	1	0
yellow cooked	½ cup	22	—	0
yellow raw	½ cup	17	—	0
FROZEN				
green cooked	½ cup	18	—	0
italian cooked	½ cup	18	—	0
yellow cooked	½ cup	18	—	0
SNAPPER				
cooked	1 fillet (6 oz)	217	—	80
cooked	3 oz	109	—	40
raw	3 oz	85	—	31
SODA				
(see also DRINK MIXERS, MINERAL/BOTTLED WATER)				
7 Up	1 oz	12	—	0
Cherry	1 oz	13	—	0
Cherry Diet	1 oz	tr	—	0
Diet	1 oz	tr	—	0
Gold	1 oz	13	—	0
Gold Diet	1 oz	tr	—	0
Barrelhead				
Root Beer	8 fl oz	110	0	0
Burst				
Cola Strawberry	8 fl oz	117	—	0
Canada Dry				
Birch Beer Brown	8 fl oz	110	0	0
Birch Beer Clear	8 fl oz	110	0	0
Black Cherry Wishniak	8 fl oz	130	0	0
Cactus Cooler	8 fl oz	110	0	0
California Strawberry	8 fl oz	110	0	0
Club	8 fl oz	0	0	0
Club Sodium Free	8 fl oz	0	0	0
Concord Grape	8 fl oz	120	0	0
Diet Ginger Ale	8 fl oz	0	0	0
Diet Ginger Ale Cherry	8 fl oz	0	0	0
Diet Ginger Ale Cranberry	8 fl oz	0	0	0
Diet Ginger Ale Lemon	8 fl oz	5	0	0
Diet Tonic Water	8 fl oz	0	0	0

FOOD	PORTION	CALS.	FIB.	CHOL.
Canada Dry (CONT.)				
Diet Tonic Water Twist Of Lime	8 fl oz	0	0	0
Ginger Ale	8 fl oz	100	0	0
Ginger Ale Cherry	8 fl oz	110	0	0
Ginger Ale Cranberry	8 fl oz	100	0	0
Ginger Ale Golden	8 fl oz	100	0	0
Ginger Ale Lemon	8 fl oz	100	0	0
Half & Half	8 fl oz	110	0	0
Hi-Spot	8 fl oz	110	0	0
Island Lime	8 fl oz	140	0	0
Jamaica Cola	8 fl oz	110	0	0
Lemon Sour	8 fl oz	100	0	0
Peach	8 fl oz	120	0	0
Pina Pineapple	8 fl oz	110	0	0
Seltzer	8 fl oz	0	0	0
Seltzer Cherry	8 fl oz	0	0	0
Seltzer Cranberry Lime	8 fl oz	0	0	0
Seltzer Grapefruit	8 fl oz	0	0	0
Seltzer Lemon Lime	8 fl oz	0	0	0
Seltzer Mandarin Orange	8 fl oz	0	0	0
Seltzer Peach	8 fl oz	0	0	0
Seltzer Raspberry	8 fl oz	0	0	0
Seltzer Strawberry	8 fl oz	0	0	0
Seltzer Tropical	8 fl oz	0	0	0
Sunripe Orange	8 fl oz	140	0	0
Tahitian Treat	8 fl oz	150	0	0
Tonic Water	8 fl oz	100	0	0
Tonic Water Twist Of Lime	8 fl oz	100	0	0
Vanilla Cream	8 fl oz	120	0	0
Vichy Water	8 fl oz	0	0	0
Wild Cherry	8 fl oz	110	0	0
Clearly Canadian	8 fl oz	0	—	0
Coca-Cola				
Cherry	8 fl oz	104	—	0
Classic	8 fl oz	97	—	0
Classic Caffeine-Free	8 fl oz	97	—	0
Coke II	8 fl oz	105	—	0
Diet Cherry	8 fl oz	1	—	0
Diet Coke	8 fl oz	1	—	0
Diet Coke Caffeine-Free	8 fl oz	1	—	0
Cott				
Cola	8 fl oz	110	0	0
Ginger Ale	8 fl oz	90	0	0
Grape	8 fl oz	130	0	0

FOOD	PORTION	CALS.	FIB.	CHOL.
Cott (CONT.)				
Orange	8 fl oz	140	0	0
Pineapple	8 fl oz	130	0	0
Punch	8 fl oz	130	0	0
Seltzer	8 fl oz	0	0	0
Crush				
Cherry	8 fl oz	140	0	0
Grape	8 fl oz	110	0	0
Orange	8 fl oz	140	0	0
Orange Diet	8 fl oz	0	0	0
Pineapple	8 fl oz	140	0	0
Strawberry	8 fl oz	130	0	0
Tropical Fruit Punch	1 bottle (10 fl oz)	180	0	0
Tropical Fruit Punch	1 can (11.5 fl oz)	200	—	0
Diet Pepsi	8 fl oz	1	—	0
Diet Rite				
Black Cherry Salt/Sodium Free	8 fl oz	2	—	0
Cola	8 fl oz	1	—	0
Cola Caffeine/Sugar Free	8 fl oz	1	—	0
Cola Salt/Sodium Free	8 fl oz	1	—	0
Fruit Punch Salt/Sodium Free	8 fl oz	2	—	0
Golden Peach Salt/Sodium Free	8 fl oz	2	—	0
Key Lime Salt/Sodium Free	8 fl oz	7	—	0
Pink Grapefruit Salt/Sodium Free	8 fl oz	2	—	0
Red Raspberry Salt/Sodium Free	8 fl oz	3	—	0
Tangerine Salt/Sodium Free	8 fl oz	2	—	0
White Grape Salt/Sodium Free	8 fl oz	1	—	0
Dr Pepper	1 oz	13	—	0
Diet	1 oz	tr	—	0
Pepper Free	1 oz	12	—	0
Pepper Free Diet	1 oz	tr	—	0
Dr. Nehi	8 fl oz	100	—	0
Fanta				
Ginger Ale	8 fl oz	86	—	0
Grape	8 fl oz	117	—	0
Orange	8 fl oz	118	—	0
Root Beer	8 fl oz	111	—	0
Fresca	8 fl oz	3	—	0
Health Valley				
Ginger Ale	12 oz	153	0	0
Rootbeer Old Fashioned	12 oz	120	—	0
Sarsaparilla Rootbeer	12 oz	153	—	0

FOOD	PORTION	CALS.	FIB.	CHOL.
Health Valley (CONT.)				
Wild Berry	12 oz	142	—	0
Hires				
Cream	8 fl oz	130	0	0
Cream Soda Diet	8 fl oz	0	0	0
Original Mocha	8 fl oz	100	0	0
Original Mocha Diet	8 fl oz	5	0	0
Root Beer	8 fl oz	130	0	0
Root Beer Diet	8 fl oz	0	0	0
Kick	8 fl oz	120	—	0
Like				
Cola	1 oz	13	—	0
Cola Sugar Free	1 oz	tr	—	0
Lucozade	7 oz	136	0	0
Manischewitz				
Seltzer No Salt Added No Calories	8 fl oz	0	—	0
Mello Yellow	8 fl oz	119	—	0
Diet	8 fl oz	4	—	0
Minute Maid	8 fl oz	110	—	0
Berry	8 fl oz	111	—	0
Diet Orange	8 fl oz	2	—	0
Fruit Punch	8 fl oz	117	—	0
Grape	8 fl oz	121	—	0
Grapefruit	8 fl oz	108	—	0
Orange	8 fl oz	118	—	0
Peach	8 fl oz	110	—	0
Pineapple	8 fl oz	109	—	0
Raspberry	8 fl oz	111	—	0
Strawberry	8 fl oz	122	—	0
Mountain Dew	8 fl oz	118	—	0
Diet	8 fl oz	2	—	0
Mr. PiBB	6 oz	97	—	0
Diet	8 fl oz	1	—	0
Mug				
Cream	8 fl oz	122	—	0
Diet Cream	8 fl oz	2	—	0
Diet Root Beer	8 fl oz	1	—	0
Root Beer	8 fl oz	141	—	0
Nehi				
Cream	8 fl oz	120	—	0
Fruit Punch	8 fl oz	120	—	0
Ginger Ale	8 fl oz	90	—	0
Grape	8 fl oz	120	—	0

FOOD	PORTION	CALS.	FIB.	CHOL.
Nehi (CONT.)				
Orange	8 fl oz	130	—	0
Peach	8 fl oz	130	—	0
Pineapple	8 fl oz	130	—	0
Quinine Water	8 fl oz	90	—	0
Root Beer	8 fl oz	120	—	0
Strawberry	8 fl oz	120	—	0
Wild Red	8 fl oz	120	—	0
Old Colony				
Grape	8 fl oz	140	0	0
Orangina	6 fl oz	80	—	0
Pepsi-Cola	8 fl oz	105	—	0
Caffeine Free	8 fl oz	105	—	0
Diet Caffeine Free	8 fl oz	1	—	0
Ramblin' Root Beer	8 fl oz	120	—	0
Razing Razberry				
Cola	8 fl oz	117	—	0
Royal Crown				
Caffeine Free Cola	8 fl oz	110	—	0
Cherry	8 fl oz	110	—	0
Cola	8 fl oz	100	—	0
Diet	8 fl oz	1	—	0
Diet	8 fl oz	1	—	0
Diet Caffeine Free	8 fl oz	1	—	0
Diet Cranberry Apple Salt/ Sodium Free	8 fl oz	2	—	0
Diet Cranberry Salt/Sodium Free	8 fl oz	2	—	0
Royal Mistic				
'N Juice Black Cherry	12 fl oz	146	—	0
'N Juice Peach Vanilla	12 fl oz	146	—	0
'N Juice Tangerine Orange	12 fl oz	146	—	0
'N Juice Tropical Supreme	12 fl oz	152	—	0
'N Juice Wild Berry	12 fl oz	156	—	0
Caribbean Fruit Punch	16 fl oz	230	—	0
Grape Strawberry	16 fl oz	230	—	0
Sparkling With Raspberry Boysenberry	11.1 fl oz	112	—	0
Sparkling Diet With Lime Kiwi	11.1 fl oz	0	—	0
Sparkling Diet With Raspberry Boysenberry	11.1 fl oz	0	—	0
Sparkling Diet With Royal Peach	11.1 fl oz	0	—	0
Sparkling Diet With Wild Cherry	11.1 fl oz	0	—	0

FOOD	PORTION	CALS.	FIB.	CHOL.
Royal Mistic (CONT.)				
Sparkling With Lime Kiwi	11.1 fl oz	112	—	0
Sparkling With Mandarin Orange Pineappple	11.1 fl oz	120	—	0
Sparkling With Mango Passion	11.1 fl oz	112	—	0
Sparkling With Royal Peach	11.1 fl oz	112	—	0
Sparkling With Wild Cherry	11.1 fl oz	112	—	0
Schweppes				
Bitter Lemon	8 fl oz	110	0	0
Club	8 fl oz	0	0	0
Club Sodium Free	8 fl oz	0	0	0
Diet Ginger Ale Dry Grape	8 fl oz	2	0	0
Diet Ginger Ale Raspberry	8 fl oz	0	0	0
Ginger Ale	8 fl oz	90	0	0
Ginger Ale Dry Grape	8 fl oz	100	0	0
Ginger Ale Raspberry	8 fl oz	100	0	0
Ginger Ale Diet	8 fl oz	0	0	0
Ginger Beer	8 fl oz	100	0	0
Grape	8 fl oz	130	0	0
Grapefruit	8 fl oz	110	0	0
Lemon Sour	8 fl oz	110	0	0
Lemon-Lime	8 fl oz	100	0	0
Seltzer Black Berry	8 fl oz	0	0	0
Seltzer Lemon	8 fl oz	0	0	0
Seltzer Lemon Lime	8 fl oz	0	0	0
Seltzer Lime	8 fl oz	0	0	0
Seltzer Orange	8 fl oz	0	0	0
Seltzer Peaches & Cream	8 fl oz	0	0	0
Seltzer Raspberry	8 fl oz	0	0	0
Tonic Citrus	8 fl oz	90	0	0
Tonic Cranberry	8 fl oz	90	0	0
Tonic Raspberry	8 fl oz	90	0	0
Tonic Water Diet	8 fl oz	0	0	0
Shasta				
Black Cherry	12 oz	162	—	0
Cherry Cola	12 oz	140	—	0
Citrus Mist	12 oz	170	—	0
Club	12 oz	0	—	0
Cola	8 oz	98	—	0
Cola	12 oz	147	—	0
Collins	12 oz	118	—	0
Creme	12 oz	154	—	0
Diet Birch Beer	12 oz	4	—	0
Diet Cola	8 oz	0	—	0

FOOD	PORTION	CALS.	FIB.	CHOL.
Shasta (CONT.)				
Diet Ginger Ale	8 oz	0	—	0
Diet Lemon Lime	8 oz	0	—	0
Dr. Diablo	12 oz	140	—	0
Free Cola	12 oz	151	—	0
Fruit Punch	12 oz	173	—	0
Ginger Ale	8 oz	80	—	0
Ginger Ale	12 oz	120	—	0
Grape	12 oz	177	—	0
Lemon Lime	12 oz	146	—	0
Lemon Lime	8 oz	97	—	0
Orange	12 oz	177	—	0
Red Berry	12 oz	158	—	0
Red Pop	12 oz	158	—	0
Root Beer	12 oz	154	—	0
Strawberry	12 oz	147	—	0
Tonic Water	12 oz	0	—	0
Slice				
Diet Lemon Lime	8 fl oz	5	—	0
Diet Mandarin	8 fl oz	5	—	0
Lemon Lime	8 fl oz	100	—	0
Mandarin Orange	8 fl oz	128	—	0
Red	8 fl oz	128	—	0
Snapple				
Amazin' Grape	8 fl oz	120	—	0
Cherry Lime Ricky	8 fl oz	110	—	0
Creme D'Vanilla	8 fl oz	130	—	0
French Cherry	8 fl oz	120	—	0
Kiwi Peach	8 fl oz	120	—	0
Kiwi Strawberry	8 fl oz	130	—	0
Mango Madness	8 fl oz	130	—	0
Passion Supreme	8 fl oz	120	—	0
Peach Melba	8 fl oz	120	—	0
Raspberry	8 fl oz	120	—	0
Seltzer Black Cherry	8 fl oz	0	—	0
Seltzer Lemon Lime	8 fl oz	0	—	0
Seltzer Original	8 fl oz	0	—	0
Seltzer Tangerine	8 fl oz	0	—	0
Tru Rool Beer	8 fl oz	110	—	0
Sprite	8 fl oz	100	—	0
Diet	8 fl oz	3	—	0
Sundrop	8 fl oz	140	0	0
Cherry	8 fl oz	130	0	0
Diet	8 fl oz	5	0	0

FOOD	PORTION	CALS.	FIB.	CHOL.
Sunkist				
Cactus Cooler	8 fl oz	110	0	0
Cherry	8 fl oz	140	0	0
Diet Citrus	8 fl oz	0	0	0
Diet Orange	8 fl oz	5	0	0
Fruit Punch	8 fl oz	130	0	0
Orange	8 fl oz	140	0	0
Peach	8 fl oz	120	0	0
Pineapple	8 fl oz	140	0	0
Strawberry	8 fl oz	140	0	0
TAB	8 fl oz	1	—	0
Tropical Chill				
Cola	8 fl oz	117	—	0
Diet	8 fl oz	1	—	0
Upper 10	8 fl oz	100	—	0
Diet Salt/Sodium Free	8 fl oz	3	—	0
Salt Free	8 fl oz	100	—	0
Welch's				
Sparkling Apple	12 oz	180	—	0
Sparkling Grape	12 oz	180	—	0
Sparkling Orange	12 oz	180	—	0
Sparkling Strawberry	12 oz	180	—	0
Wink	8 fl oz	130	0	0
Diet	8 fl oz	5	0	0
Yoo-Hoo	9 fl oz	150	tr	0
club	12 oz	0	—	0
cola	12 oz	151	—	0
cream	12 oz	191	—	0
diet cola	12 oz	2	—	0
diet cola w/ nutrasweet	12 oz	2	—	0
diet cola w/ saccharin	12 oz	2	—	0
ginger ale	12 oz can	124	—	0
grape	12 oz	161	—	0
lemon lime	12 oz	149	—	0
orange	12 oz	177	—	0
pepper type	12 oz	151	—	0
quinine	12 oz	125	—	0
root beer	12 oz	152	—	0
tonic water	12 oz	125	—	0
SOLDIER BEANS				
DRIED				
Bean Cuisine	½ cup	115	5	0

FOOD	PORTION	CALS.	FIB.	CHOL.
SOLE				
FRESH				
cooked	3 oz	99	—	58
cooked	1 fillet (4.5 oz)	148	—	86
raw	3½ oz	90	—	50
FROZEN				
Gorton's				
Microwave Entree In Lemon Butter	1 pkg	380	—	120
Microwave Entree In Wine Sauce	1 pkg	180	—	90
Mrs. Paul's				
Light Fillets	1 fillet	240	—	50
Van De Kamp's				
Light Fillets	1 piece	250	—	25
Natural Fillets	4 oz	100	—	35
TAKE-OUT				
battered & fried	3.2 oz	211	—	31
breaded & fried	3.2 oz	211	—	31
SORBET				
(*see* ICES AND ICE POPS)				
SORGHUM				
sorghum	½ cup	325	—	0
SOUFFLE				
HOME RECIPE				
grand marnier	1 cup	109	—	139
lemon chilled	1 cup	176	—	2
raspberry chilled	1 cup	173	—	3
spinach	1 cup	218	—	184
SOUP				
CANNED				
American Original Foods				
New England Chowder	4 oz	64	—	5
Campbell				
Healthy Request Bean With Bacon as prep	8 oz	140	—	5
Healthy Request Chicken Noodle as prep	8 oz	60	—	15
Healthy Request Chicken With Rice as prep	8 oz	60	—	10
Healthy Request Cream Of Mushroom as prep	8 oz	60	—	<5

FOOD	PORTION	CALS.	FIB.	CHOL.
Campbell (cont.)				
Healthy Request Cream Of Chicken	8 oz	70	—	10
Healthy Request Hearty Chicken Vegetable	8 oz	120	—	20
Healthy Request Ready-To-Serve Chicken Broth	8 oz	10	—	0
Healthy Request Ready-To-Serve Hearty Minestrone	8 oz	90	—	<2
Healthy Request Ready-To-Serve Hearty Chicken Noodle	8 oz	80	—	25
Healthy Request Ready-To-Serve Hearty Chicken Rice	8 oz	110	—	20
Healthy Request Ready-To-Serve Hearty Vegetable	8 oz	110	—	0
Healthy Request Ready-To-Serve Hearty Vegetable Beef	8 oz	120	—	15
Healthy Request Tomato as prep	8 oz	90	—	0
Healthy Request Tomato as prep w/ skim milk	8 oz	130	—	<5
Healthy Request Vegetable as prep	8 oz	90	—	<5
Healthy Request Vegetable Beef as prep	8 oz	70	—	5
College Inn				
Beef Broth	½ can (7 oz)	16	—	0
Chicken Broth	½ can (7 oz)	35	0	5
Chicken Broth Lower Salt	½ can (7 oz)	20	0	5
Gold's				
Borscht	8 oz	100	—	0
Borscht Lo-Cal	8 oz	20	—	0
Schav	8 oz	25	—	15
Gorton's				
New England Clam Chowder as prep w/ whole milk	¼ can	140	—	15
Goya				
Black Bean	7.5 oz	160	9	0
Hain				
Chicken Broth	8¾ fl oz	70	—	5
Chicken Broth No Salt Added	8¾ fl oz	60	—	5
Chicken Noodle	9½ fl oz	120	—	20
Chicken Noodle No Salt Added	9½ fl oz	120	—	25
Creamy Mushroom	9¼ fl oz	110	—	15

FOOD	PORTION	CALS.	FIB.	CHOL.
Hain (CONT.)				
Italian Vegetable Pasta	9½ fl oz	160	—	20
Italian Vegetable Pasta Low Sodium	9½ fl oz	140	—	20
Minestrone	9½ fl oz	170	—	0
Minestrone No Salt Added	9½ fl oz	160	—	0
Mushroom Barley	9½ fl oz	100	—	10
New England Clam Chowder	9¼ fl oz	180	—	25
Split Pea	9½ fl oz	170	—	0
Split Pea No Salt Added	9½ fl oz	170	—	0
Turkey Rice	9½ fl oz	100	—	20
Turkey Rice No Salt Added	9½ fl oz	120	—	15
Vegetable Chicken	9½ fl oz	120	—	15
Vegetable Chicken No Salt Added	9½ fl oz	130	—	20
Vegetable Broth	9½ fl oz	45	—	0
Vegetable Broth Low Sodium	9½ fl oz	40	—	0
Vegetable Split Pea	9½ fl oz	170	—	0
Vegetable Split Pea No Salt Added	9½ fl oz	170	—	0
Vegetarian Lentil	9½ fl oz	160	—	5
Vegetarian Lentil No Salt Added	9½ fl oz	160	—	5
Vegetarian Vegetable	9½ fl oz	140	—	0
Vegetarian Vegetable No Salt Added	9½ fl oz	150	—	0
Health Valley				
Beef Broth	7.5 oz	10	0	1
Beef Broth No Salt Added	7.5 oz	10	0	1
Black Bean	7.5 oz	150	16	0
Black Bean No Salt Added	7.5 oz	150	16	0
Chicken Broth	7.5 oz	35	0	2
Chicken Broth No Salt Added	7.5 oz	35	0	2
Chunky Chicken Vegetable	7.5 oz	125	4	12
Chunky Five Bean Vegetable	7.5 oz	110	11	0
Chunky Five Bean Vegetable No Salt Added	7.5 oz	110	11	0
Chunky Vegetable Chicken No Salt Added	7.5 oz	125	4	12
Green Split Pea	7.5 oz	180	15	0
Green Split Pea No Salt Added	7.5 oz	180	15	0
Lentil	7.5 oz	220	10	0
Lentil No Salt Added	7.5 oz	220	10	0
Manhattan Clam Chowder	7.5 oz	110	2	15
Manhattan Clam Chowder No Salt Added	7.5 oz	110	2	15

FOOD	PORTION	CALS.	FIB.	CHOL.
Health Valley (CONT.)				
Minestrone	7.5 oz	130	13	0
Minestrone No Salt Added	7.5 oz	130	13	0
Mushroom Barley	7.5 oz	100	9	0
Mushroom Barley No Salt Added	7.5 oz	100	9	0
Potato Leek	7.5 oz	130	7	0
Potato Leek No Salt Added	7.5 oz	130	7	0
Tomato	7.5 oz	130	1	0
Tomato No Salt Added	7.5 oz	130	1	0
Vegetable	7.5 oz	110	8	0
Vegetable No Salt Added	7.5 oz	110	8	0
Healthy Choice				
Bean And Ham	1 cup (8.7 oz)	180	10	5
Chicken With Noodle	1 cup (8.8 oz)	130	2	10
Chicken With Pasta	1 cup (8.6 oz)	120	1	5
Chicken With Rice	1 cup (8.4 oz)	100	3	5
Country Vegetable	1 cup (8.6 oz)	100	6	0
Garden Vegetable	1 cup (8.6 oz)	110	6	0
Hearty Beef	1 cup (8.6 oz)	140	4	10
Lentil	1 cup (8.7 oz)	140	5	0
Minestrone	1 cup (8.6 oz)	110	3	<5
Split Pea With Ham	1 cup (8.8 oz)	160	5	5
Tomato Garden	1 cup (8.6 oz)	110	3	0
Turkey Vegetable	1 cup (8.5 oz)	120	2	10
Turkey With White And Wild Rice	1 cup (8.4 oz)	110	3	0
Hormel				
Bean & Ham	1 cup (7.5 oz)	190	7	25
Beef Vegetable	1 cup (7.5 oz)	90	2	10
Broccoli Cheese With Ham	1 cup (7.5 oz)	170	1	60
Chicken & Rice	1 cup (7.5 oz)	110	1	10
Chicken Noodle	1 cup (7.5 oz)	110	1	20
New England Clam Chowder	1 cup (7.5 oz)	130	1	25
Potato Cheese With Ham	1 cup (7.5 oz)	190	1	60
Manischewitz				
Borscht Low Calorie	8 fl oz	20	—	0
Borscht With Beets	8 fl oz	80	—	0
Schav	1 cup	11	—	0
Old El Paso				
Black Bean With Bacon	1 cup	160	7	5
Chicken Vegetable	1 cup	110	0	15
Chicken With Rice	1 cup	90	0	15
Garden Vegetable	1 cup	110	0	<5

FOOD	PORTION	CALS.	FIB.	CHOL.
Old El Paso (CONT.)				
Hearty Beef	1 cup	120	0	25
Hearty Chicken Noodle	1 cup	110	0	25
Pritikin				
Chicken & Rice	1 cup (8.8 oz)	80	—	5
Chicken Broth	1 cup (8.5 oz)	15	—	0
Chicken Pasta	1 cup (8.6 oz)	100	—	5
Hearty Vegetable	1 cup (8.8 oz)	90	—	0
Lentil	1 cup (8.4 oz)	130	—	0
Minestrone	1 cup (8.8 oz)	90	—	0
Split Pea	1 cup (9.2 oz)	140	—	0
Three Bean Chili	½ cup (4.5 oz)	90	—	0
Vegetable Broth	1 cup (8.3 oz)	20	—	0
Vegetarian Vegetables	1 cup (9 oz)	100	—	0
Progresso				
Beef	1 can (10.5 fl oz)	180	—	35
Beef Barley	1 can (10.5 fl oz)	150	—	30
Beef Minestrone	1 can (10.5 fl oz)	180	—	35
Beef Noodle	9.5 fl oz	170	—	40
Beef Vegetable	1 can (10.5 fl oz)	170	—	40
Chickarina	9.5 fl oz	130	—	20
Chicken Minestrone	1 can (10.5 fl oz)	140	—	20
Chicken Vegetable	1 can (10.5 fl oz)	150	—	25
Chicken Barley	9.25 fl oz	100	4	20
Chicken Broth	4 fl oz	8	—	<5
Chicken Cream Of	9.5 fl oz	190	—	35
Chicken Noodle	1 can (10.5 fl oz)	120	—	40
Chicken Rice	1 can (10.5 fl oz)	120	—	25
Corn Chowder	9.25 fl oz	200	—	10
Escarole In Chicken Broth	9.25 fl oz	30	—	<5
Ham & Bean	9.5 fl oz	140	8	10
Hearty Minestrone	9.25 fl oz	110	—	<5
Hearty Beef	9.5 fl oz	160	—	35
Hearty Chicken	1 can (10.5 fl oz)	130	—	30
Homestyle Chicken	9.5 fl oz	110	—	20
Lentil	1 can (10.5 fl oz)	140	—	0
Lentil With Sausage	9.5 fl oz	170	5	20
Macaroni & Bean	1 can (10.5 fl oz)	150	—	0
Manhattan Clam Chowder	9.5 fl oz	120	—	10
Minestrone	1 can (10.5 fl oz)	120	—	10
Mushroom Cream Of	9.25 fl oz	160	—	15
New England Style Clam Chowder	1 can (10.5 fl oz)	220	—	20
Seasoned Beef Broth	4 fl oz	40	—	0

FOOD	PORTION	CALS.	FIB.	CHOL.
Progresso (CONT.)				
Split Pea With Ham	1 can (10.5 fl oz)	160	6	15
Tomato	9.5 fl oz	120	—	0
Tomato Tortellini	9.5 fl oz	130	—	10
Tomato Beef With Rotini	9.5 fl oz	170	—	30
Tortellini	9.5 fl oz	90	—	10
Tortellini Creamy	9.25 fl oz	240	—	35
Vegetable	1 can (10.5 fl oz)	80	—	<5
Zesty Minestrone	9.5 fl oz	150	—	10
Weight Watchers				
Chicken Noodle	10.5 oz	80	—	20
asparagus cream of as prep w/ milk	1 cup	161	—	22
asparagus cream of as prep w/ water	1 cup	87	—	5
beef broth ready-to-serve	1 can (14 oz)	27	—	1
beef broth ready-to-serve	1 cup	16	—	tr
beef noodle as prep w/water	1 cup	84	—	5
black bean turtle soup	1 cup	218	—	0
black bean as prep w/water	1 cup	116	—	0
celery cream of as prep w/ milk	1 cup	165	—	32
celery cream of as prep w/ water	1 cup	90	—	15
celery cream of not prep	1 can (10¾ oz)	219	—	34
cheese as prep w/ milk	1 cup	230	—	48
cheese as prep w/ water	1 cup	155	—	30
cheese not prep	1 can (11 oz)	377	—	72
chicken broth as prep w/ water	1 cup	39	—	1
chicken cream of as prep w/ milk	1 cup	191	—	27
chicken cream of as prep w/ water	1 cup	116	—	10
chicken gumbo as prep w/water	1 cup	56	—	5
chicken noodle as prep w/ water	1 cup	75	—	7
chicken rice as prep w/ water	1 cup	251	—	7
clam chowder manhattan as prep w/ water	1 cup	77	—	3
clam chowder new england as prep w/ water	1 cup	95	—	5
clam chowder new england as prep w/ milk	1 cup	163	—	22
consomme w/ gelatin not prep	1 can (10½ oz)	71	—	0
consomme w/ gelatin as prep w/ water	1 cup	29	—	0
escarole ready-to-serve	1 cup	27	—	2
french onion as prep w/ water	1 cup	57	—	0
gazpacho ready-to-serve	1 cup	57	—	0

FOOD	PORTION	CALS.	FIB.	CHOL.
minestrone as prep w/water	1 cup	83	—	2
mushroom cream of as prep w/ milk	1 cup	203	—	20
mushroom cream of as prep w/ water	1 cup	129	—	2
oyster stew as prep w/ milk	1 cup	134	—	32
oyster stew as prep w/ water	1 cup	59	—	14
pepperpot as prep w/ water	1 cup	103	—	10
potato cream of as prep w/ milk	1 cup	148	—	22
potato cream of as prep w/ water	1 cup	73	—	5
scotch broth as prep w/ water	1 cup	80	—	5
split pea w/ ham as prep w/ water	1 cup	189	—	8
tomato as prep w/ milk	1 cup	160	—	17
tomato as prep w/water	1 cup	86	—	0
vegetarian vegetable as prep w/ water	1 cup	72	—	0
vichyssoise	1 cup	148	—	22
DRY				
Armour				
Bouillon Cubes Beef	1 (4 g)	5	—	0
Bouillon Cubes Chicken	1 (4 g)	5	—	0
Arrowhead				
Bean & Barley	¼ cup (1.9 oz)	170	7	0
Bean Cuisine				
Bean Bouillabisse	1 cup (7.5 fl oz)	174	5	0
Island Black Bean	1 cup (8.6 fl oz)	202	8	0
Lots of Lentil	1 cup (7.7 oz)	166	6	0
Mesa Maize	1 cup (9.2 fl oz)	179	6	0
Rocky Mountain Red Bean	1 cup (8.6 oz)	202	8	0
Sante Fe Corn Chowder	1 cup (9.2 oz)	179	6	0
Thick As Fog Split Pea	1 cup (8.6 fl oz)	189	1	0
Ultima Pasta E Fagioli	1 cup (8.6 fl oz)	179	4	0
White Bean Provencal	1 cup (7.7 fl oz)	166	6	0
Casbah				
Black Bean	1 pkg (1.7 oz)	170	9	0
Split Pea	1 pkg (2.3 oz)	230	10	0
Sweet Corn Chowder	1 pkg (1.2 oz)	125	2	0
Vegetarian Chili	1 pkg (1.8 oz)	170	7	0
Cup-A-Soup				
Chicken Vegetable	6 oz	47	—	8
Chicken Broth	6 oz	19	0	1
Onion	6 oz	27	tr	0
Emes				
Beef Base	1 tsp	18	—	0

FOOD	PORTION	CALS.	FIB.	CHOL.
Emes (CONT.)				
Chicken Base	1 tsp	18	—	0
Fantastic				
Cha-Cha Chili Low Fat	1 pkg	220	13	0
Golden Dipt				
Lobster Bisque	¼ pkg	30	—	2
Manhattan Clam Chowder	¼ pkg	80	—	3
New England Clam Chowder	¼ pkg	24	—	2
Seafood Chowder	¼ pkg	70	—	2
Shrimp Bisque	¼ pkg	30	—	2
Goodman's				
Cup Of Soup Beef	1 pkg (1½ cups)	180	2	45
Cup Of Soup Chicken Noodle	1 pkg (1½ cups)	180	2	45
Cup Of Soup Vegetable	1 pkg (1½ cups)	180	2	40
Matzo Ball & Soup	1 cup	40	1	0
Matzo Ball & Soup 50% Less Salt	1 serv	50	1	0
Noodleman	1 cup	45	0	10
Noodleman Low Sodium	1 cup	50	1	10
Onion	1 cup	30	1	0
Onion Low Sodium	1 cup	30	1	0
Herb-Ox				
Beef Bouillon	1 cube (3.5 g)	10	0	0
Beef Instant Bouillon Powder	1 tsp (4 g)	10	0	0
Beef Instant Broth & Seasoning Pack	1 pkg (4.5 g)	10	0	0
Beef Instant Broth & Seasoning Pack Low Sodium	1 pkg (4 g)	15	0	0
Chicken Bouillon	1 cube (4 g)	10	0	0
Chicken Instant Bouillon Powder	1 tsp (4 g)	10	0	0
Chicken Instant Broth & Seasoning Pack	1 pkg (5 g)	10	0	0
Chicken Instant Broth & Seasoning Pack Low Sodium	1 pkg (4 g)	15	0	0
Vegetable Bouillon	1 cube (4 g)	10	0	0
Hodgson Mill				
13 Bean not prep	1.5 oz	100	12	0
Hurst				
15 Bean Soup Beef	1 serv (1.7 oz)	160	1	0
15 Bean Soup Cajun	1 serv (1.7 oz)	160	9	0
15 Bean Soup Chicken	1 serv (1.7 oz)	160	1	0
15 Bean Soup Chili	1 serv (1.7 oz)	160	1	0
15 Bean Soup Ham	1 serv (1.7 oz)	160	1	0

FOOD	PORTION	CALS.	FIB.	CHOL.
Hurst (CONT.)				
Spanish-American Black Bean	1 serv (1.3 oz)	120	8	0
Ka-Me				
Won Ton Chicken not prep	1 pkg (1.25 oz)	180	1	0
Won Ton Pork not prep	1 pkg (1.25 oz)	180	1	0
Knorr				
Black Bean Cup-A-Soup as prep	1 pkg	200	9	0
Chicken Noodle Instant as prep	6 fl oz	25	—	5
Hearty Minestrone Cup-A-Soup as prep	1 pkg	150	1	2
Lentil Cup-A-Soup as prep	1 pkg	220	6	0
Navy Bean Cup-A-Soup as prep	1 pkg	140	5	0
Potato Leek Cup-A-Soup as prep	1 pkg	120	1	0
Vegetable Cup-A-Soup as prep	1 pkg	100	0	0
Kojel				
Hearty Potato With Vegetables Instant	1 serv (6 fl oz)	60	2	0
Noodle Soup Chicken Flavor Instant	1 serv (6 fl oz)	70	2	0
Split Pea Instant	1 serv (6 fl oz)	60	3	0
Tomato Instant	1 serv 6 fl oz)	50	1	0
Vegetable Chicken Couscous Instant	1 serv (6 fl oz)	80	2	0
Lipton				
Beefy Onion	8 oz	27	—	0
Country Vegetable	8 oz	80	—	0
Onion Mushroom	8 oz	41	0	0
Manischewitz				
Minestrone as prep	6 fl oz	50	—	0
Split Pea as prep	6 fl oz	45	—	0
Vegetable as prep	6 fl oz	50	—	0
Maruchan				
Instant Lunch Oriental Noodles Beef	1 pkg (2.25 oz)	290	—	1
Instant Lunch Oriental Noodles Chicken	1 pkg (2.25 oz)	290	2	4
Instant Lunch Oriental Noodles Chicken Mushroom	1 pkg (2.25 oz)	280	—	0
Instant Lunch Oriental Noodles Mushroom	1 pkg (2.25 oz)	290	—	0
Instant Lunch Oriental Noodles Pork	1 pkg (2.25 oz)	290	—	0
Instant Lunch Oriental Noodles Shrimp	1 pkg (2.25 oz)	290	—	8

FOOD	PORTION	CALS.	FIB.	CHOL.
Maruchan (CONT.)				
Instant Lunch Oriental Noodles Toast Onion	1 pkg (2.25 oz)	270	—	0
Instant Lunch Oriental Noodles Vegetable Beef	1 pkg (2.25 oz)	290	—	0
Instant Wonton Chicken	1 pkg (1.49 oz)	200	—	5
Instant Wonton Hot & Sour	1 pkg (1.49 oz)	200	—	0
Instant Wonton Oriental	1 pkg (1.49 oz)	190	—	0
Instant Wonton Pork	1 pkg (1.49 oz)	200	—	0
Instant Wonton Shrimp	1 pkg (1.49 oz)	200	—	10
Oriental Noodle Picante Style Beef	1 pkg (2.25 oz)	290	—	0
Oriental Noodle Picante Style Chicken	1 pkg (2.25 oz)	290	—	5
Oriental Noodle Picante Style Shrimp	1 pkg (2.25 oz)	300	—	5
Ramen Beef	½ pkg (1.5 oz)	190	—	0
Ramen Chicken	½ pkg (1.5 oz)	190	—	0
Ramen Chicken Mushroom	½ pkg (1.5 oz)	190	—	0
Ramen Chili	½ pkg (1.5 oz)	190	—	0
Ramen Mushroom	½ pkg (1.5 oz)	190	—	0
Ramen Oriental	½ pkg (1.5 oz)	190	—	0
Ramen Pork	½ pkg (1.5 oz)	190	—	0
Ramen Shrimp	½ pkg (1.5 oz)	190	—	tr
Wonton Beef	⅓ pkg (0.68 oz)	90	—	0
Wonton Chicken	⅓ pkg (0.67 oz)	90	—	0
Wonton Pork	⅓ pkg (0.68 oz)	90	—	0
Wonton Vegetable	⅓ pkg (0.7 oz)	90	—	0
Nile Spice				
Couscous Almondine	1 pkg	200	2	0
Couscous Garbanzo	1 pkg	220	2	0
Couscous Lentil Curry	1 pkg	200	4	0
Couscous Minestrone	1 pkg	180	2	0
Couscous Parmesan	1 pkg	200	2	10
Homestyle Black Bean	1 pkg	190	2	0
Homestyle Chicken Flavored Vegetable	1 pkg	120	4	5
Homestyle Lentil	1 pkg	180	3	0
Homestyle Minestrone	1 pkg	160	4	0
Homestyle Red Beans & Rice	1 pkg	190	3	0
Homestyle Split Pea	1 pkg	200	6	0
Homestyle Sweet Corn Chowder	1 pkg	120	0	0
Italian Tomato	1 pkg	140	2	10

FOOD	PORTION	CALS.	FIB.	CHOL.
Nile Spice (CONT.)				
Potato Leek	1 pkg	150	2	20
Potato Romano	1 pkg	140	3	15
Ultra Slim-Fast				
Beef Noodle	6 oz	45	2	5
Chicken Leek	6 oz	50	2	<2
Chicken Noodle	6 oz	45	2	5
Creamy Broccoli	6 oz	75	2	0
Creamy Tomato	6 oz	60	2	0
Hearty Vegetable	6 oz	50	2	0
Onion	6 oz	45	2	0
Potato Leek	6 oz	80	2	0
Weight Watchers				
Chicken Noodle	7.5 oz	90	—	15
Chunky Beef Stew	7.5 oz	120	—	20
New England Clam Chowder	7.5 oz	90	—	5
Vegetable Beef	7.5 oz	90	—	10
asparagus cream of as prep w/ water	1 cup	59	—	tr
beef broth	1 pkg (0.2 oz)	14	—	1
beef broth as prep w/ water	1 cup	19	—	1
beef broth cube	1 cube (3.6 g)	6	—	tr
beef broth cube as prep w/water	1 cup	8	—	tr
celery cream of as prep w/ water	1 cup	63	—	1
chicken broth	1 pkg (0.2 oz)	16	—	1
chicken broth as prep w/water	1 cup	21	—	1
chicken broth cube	1 cube (4.8 g)	9	—	1
chicken broth cube, as prep w/ water	1 cup	13	—	1
chicken cream of as prep w/ water	1 cup	107	—	3
chicken noodle as prep w/ water	1 cup	53	—	3
french onion not prep	1 pkg (1.4 oz)	115	—	2
leek as prep w/ water	1 cup	71	—	3
onion as prep w/ water	1 cup	28	—	0
tomato as prep w/ water	1 cup	102	—	1
FROZEN				
Jaclyn's				
Barley & Mushroom	7.5 fl oz	90	—	0
Split Pea	7.5 fl oz	180	—	0
Vegetable	7.5 fl oz	90	—	0
Kettle Ready				
New England Clam Chowder	6 oz	116	tr	tr
Potato Cream Of	6 oz	121	0	0
Split Pea With Ham	6 oz	155	0	0

FOOD	PORTION	CALS.	FIB.	CHOL.
Tabatchnick				
Barley Mushroom	1 serv (7.5 oz)	70	3	0
Barley Mushroom No Salt Added	1 serv (7.5 oz)	70	3	0
Broccoli Cream Of	1 serv (7.5 oz)	90	3	5
Cabbage	1 serv (7.5 oz)	60	2	0
Chicken With Dumplings	1 serv (7.5 oz)	70	1	20
Corn Chowder	1 serv (7.5 oz)	150	1	5
Minestrone	1 serv (7.5 oz)	150	10	3
New England Potato	1 serv (7.5 oz)	150	2	9
New York Chicken	1 serv (7.5 oz)	35	0	0
Old Fashion Potato	1 serv (7.5 oz)	70	2	0
Pea	1 serv (7.5 oz)	180	11	0
Pea No Salt Added	1 serv (7.5 oz)	180	11	0
Spinach Cream Of	1 serv (7.5 oz)	90	2	5
Vegetable	1 serv (7.5 oz)	110	4	0
Vegetable No Salt Added	1 serv (7.5 oz)	110	4	0
Wisconsin Cheddar Vegetable	1 serv (7.5 oz)	140	1	13
Yankee Bean	1 serv (7.5 oz)	160	11	0
SHELF-STABLE				
Lunch Bucket				
Chicken Noodle	1 pkg (7.25 oz)	90	—	25
Country Vegetable	1 pkg (7.25 oz)	70	—	0
TAKE-OUT				
beef stew soup	1 cup (8.8 oz)	221	—	60
black bean turtle soup	1 cup	241	—	0
brunswick stew soup	1 cup (8.5 oz)	232	—	71
corn & cheese chowder	¾ cup	215	3	66
gazpacho	1 cup	46	—	0
greek	¾ cup	63	2	83
hot & sour	1 cup	74	—	70
pasta e fagioli	1 cup (8.8 oz)	194	—	3
ratatouille	1 cup (7.5 oz)	266	—	0
SOUR CREAM				
(*see also* SOUR CREAM SUBSTITUTES)				
Breakstone	2 tbsp (1 oz)	60	0	25
Free	2 tbsp (1.1 oz)	35	0	<5
Half & Half	2 tbsp (1.1 oz)	45	0	15
Cabot	1 oz	60	—	13
Light	1 oz	33	—	7
Friendship	2 tbsp (1 oz)	60	0	20
Light	2 tbsp (1 oz)	35	0	10
Heluva Good Cheese				
Fat-Free	2 tbsp (1.1 oz)	20	0	0

FOOD	PORTION	CALS.	FIB.	CHOL.
Heluva Good Cheese (CONT.)				
Light	2 tbsp (1.1 oz)	40	0	10
Sour Cream	2 tbsp (1.1 oz)	60	0	20
Hood	2 tbsp (1 oz)	60	0	20
Fat Free	2 tbsp (1 oz)	20	0	0
Light	2 tbsp (1 oz)	40	0	10
Knudsen				
Free	2 tbsp (1.1 oz)	35	0	0
Hampshire	2 tbsp (1 oz)	60	0	25
Light	2 tbsp (1.1 oz)	40	0	10
Naturally Yours				
No Fat	2 tbsp (1 fl oz)	15	—	0
Sealtest	2 tbsp (1 oz)	60	0	20
Free	2 tbsp (1.1 oz)	35	0	<5
Light	2 tbsp (1.1 oz)	40	0	10
sour cream	1 cup	493	—	102
sour cream	1 tbsp	26	—	5

SOUR CREAM SUBSTITUTES

Pet				
Imitation	1 tbsp	25	—	tr
Tofutti				
Better Than Sour Cream Sour Supreme	1 oz	50	—	0
nondairy	1 oz	59	—	0
nondairy	1 cup	479	—	0

SOURSOP

fresh	1	416	—	0
fresh cut up	1 cup	150	—	0

SOY

(*see also* ICE CREAM AND FROZEN DESSERTS, MILK SUBSTITUTES, MISO, SOY SAUCE, SOYBEANS, TEMPEH AND TOFU)

Eden				
Tamari Organic Domestic	1 tbsp (0.5 oz)	15	0	0
Tamari Organic Imported	1 tbsp (0.5 oz)	15	0	0
LaLoma				
Soyagen All Purpose	¼ cup	130	—	0
Soyagen Carob	¼ cup	140	—	0
Soyagen No Sucrose	¼ cup	130	—	0
Tree Of Life				
Shoyu	1 tbsp (0.5 oz)	15	—	0
Tamari Reduced Sodium	1 tbsp (0.5 oz)	20	—	0
Tamari Wheat Free	1 tbsp (0.5 oz)	15	—	0

FOOD	PORTION	CALS.	FIB.	CHOL.
lecithin	1 tbsp	104	—	0
roasted & toasted	1 cup	490	—	0
soy milk	1 cup	79	—	0

SOY SAUCE
(see also SAUCE, SOY)

Eden

Shoyu Organic	1 tbsp (0.5 oz)	15	0	0
Shoyu Traditional	1 tbsp (0.5 oz)	15	0	0

House Of Tsang

Dark	1 tbsp (0.6 oz)	10	0	0
Ginger Flavored Low Sodium	1 tbsp (0.6 oz)	10	0	0
Ginger Flavored	1 tbsp (0.6 oz)	20	0	0
Light	1 tbsp (0.6 oz)	5	0	0
Low Sodium	1 tbsp (0.6 oz)	5	0	0
Mushroom Flavored Low Sodium	1 tbsp (0.6 oz)	10	0	0

Ka-Me

Chinese Dark	1 tbsp (0.5 fl oz)	10	0	0
Chinese Light	1 tbsp (0.5 fl oz)	5	0	0
Dark	1 tbsp (0.5 fl oz)	10	0	0
Japanese	1 tbsp (0.5 fl oz)	5	0	0
Light	1 tbsp (0.5 oz)	5	0	0
Mild	1 tbsp (0.5 fl oz)	5	0	0

Kikkoman

	1 tbsp	12	0	0
Lite	1 tbsp	13	—	0

La Choy

	½ tsp	2	tr	0
Lite	½ tsp	1	tr	0

Trappey

Chef Magic	1 tbsp (0.5 oz)	23	tr	0
shoyu	1 tbsp	9	—	0
soy sauce	1 tbsp	7	—	0
tamari	1 tbsp	11	—	0

SOYBEANS
(see also MILK SUBSTITUTES, MISO, SOY, TEMPEH, AND TOFU)

dried cooked	1 cup	298	—	0
dry-roasted	½ cup	387	—	0
roasted	½ cup	405	—	0
roasted & toasted	1 oz	129	—	0
roasted & toasted salted	1 cup	490	—	0
roasted & toasted salted	1 oz	129	—	0
sprouts raw	½ cup	43	—	0
sprouts steamed	½ cup	38	—	0
sprouts stir fried	1 cup	125	—	0

FOOD	PORTION	CALS.	FIB.	CHOL.
FRESH				
green cooked	½ cup	127	4	0

SPAGHETTI
(see PASTA, PASTA DINNERS, PASTA SALAD, SPAGHETTI SAUCE)

SPAGHETTI SAUCE
(see also PIZZA, TOMATO)
JARRED

FOOD	PORTION	CALS.	FIB.	CHOL.
Classico				
Beef & Pork	4 fl oz	80	—	10
Four Cheese	4 fl oz	70	—	<5
Spicy Red Pepper	4 fl oz	50	—	0
Sweet Peppers & Onions	4 fl oz	50	—	0
Tomato & Basil	4 fl oz	60	—	0
Ripe Olives & Mushrooms	4 fl oz	50	—	0
Contadina				
Italian	¼ cup	15	1	0
Thick & Zesty	¼ cup	15	1	0
Del Monte				
Traditional	½ cup (4.4 oz)	80	tr	0
Traditional No Sugar Added	½ cup (4.4 oz)	60	tr	0
With Garlic & Onion	½ cup (4.4 oz)	70	tr	0
With Green Peppers & Mushrooms	½ cup (4.4 oz)	70	tr	0
With Meat	½ cup (4.4 oz)	40	tr	0
With Mushrooms	½ cup (4.4 oz)	80	tr	0
Eden				
Organic	½ cup (4.4 oz)	80	3	0
Organic No Salt Added	½ cup (4.4 oz)	80	3	0
Enrico's				
Fat Free Organic Basil	½ cup (4 oz)	50	4	0
Fat Free Organic Garlic	½ cup (4 oz)	50	5	0
Fat Free Organic Hot Pepper	½ cup (4 oz)	50	5	0
Fat Free Organic Mushroom	½ cup (4 oz)	60	7	0
Fat Free Organic Traditional	½ cup (4 oz)	45	6	0
Healthy Choice				
Extra Chunky Garlic & Onions	½ cup (4.4 oz)	50	2	0
Extra Chunky Italian Style Vegetable	½ cup (4.4 oz)	50	2	0
Extra Chunky Mushrooms	½ cup (4.4 oz)	50	2	0
Original Garlic & Herbs	½ cup (4.4 oz)	50	2	0
Original Mushrooms	½ cup (4.4 oz)	50	2	0
Original Traditional	½ cup (4.4 oz)	50	2	0
Original With Meat	½ cup (4.4 oz)	50	2	0

FOOD	PORTION	CALS.	FIB.	CHOL.
Hunt's				
Chunky	¼ cup (2.2 fl oz)	30	1	0
Classic Italian With Parmesan	½ cup (4.4 fl oz)	50	2	0
Homestyle Traditional No Sugar Added	½ cup (4.4 fl oz)	60	2	0
Traditional	4 oz	70	2	0
Traditional Light	½ cup (4 oz)	40	3	0
With Meat	4 oz	70	2	2
With Mushrooms	4 oz	70	2	0
Mama Rizzo's				
Mushroom Onion	½ cup (4.3 oz)	60	1	0
Pepper Mushroom Onion	½ cup (4.3 oz)	60	1	0
Pepper Primavera Vegetable	½ cup (4.2 oz)	50	2	0
Pepper Tomato Basil Garlic	½ cup (4.7 oz)	60	1	0
Primavera Vegetable	½ cup (4.2 oz)	50	2	0
Tomato Basil Garlic	½ cup (4.6 oz)	60	2	0
Newman's Own				
Marinara	4 oz	70	—	0
Marinara With Mushrooms	4 oz	70	—	0
Sockarooni	4 oz	70	—	0
Pritikin				
Chunky Garden	½ cup (4 oz)	50	—	0
Marinara	½ cup (4 oz)	60	—	0
Original	½ cup (4 oz)	60	—	0
Progresso	½ cup	110	—	2
Bolognese	½ cup	150	3	20
Marinara	½ cup	90	—	1
Meat Flavored	½ cup	110	—	5
Mushroom	½ cup	110	—	5
Sicilian	½ cup	30	tr	0
Ragu	4 fl oz	80	—	0
Fino Italian Parmesan	½ cup (4.5 oz)	100	2	<5
Fino Italian Garden Medley	½ cup (4.5 oz)	90	2	0
Fino Italian Garlic & Basil	½ cup (4.5 oz)	90	2	0
Fino Italian Sliced Mushroom	½ cup (4.5 oz)	90	2	0
Fino Italian Tomato & Herb	½ cup (4.5 oz)	90	2	0
Fino Italian Zesty Tomato	½ cup (4.5 oz)	90	2	0
Gardenstyle Chunky Graden Combination	½ cup (4.5 oz)	120	3	0
Gardenstyle Chunky Green & Red Pepper	½ cup (4.5 oz)	120	2	0
Gardenstyle Chunky Mushroom & Green Pepper	½ cup (4.5 oz)	120	3	0
Gardenstyle Chunky Mushroom & Onion	½ cup (4.5 oz)	120	3	0

FOOD	PORTION	CALS.	FIB.	CHOL.
Ragu (CONT.)				
Gardenstyle Chunky Tomato Garlic & Onion	½ cup (4.5 oz)	120	3	0
Gardenstyle Super Mushroom	½ cup (4.5 oz)	120	3	0
Gardenstyle Super Vegetable Primavera	½ cup (4.5 oz)	110	4	0
Homestyle Mushroom	½ cup (4.5 oz)	120	3	0
Homestyle Tomato & Herb	½ cup (4.5 oz)	120	3	0
Homestyle With Meat	½ cup (4.5 oz)	130	3	<5
Light Chunky Mushroom	½ cup (4.4 oz)	50	2	0
Light Garden Harvest	½ cup (4.4 oz)	50	2	0
Light No Sugar Added	½ cup (4.4 oz)	60	3	0
Light Tomato & Herb	½ cup (4.4 oz)	50	2	0
Old World Style Marinara	½ cup (4.4 oz)	90	3	0
Old World Style Mushrooms	½ cup (4.4 oz)	80	3	0
Old World Style Traditional	½ cup (4.4 oz)	80	3	0
Old World Style With Meat	½ cup (4.4 oz)	90	3	<5
Thick & Hearty Mushroom	½ cup (4.5 oz)	120	3	0
Thick & Hearty Spaghetti Sauce	4 oz	100	—	0
Thick & Hearty Tomato & Herb	½ cup (4.5 oz)	120	3	0
Thick & Hearty With Meat	1.2 cup (4.5 oz)	130	3	<5
Tree Of Life				
Pasta Sauce	½ cup (4 oz)	50	—	0
Pasta Sauce Fat Free Classic	½ cup (3.9 oz)	40	0	0
Pasta Sauce Fat Free Mushroom & Basil	½ cup (3.9 oz)	30	0	0
Pasta Sauce Fat Free Onion & Garlic	½ cup (3.9 oz)	30	0	0
Pasta Sauce Fat Free Sweet Pepper	½ cup (3.9 oz)	30	0	0
Pasta Sauce No Salt	½ cup (3.9 oz)	50	—	0
Weight Watchers				
With Mushrooms	⅓ cup	35	—	0
marinara sauce	1 cup	171	—	0
spaghetti sauce	1 cup	272	—	0
REFRIGERATED				
Contadina				
Alfredo	½ cup (4.2 fl oz)	400	0	80
Four Cheese Sauce With White Wine & Shallots	½ cup (4.2 fl oz)	320	0	70
Light Alfredo	½ cup (4.2 fl oz)	190	0	40
Light Chunky Tomato	½ cup (4.4 fl oz)	45	3	0
Light Garden Vegetable	½ cup (4.4 fl oz)	45	3	0
Marinara	½ cup (4.4 fl oz)	80	2	0

FOOD	PORTION	CALS.	FIB.	CHOL.
Contadina (CONT.)				
Pesto With Basil	¼ cup (2 oz)	310	0	10
Pesto With Sun Dried Tomatoes	¼ cup (2 oz)	250	3	0
Plum Tomato With Basil	½ cup (4.4 fl oz)	70	3	0
Spicy Italian Sausage & Bell Pepper	½ cup (4.4 fl oz)	100	3	40
Di Giorno				
Alfredo	¼ cup (2.2 oz)	230	0	45
Four Cheese	¼ cup (2.2 oz)	200	0	45
Light Chunky Tomato With Basil	½ cup (4.5 oz)	70	2	0
Light Reduced Fat Alfredo	¼ cup (2.4 oz)	170	0	30
Marinara	½ cup (4.5 oz)	100	3	<5
Olive Oil & Garlic With Grated Cheese	¼ cup (2.1 oz)	370	0	20
Pesto	¼ cup (2.2 oz)	320	0	15
Plum Tomato & Mushroom	½ cup (4.4 oz)	70	2	0
Traditional Meat	½ cup (4.5 oz)	120	3	15

SPANISH FOOD

(*see also* BEANS, CHIPS, DINNER, PEPPERS, SALSA, SNACKS, SAUCE, TORTILLA)

CANNED

FOOD	PORTION	CALS.	FIB.	CHOL.
Chi-Chi's				
Picante Hot	2 tbsp (1 oz)	10	0	0
Picante Medium	2 tbsp (1 oz)	10	0	0
Picante Mild	2 tbsp (1 oz)	10	0	0
Pico De Gallo	2 tbsp (1.2 oz)	10	0	0
Derby				
Tamales	2	160	1	24
El Molino				
Green Chili Sauce Mild	2 tbsp	10	—	0
Gebhardt				
Enchiladas	2	310	2	58
Tamales	2	290	2	54
Tamales Jumbo	2	400	3	75
Guiltless Gourmet				
Picante Mild	1 oz	6	tr	0
Queso Mild Cheddar	1 oz	22	tr	tr
Hormel				
Tamales Beef	3 (7.5 oz)	280	3	35
Tamales Chicken	3 (7.5 oz)	210	2	60
Tamales Hot Spicy Beef	3 (7.5 oz)	280	3	35
Tamales Jumbo Beef	2 (6.9 oz)	270	3	35

FOOD	PORTION	CALS.	FIB.	CHOL.
Hormel (CONT.)				
Tamales Beef	1 can (7.5 oz)	290	3	35
Old El Paso				
Tamales	2	190	—	20
Rosarita				
Enchilada Sauce Mild	2.5 oz	25	tr	0
Picante Chunky Hot	3 tbsp (2 fl oz)	18	tr	0
Picante Chunky Medium	3 tbsp (2 fl oz)	16	tr	0
Picante Chunky Mild	3 tbsp (2 oz)	25	tr	0
Van Camp's				
Tamales	2 (5.1 oz)	210	3	20
FROZEN				
Banquet				
Beef & Bean Burrito	9.5 oz	390	—	15
Beef Enchilada & Tamale w/ Chili Gravy	10 oz	300	—	20
Chimichanga	9.5 oz	480	—	15
Enchilada Chicken	11 oz	340	—	20
Enchilada Beef	11 oz	370	—	15
Enchilada Cheese	11 oz	340	—	15
Tamale Beef	11 oz	420	—	25
El Charrito				
Burrito Grande B&B	1 pkg (6 oz)	430	—	25
Burrito Grande Green Chili B&B	1 pkg (6 oz)	410	—	20
Burrito Grande Jalapeno	1 pkg (6 oz)	410	—	25
Burrito Grande Red Chili B&B	1 pkg (6 oz)	410	—	25
Burrito Green Chili B&B	1 pkg (5 oz)	370	—	20
Burrito Red Chili B&B	1 pkg (5 oz)	380	—	20
Burrito Red Hot B&B	1 pkg (5 oz)	540	—	20
Burrito Red Hot Beef	1 pkg (5 oz)	340	—	20
Enchilada Chicken Dinner	1 pkg (13.75 oz)	510	—	50
Enchilada Beef Dinner	1 pkg (13.75 oz)	620	—	45
Enchilada Cheese Dinner	1 pkg (13.75 oz)	570	—	30
Enchilada Grande Beef Dinner	1 pkg (21 oz)	950	—	70
Enchiladas 3 Beef	1 pkg (11 oz)	560	—	55
Enchiladas 3 Cheese	1 pkg (11 oz)	470	—	30
Enchiladas 3 Chicken	1 pkg (11 oz)	440	—	60
Enchiladas 4 Grande Beef	1 pkg (16.5 oz)	890	—	65
Enchiladas 6 Beef	1 pkg (16.25 oz)	880	—	75
Enchiladas 6 Beef & Cheese	1 pkg (16.25 oz)	880	—	70
Enchiladas 6 Cheese	1 pkg (16.25 oz)	780	—	45
Grande Mexican Dinner	1 pkg (20 oz)	850	—	65
Mexican Dinner	1 pkg (14.25 oz)	690	—	45
Queso Dinner	1 pkg (13.25 oz)	490	—	15

FOOD	PORTION	CALS.	FIB.	CHOL.
El Charrito (CONT.)				
Satillo Dinner	1 pkg (13.5 oz)	570	—	30
Satillo Grande Dinner	1 pkg (20.75 oz)	820	—	45
Healthy Choice				
Burrito Con Queso Chicken	1 (5.4 oz)	280	5	10
Burrito Ranchero Beef Medium	1 (5.4 oz)	290	6	15
Burrito Ranchero Beef Mild	1 (5.4 oz)	300	7	15
Enchilada Suprema Chicken	1 meal (13.4 oz)	390	8	30
Enchilada Beef Rio Grande	1 meal (13.4 oz)	410	9	15
Enchiladas Suiza Chicken	1 meal (10 oz)	270	5	25
Feista Fajitas Chicken	1 meal (7 oz)	260	5	30
Jimmy Dean				
Burrito Breakfast Bacon	1 (4 oz)	260	1	70
Burrito Breakfast Sausage	1 (4 oz)	250	2	45
Le Menu				
Entree LightStyle Enchilada Chicken	8 oz	280	—	35
Lean Cuisine				
Enchanadas Chicken	1 pkg (9.9 oz)	220	4	30
Enchilada Suiza Chicken	1 pkg (9 oz)	290	5	25
Lightlife				
Vegetarian Taco	2 oz	51	—	0
Old El Paso				
Burrito Beef & Bean Hot	1	320	—	15
Burrito Beef & Bean Medium	1	320	—	15
Burrito Beef & Bean Mild	1	330	—	15
Burrito Bean & Cheese	1	290	3	15
Chimichangas Beef	1	310	—	10
Chimichangas Chicken	1	350	—	20
Patio				
Britos Beef & Bean	1 (3 oz)	210	—	15
Britos Nacho Beef	1 (3 oz)	220	—	25
Britos Nacho Cheese	1 (3.63 oz)	250	—	20
Britos Spicy Chicken & Cheese	1 (3 oz)	210	—	25
Burritos Hot Beef & Bean Red Chili	1 (5 oz)	340	—	20
Burritos Medium Beef & Bean	1 (5 oz)	370	—	25
Burritos Mild Beef & Bean Green Chili	1 (5 oz)	330	—	30
Enchilada Beef Dinner	13.25 oz	520	—	40
Enchilada Cheese Dinner	12 oz	370	—	20
Fiesta Dinner	12 oz	460	—	30
Mexican Dinner	13.25	540	—	45
Tamale Dinner	13 oz	470	—	35

FOOD	PORTION	CALS.	FIB.	CHOL.
Rudy's Farm				
Burrito Beef/Bean	1 (5 oz)	326	5	15
Burrito Hot Beef/Bean	1 (5 oz)	305	5	11
Senor Felix's				
Burritos Charbroiled Chicken	1 + 4 tsp sauce (6.7 oz)	320	7	20
Burrito Black Bean	1 (10 oz)	540	7	40
Burrito Black Bean Soy	1 (5 oz)	240	3	0
Burrito Chicken	1 (10 oz)	520	3	65
Burrito Hot Potato	1 (10 oz)	560	5	40
Burrito Soy Hot	1 (10 oz)	520	5	0
Burritos Sonora Style	1 + 4 tsp sauce (6.7 oz)	280	3	10
Burritos Yucatan Style	1 + 4 tsp sauce (6.7 oz)	310	5	10
Empanadas Chicken	1 (4.7 oz)	340	13	30
Empanadas Corn & Rice	1 (4.7 oz)	280	6	25
Empanadas Pumpkin & Mushroom	1 (4.7 oz)	260	6	25
Empanadas Spinach & Ricotta	1 (4.7 oz)	260	6	30
Enchilada Red Pepper	1 (10 oz)	420	8	25
Enchilada Soy Verda	1 (10 oz)	430	6	0
Enchilada Supreme Soy Cheese	1 (10 oz)	460	6	0
Enchilada Verde	1 (5 oz)	423	6	25
Tamales Blue Corn & Soy Cheese	2 + 4 tsp sauce (5.7 oz)	240	3	15
Tamales Chicken	2 + 4 tsp sauce (5.7 oz)	240	8	20
Tamales Gourmet Vegetarian	2 + 4 tsp sauce	240	8	20
Taquitos Blue Corn Soy	3 + 4 tsp sauce (5.2 oz)	230	3	0
Taquitos Chicken	2 + 4 tsp sauce (5.7 oz)	240	3	15
Stouffer's				
Cheese Enchilada	1 pkg (9.75 oz)	370	5	25
Chicken Enchilada	1 pkg (10 oz)	370	3	30
Today's Tamales				
Cheese & Chili	1 pkg (7 oz)	390	6	30
Del Sol	1 pkg (6.5 oz)	310	15	0
Original Bean	1 pkg (7 oz)	330	10	0
Spicy Taco	1 pkg (7 oz)	310	10	0
Weight Watchers				
Enchiladas Ranchero Beef	9.12 oz	190	—	20
Enchiladas Ranchero Cheese	8.87 oz	260	—	25

FOOD	PORTION	CALS.	FIB.	CHOL.
Weight Watchers (CONT.)				
Enchiladas Suiza Chicken	9 oz	230	—	40
Fajitas Chicken	6.75 oz	210	—	25
MIX				
Gebhardt				
Menudo Mix	1 tsp	5	tr	0
Hain				
Taco Seasoning Mix	1/10 pkg	10	—	0
Old El Paso				
Burrito Seasoning Mix	⅛ pkg	17	1	0
Burrito Dinner (with filling)	1 serv	299	4	23
Enchilada Seasoning Mix	1/18 pkg	6	0	0
Guacamole Seasoning Mix	½ pkg	7	0	0
Taco Seasoning Mix	1/12 pkg	8	—	0
Ortega				
Taco Meat Seasoning Mix Mild	1 filled taco	90	—	0
Quaker				
Masa Trigo	2 tortillas	149	1	0
READY-TO-USE				
Chi-Chi's				
Taco Shells White Corned	2 (1 oz)	130	2	0
Gebhardt				
Taco Shells	1	50	tr	0
Old El Paso				
Taco Shells	1	55	1	0
Taco Shells Mini	3	70	1	0
Taco Shells Super	1	100	2	0
Tastaco Shells	1	100	1	0
Tostada Shells	1	55	1	0
Rosarita				
Taco Shells	1 shell (11 g)	50	tr	0
Tostada Shells	1 shell (14 g)	60	tr	0
taco shell baked	1 med (½ oz)	61	tr	0
taco shell baked w/o salt	1 med (½ oz)	61	tr	0
TAKE-OUT				
burrito w/ apple	1 lg (5.4 oz)	484	—	7
burrito w/ apple	1 sm (2.6 oz)	231	—	3
burrito w/ beans	2 (7.6 oz)	448	—	5
burrito w/ beans & cheese	2 (6.5 oz)	377	—	27
burrito w/ beans & chili peppers	2 (7.2 oz)	413	—	33
burrito w/ beans & meat	2 (8.1 oz)	508	—	48
burrito w/ beans cheese & beef	2 (7.1 oz)	331	—	125
burrito w/ beans cheese & chili peppers	2 (11.8 oz)	663	—	158

FOOD	PORTION	CALS.	FIB.	CHOL.
burrito w/ beef	2 (7.7 oz)	523	—	65
burrito w/ beef & chili peppers	2 (7.1 oz)	426	—	54
burrito w/ beef cheese & chili peppers	2 (10.7 oz)	634	—	170
burrito w/ cherry	1 sm (2.6 oz)	231	—	3
burrito w/ cherry	1 lg (5.4 oz)	484	—	7
chimichanga w/ beef	1 (6.1 oz)	425	—	9
chimichanga w/ beef & cheese	1 (6.4 oz)	443	—	51
chimichanga w/ beef & red chili peppers	1 (6.7 oz)	424	—	9
chimichanga w/ beef cheese & red chili peppers	1 (6.3 oz)	364	—	50
enchilada w/ cheese	1 (5.7 oz)	320	—	44
enchilada w/ cheese & beef	1 (6.7 oz)	324	—	40
enchiladas eggplant	1	142	—	7
enchirito w/ cheese beef & beans	1 (6.8 oz)	344	—	49
frijoles w/ cheese	1 cup (5.9 oz)	226	—	36
nachos w/ cheese	6 to 8 (4 oz)	345	—	18
nachos w/ cheese & jalapeno peppers	6 to 8 (7.2 oz)	607	—	83
nachos w/ cheese beans ground beef & peppers	6 to 8 (8.9 oz)	568	—	21
nachos w/ cinnamon & sugar	6 to 8 (3.8 oz)	592	—	39
taco	1 sm (6 oz)	370	—	57
taco salad	1½ cups	279	—	44
taco salad w/ chili con carne	1½ cups	288	—	4
tostada w/ beans & cheese	1 (5.1 oz)	223	—	30
tostada w/ beans beef & cheese	1 (7.9 oz)	334	—	75
tostada w/ beef & cheese	1 (5.7 oz)	315	—	41
tostada w/ guacamole	2 (9.2 oz)	360	—	39

SPARE RIBS
(see PORK)

SPICES
(see HERBS/SPICES, INDIVIDUAL NAMES)

SPINACH
CANNED
Del Monte

50% Less Salt	½ cup (4 oz)	30	2	0
Chopped	½ cup (4 oz)	30	2	0
No Salt Added	½ cup (4 oz)	30	2	0
Whole Leaf	½ cup (4 oz)	30	2	0

Popeye

Chopped	½ cup (4.1 oz)	40	4	0

FOOD	PORTION	CALS.	FIB.	CHOL.
Popeye (CONT.)				
Leaf	½ cup (4.2 oz)	45	4	0
Low Sodium	½ cup (4.2 oz)	35	3	0
S&W				
Northwest Premium	½ cup	25	—	0
Sunshine				
Chopped	½ cup (4.1 oz)	40	4	0
spinach	½ cup	25	—	0
FRESH				
Dole	3 oz	9	8	0
Fresh Express	1½ cups (3 oz)	40	5	0
cooked	½ cup	21	2	0
mustard chopped cooked	½ cup	14	—	0
mustard raw chopped	½ cup	17	—	0
new zealand chopped cooked	½ cup	11	—	0
new zealand raw	½ cup	4	—	0
raw chopped	½ cup	6	1	0
raw chopped	1 pkg (10 oz)	46	—	0
FROZEN				
Birds Eye				
Chopped	½ cup	20	3	0
Creamed	½ cup	90	1	15
Leaf	½ cup	20	3	0
Budget Gourmet				
Au Gratin	1 pkg (5.5 oz)	160	—	25
Green Giant				
Creamed	½ cup	25	5	0
Creamed	½ cup	70	—	2
Cut Leaf In Butter Sauce	½ cup	40	4	5
Harvest Fresh	½ cup	25	3	0
Stouffer's				
Creamed	½ cup (2.25 oz)	150	2	15
Souffle	½ cup (4 oz)	150	—	120
Tabatchnick				
Creamed	7.5 oz	60	2	5
cooked	½ cup	27	—	0

SPINACH JUICE

juice	3½ oz	7	—	0

SPORTS DRINKS

Gatorade				
Orange	1 cup (8 fl oz)	50	—	0
PowerAde				
Fruit Punch	8 fl oz	72	—	0
Grape	8 fl oz	73	—	0

FOOD	PORTION	CALS.	FIB.	CHOL.
PowerAde (CONT.)				
Lemon-Lime	8 fl oz	72	—	0
Orange	8 fl oz	72	—	0
Slice				
All Sport Diet Lemon Lime	8 fl oz	1	—	0
All Sport Lemon Lime	8 fl oz	72	—	0
All Sport Orange	8 fl oz	74	—	0
All Sport Punch	8 fl oz	81	—	0
Snapple				
Sport Fruit	1 bottle	80	—	0
SQUAB				
breast w/o skin raw	1 (3.5 oz)	135	—	91
SQUASH				
(see also ZUCCHINI)				
CANNED				
Allen				
Yellow	½ cup (4.2 oz)	25	2	0
Sunshine				
Yellow	½ cup (4.2 oz)	25	2	0
crookneck sliced	½ cup	14	—	0
FRESH				
Nature's Pasta				
Spaghetti Squash	1 cup (5.5 oz)	20	2	0
acorn cooked mashed	½ cup	41	3	0
acorn cubed baked	½ cup	57	2	0
butternut baked	½ cup	41	2	0
crookneck raw sliced	½ cup	12	1	0
crookneck sliced cooked	½ cup	18	1	0
hubbard baked	½ cup	51	3	0
hubbard cooked mashed	½ cup	35	3	0
scallop raw sliced	½ cup	12	1	0
scallop sliced cooked	½ cup	14	1	0
spaghetti cooked	½ cup	23	2	0
FROZEN				
Birds Eye				
Winter Cooked	½ cup	45	2	0
Southland				
Butternut	4 oz	45	—	0
butternut cooked mashed	½ cup	47	3	0
crookneck sliced cooked	½ cup	24	—	0
SEEDS				
dried	1 oz	154	—	0
dried	1 cup	747	—	0

FOOD	PORTION	CALS.	FIB.	CHOL.
roasted	1 oz	148	—	0
roasted	1 cup	1184	—	0
salted & roasted	1 oz	148	—	0
salted & roasted	1 cup	1184	—	0
whole roasted	1 oz	127	—	0
whole roasted	1 cup	285	—	0
whole salted roasted	1 cup	285	—	0
whole salted roasted	1 oz	127	—	0

SQUID

fried	3 oz	149	—	221
raw	3 oz	78	—	198

SQUIRREL

roasted	3 oz	147	—	103

STRAWBERRIES
CANNED

in heavy syrup	½ cup	117	—	0
FRESH				
Dole	8	50	3	0
strawberries	1 pint	97	—	0
strawberries	1 cup	45	4	0
FROZEN				
Big Valley	⅔ cup (4.9 oz)	50	2	0
Birds Eye				
Halved In Delicious Syrup	½ cup	120	2	0
Halved In Lite Syrup	½ cup	90	2	0
Whole In Lite Syrup	½ cup	80	2	0
sweetened sliced	1 pkg (10 oz)	273	—	0
sweetened sliced	1 cup	245	—	0
unsweetened	1 cup	52	—	0
whole sweetened	1 pkg (10 oz)	223	—	0
whole sweetened	1 cup	200	—	0

STRAWBERRY JUICE

Juice Works	6 oz	100	—	0
Kern's				
Nectar	6 fl oz	110	—	0
Libby				
Nectar	1 can (11.5 fl oz)	210	—	0
Smucker's	8 oz	130	—	0
Tang				
Strawberry	8.45 fl oz	121	—	0

FOOD	PORTION	CALS.	FIB.	CHOL.
Wylers				
Drink Mix Unsweetened Strawberry Split	8 oz	2	—	0

STUFFING/DRESSING
HOME RECIPE

FOOD	PORTION	CALS.	FIB.	CHOL.
bread as prep w/ water & fat	½ cup	251	—	tr
bread as prep w/ water egg & fat	½ cup	107	—	75
MIX				
Arnold				
All Purpose Seasoned	½ oz	50	1	0
Corn	½ oz	50	1	0
Herb Seasoned	½ oz	50	1	0
Sage & Onion	½ oz	50	1	0
Brownberry				
Corn	1 oz	103	2	0
Herb	1 oz	100	2	0
Sage & Onion	1 oz	97	2	0
Kellogg's				
Croutettes	1 cup (1.2 oz)	120	0	0
Stove Top				
Beef as prep	½ cup	178	—	tr
Chicken as prep	½ cup	176	—	1
Chicken With Rice as prep	½ cup	182	—	1
Cornbread as prep	½ cup	175	—	tr
Flex Serve Chicken as prep	½ cup	173	—	1
Flex Serve Cornbread as prep	½ cup	181	—	tr
Flex Serve Homestyle Herb as prep	½ cup	173	—	1
Long Grain & Wild Rice as prep	½ cup	182	—	1
Select Wild Rice & Mushroom	½ cup	172	—	21
Wonder				
Seasoned Stuffing	1 cup (0.9 oz)	60	tr	0
cornbread as prep	½ cup	179	—	0
TAKE-OUT				
bread	½ cup (3½ oz)	195	3	0
sausage	½ cup	292	1	12

SUCKER

FOOD	PORTION	CALS.	FIB.	CHOL.
white baked	3 oz	101	—	45

SUGAR
(*see also* FRUCTOSE, SUGAR SUBSTITUTES, SYRUP)

FOOD	PORTION	CALS.	FIB.	CHOL.
C&H				
White	1 tsp	16	—	0

FOOD	PORTION	CALS.	FIB.	CHOL.
Domino				
White	1 tsp	16	—	0
Hain				
Turbinado	1 tbsp	50	—	0
Hollywood				
Turbinado	1 tbsp	50	—	0
brown packed	1 cup (7.7 oz)	828	—	0
brown unpacked	1 cup (5.1 oz)	546	—	0
maple	1 piece (1 oz)	100	—	0
powdered	1 tbsp (0.3 oz)	31	—	0
powdered unsifted	1 cup (4.2 oz)	467	—	0
white	1 tbsp	45	—	0
white	1 packet (6 g)	25	—	0
white	1 cup (7 oz)	773	—	0
white	1 tsp (4 g)	15	—	0

SUGAR SUBSTITUTES
(see also FRUCTOSE)

FOOD	PORTION	CALS.	FIB.	CHOL.
Equal	1 pkg	4	—	0
NatraTaste	1 pkg (1 g)	0	—	0
S&W				
Liquid Table Sweetener	⅛ tsp	0	—	0
Sprinkle Sweet	1 tsp	2	—	0
SugarTwin	1 pkg (0.8 g)	3	—	0
Brown	1 tsp (0.4 g)	2	—	0
Sweet One	1 pkg (1 g)	4	—	0
Sweet'N Low				
Granulated	1 pkg (1g)	4	—	0
*Sweet*10*	⅛ tsp	0	—	0
Weight Watchers				
Sweet'ner	1 pkg	4	—	0

SUGAR-APPLE

FOOD	PORTION	CALS.	FIB.	CHOL.
fresh	1	146	—	0
fresh cut up	1 cup	236	—	0

SUNDAE TOPPINGS
(see ICE CREAM TOPPINGS)

SUNFISH

FOOD	PORTION	CALS.	FIB.	CHOL.
pumpkinseed baked	3 oz	97	—	73

SUNFLOWER

FOOD	PORTION	CALS.	FIB.	CHOL.
Fisher				
Seeds Oil Roasted	1 oz	170	—	0
Seeds Salted In Shell shelled	1 oz	160	—	0

FOOD	PORTION	CALS.	FIB.	CHOL.
Fisher (CONT.)				
Seeds Salted in Shell unshelled	1 oz	170	—	0
Frito Lay	1 oz	160	—	0
Planters				
Sunflower Nuts Dry Roasted Unsalted	1 oz	170	—	0
Sunflower Seeds	1 oz	160	—	0
Stone-Buhr				
Seeds Raw	4 tsp (1 oz)	170	6	0
dried	1 oz	162	—	0
dried	1 cup	821	—	0
dry roasted	1 cup	745	—	0
dry roasted	1 oz	165	—	0
dry roasted salted	1 cup	745	—	0
dry roasted salted	1 oz	165	—	0
oil roasted	1 cup	830	—	0
oil roasted salted	1 oz	175	—	0
oil roasted salted	1 cup	830	—	0
sunflower butter	1 tbsp	93	—	0
sunflower butter w/o salt	1 tbsp	93	—	0
toasted	1 cup	826	—	0
toasted	1 oz	176	—	0
toasted salted	1 oz	176	—	0
toasted salted	1 cup	826	—	0

SURF
CANNED

American Original	4 oz	100	—	20
FRESH				
American Original	4 oz	90	—	40

SUSHI
TAKE-OUT

california roll	1 piece (0.8 oz)	28	—	1
kim chi	½ cup (5.8 oz)	18	—	0
sashimi	1 serving (6 oz)	198	—	63
tuna roll	1 piece (0.7 oz)	23	—	3
vegetable roll	1 piece (1.2 oz)	27	—	0
vinegared ginger	⅓ cup (1.6 oz)	48	—	0
wasabi	2 tsp (0.3 oz)	5	—	0
yellowtail roll	1 piece (0.6 oz)	25	—	0

SWAMP CABBAGE

chopped cooked	½ cup	10	—	0
raw chopped	1 cup	11	—	0

FOOD	PORTION	CALS.	FIB.	CHOL.
SWEET POTATO				
(see also YAM)				
CANNED				
Princella				
Mashed	⅔ cup (5.1 oz)	120	3	0
Royal Prince				
Candied	½ cup (4.9 oz)	210	2	0
Halves	3 pieces (5.7 oz)	190	4	0
Orange Pineapple	½ cup (4.8 oz)	210	3	0
Sugary Sam				
Mashed	⅔ cup (5.1 oz)	120	3	0
in syrup	½ cup	106	—	0
pieces	1 cup	183	—	0
FRESH				
baked w/ skin	1 (3½ oz)	118	3	0
leaves cooked	½ cup	11	—	0
mashed	½ cup	172	3	0
FROZEN				
cooked	½ cup	88	—	0
TAKE-OUT				
candied	3½ oz	144	—	0
SWEETBREADS				
lamb braised	3 oz	199	—	340
SWISS CHARD				
cooked	½ cup	18	—	0
raw chopped	½ cup	3	—	0
SWORDFISH				
cooked	3 oz	132	—	43
raw	3 oz	103	—	33
SYRUP				
(see also ICE CREAM TOPPINGS, PANCAKE/WAFFLE SYRUP)				
Eden				
Barley Malt Organic Syrup	1 tbsp (0.7 fl oz)	60	0	0
Estee				
Blueberry Lite	¼ cup (2.4 oz)	80	—	0
Home Brands				
Maple Rich	1 oz	110	—	0
Karo				
Corn Syrup Dark	1 tbsp (21 g)	60	—	0
Corn Syrup Dark	1 cup (331 g)	975	—	0
Corn Syrup Light	1 tbsp (21 g)	60	—	0
Corn Syrup Light	1 cup (331 g)	960	—	0

FOOD	PORTION	CALS.	FIB.	CHOL.
McIlhenny				
Cane	2 tbsp (1.4 oz)	130	tr	0
Red Wing				
Strawberry	2 tbsp (1.4 oz)	110	0	0
S&W				
Blueberry Diet	1 tbsp	4	—	0
Maple Flavored Diet	1 tbsp	4	—	0
Strawberry Diet	1 tbsp	4	—	0
Smucker's				
All Flavors Fruit Syrup	2 tbsp	100	—	0
Tree Of Life				
Maple	¼ cup (2.1 oz)	200	—	0
corn	2 tbsp	122	—	0
corn dark	1 tbsp (0.7 oz)	56	—	0
corn dark	1 cup (11.5 oz)	925	—	0
corn light	1 cup (11.5 oz)	925	—	0
corn light	1 tbsp (0.7 oz)	56	—	0
malt	1 tbsp (0.8 oz)	76	—	0
malt	1 cup (13 oz)	1222	—	0
maple	1 tbsp (0.8 oz)	52	—	0
maple	1 cup (11.1 oz)	824	—	0
raspberry	3½ oz	267	—	0
sorghum	1 tbsp (0.7 oz)	61	—	0
sorghum	1 cup (11.6 oz)	957	—	0

TACO
(*see* SPANISH FOOD)

TAHINI
(*see* SESAME)

TAMARIND

fresh	1	5	—	0
fresh cut up	1 cup	287	—	0

TANGERINE
CANNED

in light syrup	½ cup	76	—	0
juice pack	½ cup	46	—	0
FRESH				
Dole	2	70	2	0
sections	1 cup	86	—	0
tangerine	1	37	—	0

TANGERINE JUICE
Dole

Mandarin frzn as prep	8 fl oz	140	0	0

FOOD	PORTION	CALS.	FIB.	CHOL.
Minute Maid				
Frozen	8 fl oz	120	—	0
canned sweetened	1 cup	125	—	0
fresh	1 cup	106	—	0
frzn sweetened as prep	1 cup	110	—	0
frzn sweetened not prep	6 oz	344	—	0

TAPIOCA
General Foods

Minute Tapioca	1 tbsp	32	—	0
pearl dry	⅓ cup	174	1	0

TARO

chips	1 oz	141	—	0
chips	10 (0.8 oz)	115	—	0
leaves cooked	½ cup	18	—	0
raw sliced	½ cup	56	—	0
shoots sliced cooked	½ cup	10	—	0
sliced cooked	½ cup (2.3 oz)	94	—	0
tahitian sliced cooked	½ cup	30	—	0

TARRAGON

ground	1 tsp	5	—	0

TEA/HERBAL TEA
HERBAL
Bigelow

Almond Orange	5 fl oz	tr	—	0
Apple Orchard	5 fl oz	5	—	0
Apple Spice	5 fl oz	tr	—	0
Chamomile	5 fl oz	tr	—	0
Chamomile Mint	5 fl oz	tr	—	0
Cinnamon Orange	5 fl oz	tr	—	0
Early Riser	5 fl oz	3	—	0
Feeling Free	5 fl oz	1	—	0
Fruit & Almond	5 fl oz	1	—	0
Hibiscus & Rose Hips	5 fl oz	1	—	0
I Love Lemon	5 fl oz	1	—	0
Lemon & C	5 fl oz	tr	—	0
Looking Good	5 fl oz	1	—	0
Mint Blend	5 fl oz	tr	—	0
Mint Medley	5 fl oz	1	—	0
Orange & C	5 fl oz	tr	—	0
Orange & Spice	5 fl oz	tr	—	0
Peppermint	5 fl oz	tr	—	0
Roasted Grains & Carob	5 fl oz	3	—	0

FOOD	PORTION	CALS.	FIB.	CHOL.
Bigelow (CONT.)				
Spearmint	5 fl oz	tr	—	0
Sweet Dreams	5 fl oz	1	—	0
Take-A-Break	5 fl oz	3	—	0
Celestial Seasonings				
Almond Sunset	8 fl oz	3	—	0
Bengal Spice	8 fl oz	5	—	0
Caffeine Free	8 fl oz	2	—	0
Chamomile	8 fl oz	2	—	0
Cinnamon Apple Spice	8 fl oz	<3	—	0
Cinnamon Rose	8 fl oz	<4	—	0
Country Peach Spice	8 fl oz	3	—	0
Cranberry Cove	8 fl oz	2	—	0
Emperor's Choice	8 fl oz	4	—	0
Ginseng Plus	8 fl oz	3	—	0
Grandma's Tummy Mint	8 fl oz	2	—	0
Lemon Mist	8 fl oz	3	—	0
Lemon Zinger	8 of oz	4	—	0
Mama Bear's Cold Care	8 fl oz	6	—	0
Mandarin Orange Spice	8 fl oz	5	—	0
Mellow Mint	8 fl oz	2	—	0
Mint Magic	8 fl oz	1	—	0
Orange Zinger	8 fl oz	6	—	0
Peppermint	8 fl oz	2	—	0
Raspberry Patch	8 fl oz	4	—	0
Red Zinger	8 fl oz	4	—	0
Roastaroma	8 fl oz	10	—	0
Sleepytime	8 fl oz	4	—	0
Spearmint	8 fl oz	5	—	0
Strawberry Fields	8 fl oz	4	—	0
Sunburst C	8 fl oz	3	—	0
Tropical Escape	8 fl oz	1	—	0
Wild Forest Blackberry	8 fl oz	2	—	0
ICED				
Arizona				
Raspberry	8 fl oz	95	—	0
Bigelow				
Nice Over Ice	5 fl oz	1	—	0
Celestial Seasonings				
Iced Delight	8 fl oz	4	—	0
Crystal Light				
Decaffeinated Sugar Free	8 oz	2	—	0
Sugar Free	8 oz	3	—	0

FOOD	PORTION	CALS.	FIB.	CHOL.
Lipton				
Instant	6 oz	0	—	0
Instant Decaffeinated	6 oz	0	—	0
Instant Lemon	8 oz	3	—	0
Instant Raspberry	8 oz	3	—	0
Lemon	6 oz	55	—	0
Lemon w/ Vitamin C	6 oz	58	0	0
Sugar Free	8 oz	1	—	0
Sugar Free Peach	8 oz	5	—	0
Sugar Free Raspberry	8 oz	5	—	0
With Nutrasweet	8 oz	3	—	0
With Nutrasweet Decaffeinated	8 oz	3	—	0
Nestea				
100% Instant Tea as prep	8 oz	2	—	0
Ice Tea Mix Sugarfree	8 oz	4	—	0
Ice Teasers Citrus	8 oz	6	—	0
Ice Teasers Lemon	8 oz	6	—	0
Ice Teasers Orange	8 oz	6	—	0
Ice Teasers Tropical	8 oz	6	—	0
Ice Teasers Wild Cheery	8 oz	6	—	0
Lemon	8 oz	6	—	0
Mix With Sugar & Lemon as prep	8 oz	70	—	0
Peach	8 fl oz	88	—	0
Raspberry	8 fl oz	88	—	0
With Sugar & Lemon	1 can (11.5 fl oz)	127	—	0
With Sugar & Lemon	1 bottle (16 fl oz)	176	—	0
Royal Mistic				
Diet	12 fl oz	8	—	0
Lemon	12 fl oz	144	—	0
Orange	12 fl oz	144	—	0
Wild Berry	12 fl oz	144	—	0
Schweppes	8 fl oz	90	0	0
Shasta	12 oz	124	—	0
Sipps	8.45 oz	100	—	0
Snapple				
Cranberry	8 fl oz	110	—	0
Diet	8 fl oz	0	—	0
Diet Peach	8 fl oz	0	—	0
Diet Raspberry	8 fl oz	0	—	0
Lemon	8 fl oz	110	—	0
Mango	8 fl oz	110	—	0
Mint	8 fl oz	120	—	0
Old Fashioned	8 fl oz	80	—	0

FOOD	PORTION	CALS.	FIB.	CHOL.
Snapple (CONT.)				
Orange	8 fl oz	110	—	0
Peach	8 fl oz	110	—	0
Raspberry	8 fl oz	120	—	0
Strawberry	8 fl oz	100	—	0
Tropicana				
Diet Lemon Fruit	8 fl oz	15	—	0
Lemon Fruit	8 fl oz	100	—	0
Peach Fruit	1 bottle (10 fl oz)	140	—	0
Peach Fruit	1 can (11.5 fl oz)	160	—	0
Peach Fruit	8 fl oz	120	—	0
Raspberry Fruit	8 fl oz	120	—	0
Raspberry Fruit	1 can (11.5 fl oz)	160	—	0
Raspberry Fruit	1 bottle (10 fl oz)	140	—	0
Tangerine Fruit	1 can (11.5 fl oz)	170	—	0
Tangerine Fruit	8 fl oz	110	—	0
Tangerine Fruit	1 bottle (10 fl oz)	140	—	0
Twister Apple Berry	8 fl oz	100	—	0
Twister Lemon Citrus	8 fl oz	110	—	0
Veryfine				
With Lemon	8 oz	80	—	0
instant artificially sweetened lemon flavored as prep w/ water	8 oz	5	—	0
instant sweetened lemon flavor as prep w/ water	9 oz	87	—	0
instant unsweetened lemon flavor as prep w/ water	8 oz	4	—	0
REGULAR				
Bigelow				
Chinese Fortune	5 fl oz	1	—	0
Cinnamon Stick	5 fl oz	1	—	0
Constant Comment	5 fl oz	1	—	0
Darjeeling Blend	5 fl oz	1	—	0
Earl Gray	5 fl oz	1	—	0
English Teatime	5 fl oz	1	—	0
Lemon Lift	5 fl oz	1	—	0
Orange Pekoe	5 fl oz	1	—	0
Peppermint Stick	5 fl oz	1	—	0
Plantation Mint	5 fl oz	1	—	0
Raspberry Royale	5 fl oz	1	—	0
Celestial Seasonings				
Cinnamon Vienna	8 fl oz	2	—	0
Earl Grey Extraordinary	8 fl oz	3	—	0

FOOD	PORTION	CALS.	FIB.	CHOL.
Celestial Seasonings (CONT.)				
English Breakfast Classic	8 fl oz	3	—	0
Lemon	8 fl oz	7	—	0
Mint	8 fl oz	4	—	0
Morning Thunder	8 fl oz	3	—	0
Naturally Decaffeinated	8 fl oz	10	—	0
Orange Spice	8 fl oz	7	—	0
Orange Spice Decaff	8 fl oz	7	—	0
Organically Grown	8 fl oz	12	—	0
Raspberry	8 fl oz	7	—	0
Natural Touch				
Kaffree	8 fl oz	0	—	0
Nestea				
Tea Bag as prep	6 oz	0	—	0
brewed tea	6 oz	2	—	0
instant unsweetened as prep w/ water	8 oz	2	—	0
TEFF				
Arrowhead				
Whole Grain	¼ cup (1.6 oz)	160	6	0
TEMPEH				
Lightlife	4 oz	182	—	0
White Wave				
Burger	1 patty (3 oz)	110	6	0
Lemon Broil	1 patty (2 oz)	130	4	0
Organic Wild Rice	⅓ block (2.7 oz)	140	6	0
Teriyaki Burger	1 patty (3 oz)	110	6	0
tempeh	½ cup	165	—	0
THYME				
Watkins	¼ tsp (0.5 oz)	0	0	0
ground	1 tsp	4	—	0
TOFU				
Casbah				
Gyro as prep w/ tofu	1 patty (2 oz)	105	tr	0
Jaclyn's				
Grilled In Black Bean Sauce	10.75 oz	270	—	0
Grilled In Peanut Sauce	10.75 oz	260	—	0
Mori-Nu				
Extra Firm	1 in slice (3 oz)	55	—	0
Firm	1 in slice (3 oz)	50	—	0
Lite Extra Firm	1 in slice (3 oz)	35	—	0
Lite Firm	1 in slice (3 oz)	35	—	0

FOOD	PORTION	CALS.	FIB.	CHOL.
Mori-Nu (CONT.)				
Soft	1 in slice (3 oz)	45	—	0
Nasoya				
Extra Firm	⅕ block (3 oz)	90	0	0
Firm	⅕ block (3 oz)	80	0	0
Silken	⅙ block (3 oz)	50	0	0
Soft	⅕ block (3 oz)	60	0	0
Spring Creek				
Baked Barbeque	2 oz	88	—	0
Baked Cajun	2 oz	87	—	0
Baked Teriyaki	2 oz	84	—	0
Great Balls Of Tofu!	2 (3 oz)	107	—	0
Nigari Firm	4 oz	140	3	0
Tofu Salads !Onion Dip	2 oz	46	—	0
Tofu Salads !Taco Dip	2 oz	46	—	0
Tofu Salads Missing Egg	2 oz	49	—	0
Tree Of Life				
Baked	⅕ block (3.2 oz)	150	0	0
Firm	⅕ block (3.2 oz)	100	0	0
Raw Firm	⅕ block (3.2 oz)	100	0	0
Ready Ground Hot & Spicy	⅓ pkg (3 oz)	60	0	0
Ready Ground Original	⅓ pkg (3 oz)	60	0	0
Ready Ground Savory Garlic	⅓ pkg (3 oz)	60	0	0
Reduced Fat	⅕ block (3.2 oz)	90	2	0
Savory Baked	⅕ block (3.2 oz)	140	0	0
Smoked Hot 'N Spicy	½ block (3 oz)	120	0	0
Smoked Original	½ block (3 oz)	120	0	0
White Wave				
Baked Tofus Teriyaki Oriental Style	¼ block (2 oz)	120	1	0
Hard	4 oz	120	—	0
International Baked Italian Garlic Herb	¼ pkg (2 oz)	120	1	0
International Baked Mexican Jalapeno	¼ pkg (2 oz)	120	1	0
International Baked Oriental Teriyaki	¼ pkg (2 oz)	120	1	0
International Baked Thai Sesame Peanut	¼ pkg (2 oz)	120	1	0
Soft	4 oz	120	—	0
firm	½ cup	183	2	0
firm	¼ block (3 oz)	118	1	0
fresh fried	1 piece (½ oz)	35	tr	0
fuyu salted & fermented	1 block (⅓ oz)	13	tr	0

FOOD	PORTION	CALS.	FIB.	CHOL.
koyadofu dried frozen	1 piece (½ oz)	82	tr	0
okara	½ cup	47	1	0
regular	¼ block (4 oz)	88	1	0
regular	½ cup	94	1	0

TOFUTTI
(*see* ICE CREAM AND FROZEN DESSERTS)

TOMATILLO
fresh	1 (1.2 oz)	11	—	0
fresh chopped	½ cup	21	—	0

TOMATO
(*see also* PIZZA, SPAGHETTI SAUCE)

CANNED

Claussen

Kosher	1	9	—	0

Contadina

Crushed	¼ cup	20	1	0
Italian Style Pear	½ cup	25	1	0
Italian Style Stewed	½ cup	40	1	0
Mexican Style Stewed	½ cup	40	1	0
Pasta Ready With Three Cheeses	½ cup	70	tr	<5
Paste	2 tbsp	30	1	0
Peeled Whole	½ cup	25	1	0
Puree	¼ cup	20	tr	0
Recipe Ready	½ cup	25	3	0
Stewed	½ cup	40	1	0

Del Monte

Paste	2 tbsp (1.2 oz)	30	2	0
Peeled Diced	½ cup (4.4 oz)	25	2	0
Puree	¼ cup (2.2 oz)	30	1	0
Sauce	¼ cup (2.1 oz)	20	tr	0
Sauce No Salt Added	¼ cup (2.1 oz)	20	tr	0
Stewed Cajun Style	½ cup (4.4 oz)	35	2	0
Stewed Chunky Chili	½ cup (4.5 oz)	30	2	0
Stewed Chunky Pasta	½ cup (4.5 oz)	45	2	0
Stewed Chunky Pizza	½ cup (4.5 oz)	35	2	0
Stewed Chunky Salsa	½ cup (4.5 oz)	35	2	0
Stewed Italian Style	½ cup (4.4 oz)	30	2	0
Stewed Mexican Style	½ cup (4.4 oz)	35	2	0
Stewed Original	½ cup (4.4 oz)	35	2	0
Stewed Original No Salt Added	½ cup (4.4 oz)	35	2	0
Wedges	½ cup (4.4 oz)	35	2	0

FOOD	PORTION	CALS.	FIB.	CHOL.
Del Monte (CONT.)				
Whole Peeled	½ cup (4.4 oz)	25	2	0
Eden				
Crushed Organic	¼ cup (2.1 oz)	20	1	0
Sauce Lightly Seasoned	¼ cup (2.1 oz)	25	1	0
Health Valley				
Sauce	1 cup	70	tr	0
Sauce Low Sodium	1 cup	70	1	0
Hebrew National				
Pickled	⅓ tomato (1 oz)	4	—	0
Hunt's				
All Natural Sauce	¼ cup (2.2 fl oz)	15	tr	0
Crushed Angela Mia	4 oz	35	tr	0
Crushed Italian	4 oz	40	tr	0
Italian Pear Shaped	4 oz	20	tr	0
Paste	1 oz	25	1	0
Paste Italian Style	2 oz	50	2	0
Paste No Salt Added	2 oz	45	2	0
Paste With Garlic	2 oz	50	2	0
Peeled Choice-Cut	4 oz	20	1	0
Puree	4 oz	45	2	0
Sauce Herb	4 oz	70	2	tr
Sauce Italian	4 oz	60	2	tr
Sauce Meatloaf Fixin's	4 oz	20	tr	0
Sauce No Salt Added	4 oz	35	2	0
Sauce Special	4 oz	35	2	0
Sauce With Bits	4 oz	30	2	0
Sauce With Garlic	4 oz	70	2	0
Sauce With Mushrooms	4 oz	25	2	0
Stewed	4 oz	35	tr	0
Stewed Italian	4 oz	40	tr	0
Stewed No Salt Added	4 oz	35	tr	0
Whole	4 oz	20	tr	0
Whole Italian	4 oz	25	tr	0
Whole No Salt Added	4 oz	20	tr	0
Rosoff's				
Pickled	⅓ tomato (1 oz)	5	—	0
S&W				
Aspic Supreme	½ cup	60	—	0
Diced In Rich Puree	½ cup	35	—	0
Italian Stewed Sliced	½ cup	35	—	0
Italian Style w/ Basil	½ cup	25	—	0
Paste	6 oz	150	—	0
Peeled Ready Cut	½ cup	25	—	0

FOOD	PORTION	CALS.	FIB.	CHOL.
S&W (cont.)				
Puree	½ cup	60	—	0
Sauce	½ cup	40	—	0
Sauce Chunky	½ cup	45	—	0
Stewed 50% Salt Reduced	½ cup	35	—	0
Stewed Mexican Style	½ cup	40	—	0
Stewed Sliced	½ cup	35	—	0
Whole Diet	½ cup	25	—	0
Whole Peeled	½ cup	25	—	0
Schorr's				
Pickled	⅓ tomato (1 oz)	4	—	0
paste	½ cup	110	6	0
puree	1 cup	102	6	0
puree w/o salt	1 cup	102	6	0
red whole	½ cup	24	—	0
sauce	½ cup	37	2	0
sauce spanish style	½ cup	40	2	0
sauce w/ mushrooms	½ cup	42	—	0
sauce w/ onion	½ cup	52	—	0
stewed	½ cup	34	—	0
w/ green chiles	½ cup	18	—	0
wedges in tomato juice	½ cup	34	—	0
DRIED				
sun dried	1 piece	5	—	0
sun dried	1 cup	140	—	0
sun dried in oil	1 piece (3 g)	6	—	0
sun dried in oil	1 cup (4 oz)	235	—	0
FRESH				
cooked	½ cup	32	—	0
green	1	30	—	0
red	1 (4½ oz)	26	2	0
red chopped	1 cup	35	2	0
TAKE-OUT				
stewed	1 cup	80	—	0
TOMATO JUICE				
Campbell	6 oz	40	—	0
Del Monte				
Snap-E-Tom	8 fl oz	50	2	0
Snap-E-Tom	6 fl oz	40	1	0
Snap-E-Tom	10 fl oz	60	2	0
Hunt's	6 oz	30	—	0
No Salt Added	6 oz	35	2	0
Libby	6 oz	35	—	0

FOOD	PORTION	CALS.	FIB.	CHOL.
Mott's				
Beefamato	8 fl oz	80	1	0
Clamato	8 fl oz	100	2	0
Clamato Ceasar	8 fl oz	100	0	0
S&W				
California	6 oz	35	—	0
Diet	½ cup	35	—	0
tomato juice	6 oz	32	—	0
tomato juice	½ cup	21	—	0

TONGUE

beef simmered	3 oz	241	—	91
lamb braised	3 oz	234	—	161
pork braised	3 oz	230	—	124

TOPPINGS
(*see* ICE CREAM TOPPINGS)

TORTILLA
(*see also* CHIPS TORTILLA, SPANISH FOOD)

Alvarado St. Bakery				
Burrito Size	1 (2.2 oz)	170	1	0
Fajita Size	1 (1.6 oz)	130	1	0
El Charrito				
Corn	2	95	—	0
Flour	2	170	—	0
Tyson				
Burrito Style Flour	1	170	—	0
Burrito Style Hand Stretched Small Flour	1	106	—	0
Burrito Style Heat Pressed Large Flour	1	182	—	0
Enchilada Style Corn	1	54	—	0
Fajita Style Flour	1	89	—	0
Soft Taco Flour	1	121	—	0
Whole Wheat	1	120	—	0
Wonder				
Low Fat Wheat	1 (1.4 oz)	120	1	0
Low Fat White	1 (1.4 oz)	110	1	0
corn	1 (6 in diam)	56	1	0
corn w/o salt	1-6 in diam (.9 oz)	56	1	0
flour w/o salt	1-8 in diam (1.2 oz)	114	1	0

TORTILLA CHIPS
(*see* CHIPS)

TREE FERN

chopped cooked	½ cup	28	—	0

FOOD	PORTION	CALS.	FIB.	CHOL.
TRITICALE				
(see also FLOUR)				
dry	½ cup	323	17	0
TROUT				
Clear Springs				
Rainbow	3.5 oz	140	—	75
baked	3 oz	162	—	63
rainbow cooked	3 oz	129	—	62
seatrout baked	3 oz	113	—	90
TRUFFLES				
fresh	3½ oz	25	—	0
TUNA				
(see also TUNA DISHES)				
CANNED				
Bumble Bee				
Chunk Light In Oil	2 oz	160	—	30
Chunk Light In Water	2 oz	60	—	30
Chunk White In Oil	2 oz	160	—	30
Chunk White In Water	2 oz	70	—	30
Solid White In Oil	2 oz	130	—	30
Solid White In Water	2 oz	70	—	30
Tree Of Life				
Tongol In Spring Water	2 oz	60	0	30
light in oil	3 oz	169	—	15
light in oil	1 can (6 oz)	399	—	30
light in water	1 can (5.8 oz)	192	—	49
light in water	3 oz	99	—	25
white in oil	1 can (6.2 oz)	331	—	55
white in oil	3 oz	158	—	26
white in water	3 oz	116	—	35
white in water	1 can (6 oz)	234	—	72
FRESH				
bluefin cooked	3 oz	157	—	42
bluefin raw	3 oz	122	—	32
skipjack baked	3 oz	112	—	51
yellowfin baked	3 oz	118	—	49
TUNA DISHES				
FROZEN				
Chefwich				
Tuna Melt	5 oz	360	—	23
MIX				
Bumble Bee				
Tuna Mix-ins Classic Italian	⅓ pkg (0.17 oz)	25	—	0

FOOD	PORTION	CALS.	FIB.	CHOL.
Bumble Bee (CONT.)				
Tuna Mix-ins Garden & Herb	⅓ pkg (0.17 oz)	25	—	0
Tuna Mix-ins Lemon Herb	⅓ pkg (0.17 oz)	25	—	0
Tuna Mix-ins Zesty Tomato	⅓ pkg (0.17 oz)	25	—	0
READY-TO-USE				
The Spreadables				
Tuna Salad	¼ can	90	—	13
Wampler Longacre				
Salad	1 oz	60	—	5
TAKE-OUT				
tuna salad	1 cup	383	—	27
tuna salad	3 oz	159	—	11
tuna salad submarine sandwich w/ lettuce & oil	1	584	—	47

TURKEY
(see also DINNER, HOT DOG, TURKEY DISHES, TURKEY SUBSTITUTES)

FOOD	PORTION	CALS.	FIB.	CHOL.
CANNED				
Armour				
Turkey Loaf	2 oz	110	—	40
Hormel				
Chunk	2 oz	70	0	35
Chunk Turkey Ham	2 oz	70	0	40
Chunk White	2 oz	60	0	25
Underwood				
Chunky Light	2.08 oz	75	—	25
FRESH				
Butterball				
Ground All White Meat	3 oz	100	—	45
Louis Rich				
Ground	3 oz	140	0	70
Mr. Turkey				
Ground 85% Fat Free	3.5 oz	210	—	110
Ground 91% Fat Free	3.5 oz	170	—	95
Perdue				
Breast Tenderloins Skinless & Boneless cooked	1 oz	29	—	13
Breast Cutlets Thin-Sliced Skinless & Boneless	1 oz	28	—	15
Breast Fillets Skinless & Boneless Fit 'n Easy cooked	1 oz	28	—	15
Breast Hotel Style Prime w/ Skin cooked	1 oz	43	—	16
Breast Skinless Boneless Fit'n Easy cooked	1 oz	28	—	15

FOOD	PORTION	CALS.	FIB.	CHOL.
Perdue (CONT.)				
Breast w/ Skin Fresh Young cooked	1 oz	44	—	17
Drumsticks w/ Skin Fresh Young cooked	1 oz	36	—	22
Ground cooked	1 oz	35	—	25
Ground Breast Meat cooked	1 oz	28	—	15
Thighs Skinless & Boneless Fit 'n Fresh cooked	1 oz	36	—	22
Thighs w/ Skin Fresh Young cooked	1 oz	48	—	23
Whole Dark Meat w/ skin cooked	1 oz	48	—	21
Whole White Meat Fresh Young w/ Skin cooked	1 oz	44	—	17
Wings Drummettes w/ Skin Fresh Young cooked	1 oz	43	—	23
Wings Portions w/ Skin Fresh Young cooked	1 oz	51	—	25
Wings w/ Skin Fresh Young cooked	1 oz	45	—	24
Swift-Eckrich				
Ground All White	3 oz	100	—	45
Wampler Longacre				
Ground raw	1 oz	60	—	30
back w/ skin roasted	½ back (9 oz)	637	—	238
breast w/ skin roasted	4 oz	212	—	83
dark meat w/ skin roasted	3.6 oz	230	—	93
dark meat w/o skin roasted	3 oz	170	—	78
dark meat w/o skin roasted	1 cup (5 oz)	262	—	119
ground cooked	3 oz	188	—	57
leg w/ skin roasted	2.5 oz	147	—	61
leg w/ skin roasted	1 (1.2 lbs)	1133	—	466
light meat w/ skin roasted	from ½ turkey (2.3 lbs)	2069	—	794
light meat w/ skin roasted	4.7 oz	268	—	103
light meat w/o skin roasted	4 oz	183	—	81
neck simmered	1 (5.3 oz)	274	—	186
skin roasted	from ½ turkey (9 oz)	1096	—	281
skin roasted	1 oz	141	—	36
w/ skin roasted	8.4 oz	498	—	196
w/ skin roasted	½ turkey (4 lbs)	3857	—	1514
w/ skin neck & giblets roasted	½ turkey (8.8 lbs)	4123	—	1920

FOOD	PORTION	CALS.	FIB.	CHOL.
w/o skin roasted	1 cup (5 oz)	238	—	107
w/o skin roasted	7.3 oz	354	—	159
wing w/ skin roasted	1 (6.5 oz)	426	—	150
FROZEN				
roast boneless seasoned light & dark meat roasted	1 pkg (1.7 lbs)	1213	—	413
FROZEN PREPARED				
Empire				
Patties	1 (3.1 oz)	200	1	5
READY-TO-USE				
Carl Buddig	1 oz	50	0	15
Honey Turkey	1 oz	40	—	15
Turkey Ham	1 oz	40	0	15
Empire				
Barbecue Whole	5 oz	250	0	100
Bologna	3 slices (1.8 oz)	90	0	30
Oven Prepared Breast Slices	3 slices (1.8 oz)	50	0	15
Pastrami	3 slices (1.8 oz)	60	1	30
Salami	3 slices (1.8 oz)	70	0	35
Smoked Breast Slices	3 slices (1.8 oz)	40	0	15
Falls				
BBQ	3 oz	140	—	55
Gourmet Breast	3 oz	80	—	35
Premium Cooked Breast	3 oz	100	—	40
Hansel n'Gretel				
Breast Gourmet	1 oz	28	—	9
Breast Gourmet Smoked	1 oz	31	—	11
Breast Honey	1 oz	28	—	9
Breast Lessalt Cooked	1 oz	25	—	9
Breast Oven Cooked	1 oz	26	—	8
Doubledecker Turkey Corned Beef	1 oz	30	—	12
Doubledecker Turkey Ham	1 oz	30	—	11
Healthy Choice				
Deli-Thin Variety Pack Honey Roast & Smoked	1.9 oz	60	0	25
Deli-Thin Variety Pack Breast	2.2 oz	70	0	30
Honey Roasted & Smoked	1 slice (1 oz)	35	0	15
Oven Roasted Breast	1 slice (1 oz)	35	0	15
Smoked Breast	1.9 oz	60	0	25
Hebrew National				
Deli Thin Hickory Smoked	1.8 oz	55	—	25
Deli Thin Lemon Garlic	1.8 oz	50	—	20
Deli Thin Oven Roasted	1.8 oz	80	—	20

FOOD	PORTION	CALS.	FIB.	CHOL.
Hormel				
Light & Lean 97 Breast Sliced	1 slice (1 oz)	30	0	10
Light & Lean 97 Breast Smoked	3 oz	80	0	35
Light & Lean 97 Cuts	16 pieces (1 oz)	30	0	15
Light & Lean 97 Cuts Smoked	16 pieces (1 oz)	30	0	15
Louis Rich				
Bologna	1 slice (28 g)	50	0	20
Breaded Nuggets	4 (3.2 oz)	260	0	35
Breaded Patties	1 (3 oz)	220	0	35
Breaded Sticks	3 (3 oz)	230	0	35
Carving Board Oven Roasted Breast	2 slices (1.6 oz)	40	0	20
Carving Board Oven Roasted Thin Carved Breast	6 slices (2.1 oz)	60	0	25
Carving Board Smoked Breast	2 slices (1.6 oz)	40	0	20
Chopped Ham	1 slice (1 oz)	46	0	20
Cotto Salami	1 slice (28 g)	40	0	25
Deli-Thin Smoked Breast	4 slices (1.8 oz)	50	0	20
Fat Free Hickory Smoked Breast	1 slice (1 oz)	25	0	10
Fat Free Oven Roasted Breast	1 slice (28 g)	25	0	10
Ham Round	1 slice (28 g)	34	0	20
Ham Square	3 slices (2.2 oz)	70	0	45
Hickory Smoked Dinner Slices Breast	1 slice (2.8 oz)	80	0	35
Honey Cured Turkey Ham	3 slices (2.2 oz)	70	0	45
Honey Roasted Breast	1 slice (1 oz)	30	0	10
Honey Roasted Dinner Slices Breast	1 slice (2.8 oz)	80	0	35
Oven Roasted Breast	2 oz	60	0	25
Oven Roasted Breast	1 slice (1 oz)	30	0	10
Oven Roasted Deli-Thin Breast	4 slices (1.8 oz)	50	0	20
Oven Roasted Dinner Slices Breast	1 slice (2.8 oz)	70	0	35
Pastrami	2 slices (1.6 oz)	45	0	30
Salami	1 slice (28 g)	45	0	20
Skinless Barbecued Breast	2 oz	60	0	25
Skinless Hickory Smoked Breast	2 oz	60	0	25
Skinless Honey Roasted Breast	2 oz	60	0	25
Skinless Oven Roasted Breast	2 oz	50	0	25
Smoked Breast	1 slice (1 oz)	25	0	10
Smoked White	1 slice (1 oz)	30	0	15
Turkey Ham	4 slices (1.8 oz)	60	0	35

FOOD	PORTION	CALS.	FIB.	CHOL.
Mr. Turkey				
Deli Cuts Hardwood Smoked Breast	3 slices	30	—	13
Deli Cuts Honey Roasted Breast	3 slices	30	—	15
Deli Cuts Oven Roasted Breast	3 slices	30	—	13
Deli Cuts Turkey Ham	3 slices	35	—	20
Deli Cuts Turkey Pastrami	3 slices	35	—	20
Hardwood Smoked Breast	1 slice	30	—	15
Hardwood Smoked Turkey Ham	1 slice	35	—	20
Honey Cured Turkey Ham	1 slice	30	—	20
Oven Roasted Breast	1 slice	30	—	15
Smoked Breakfast Turkey Ham	1 oz	30	—	18
Turkey Cotto Salami	1 slice	50	—	20
Turkey Ham	1 slice	35	—	20
Turkey Pastrami	1 slice	30	—	15
Turkey Bologna	1 slice	70	—	25
Oscar Mayer				
Deli-Thin Roast	4 slices (1.8 oz)	50	0	20
Deli-Thin Smoked Honey Roasted	4 slices (1.8 oz)	60	0	20
Free Oven Roasted Breast	4 slices (1.8 oz)	40	—	15
Free Smoked Breast	4 slices (1.8 oz)	40	—	15
Healthy Favorites Oven Roasted Breast	4 slices (1.8 oz)	40	0	15
Healthy Favorites Smoked Breast	4 slices (1.8 oz)	40	0	15
Lunchables Fun Pack Turkey/ Pacific Cooler	1 pkg (11.2 oz)	460	tr	50
Lunchables Fun Pack Turkey/ Surger Cooler	1 pkg (11.2 oz)	440	0	45
Lunchables Turkey Oven Roasted/Green Onion Cheese	1 pkg (4.5 oz)	380	1	40
Lunchables Turkey Smoked/ Ranch & Herb Cheese	1 pkg (4.5 oz)	380	1	45
Lunchables Turkey/Cheddar	1 pkg (4.5 oz)	360	1	70
Perdue				
Nuggets	1 (.67 oz)	54	—	7
Sara Lee				
Hardwood Smoked Breast Of Turkey	2 oz	60	—	20
Hardwood Smoked Turkey Ham	2 oz	60	—	40
Honey Roasted Breast Of Turkey	2 oz	60	—	20
Honey Roasted Turkey Ham	2 oz	70	—	40

FOOD	PORTION	CALS.	FIB.	CHOL.
Sara Lee (CONT.)				
Mesquite Smoked Breast Of Turkey	2 oz	60	—	30
Oven Roasted Breast Of Turkey	2 oz	60	—	25
Peppered Breast Of Turkey	2 oz	50	—	20
Seasoned Breast Of Turkey Pastrami	2 oz	60	—	30
Wampler Longacre				
Bologna	1 oz	60	—	20
Breast Chops	1 serv (4 oz)	120	—	50
Breast Sliced	1 slice (1 oz)	35	—	30
Breast Sliced Smoked	1 slice (0.75 oz)	20	—	10
Burger	1 (4 oz)	230	—	120
Burger	1 (3 oz)	170	—	90
Burger Barbecue	1 (4 oz)	240	—	120
Chef Select Breast Skinless	1 oz	35	—	15
Chef's Select Breast Smoked	1 oz	35	—	15
Chunk Dark Smoked Cured	1 oz	45	—	25
Chunk Ham 12% Water Smoked	1 oz	45	—	15
Chunk Ham 20% Water	1 oz	40	—	20
Chunk Pastrami	1 oz	35	—	20
Cook-In-The-Bag Breast	1 oz	30	—	15
Cook-In-The-Bag Breast Mini	1 oz	30	—	10
Cook-In-The-Bag Combo Roast	1 oz	35	—	15
Cook-In-The-Bag Thigh Roast	1 oz	40	—	15
Dark Smoked Cured	1 oz	45	—	25
Deli Chef Breast And White Meat No Skin	1 oz	40	—	15
Gourmet Breast	1 oz	35	—	15
Gourmet Breast Mini	1 oz	35	—	15
Gourmet Breast Mini Smoked	1 oz	35	—	15
Gourmet Breast Smoked	1 oz	30	—	15
Gourmet Brown & Glazed Breast	1 oz	35	—	15
Gourmet Brown & Roasted Breast	1 oz	35	—	15
Gourmet Honey Cured Breast	1 oz	30	—	15
Lean-Lite Breast Skinless	1 oz	35	—	15
Lean-Lite Deli Breast	1 oz	35	—	15
Lean-Lite Deli Breast Smoked	1 oz	35	—	15
Old Fashioned Brown & Roasted Breast	1 oz	35	—	15
Pastrami	1 oz	35	—	20

FOOD	PORTION	CALS.	FIB.	CHOL.
Wampler Longacre (CONT.)				
Premium Breast Skinless	1 oz	30	—	15
Premium Brown & Roasted Breast Skinless	1 oz	16	—	15
Roll Combo	1 oz	44	—	17
Roll Sliced Breast	1 slice (0.75 oz)	30	—	30
Roll White	1 oz	45	—	15
Salami	1 oz	50	—	20
Salt Watchers Breast Skinless	1 oz	35	—	15
Seasoned Roast	1 oz	40	—	15
Sliced Salami	1 slice (0.8 oz)	45	—	20
Tenderlings BBQ	1 serv (4 oz)	110	—	40
Tenderlings Cajun	1 serv (4 oz)	110	—	40
Tenderlings Garlic & Pepper	1 serv (4 oz)	110	—	40
Tenderlings Original	1 serv (4 oz)	110	—	40
Turkey Ham 12% Water Baked	1 oz	45	—	15
Turkey Ham 20% Water Baked	1 oz	40	—	20
Unseasoned Roast	1 oz	40	—	15
Whole Browned & Roasted	1 oz	60	—	20
Weight Watchers				
Deli Thin Smoked Breast	5 slices (⅓ oz)	10	—	5
Oven Roasted Breast	2 slices (¾ oz)	25	—	10
Oven Roasted Turkey Ham	2 slices (¾ oz)	25	—	10
Roasted & Smoked Breast	2 slices (¾ oz)	25	—	10
bologna	1 oz	57	—	28
breast	1 slice (¾ oz)	23	—	9
poultry salad sandwich spread	1 oz	238	—	9
poultry salad sandwich spread	1 tbsp	109	—	4
prebasted breast w/ skin roasted	1 breast (3.8 lbs)	2175	—	718
prebasted breast w/ skin roasted	½ breast (1.9 lbs)	1087	—	359
prebasted thigh w/ skin roasted	1 thigh (11 oz)	494	—	194
roll light & dark meat	1 oz	42	—	16
roll light meat	1 oz	42	—	12
salami cooked	2 oz	111	—	46
salami cooked	1 pkg (8 oz)	446	—	186
turkey loaf breast meat	1 pkg (6 oz)	187	—	69
turkey loaf breast meat	2 slices (1.5 oz)	47	—	17

TURKEY DISHES

(*see also* DINNER, TURKEY SUBSTITUTES)

CANNED

Dinty Moore

| American Classics Chicken With Mashed Potatoes | 1 bowl (10 oz) | 250 | 3 | 25 |

FOOD	PORTION	CALS.	FIB.	CHOL.
Dinty Moore (CONT.)				
American Classics Turkey & Dressing With Gravy	1 bowl (10 oz)	280	4	35
FROZEN				
Luigino's				
Gravy Dressing & Turkey	1 pkg (8 oz)	340	2	40
READY-TO-USE				
Spreadables				
Turkey Salad	¼ can	100	—	20
Wampler Longacre				
Meatloaf Italian	1 serv (4 oz)	114	—	56
Meatloaf Mexican	1 serv (4 oz)	114	—	56
Meatloaf Original	1 serv (4 oz)	126	—	80
Salad	1 oz	60	—	10
Salad Turkey Ham	1 oz	50	—	10
Teriyaki	1 serv (4 oz)	112	—	25

TURKEY SUBSTITUTES

Harvest Direct				
TVP Poultry Chunks	3.5 oz	280	18	0
TVP Poultry Ground	3.5 oz	280	18	0
White Wave				
Meatless Sandwich Slices	2 slices (1.6 oz)	80	1	0

TURMERIC

ground	1 tsp	8	—	0

TURNIPS

CANNED				
Allen				
Chopped Greens And Diced Turnip	½ cup (4.2 oz)	30	tr	0
Greens	½ cup (4.2 oz)	25	2	0
Sunshine				
Chopped Greens And Diced Turnip	½ cup (4.2 oz)	30	tr	0
Greens	½ cup (4.2 oz)	25	2	0
greens	½ cup	17	—	0
FRESH				
cooked mashed	½ cup (4.2 oz)	47	—	0
cubed cooked	½ cup (3 oz)	33	—	0
greens chopped cooked	½ cup	15	2	0
greens raw chopped	½ cup	7	1	0
raw cubed	½ cup (2.4 oz)	25	—	0

FOOD	PORTION	CALS.	FIB.	CHOL.
FROZEN				
Southland				
Rutabaga Yellow Turnips	4 oz	50	—	0
greens cooked	½ cup	24	2	0
VANILLA				
Virginia Dare				
Vanilla Extract	1 tsp	10	—	0
VEAL				
(see also BEEF, DINNER, VEAL DISHES)				
FRESH				
cutlet lean only braised	3 oz	172	—	115
cutlet lean only fried	3 oz	156	—	91
ground broiled	3 oz	146	—	87
loin chop w/ bone lean & fat braised	1 chop (2.8 oz)	227	—	94
loin chop w/ bone lean only braised	1 chop (2.4 oz)	155	—	86
shoulder w/ bone lean only braised	3 oz	169	—	110
sirloin w/ bone lean & fat roasted	3 oz	171	—	87
sirloin w/ bone lean only roasted	3 oz	143	—	89
VEAL DISHES				
TAKE-OUT				
parmigiana	4.2 oz	279	2	136
VEGETABLE JUICE				
Mott's				
Vegetable Juice as prep	8 fl oz	60	2	0
Odwalla				
Vegetable Cocktail	8 fl oz	70	2	0
V8				
No Salt Added	6 fl oz	35	—	0
Spicy Hot	6 fl oz	35	—	0
vegetable juice cocktail	6 fl oz	34	—	0
vegetable juice cocktail	½ cup	22	—	0
VEGETABLES MIXED				
(see also individual vegetables, VEGETABLE JUICES)				
CANNED				
Allen				
Green Beans And Pototoes	½ cup (4.2 oz)	35	2	0
Okra & Tomatoes	½ cup (4 oz)	25	3	0
Okra Tomatoes & Corn	½ cup (4.1 oz)	30	4	0

FOOD	PORTION	CALS.	FIB.	CHOL.
Chi-Chi's				
Diced Tomatoes & Green Chilies	¼ cup (2.5 oz)	20	0	0
Del Monte				
Mixed	½ cup (4.4 oz)	40	2	0
Peas And Carrots	½ cup (4.5 oz)	60	2	0
Green Giant				
Garden Medley	½ cup	40	1	0
Hanover				
Mixed	½ cup	110	—	0
Vegetable Salad	½ cup	90	—	0
House Of Tsang				
Vegetables & Sauce Cantonese Classic	½ cup (4.2 oz)	70	1	0
Vegetables & Sauce Hong Kong Sweet & Sour	½ cup (4.5 oz)	160	0	0
Vegetables & Sauce Szechuan Hot & Spicy	½ cup (4.2 oz)	70	1	0
Vegetables & Sauce Tokyo Teriyaki	½ cup (4.4 oz)	100	0	0
Ka-Me				
Stir Fry	½ cup (4.5 oz)	20	2	0
La Choy				
Chop Suey Vegetables	½ cup	10	tr	0
S&W				
Garden Salad Marinated	½ cup	60	—	0
Mixed Vegetables Old Fashion Harvest Time	½ cup	35	—	0
Peas & Carrots Water Pack	½ cup	35	—	0
Succotash Country Style	½ cup	80	—	0
Sweet Peas & Diced Carrots	½ cup	50	—	0
Sweet Peas w/ Tiny Pearl Onions	½ cup	60	—	0
Seneca				
Peas & Carrots	½ cup	60	4	0
Succotash	½ cup	90	2	0
Sunshine				
Green Beans And Pototoes	½ cup (4.2 oz)	35	2	0
Trappey				
Okra & Tomatoes	½ cup (4 oz)	25	3	0
Okra Tomatoes & Corn	½ cup (4.1 oz)	30	4	0
mixed vegetables	½ cup	39	—	0
peas & carrots	½ cup	48	—	0
peas & carrots low sodium	½ cup	48	—	0

FOOD	PORTION	CALS.	FIB.	CHOL.
peas & onions	½ cup	30	—	0
succotash	½ cup	102	—	0
FROZEN				
Big Valley				
California Blend	¾ cup (3 oz)	25	3	0
Italian Blend	¾ cup (3 oz)	30	2	0
Oriental Blend	¾ cup (3 oz)	25	3	0
Stew Vegetables	⅔ cup (3 oz)	40	2	0
Winter Blend	¾ cup (3 oz)	25	2	0
Birds Eye				
Broccoli Cauliflower And Carrots With Cheese Sauce	½ pkg	80	4	10
Farm Fresh Broccoli Carrots And Water Chestnuts	¾ cup	40	3	0
Farm Fresh Broccoli Cauliflower And Carrots	¾ cup	35	3	0
Farm Fresh Broccoli Cauliflower And Red Peppers	¾ cup	30	3	0
Farm Fresh Broccoli And Cauliflower	¾ cup	30	3	0
Farm Fresh Broccoli Corn And Red Peppers	⅔ cup	60	3	0
Farm Fresh Broccoli Green Beans Pearl Onions and Red Peppers	¾ cup	35	3	0
Farm Fresh Broccoli Red Peppers Onions And Mushrooms	¾ cup	30	3	0
Farm Fresh Brussels Sprouts Cauliflower And Carrots	¾ cup	40	4	0
Farm Fresh Cauliflower Carrots And Snow Peas	⅔ cup	35	4	0
In Butter Sauce Broccoli Cauliflower And Carrots	½ cup	40	2	5
In Sauce Peas And Pearl Onions With Seasonings	½ cup	70	3	0
Internationals Austrian	3.3 oz	70	1	10
Internationals Bavarian	3.3 oz	90	2	25
Internationals California	3.3 oz	90	3	10
Internationals French Country	3.3 oz	70	2	10
Internationals Japanese	3.3 oz	60	2	10
Internationals New England	3.3 oz	100	2	10
Internationals Italian	3.3 oz	80	2	20
Mixed	½ cup	60	2	0

FOOD	PORTION	CALS.	FIB.	CHOL.
Birds Eye (CONT.)				
Peas And Potatoes With Cream Sauce	½ cup	100	1	10
Polybag	½ cup	60	2	0
Budget Gourmet				
Mandarin Vegetables	1 pkg (5.25 oz)	160	—	10
New England Recipe Vegetables	1 pkg (5.5 oz)	230	—	25
Spring Vegetables In Cheese Sauce	1 pkg (5 oz)	130	—	20
Green Giant				
American Mixtures California	½ cup	25	2	0
American Mixtures Heartland	½ cup	25	2	0
American Mixtures New England	½ cup	70	4	0
American Mixtures San Francisco	½ cup	25	—	0
American Mixtures Sante Fe	½ cup	70	—	0
American Mixtures Seattle	½ cup	25	—	0
Broccoli Cauliflower And Carrots In Cheese Sauce	½ cup	60	2	2
Broccoli Cauliflower And Carrots In Butter Sauce	½ cup	30	—	5
Harvest Fresh Mixed Vegetables	½ cup	40	2	0
Mixed	½ cup	40	2	0
Mixed In Butter Sauce	½ cup	60	2	5
One Serve Broccoli Carrots & Rotini In Cheese Sauce	1 pkg	120	—	5
One Serve Broccoli Cauliflower And Carrots	1 pkg	25	3	0
Valley Combinations Broccoli & Cauliflower	½ cup	60	—	0
Hanover				
Broccoli Cut & Cauliflower Cut	½ cup	20	—	0
Caribbean Blend	½ cup	20	—	0
Garden Medley	½ cup	20	—	0
Mixed	½ cup	50	—	0
Oriental Blend	½ cup	25	—	0
Succotash	½ cup	80	—	0
Summer Vegetables	½ cup	35	—	0
Vegetables For Soup	½ cup	60	—	0
La Choy				
Mixed Fancy	½ cup	12	1	0

FOOD	PORTION	CALS.	FIB.	CHOL.
Ore Ida				
Stew Vegetables	⅔ cup (3 oz)	50	tr	0
Soglowek				
Golden Vegetarian Nuggets	4 pieces (2.5 oz)	190	1	0
Southland				
Peppers & Onions	2 oz	15	—	0
Soup Mix Vegetables	3.2 oz	50	—	0
Stew Vegetables	4 oz	60	—	0
Tree Of Life				
Mixed	½ cup (3 oz)	65	3	0
mixed vegetables cooked	½ cup	54	2	0
peas & carrots cooked	½ cup	38	—	0
peas & onions cooked	½ cup	40	—	0
succotash cooked	½ cup	79	—	0
SHELF-STABLE				
Pantry Express				
Corn Green Beans Carrots Pasta In Tomato Sauce	½ cup	80	3	0
Green Beans Potatoes And Mushrooms In A Seasoned Sauce	½ cup	50	2	0
Mixed Vegetables	½ cup	35	1	0
TAKE-OUT				
caponata	¼ cup	28	—	0
succotash	½ cup	111	—	0

VENISON
Broken Arrow Ranch

FOOD	PORTION	CALS.	FIB.	CHOL.
Antelope Chili Meat	3.5 oz	115	—	70
Antelope Ground Venison	3.5 oz	110	—	73
Antelope Stew Meat	3.5 oz	110	—	72
Nilgai Chili Meat	3.5 oz	115	—	70
Nilgai Leg	3.5 oz	100	—	65
Nilgai Stew Meat	3.5 oz	110	—	72
roasted	3 oz	134	—	95

VINEGAR
Hain

FOOD	PORTION	CALS.	FIB.	CHOL.
Cider	1 tbsp	2	—	0
Ka-Me				
Chinese Seasoned	1 tbsp (0.5 fl oz)	5	0	0
Rice Wine Chinese	1 tbsp (0.5 fl oz)	5	0	0
Rice Wine Japanese	1 tbsp (0.5 oz)	0	0	0
Seasoned Rice Japanese	1 tbsp (0.5 fl oz)	10	0	0
Nakano				
Rice	1 tbsp	0	—	0

FOOD	PORTION	CALS.	FIB.	CHOL.
Regina				
Red Wine	1 oz	4	—	0
Tree Of Life				
Apple Cidar Organic	1 tbsp (0.5 oz)	0	—	0
Brown Rice	1 tbsp (0.5 oz)	2	—	0
White House				
Apple Cider	2 tbsp	2	0	0
Red Wine	2 tbsp	4	—	0
cider	1 tbsp	tr	—	0

WAFFLES

FROZEN

FOOD	PORTION	CALS.	FIB.	CHOL.
Aunt Jemima				
Blueberry	2 (2.5 oz)	190	1	10
Buttermilk	2 (2.5 oz)	170	1	10
Cinnamon	2 (2.5 oz)	180	1	10
Oatmeal	2 (2.5 oz)	170	3	0
Whole Grain	2 (2.5 oz)	170	2	0
Belgian Chef				
Belgian	2 (2.5 oz)	140	1	0
Downyflake				
Blueberry	2	180	—	0
Buttermilk	2	190	—	0
Multi-Grain	2	250	4	0
Oat Bran	2	260	3	0
Regular	2	120	—	0
Regular Jumbo	2	170	—	0
Rice Bran	2	210	4	0
Roman Meal	2	280	3	4
Eggo				
Apple Cinnamon	2 (2.7 oz)	220	0	20
Blueberry	2 (2.7 oz)	220	0	20
Buttermilk	2 (2.7 oz)	220	0	25
Common Sense Oat Bran	2 (2.7 oz)	200	3	0
Common Sense Oat Bran With Fruit & Nut	2 (2.9 oz)	220	4	0
Homestyle	2 (2.7 oz)	220	0	25
Minis Blueberry	12 (3 oz)	240	0	25
Minis Cinnamon Toast	12 (3.2 oz)	280	0	25
Minis Homestyle	12 (1.8 oz)	240	0	25
Nut & Honey	2 (2.7 oz)	240	0	25
Nutri-Grain	2 (2.7 oz)	190	4	0
Nutri-Grain Multi-Bran	2 (2.7 oz)	180	6	0
Nutri-Grain Raisin & Bran	2 (3 oz)	210	5	0

FOOD	PORTION	CALS.	FIB.	CHOL.
Eggo (CONT.)				
Special K	2 (2 oz)	140	0	0
Strawberry	2 (2.7 oz)	220	0	20
Van's				
Belgian 7 Grain	1	80	—	0
Belgian Original	1	73	—	0
Toaster Apple Cinnamon	1	75	3	0
Toaster Honey Almond	1	75	3	0
Toaster Multigrain	1	75	3	0
Toaster Wheat Free	1	110	3	0
Toaster Wheat Free Cinnamon Apple	1	110	3	0
Weight Watchers				
Belgian	1 (1.5 oz)	120	—	5
Multi-Grain Belgian	1 (1.5 oz)	120	—	5
HOME RECIPE				
plain	1 (7 in diam)	218	—	52
MIX				
plain as prep	1-7 in diam (2.6 oz)	218	1	39
WALNUTS				
Planters				
Black	1 oz	180	—	0
English Halves	1 oz	190	—	0
black dried	1 oz	172	1	0
black dried chopped	1 cup	759	—	0
english dried	1 oz	182	1	0
english dried chopped	1 cup	770	6	0
WATER CHESTNUTS				
CANNED				
Empress				
Sliced	2 oz	14	—	0
Whole	2 oz	14	—	0
Ka-Me				
Whole in Water	½ cup (4.5 oz)	45	4	0
La Choy				
Sliced	¼ cup	18	tr	0
Whole	4	14	tr	0
chinese sliced	½ cup	35	—	0
FRESH				
sliced	½ cup	66	—	0
WATERCRESS				
(see also CRESS)				
FRESH				
raw chopped	½ cup	2	tr	0

FOOD	PORTION	CALS.	FIB.	CHOL.
WATERMELON				
cut up	1 cup	50	1	0
wedge	1/16	152	2	0
SEEDS				
dried	1 oz	158	—	0
dried	1 cup	602	—	0
WAX BEANS				
CANNED				
Del Monte				
Cut Golden	½ cup (4.3 oz)	20	2	0
Owatonna				
Cut	½ cup	20	—	0
S&W				
Golden Cut Premium	½ cup	20	—	0
Seneca				
Cuts Natural Pack	½ cup	25	2	0
Wax Beans	½ cup	25	2	0
WHEAT				
(see also BULGUR, BRAN, CEREAL, COUSCOUS, FLOUR, WHEAT GERM)				
Arrowhead				
Kamut Grain	¼ cup (1.7 oz)	140	5	0
Seitan Quick Mix	⅓ cup (1.4 oz)	150	2	0
Hodgson Mill				
Vital Wheat Gluten Plus Ascorbic Acid	1 tbsp (0.3 oz)	30	1	0
Near East				
Taboule Salad Mix as prep	⅔ cup	120	3	0
Wheat Pilaf as prep	1 cup	220	5	0
White Wave				
Seitan	½ pkg (4 oz)	140	1	0
Seitan Fajita Strips	⅓ cup (1.8 oz)	60	1	0
Seitan Marinated Slices	3 slices (1.8 oz)	60	1	0
sprouted	⅓ cup	71	—	0
WHEAT GERM				
Arrowhead	3 tbsp (0.5 oz)	50	2	0
Hodgson Mill	2 tbsp (0.5 oz)	55	4	0
Kretschmer	¼ cup	103	3	0
Honey Crunch	¼ cup	105	3	0
Stone-Buhr				
Untoasted	2 tbsp (0.5 oz)	58	2	0
plain toasted	¼ cup	108	4	0
plain toasted	1 cup	431	—	0
plain untoasted	¼ cup	104	4	0

FOOD	PORTION	CALS.	FIB.	CHOL.
WHIPPED TOPPINGS				
(see also CREAM)				
Cool Whip				
Extra Creamy	1 tbsp	13	—	tr
Lite	1 tbsp	9	—	tr
Non Dairy	1 tbsp	11	—	tr
D-Zerta				
D-Zerta as prep	1 tbsp	7	—	tr
Dream Whip				
as prep	1 tbsp	9	—	1
Hood				
Instant	2 tbsp	20	0	<5
Light Instant	2 tbsp	15	0	<5
Kraft				
Real Cream	2 tbsp (0.4 oz)	20	0	5
Whipped Topping	2 tbsp (0.4 oz)	20	0	0
La Creme	1 tbsp	16	—	tr
Pet				
Whip	1 tbsp	14	—	0
Reddiwip				
Lite	2 tbsp (8 g)	15	—	0
Non-Dairy	2 tbsp (8 g)	20	—	0
Real Whipped Heavy Cream	2 tbsp (8 g)	30	—	10
Real Whipped Light Cream	2 tbsp (8 g)	20	—	<5
cream pressurized	1 cup	154	—	46
cream pressurized	1 tbsp	8	—	2
nondairy powdered as prep w/ whole milk	1 cup	151	—	8
nondairy powdered as prep w/ whole milk	1 tbsp	8	—	tr
nondairy pressurized	1 tbsp	11	—	0
nondairy pressurized	1 cup	184	—	0
nondairy frzn	1 tbsp	13	—	0
WHITE BEANS				
CANNED				
Goya				
Spanish Style	7.5 oz	130	12	0
Progresso				
Cannellini	½ cup	80	7	0
white beans	1 cup	306	—	0
DRIED				
regular cooked	1 cup	249	—	0
small cooked	1 cup	253	—	0

FOOD	PORTION	CALS.	FIB.	CHOL.

WHITEFISH
baked	3 oz	146	—	65
smoked	3 oz	92	—	28
smoked	1 oz	39	—	9

WHITING
cooked	3 oz	98	—	71
raw	3 oz	77	—	57

WILD RICE
cooked	½ cup	83	—	0

WINE
(see also CHAMPAGNE, WINE COOLERS)

FOOD	PORTION	CALS.	FIB.	CHOL.
Boone's				
Country Kwencher	1 fl oz	24	—	0
Delicious Apple	1 fl oz	21	—	0
Sangria	1 fl oz	22	—	0
Snow Creek Berry	1 fl oz	18	—	0
Strawberry Hill	1 fl oz	22	—	0
Sun Peak Peach	1 fl oz	18	—	0
Wild Island	1 fl oz	18	—	0
Carlo Rossi				
Blush	1 fl oz	21	—	0
Burgundy	1 fl oz	22	—	0
Chablis	1 fl oz	21	—	0
Paisano	1 fl oz	23	—	0
Red Sangria	1 fl oz	24	—	0
Rhine	1 fl oz	21	—	0
Vin Rosé	1 fl oz	21	—	0
White Grenache	1 fl oz	20	—	0
Fairbanks				
Cream Sherry	1 fl oz	42	—	0
Port	1 fl oz	44	—	0
Sherry	1 fl oz	34	—	0
White Port	1 fl oz	44	—	0
Gallo				
Blush Chablis	1 fl oz	22	—	0
Burgundy	1 fl oz	22	—	0
Cabernet Sauvignon	1 fl oz	22	—	0
Chablis Blanc	1 fl oz	20	—	0
Chardonnay	1 fl oz	23	—	0
Classic Burgundy	1 fl oz	21	—	0
French Colombard	1 fl oz	21	—	0
Hearty Burgundy	1 fl oz	22	—	0

FOOD	PORTION	CALS.	FIB.	CHOL.
Gallo (CONT.)				
Johannesburg Riesling '88	1 fl oz	20	—	0
Pink Chablis	1 fl oz	20	—	0
Red Rosé	1 fl oz	23	—	0
Rhine	1 fl oz	22	—	0
Sauvignon Blanc '90	1 fl oz	20	—	0
White Grenache '92	1 fl oz	20	—	0
White Grenache New Vintage	1 fl oz	20	—	0
White Zinfandel '91	1 fl oz	18	—	0
White Zinfandel New Vintage	1 fl oz	18	—	0
Zinfandel '87	1 fl oz	23	—	0
Ka-Me				
Chinese Cooking	2 tbsp (1 fl oz)	20	0	0
Sheffield Cellars				
Sherry	1 fl oz	44	—	0
Tawny Port	1 fl oz	45	—	0
Vermouth Extra Dry	1 fl oz	28	—	0
Vermouth Sweet	1 fl oz	43	—	0
Very Dry Sherry	1 fl oz	32	—	0
red	3½ oz	74	—	0
rose	3½ oz	73	—	0
sherry	2 oz	84	—	0
sweet dessert	2 oz	90	—	0
vermouth dry	3½ oz	105	—	0
vermouth sweet	3½ oz	167	—	0
white	3½ oz	70	—	0

WINE COOLERS

Bartles & Jaymes				
Berry	12 fl oz	210	—	0
Margarita	12 fl oz	260	—	0
Original	12 fl oz	190	—	0
Peach	12 fl oz	210	—	0
Pina Colada	12 fl oz	280	—	0
Planter's Punch	12 fl oz	230	—	0
Strawberry	12 fl oz	210	—	0
Strawberry Daiquiri	12 fl oz	230	—	0
Tropical	12 fl oz	230	—	0

WINGED BEANS

dried cooked	1 cup	252	—	0

WOLFFISH

atlantic baked	3 oz	105	—	50

FOOD	PORTION	CALS.	FIB.	CHOL.
YAM				
(see also SWEET POTATO)				
CANNED				
Allen				
Cut	⅔ cup (5.8 oz)	160	3	0
Princella				
Cut	⅔ cup (5.8 oz)	160	3	0
Royal Prince				
Whole	4 pieces (5.9 oz)	200	4	0
S&W				
Candied	½ cup	180	—	0
Southern Whole In Extra Heavy Syrup	½ cup	139	—	0
Sugary Sam				
Cut	⅔ cup (5.8 oz)	160	3	0
Trappey				
Whole	4 pieces (5.9 oz)	200	4	0
FRESH				
mountain yam hawaii cooked	½ cup	59	—	0
yam cubed cooked	½ cup	79	—	0
YAMBEAN				
cooked	¾ cup	38	—	0
YARDLONG BEANS				
dried cooked	1 cup	202	—	0
YEAST				
Fleischmann's				
Active Dry	1 pkg (¼ oz)	20	—	0
Fresh Active	1 pkg (0.6 oz)	15	—	0
Household Yeast	½ oz	15	—	0
RapidRise	1 pkg (¼ oz)	20	—	0
Red Star				
Small Flakes	4 tbsp (0.5 oz)	47	4	0
Yeast Flakes	3 tbsp (0.5 oz)	47	4	0
	3 tbsp (0.5 oz)	47	4	0
baker's compressed	1 cake (0.6 oz)	18	2	0
baker's dry	1 tbsp	35	3	0
baker's dry	1 pkg (¼ oz)	21	—	0
brewer's dry	1 tbsp	25	—	0
YELLOW BEANS				
CANNED				
B&M				
Baked Beans	8 oz	326	—	4

FOOD	PORTION	CALS.	FIB.	CHOL.
DRIED				
cooked	1 cup	254	—	0
YELLOWEYE BEANS				
DRIED				
Bean Cuisine	½ cup	115	5	0
YOGURT				
(see also YOGURT FROZEN)				
Breyers				
1% Fat Black Cherry	8 oz	260	0	15
1% Fat Blueberry	8 oz	250	0	15
1% Fat Mixed Berry	8 oz	250	0	15
1% Fat Peach	8 oz	250	0	15
1% Fat Pineapple	8 oz	250	0	15
1% Fat Red Raspberry	8 oz	250	2	15
1% Fat Strawberry	8 oz	250	0	15
1% Fat Strawberry Banana	8 oz	250	tr	15
1.5% Fat Coffee	8 oz	220	0	20
1.5% Fat Plain	8 oz	130	0	20
1.5% Fat Vanilla	8 oz	220	0	20
Cabot				
All Flavors	8 oz	220	—	10
Plain	8 oz	140	—	14
Colombo				
Banana Strawberry	8 oz	210	0	15
Black Cherry	8 oz	200	0	15
Blueberry	8 oz	200	0	15
Fat Free Apples 'n Spice	8 oz	190	0	5
Fat Free Apricot	8 oz	190	0	5
Fat Free Banana Strawberry	8 oz	200	0	5
Fat Free Blueberry	8 oz	190	0	5
Fat Free Cappuccino	8 oz	180	0	<5
Fat Free Cherry	8 oz	190	0	5
Fat Free Cranberry Strawberry	8 oz	200	0	5
Fat Free French Roast	8 oz	180	0	<5
Fat Free Fruit Cocktail	8 oz	190	0	5
Fat Free Lemon	8 oz	170	0	<5
Fat Free Peach	8 oz	190	0	5
Fat Free Plain	8 oz	110	0	5
Fat Free Raspberry	8 oz	190	0	5
Fat Free Strawberry	8 oz	190	0	5
Fat Free Strawberry Pineapple Orange	8 oz	190	0	5
Fat Free Vanilla	8 oz	170	0	5

FOOD	PORTION	CALS.	FIB.	CHOL.
Colombo (CONT.)				
French Vanilla	8 oz	180	0	20
Light 100 Blueberry	8 oz	100	0	<5
Light 100 Cherry Vanilla	8 oz	100	0	<5
Light 100 Coffee & Cream	8 oz	100	0	<5
Light 100 Creamy Vanilla	8 oz	100	0	<5
Light 100 Fruit Medley	8 oz	100	0	<5
Light 100 Juicy Peach	8 oz	100	0	<5
Light 100 Lemon Creme	8 oz	100	0	<5
Light 100 Mandarin Orange	8 oz	100	0	<5
Light 100 Mixed Berries	8 oz	100	0	<5
Light 100 Raspberry	8 oz	100	0	<5
Light 100 Strawberry	8 oz	100	0	<5
Peach Melba	8 oz	200	0	15
Plain	8 oz	120	0	20
Raspberry	8 oz	200	0	15
Sprinkl'ns All Flavors	1 pkg (4.1 oz)	145	—	5
Strawberry	8 oz	200	0	15
Dannon				
Blended Nonfat Blueberry	6 oz	160	0	<5
Blended Nonfat French Vanilla	6 oz	160	0	<5
Blended Nonfat Lemon Chiffon	6 oz	150	0	<5
Blended Nonfat Peach	6 oz	150	0	<5
Blended Nonfat Raspberry	6 oz	160	0	<5
Blended Nonfat Strawberry	6 oz	150	0	<5
Blended Nonfat Strawberry Banana	6 oz	150	0	<5
Danimals Lowfat Tropical Punch	4.4 oz	140	0	10
Danimals Lowfat Blueberry	4.4 oz	140	0	10
Danimals Lowfat Grape Lemonade	4.4 oz	130	0	10
Danimals Lowfat Lemon Ice	4.4 oz	130	0	10
Danimals Lowfat Orange Banana	4.4 oz	140	0	10
Danimals Lowfat Strawberry	4.4 oz	140	0	10
Danimals Lowfat Vanilla	4.4 oz	140	0	10
Danimals Lowfat Wild Raspberry	4.4 oz	130	0	10
Fruit On The Bottom Lowfat Apple Cinnamon	8 oz	240	1	15
Fruit On The Bottom Lowfat Blueberry	8 oz	240	1	15
Fruit On The Bottom Lowfat Boysenberry	8 oz	240	1	15

FOOD	PORTION	CALS.	FIB.	CHOL.
Dannon (CONT.)				
Fruit On The Bottom Lowfat Cherry	8 oz	240	1	15
Fruit On The Bottom Lowfat Mixed Berries	8 oz	240	1	15
Fruit On The Bottom Lowfat Orange	8 oz	240	0	15
Fruit On The Bottom Lowfat Peach	8 oz	240	1	15
Fruit On The Bottom Lowfat Pear	8 oz	240	1	15
Fruit On The Bottom Lowfat Raspberry	8 oz	240	1	15
Fruit On The Bottom Lowfat Strawberry	8 oz	240	1	15
Fruit On The Bottom Lowfat Strawberry Banana	8 oz	240	1	15
Light Nonfat Banana Cream Pie	4.4 oz	60	0	0
Light Nonfat Cherry Vanilla	1 cup (3.5 oz)	110	0	<5
Light Nonfat Lemon Chiffon	4.4 oz	60	0	0
Light Nonfat Peach	4.4 oz	50	0	0
Light Nonfat Strawberry	1 cup (3.5 oz)	110	0	<5
Light Nonfat Strawberry	4.4 oz	50	0	0
Light Nonfat Vanilla	1 cup (3.5 oz)	110	0	<5
Light 'N Crunchy Nonfat Cappuccino w/ Chocolate	1 pkg	150	0	<5
Light 'N Crunchy Nonfat Caramel Apple Crunch	1 pkg	150	0	<5
Light 'N Crunchy Nonfat Raspberry w/ Granola	1 pkg	150	0	<5
Light 'N Crunchy Nonfat Vanilla w/ Chocolate	1 pkg	150	0	<5
Light 'n Crunchy Nonfat Lemon Chiffon w/ Blueberry	1 pkg	140	0	<5
Light Nonfat Banana Cream Pie	8 oz	100	0	<5
Light Nonfat Blueberry	8 oz	100	0	<5
Light Nonfat Creme Caramel	8 oz	100	0	<5
Light Nonfat Lemon	8 oz	100	0	<5
Light Nonfat Peach	8 oz	100	0	<5
Light Nonfat Raspberry	8 oz	100	0	<5
Light Nonfat Strawberry	8 oz	100	0	<5
Light Nonfat Strawberry Banana	8 oz	100	0	<5
Light Nonfat Tropical Fruit	8 oz	100	0	<5

FOOD	PORTION	CALS.	FIB.	CHOL.
Dannon (CONT.)				
Light Nonfat Vanilla	8 oz	100	0	<5
Lowfat Coffee	1 cup (8.7 oz)	230	0	20
Lowfat Coffee	8 oz	210	0	15
Lowfat Cranberry Raspberry	8 oz	210	0	15
Lowfat Lemon	1 cup (8.7 oz)	230	0	20
Lowfat Lemon	8 oz	210	0	15
Lowfat Plain	1 cup (8.7 oz)	150	0	20
Lowfat Plain	8 oz	140	0	20
Lowfat Vanilla	1 cup (8.7 oz)	230	0	20
Lowfat Vanilla	8 oz	210	0	15
Minipack Blended Nonfat Blueberry	4.4 oz	120	0	<5
Minipack Blended Nonfat Cherry	4.4 oz	110	0	<5
Minipack Blended Nonfat Peach	4.4 oz	110	0	<5
Minipack Blended Nonfat Raspberry	4.4 oz	120	0	<5
Minipack Blended Nonfat Strawberry	4.4 oz	110	0	<5
Minipack Blended Nonfat Strawberry Banana	4.4 oz	110	0	<5
Nonfat Plain	8 oz	110	0	5
Nonfat Plain	1 cup (8.7 oz)	120	0	0
Nonfat Light Cherry Vanilla	8 oz	100	0	<5
Nonfat Light Strawberry Fruit Cup	8 oz	100	0	<5
Sprinkl'ins Banana	4.1 oz	140	0	10
Sprinkl'ins Cherry Vanilla	4.1 oz	140	0	10
Sprinkl'ins Crazy Crunch Cherry w/ Honey Grahams	4.4 oz	170	0	10
Sprinkl'ins Crazy Crunch Grape w/ Chocolate Grahams	4.4 oz	160	0	10
Sprinkl'ins Crazy Crunch Vanilla w/ Chocolate Grahams	4.4 oz	160	0	10
Sprinkl'ins Crazy Crunch Vanilla w/ Honey Grahams	4.4 oz	170	0	10
Sprinkl'ins Strawberry	4.1 oz	140	0	10
Sprinkl'ins Strawberry Banana	4.1 oz	140	0	10
Tropifruta Nonfat Banana	6 oz	150	0	5
Tropifruta Nonfat Guava	6 oz	150	0	5
Tropifruta Nonfat Mango	6 oz	150	0	5
Tropifruta Nonfat Papaya Pineapple	6 oz	150	0	5

FOOD	PORTION	CALS.	FIB.	CHOL.
Dannon (CONT.)				
Tropifruta Nonfat Pina Colada	6 oz	150	0	5
Tropifruta Nonfat Strawberry	6 oz	150	0	5
Tropifruta Nonfat Strawberry Banana	6 oz	150	0	5
Tropifruta Nonfat Strawberry Kiwi	6 oz	150	0	5
With Fruit Toppings Banana Creme Strawberry	6 oz	170	1	10
With Fruit Toppings Bavarian Creme Raspberry	6 oz	170	0	10
With Fruit Toppings Cheesecake Cherry	6 oz	170	0	10
With Fruit Toppings Cheesecake Strawberry	6 oz	170	1	10
With Fruit Toppings Vanilla Peach & Apricot	6 oz	170	0	10
With Fruit Toppings Vanilla Strawberry	6 oz	170	1	10
Friendship				
Coffee	8 oz	210	0	20
Fruit Crunch Blueberry	6 oz	190	0	10
Fruit Crunch Peach	6 oz	190	0	10
Fruit Crunch Strawberry	6 oz	190	0	10
Fruit Crunch Strawberry Banana	6 oz	190	0	10
Plain	8 oz	150	0	20
Hood				
Fat Free Blueberry	1 (8 oz)	190	1	5
Fat Free Plain	1 (8 oz)	130	0	5
Fat Free Raspberry	1 (8 oz)	190	1	5
Fat Free Strawberry	1 (8 oz)	190	1	5
Fat Free Strawberry Banana	1 (8 oz)	190	1	5
Fat Free Vanilla	1 (8 oz)	190	1	5
Fat Free Swiss Blueberry	1 (8 oz)	210	0	5
Fat Free Swiss Lemon	1 (8 oz)	210	0	5
Fat Free Swiss Raspberry	1 (8 oz)	210	0	5
Fat Free Swiss Strawberry	1 (8 oz)	210	0	5
Fat Free Swiss Strawberry Banana	1 (8 oz)	210	0	5
Fat Free Swiss Vanilla	1 (8 oz)	210	0	5
Knudsen				
1.5% Fat Creamy Lemon	8 oz	220	0	20
70 Calories Black Cherry	6 oz	70	0	<5

FOOD	PORTION	CALS.	FIB.	CHOL.
Knudsen (CONT.)				
70 Calories Blueberry	6 oz	70	0	5
70 Calories Lemon	6 oz	70	tr	5
70 Calories Peach	6 oz	70	tr	5
70 Calories Pineapple	6 oz	70	0	5
70 Calories Red Raspberry	6 oz	70	0	5
70 Calories Strawberry	6 oz	70	0	5
70 Calories Strawberry Banana	6 oz	70	0	5
70 Calories Strawberry Fruit Basket	6 oz	70	0	5
70 Calories Vanilla	6 oz	70	0	5
Free Lemon	6 oz	160	0	5
Free Mixed Berry	6 oz	170	0	5
Free Peach	6 oz	170	0	5
Free Red Raspberry	6 oz	170	0	5
Free Strawberry	6 oz	170	0	5
Free Vanilla	6 oz	170	0	5
La Yogurt				
French Style Banana	6 oz	180	0	10
French Style Blueberry	6 oz	180	1	10
French Style Cherry	6 oz	180	0	10
French Style Cherry Vanilla	6 oz	190	0	10
French Style Guava	6 oz	180	1	10
French Style Key Lime	6 oz	180	0	10
French Style Mango	6 oz	180	0	10
French Style Mixed Berry	6 oz	180	0	10
French Style Nonfat Blueberry	6 oz	70	0	5
French Style Nonfat Cherry	6 oz	75	0	5
French Style Nonfat Raspberry	6 oz	70	0	5
French Style Nonfat Strawberry	6 oz	70	0	5
French Style Nonfat Strawberry Banana	6 oz	70	0	5
French Style Peach	6 oz	180	0	10
French Style Pina Colada	6 oz	180	0	10
French Style Raspberry	6 oz	180	1	10
French Style Strawberry	6 oz	180	0	10
French Style Strawberry Banana	6 oz	180	0	10
French Style Strawberry Fruit Cup	6 oz	180	0	10
French Style Tropical Orange	6 oz	180	0	10
French Style Vanilla	6 oz	170	0	15
Latin Style Banana	6 oz	190	0	10
Latin Style Guava	6 oz	190	0	10

FOOD	PORTION	CALS.	FIB.	CHOL.
La Yogurt (CONT.)				
Latin Style Mango	6 oz	190	0	10
Latin Style Papaya	6 oz	190	0	10
Latin Style Passion Fruit	6 oz	190	0	10
Latin Style Strawberry Kiwi	6 oz	180	0	10
Light N'Lively				
Free Blueberry	6 oz	190	0	5
Free Lemon	6 oz	170	0	5
Free Mixed Berry	6 oz	170	0	5
Free Peach	6 oz	170	0	5
Free Red Raspberry	6 oz	180	0	5
Free Strawberry	6 oz	180	0	5
Free Strawberry Fruit Cup	6 oz	170	0	5
Free Vanilla	6 oz	160	0	5
Free 50 Calories Blueberry	4.4 oz	50	0	<5
Free 50 Calories Peach	4.4 oz	50	0	<5
Free 50 Calories Red Raspberry	4.4 oz	50	0	<5
Free 50 Calories Strawberry	4.4 oz	50	0	<5
Free 50 Calories Strawberry Banana	4.4 oz	50	0	<5
Free 50 Calories Strawberry Fruit Cup	4.4 oz	50	0	<5
Free 70 Calories Black Cherry	6 oz	70	0	<5
Free 70 Calories Blueberry	6 oz	70	0	<5
Free 70 Calories Lemon	6 oz	70	0	<5
Free 70 Calories Peach	6 oz	70	0	<5
Free 70 Calories Red Raspberry	6 oz	70	0	<5
Free 70 Calories Strawberry	6 oz	70	0	<5
Free 70 Calories Strawberry Banana	6 oz	70	0	<5
Free 70 Calories Strawberry Fruit Cup	6 oz	70	0	<5
Kidpack Banana Berry	4.4 oz	130	0	10
Kidpack Berry Blue	4.4 oz	150	0	10
Kidpack Cherry	4.4 oz	140	0	10
Kidpack Grape	4.4 oz	130	0	10
Kidpack Outrageous Orange	4.4 oz	150	0	10
Kidpack Tropical Punch	4.4 oz	140	0	10
Kidpack Wild Berry	4.4 oz	140	0	10
Kidpack Wild Strawberry	4.4 oz	140	0	10
Multipack Blueberry	4.4 oz	140	0	10
Multipack Peach	4.4 oz	140	0	10
Multipack Pineapple	4.4 oz	140	0	5
Multipack Red Raspberry	4.4 oz	130	0	10

FOOD	PORTION	CALS.	FIB.	CHOL.
Light N'Lively (CONT.)				
Multipack Strawberry	4.4 oz	140	0	10
Multipack Strawberry Banana	4.4 oz	140	0	10
Multipack Strawberry Fruit Cup	4.4 oz	140	0	10
Weight Watchers				
Nonfat Plain	1 cup	90	—	5
Ultimate 90 All Flavors	1 cup	90	—	5
Yoplait				
Custard Style Banana	6 oz	190	—	20
Custard Style Blueberry	6 oz	190	—	20
Custard Style Cherry	6 oz	180	—	20
Custard Style Lemon	6 oz	190	—	20
Custard Style Mixed Berry	6 oz	180	—	20
Custard Style Raspberry	6 oz	190	—	20
Custard Style Strawberry	4 oz	130	—	15
Custard Style Strawberry	6 oz	190	—	20
Custard Style Strawberry Banana	6 oz	190	—	20
Custard Style Strawberry Banana	4 oz	130	—	15
Custard Style Vanilla	4 oz	130	—	15
Custard Style Vanilla	6 oz	180	—	20
Fat Free Blueberry	6 oz	150	—	5
Fat Free Cherry	6 oz	150	—	5
Fat Free Mixed Berry	6 oz	150	—	5
Fat Free Peach	6 oz	150	—	5
Fat Free Raspberry	6 oz	150	—	5
Fat Free Strawberry	6 oz	150	—	5
Fat Free Strawberry Banana	6 oz	150	—	5
Light Blueberry	4 oz	60	—	<5
Light Blueberry	6 oz	80	—	<5
Light Cherry	6 oz	80	—	<5
Light Cherry	4 oz	60	—	<5
Light Peach	4 oz	60	—	<5
Light Peach	6 oz	80	—	<5
Light Raspberry	6 oz	80	—	<5
Light Raspberry	4 oz	60	—	<5
Light Strawberry	6 oz	80	—	<5
Light Strawberry	4 oz	60	—	<5
Light Strawberry Banana	6 oz	80	—	<5
Light Strawberry Banana	4 oz	60	—	<5
Nonfat Plain	8 oz	120	—	5
Nonfat Vanilla	8 oz	180	—	5
Original Apple	6 oz	190	—	10

FOOD	PORTION	CALS.	FIB.	CHOL.
Yoplait (CONT.)				
Original Blueberry	6 oz	190	—	10
Original Blueberry	4 oz	120	—	5
Original Boysenberry	6 oz	190	—	10
Original Cherry	6 oz	190	—	10
Original Lemon	6 oz	190	—	10
Original Mixed Berry	6 oz	190	—	10
Original Orange	6 oz	190	—	10
Original Peach	6 oz	190	—	10
Original Peach	4 oz	120	—	5
Original Pina Colada	6 oz	190	—	10
Original Pineapple	6 oz	190	—	10
Original Plain	6 oz	130	—	15
Original Raspberry	6 oz	190	—	10
Original Raspberry	4 oz	120	—	5
Original Strawberry	6 oz	190	—	10
Original Strawberry	4 oz	120	—	5
Original Strawberry Banana	6 oz	190	—	10
Original Strawberry Rhubarb	6 oz	190	—	10
Original Vanilla	6 oz	180	—	10
coffee lowfat	8 oz	194	—	11
fruit lowfat	4 oz	113	—	5
fruit lowfat	8 oz	225	—	10
plain	8 oz	139	—	29
plain lowfat	8 oz	144	—	14
plain no fat	8 oz	127	—	4
vanilla lowfat	8 oz	194	—	11

YOGURT FROZEN
(*see also* TOFU YOGURT)

FOOD	PORTION	CALS.	FIB.	CHOL.
Bee-Lite				
Chocolate	4 oz	100	—	0
Vanilla	4 oz	110	—	0
Ben & Jerry's				
Apple Pie	½ cup (4 fl oz)	140	0	10
Banana Strawberry	½ cup (4 fl oz)	130	0	5
Blueberry Cheesecake	½ cup (4 fl oz)	130	0	10
Cherry Garcia	½ cup (4 fl oz)	150	0	10
Chocolate	½ cup (4 fl oz)	140	0	5
Chocolate	1 pop (2.5 fl oz)	150	1	0
Chocolate Fudge Brownie	½ cup (4 fl oz)	170	1	10
Coffee Almond Fudge	½ cup (4 fl oz)	180	0	10
Heath Bar Crunch	½ cup (4 fl oz)	170	0	10
Raspberry	½ cup (4 fl oz)	120	0	5

FOOD	PORTION	CALS.	FIB.	CHOL.
Bresler's				
All Flavors	5 oz	145	—	9
All Flavors Lite	5 oz	135	—	0
Breyers				
Black Cherry	½ cup (2.7 oz)	140	0	15
Chocolate	½ cup (2.7 oz)	150	1	15
Chocolate Brownie	½ cup (2.7 oz)	170	1	20
Peach	½ cup (2.7 oz)	140	0	15
Red Raspberry	½ cup (2.7 oz)	140	0	15
Strawberry	½ cup (2.7 oz)	130	0	15
Strawberry Banana	½ cup (2.7 oz)	140	0	15
Strawberry Cheesecake	½ cup (2.7 oz)	160	0	20
Toffee Bar Crunch	½ cup (2.7 oz)	160	0	15
Vanilla	½ cup (2.7 oz)	140	0	15
Vanilla Chocolate Strawberry	½ cup (2.7 oz)	140	0	15
Vanilla Raspberry Swirl	½ cup (2.7 oz)	140	0	15
Vanilla Fudge Twirl	½ cup (2.7 oz)	150	1	15
Dannon				
Coco-Nut Fudge	½ cup (3 oz)	160	0	15
Light Cappuccino	½ cup (2.8 oz)	80	0	0
Light Cherry Vanilla Swirl	½ cup (2.8 oz)	90	0	0
Light Chocolate	½ cup (2.7 oz)	80	1	0
Light Lemon Chiffon	½ cup (2.8 oz)	90	0	0
Light Peach Raspberry Melba	½ cup (2.8 oz)	90	0	0
Light Strawberry Cheesecake	½ cup (2.8 oz)	90	0	0
Light Vanilla	½ cup (2.8 oz)	80	0	0
Light Nonfat Cappuccino	8 oz	100	0	<5
Light'N Crunchy Banana Cream Pie	½ cup (2.8 oz)	110	0	0
Light'N Crunchy Mocha Chocolate Chunk	½ cup (2.8 oz)	110	0	0
Light'N Crunchy Peanut Chocolate Crunch	½ cup (2.8 oz)	110	0	0
Light'N Crunchy Triple Chocolate	½ cup (2.8 oz)	110	0	0
Light'N Crunchy Vanilla Blueberry Swirl	½ cup (2.8 oz)	110	0	0
Prue Indulgence Crunchy Expresso	½ cup (3 oz)	150	0	15
Prue Indulgence Heath Toffee Crunch	½ cup (3 oz)	150	0	5
Pure Indulgence Cherry Chocolate Cherry	½ cup (3 oz)	150	0	15
Pure Indulgence Chunky Chocolate Nut	½ cup (3 oz)	150	0	0

FOOD	PORTION	CALS.	FIB.	CHOL.
Dannon (CONT.)				
Pure Indulgence Cookies'n Cream	½ cup (3 oz)	150	0	0
Pure Indulgence Vanilla Raspberry Truffle	½ cup (3 oz)	150	1	15
Desserve				
All Flavors	4 oz	70	—	0
Dutch Chocolate	4 oz	80	—	0
Edy's				
Banana Strawberry	3 oz	80	—	5
Blueberry	3 oz	80	—	5
Cherry	3 oz	80	—	5
Chocolate	3 oz	80	—	5
Chocolate Chip	3 oz	100	—	5
Citrus Heights	3 oz	80	—	5
Cookies'N'Cream	3 oz	100	—	5
Marble Fudge	3 oz	100	—	5
Perfectly Peach	3 oz	80	—	5
Raspberry	3 oz	80	—	5
Raspberry Vanilla Swirl	3 oz	80	—	5
Strawberry	3 oz	80	—	5
Vanilla	3 oz	80	—	5
Elan				
Blueberry	4 oz	130	—	11
Caramel Almond Praline	4 oz	150	—	10
Chocolate	4 oz	130	—	10
Chocolate Almond	4 oz	160	—	10
Coffee	4 oz	130	—	11
Coffee Decaffeinated	4 oz	130	—	11
Peach	4 oz	130	—	10
Rum Raisin	4 oz	135	—	12
Strawberry	4 oz	125	—	10
Vanilla	4 oz	130	—	11
Fi-Bar				
Chocolate	1	190	4	0
Strawberry	1	190	4	0
Vanilla	1	190	4	0
Good Humor				
Creamsicle Raspberry	1 (2.8 oz)	100	0	<5
Frista Cup	1 (6.2 oz)	220	1	15
Haagen-Dazs				
Bar Peach & Vanilla	1 bar	100	—	15
Bar Raspberry & Vanilla	1 bar (2.5 oz)	90	0	15
Chocolate	3 oz	130	—	25

FOOD	PORTION	CALS.	FIB.	CHOL.
Haagen-Dazs (CONT.)				
Peach	3 oz	120	—	31
Strawberry	3 oz	120	—	30
Vanilla	3 oz	130	—	40
Vanilla Almond Crunch	3 oz	150	—	33
Hood				
Bavarian Truffle & Twist	½ cup (2.6 oz)	150	0	10
Coffee Toffee Chunk Sundae	½ cup (2.6 oz)	150	0	10
Combo Bars	1 (2.2 oz)	90	0	5
Cookies & Cream	½ cup (2.6 oz)	140	0	10
Grandma's Raisin Oatmeal Cookie Dough	½ cup (2.6 oz)	140	0	10
Mixed Berry Swirl	½ cup (2.6 oz)	120	0	10
Natural Strawberry	½ cup (2.6 oz)	110	0	10
Natural Strawberry Banana	½ cup (2.6 oz)	110	0	10
Natural Vanilla	½ cup (2.6 oz)	120	0	10
Nonfat Caramel & Brownie Sundae	½ cup (2.6 oz)	120	0	0
Nonfat Chocolate Marshmallow	½ cup (2.6 oz)	110	0	0
Nonfat Double Raspberry	½ cup (2.6 oz)	120	0	0
Nonfat Mocha Fudge	½ cup (2.6 oz)	120	0	0
Nonfat Olde Fashioned Vanilla	½ cup (2.6 oz)	110	0	0
Nonfat Peach Cobbler A La Mode	½ cup (2.6 oz)	110	0	0
Nonfat Strawberry	½ cup (2.6 oz)	100	0	0
Nonfat Vanilla Fudge	½ cup (2.6 oz)	120	0	0
Raspberry Swirl	½ cup (2.6 oz)	130	0	10
Sundae Cups Chocolate & Strawberry	1 (2.2 oz)	110	1	5
Vanilla Chocolate Strawberry	½ cup (2.6 oz)	120	0	10
Vanilla Swiss Almond Sundae	½ cup (2.6 oz)	150	0	10
Just 10				
All Flavors	1 oz	10	—	0
Kissed With Honey				
Chocolate	3.5 oz	100	—	9
Nonfat Chocolate	3.5 oz	85	—	0
Nonfat Vanilla	3.5 oz	85	—	0
Vanilla	3.5 oz	100	—	9
Pure Indulgence				
All Flavors	½ cup	160	—	20
Sealtest				
Chocolate	½ cup (2.7 oz)	120	tr	5
Mocha Fudge	½ cup (2.6 oz)	130	tr	10
Vanilla	½ cup (2.6 oz)	120	0	10

FOOD	PORTION	CALS.	FIB.	CHOL.
Tofutti				
Beter Than Yogurt Passion Island Fruit	4 fl oz	100	0	0
Better Than Yogurt Chocolate Fudge	4 fl oz	120	0	0
Better Than Yogurt Coffee Mashmallow Swirl	4 fl oz	100	0	0
Better Than Yogurt Peach Mango	4 fl oz	100	0	0
Better Than Yogurt Strawberry Banana	4 fl oz	100	0	0
Better Than Yogurt Vanilla Fudge	4 fl oz	120	0	0
Weight Watchers				
Chocolate Shake	7.5 oz	220	—	5
chocolate soft serve	½ cup (4 fl oz)	115	—	3
vanilla soft serve	½ cup (4 fl oz)	114	—	2

ZABAGLIONE
(*see* CUSTARD)

ZUCCHINI
CANNED
Del Monte				
With Italian Tomato Sauce	½ cup (4.2 oz)	30	1	0
Progresso				
Italian Style	½ cup	50	2	tr
S&W				
Italian Style	½ cup	45	—	0
italian style	½ cup	33	—	0
FRESH				
baby raw	1 (½ oz)	3	tr	0
raw sliced	½ cup	9	1	0
sliced cooked	½ cup	14	1	0
FROZEN				
Big Valley				
	¾ cup (3 oz)	10	1	0
Empire				
Breaded	1 (2.9 oz)	100	1	0
Southland				
Zucchini Sliced	3.2 oz	15	—	0
cooked	½ cup	19	—	0

PART · II

RESTAURANT,

TAKE-OUT

AND

FAST-FOOD CHAINS

FOOD	PORTION	CALS.	FIB.	CHOL.
ARBY'S				
BAKED SELECTIONS				
Cheese Cake	1 serving	306	—	95
Chocolate Chip Cookie	1	130	—	0
Turnover Blueberry	1	320	—	0
Turnover Apple	1	303	—	0
Turnover Cherry	1	280	—	0
BEVERAGES				
Chocolate Shake	12 fl oz	451	—	36
Coca-Cola Classic	12 oz	141	—	0
Coffee	8 oz	3	—	0
Diet Coke	12 oz	1	—	0
Diet Seven Up	12 oz	4	—	0
Hot Chocolate	8 oz	110	—	0
Iced Tea	16 oz	6	—	0
Jamocha Shake	11.5 fl oz	368	—	35
Milk Lo Fat 2%	8 oz	121	—	18
Nehi Orange	12 oz	190	—	0
Orange Juice	6 oz	82	—	0
Pepsi Cola	12 oz	159	—	0
R.C. Cola	12 oz	173	—	0
R.C. Diet Rite	12 oz	1	—	0
R.C. Root Beer	12 oz	173	—	0
Seven Up	12 oz	144	—	0
Sugar Substitute	1 pkg (0.8 g)	4	—	0
Upper Ten	12 oz	169	—	0
Vanilla Shake	11 fl oz	330	—	32
BREAKFAST SELECTIONS				
Biscuit Bacon	1	318	—	8
Biscuit Ham	1	323	—	21
Biscuit Plain	1	280	—	0
Biscuit Sausage	1	460	—	60
Blueberry Muffin	1	200	—	22
Cinnamon Nut Danish	1	340	—	0
Croissant Bacon/Egg	1	389	—	221
Croissant Ham/Cheese	1	345	—	90
Croissant Mushroom/Cheese	1	493	—	116
Croissant Plain	1	260	—	49
Croissant Sausage/Egg	1	519	—	271
Maple Syrup	1.5 oz	120	—	0
Platter Bacon	1	860	—	366
Platter Egg	1	460	—	346
Platter Ham	1	518	—	374

FOOD	PORTION	CALS.	FIB.	CHOL.
Platter Sausage	1	640	—	406
Toastix	1 serving	420	—	20
ICE CREAM				
Polar Swirl Butterfinger	1	457	—	28
Polar Swirl Heath	1	543	—	39
Polar Swirl Oreo	1	482	—	35
Polar Swirl P'nut Butter Cup	1	517	—	34
Polar Swirl Snickers	1	511	—	33
MAIN MENU SELECTIONS				
Arby's Sauce	0.5 oz	15	—	0
Au Jus	4 oz	7	—	0
Bac N'Cheddar Deluxe Sandwich	1	532	—	83
Baked Potato Broccoli 'N Cheddar	1	417	—	22
Baked Potato Deluxe	1	621	—	58
Baked Potato Mushroom & Cheese	1	515	—	47
Baked Potato Plain	1	240	—	0
Baked Potato With Butter/ Margarine And Sour Cream	1	463	—	40
Beef N'Cheddar Sandwich	1	451	—	52
Cheddar Fries	1 serving (5 oz)	399	—	9
Chicken Breast Sandwich	1	489	—	45
Chicken Cordon Bleu Sandwich	1	658	—	65
Chicken Fajita Pita	1	272	—	27
Curly Fries	1 serving (3.5 oz)	337	—	0
Fish Fillet Sandwich	1	537	—	79
French Dip	1	345	—	5
French Dip 'N Swiss	1	425	—	87
French Fries	1 serving	246	—	0
Grilled Chicken Barbeque Sandwich	1	378	—	44
Grilled Chicken Deluxe Sandwich	1	426	—	44
Ham 'N Cheese Sandwich	1	330	—	45
Horsey Sauce	0.5 oz	55	—	1
Ketchup	0.5 oz	16	—	0
Light Ham Deluxe	1	255	—	30
Light Roast Beef Deluxe	1	294	—	42
Light Roast Chicken Deluxe	1	263	—	39
Light Roast Turkey Deluxe	1	260	—	30
Mayonnaise Cholesterol Free	0.5 oz	90	—	0
Mustard	0.5 oz	11	—	0
Philly Beef N' Swiss Sandwich	1	498	—	91
Potato Cakes	1 serving	204	—	0
Roast Beef Sandwich Giant	1	530	—	78

FOOD	PORTION	CALS.	FIB.	CHOL.
Roast Beef Sandwich Junior	1	218	—	23
Roast Beef Sandwich Regular	1	353	—	39
Roast Beef Sandwich Super	1	529	—	47
Roast Chicken Club	1	513	—	75
Roast Chicken Salad	1	184	—	36
Sub Deluxe	1	482	—	45
Turkey Deluxe Sandwich	1	399	—	39
SALAD DRESSINGS				
Blue Cheese	2 oz	295	—	50
Buttermilk Ranch	2 oz	349	—	6
Honey French	2 oz	322	—	0
Italian Light	2 oz	23	—	0
Thousand Island	2 oz	298	—	24
Weight Watchers Creamy French	1 oz	48	—	0
Weight Watchers Creamy Italian	1 oz	29	—	0
SALADS AND SALAD BARS				
Cashew Chicken Salad	1	590	—	65
Chef Salad	1	210	—	115
Croutons	½ oz	59	—	1
Garden Salad	1	149	—	74
SOUPS				
Beef With Vegetables & Barley	8 oz	96	—	10
Boston Clam Chowder	8 oz	207	—	28
French Onion	8 oz	67	—	0
Lumberjack Mixed Vegetable	8 oz	89	—	4
Old Fashioned Chicken Noodle	8 oz	99	—	25
Pilgrim's Corn Chowder	5 oz	193	—	28
Split Pea With Ham	8 oz	200	—	30
Tomato Florentine	8 oz	244	—	2
Wisconsin Cheese	8 oz	287	—	31

AU BON PAIN
BREADS AND ROLLS

3 Seed Raisin Roll	1	250	—	0
Alpine Roll	1	220	—	0
Baguette Loaf	1	810	—	0
Braided Roll	1	387	—	34
Cheese Loaf	1	1670	—	75
Country Seed Roll	1	220	—	0
Four Grain Loaf	1	1420	—	tr
French Roll	1	320	—	0
Hearth Roll	1	250	—	0
Hearth Sandwich Roll	1	370	—	0
Multigrain	2 slices	391	—	1

FOOD	PORTION	CALS.	FIB.	CHOL.
Onion Herb Loaf	1	1430	—	0
Parisienne Loaf	1	1490	—	0
Petit Pain Roll	1	220	—	0
Pumpernickel Roll	1	210	—	0
Rye	2 slices	374	—	1
Rye Roll	1	230	—	0
Sandwich Croissant	1	300	—	35
Vegetable Roll	1	230	—	0
COOKIES				
Chocolate Chip	1	280	—	25
Chocolate Chunk Pecan	1	290	—	10
Oatmeal Raisin	1	250	—	10
Peanut Butter	1	290	—	10
White Chocolate Chunk Pecan	1	300	—	10
CROISSANTS				
Almond	1	420	—	95
Apple	1	250	—	25
Blueberry Cheese	1	380	—	60
Chocolate	1	400	—	35
Chocolate Hazelnut	1	480	—	35
Cinnamon Raisin	1	390	—	35
Coconut Pecan	1	440	—	45
Ham & Cheese	1	370	—	55
Plain	1	220	—	25
Raspberry Cheese	1	400	—	60
Spinach & Cheese	1	290	—	45
Strawberry Cheese	1	400	—	60
Sweet Cheese	1	420	—	70
Turkey & Havariti	1	410	—	70
Turkey & Cheddar	1	410	—	70
MUFFINS				
Blueberry	1	390	—	40
Bran	1	390	—	20
Carrot	1	450	—	15
Corn	1	460	—	25
Cranberry Walnut	1	350	—	15
Oat Bran Apple	1	400	—	0
Pumpkin	1	410	—	20
Whole Grain	1	440	—	30
SALAD DRESSINGS				
Balsamic Vinaigrette	1 serving (2.25 fl oz)	311	—	1
Champagne Vinaigrette	1 serving (2.25 fl oz)	251	—	2

FOOD	PORTION	CALS.	FIB.	CHOL.
County Blue Cheese	1 serving (2.25 fl oz)	325	—	46
Honey With Poppy Seed	1 serving (2.25 fl oz)	354	—	2
Italian Low Cal	1 serving (2.25 fl oz)	68	—	5
Olive Oil Ceasar	1 serving (2.25 fl oz)	255	—	tr
Parmesan & Pepper	1 serving (2.25 fl oz)	235	—	19
Sesame French	1 serving (2.25 fl oz)	339	—	3
Tomato Basil	1 serving (2.25 fl oz)	66	—	0
SALADS AND SALAD BARS				
Chicken Cracked Pepper Garden	1	100	—	25
Chicken Grilled Garden	1	110	—	30
Chicken Tarragon Garden	1	310	—	70
Garden Large	1	40	—	0
Garden Small	1	20	—	0
Shrimp Garden	1	102	—	105
Tuna Garden	1	350	—	40
SANDWICHES AND FILLINGS				
Bacon	1 serving	140	—	30
Brie	1 serving	300	—	85
Cheddar Cheese	1 serving	110	—	30
Chicken Cracked Pepper	1 serving	120	—	50
Chicken Grilled	1 serving	130	—	60
Chicken Tarragon	1 serving	270	—	70
Country Ham	1 serving	150	—	115
Herb Cheese	1 serving	290	—	90
Provolone Cheese	1 serving	155	—	36
Roast Beef	1 serving	180	—	60
Smoked Turkey	1 serving	100	—	35
Swiss	1 serving	330	—	80
Tuna Salad	1 serving	310	—	40
SOUPS				
Beef Barley	1 bowl	112	3	18
Beef Barley	1 cup	75	2	12
Chicken Noodle	1 cup	79	1	17
Chicken Noodle	1 bowl	119	2	26
Clam Chowder	1 bowl	433	2	90
Clam Chowder	1 cup	289	1	60
Cream Of Broccoli	1 bowl	302	2	54

FOOD	PORTION	CALS.	FIB.	CHOL.
Cream Of Broccoli	1 cup	201	1	36
Garden Vegetarian	1 bowl	44	3	0
Garden Vegetarian	1 cup	29	2	0
Minestrone	1 bowl	158	3	2
Minestrone	1 cup	105	2	1
Split Pea	1 cup	176	7	tr
Split Pea	1 bowl	264	10	1
Tomato Florentine	1 bowl	92	2	0
Tomato Florentine	1 cup	61	1	0
Vegetarian Chili	1 cup	139	2	0
Vegetarian Chili	1 bowl	208	3	0

BASKIN-ROBBINS

FOOD	PORTION	CALS.	FIB.	CHOL.
Sugar Cone	1	60	—	0
Waffle Cone	1	140	—	0
FROZEN YOGURT				
Cafe Mocha	½ cup (4 fl oz)	70	—	0
Chocolate Nonfat	½ cup	110	—	0
Chocolate Vanilla	½ cup	110	—	0
Dutch Chocolate Chip Bar	1	260	—	7
Pralines Vanilla Bar	1	250	—	7
Strawberry Low-Fat	½ cup (4 fl oz)	120	—	5
Strawberry Nonfat	½ cup	110	—	0
Wild Cherry	½ cup (4 fl oz)	70	—	0
ICE CREAM				
Almond Butter Crunch Light	½ cup	130	—	12
Butter Pecan	½ cup	160	—	25
Butterfinger	½ cup	170	—	15
Caramel Banana Fat Free	½ cup	100	—	1
Cherry Cordial Sugar Free	½ cup	100	—	3
Chewy Babyruth	½ cup	190	—	25
Chilly Burgers Vanilla	1	240	—	29
Chocolate	½ cup	150	—	20
Chocolate Almond	½ cup	170	—	20
Chocolate Chip	½ cup	150	—	25
Chocolate Chip Sugar Free	½ cup	100	—	4
Chocolate Fudge	½ cup	170	—	25
Chocolate Mousse Royale	½ cup	180	—	20
Chocolate Raspberry Truffle	½ cup	180	—	25
Chocolate Vanilla Fat Free	½ cup	100	—	0
Chocolate Wonder Fat Free	½ cup	120	—	1
Chunky Banana Sugar Free	½ cup	80	—	3
Coconut Caramel Nut Light	½ cup	130	—	8
Cookies N Cream	½ cup	160	—	20

FOOD	PORTION	CALS.	FIB.	CHOL.
Double Raspberry Light	½ cup	120	—	9
Espresso N Cream Light	½ cup	120	—	12
French Vanilla	½ cup	170	—	55
Fudge Brownie	½ cup	180	—	20
Gold Medal Ribbon	½ cup	150	—	20
Jamoca Swirl Fat Free	½ cup	100	—	2
Jamoca Swiss Almond Sugar Free	½ cup	90	—	4
Jamoco Almond Fudge	½ cup	150	—	20
Just Peachy Fat Free	½ cup	100	—	2
Kahula N Cream	½ cup	160	—	10
Mint Chocolate Chip	½ cup	150	—	25
Peanut Butter Chocolate	½ cup	190	—	20
Pineapple Cheesecake Fat Free	½ cup	110	—	0
Pineapple Coconut Sugar Free	½ cup	90	—	3
Pistachio Almond	½ cup	160	—	20
Praline Dream Light	½ cup	130	—	11
Pralines N Cream	½ cup	160	—	20
Reeses Peanut Butter Cup	½ cup	170	—	20
Rocky Road	½ cup	170	—	20
Strawberry Sugar Free	½ cup	80	—	3
Strawberry Royal Light	½ cup	110	—	9
Thin Mint Chip Sugar Free	½ cup	90	—	4
Tiny Toon Adventures Toonwiches Chocolate	1	330	—	33
Tiny Toon Adventures Toonwiches Vanilla	1	340	—	34
Tiny Toon Adventures Bar Mint Chocolate Chip	1	230	—	17
Tiny Toon Adventures Bar Vanilla	1	210	—	18
Vanilla	½ cup	140	—	30
Vanilla Fudge Light	½ cup	110	—	11
Very Berry Strawberry	½ cup	120	—	15
World Class Chocolate	½ cup	160	—	20
ICES AND ICE POPS				
Daiquiri Ice	1 scoop	140	—	0
Rainbow Sherbet	1 scoop	160	—	6
Sorbet Strawberry	½ cup (4 fl oz)	100	—	0

BEN & JERRY'S
FROZEN YOGURT

FOOD	PORTION	CALS.	FIB.	CHOL.
Apple Pie	½ cup (4 fl oz)	140	0	10
Banana Strawberry	½ cup (4 fl oz)	130	0	5
Blueberry Cheesecake	½ cup (4 fl oz)	130	0	10
Cherry Garcia	½ cup (4 fl oz)	150	0	10

FOOD	PORTION	CALS.	FIB.	CHOL.
Chocolate	½ cup (4 fl oz)	140	0	5
Chocolate Fudge Brownie	½ cup (4 fl oz)	170	1	10
Coffee Almond Fudge	½ cup (4 fl oz)	180	0	10
Heath Bar Crunch	½ cup (4 fl oz)	170	0	10
Pop Chocolate	1 (2.5 fl oz)	150	1	0
Raspberry	½ cup (4 fl oz)	120	0	5
ICE CREAM				
Bar Vanilla Brownie	1 (4 fl oz)	260	0	50
Cherry Garcia	½ cup (4 fl oz)	230	0	80
Chocolate	½ cup (4 fl oz)	230	0	55
Chocolate Chip Cookie Dough	½ cup (4 fl oz)	260	0	85
Chocolate Fudge Brownie	½ cup (4 fl oz)	250	1	50
Chocolate Peanut Butter Chocolate Chip Cookie Dough	½ cup (4 fl oz)	280	0	55
Chunky Monkey	½ cup (4 fl oz)	270	0	70
Coffee Heath Bar Crunch	½ cup (4 fl oz)	270	0	80
Heath Bar Crunch	½ cup (4 fl oz)	270	0	85
Mint Cookie	½ cup (4 fl oz)	250	0	85
New York Super Fudge	½ cup (4 fl oz)	290	0	45
Pop Cherry Garcia	1 (3.7 fl oz)	250	2	45
Pop Chocolate Chip Cookie Dough	1 (2.5 fl oz)	240	1	45
Pop Heath Bar Crunch	1 (2.5 fl oz)	260	0	35
Pop Heath Bar Crunch	1 (3.7 fl oz)	340	0	50
Pop Milk Chocolate Almond	1 (2.5 fl oz)	250	3	35
Pop New York Super Fudge	1 (3.7 fl oz)	330	3	25
Pop Rain Forest Crunch	1 (3.7 fl oz)	350	2	50
Rain Forest Crunch	½ cup (4 fl oz)	270	0	85
Vanilla	½ cup (4 fl oz)	215	0	95
Vanilla Chocolate Chunk	½ cup (4 fl oz)	250	0	85

BIG BOY
DESSERT

FOOD	PORTION	CALS.	FIB.	CHOL.
Frozen Yogurt	1 serving	72	—	0
Frozen Yogurt Shake	1 serving	184	—	2
No-No Frozen Dessert	1 serving	75	—	0
MAIN MENU SELECTIONS				
Baked Cod Dinner	1 serving	392	—	76
Baked Cod Dijon Dinner	1 serving	455	—	76
Baked Potato	1	163	—	0
Bran Muffin	1	367	—	0
Breast of Chicken Dinner	1 serving	358	—	68
Breast of Chicken w/ Mozzarella Dinner	1 serving	379	—	79
Breast of Chicken w/ Mozzarella Sandwich	1	390	—	71

FOOD	PORTION	CALS.	FIB.	CHOL.
Broiled Cod Dijon Dinner	1 serving	455	—	76
Broiled Cod Dinner	1 serving	392	—	76
Cajun Chicken Dinner	1 serving	358	—	68
Cajun Cod Dinner	1 serving	392	—	76
Carrots	1 serving	35	—	0
Chicken Breast Salad w/ Dijon And Pita Bread	1 serving	377	—	60
Corn	1 serving	90	—	0
Dijon Sauce	1 serving	63	—	0
Dinner Salad	1	19	—	0
Green Beans	1 serving	28	—	0
Mixed Vegetables	1 serving	27	—	0
Peas	1 serving	77	—	0
Promise Margarine	1 pat (5 g)	35	—	0
Rice	1 serving	114	—	0
Roll	1	139	—	2
Spaghetti Marinara Dinner	1 serving	450	—	8
Stir Fry Vegetable	1 serving	408	—	0
Stir Fry Dinner Chicken 'n Vegetable	1 serving	562	—	68
Turkey Pita	1	224	—	75
Vegetable Pita	1	144	—	10
SALAD DRESSINGS				
Buttermilk	1 serving	36	—	10
SOUPS				
Cabbage	1 cup	37	—	1
Cabbage	1 bowl	43	—	1

BOSTON CHICKEN

FOOD	PORTION	CALS.	FIB.	CHOL.
DESSERTS				
Brownie	1 (3.36 oz)	452	3	81
Cookie Chocolate Chip	1 (2.79 oz)	369	2	27
Cookie Oatmeal Raisin	1 (2.79 oz)	341	3	28
MAIN MENU SELECTIONS				
½ Chicken With Skin	1 serv (10.05 oz)	642	tr	307
¼ Dark Meat With Skin	1 serv (4.67 oz)	330	tr	151
¼ Dark Meat Without Skin	1 serv (3.65 oz)	218	tr	121
¼ White Meat With Skin	1 serv (5.39 oz)	332	tr	150
¼ White Meat Without Skin & Wing	1 serv (3.68 oz)	164	tr	89
BBQ Baked Beans	1 serv (7.1 oz)	290	8	7
Buttered Corn	1 serv (5.14 oz)	181	5	tr
Butternut Squash	1 serv (6.79 oz)	247	4	28
Chicken Pot Pie	1 serv (15.01 oz)	703	4	109

FOOD	PORTION	CALS.	FIB.	CHOL.
Chicken Soup	1 serv (6.8 oz)	87	tr	31
Chunky Chicken Salad	1 serv (5.57 oz)	460	tr	145
Cole Slaw	1 serv (6.49 oz)	289	2	13
Corn Bread	1 serv (2.4 oz)	253	tr	30
Creamed Spinach	1 serv (6.37 oz)	298	3	71
Fruit Salad	1 serv (4.4 oz)	49	tr	0
Homestyle Mashed Potatoes & Gravy	1 serv (6.69 oz)	205	2	25
Macaroni & Cheese	1 serv (6.76 oz)	290	2	19
Mediterranean Pasta Salad	1 serv (4.54 oz)	160	3	12
New Potatoes	1 serv (4.61 oz)	129	3	tr
Rice Pilaf	1 serv (5.13 oz)	188	tr	tr
Sandwich Chicken Breast	1 (9.13 oz)	422	3	99
Sandwich Chunky Chicken Salad	1 (12.11 oz)	763	3	170
Steamed Vegetables	1 serv (3.69 oz)	32	2	tr
Stuffing	1 serv (6.14 oz)	282	3	tr
Tortellini Salad	1 serv (5.62 oz)	430	2	55
Zucchini Marinara	1 serv (6.68 oz)	80	6	tr

BURGER KING

BEVERAGES

FOOD	PORTION	CALS.	FIB.	CHOL.
Cocoa Cola Classic	1 med (22 fl oz)	264	—	0
Coffee Black	1 (8.6 fl oz)	2	—	0
Diet Coke	1 med (22 fl oz)	1	—	0
Milk 2%	1 (8.6 fl oz)	121	—	18
Orange Juice	1 (6.4 fl oz)	82	—	0
Shake Chocolate	1 med (10 fl oz)	320	—	20
Shake Chocolate Syrup Added	1 med (11 fl oz)	400	—	20
Shake Strawberry Syrup Added	1 med (10.9 fl oz)	370	—	20
Shake Vanilla	1 med (10 fl oz)	310	—	20
Sprite	1 med (22 fl oz)	264	—	0

BREAKFAST SELECTIONS

FOOD	PORTION	CALS.	FIB.	CHOL.
A.M. Express Dip	1 oz	84	—	0
Breakfast Buddy With Sausage, Egg And Cheese	1 (2.9 oz)	255	—	127
Cream Cheese	1 serving (1 oz)	98	—	25
Croissan'wich Bacon, Egg And Cheese	1 (4.1 oz)	353	—	230
Croissan'wich Ham, Egg And Cheese	1 (5.1 oz)	351	—	236
Croissan'wich Sausage, Egg And Cheese	1 (5.6 oz)	534	—	258
French Toast Sticks	1 serving (4.9 oz)	440	—	0
Hash Browns	1 serving (2.5 oz)	213	—	0
Mini Muffins Blueberry	1 serving (3.3 oz)	292	—	72

FOOD	PORTION	CALS.	FIB.	CHOL.
DESSERTS				
Dutch Apple Pie	1 serving (4 oz)	308	—	0
Popcorn	1 serving (1 oz)	130	—	15
Snickers Ice Cream Bar	1 (2 oz)	220	—	15
MAIN MENU SELECTIONS				
American Cheese	1 slice (1 oz)	92	—	25
BK Big Fish Sandwich	1 (8.9 oz)	710	—	60
BK Broiler	1 (5.4 oz)	280	—	50
BK Broiler Sauce	1 serving (0.4 fl oz)	37	—	5
Bacon Bits	½ tsp (3 g)	16	—	5
Bacon Double Cheeseburger	1 (5.2 oz)	470	—	100
Bacon Double Cheeseburger Deluxe	1 (6.5 oz)	570	—	110
Baked Potato	1 (7 oz)	210	—	0
Bull's Eye Barbecue Sauce	0.5 fl oz	22	—	0
Butterfly Shrimp	1 serving (4.1 oz)	300	—	105
Cheeseburger	1 (4 oz)	300	—	45
Chicken Sandwich	1 (8 oz)	700	—	60
Chicken Tenders	6 pieces (3.2 oz)	236	—	38
Cocktail Sauce	1 serving (0.7 oz)	20	—	0
Croutons	1 serving (0.2 oz)	31	—	46
Dinner Roll	1 (0.9 oz)	80	—	0
Dipping Sauce Barbecue	1 oz	36	—	0
Dipping Sauce Honey	1 oz	91	—	0
Dipping Sauce Ranch	1 oz	171	—	0
Dipping Sauce Sweet & Sour	1 oz	45	—	0
Double Cheeseburger	1 (5.6 oz)	450	—	90
Double Whopper	1 (12.3 oz)	860	—	170
French Fries Salted	1 med (4.1 oz)	372	—	0
Hamburger	1 (3.6 oz)	260	—	30
Ketchup	0.5 fl oz	17	—	0
Lettuce	1 leaf (0.7 oz)	3	—	0
Mayonnaise	1 oz	210	—	20
Mustard	½ tsp (3 g)	2	—	0
Onion	0.5 oz	5	—	0
Onion Rings	1 serving (3.4 oz)	339	—	0
Pickles	0.5 oz	1	—	0
Sour Cream	1 oz	60	—	15
Tartar Sauce	1 oz	175	—	15
Tomato	1 oz	6	—	0
Whipped Classic Blend	1 serving (0.4 oz)	65	—	0
Whopper	1 (9.5 oz)	630	—	90
Whopper Double With Cheese	1 (13.2 oz)	950	—	195
Whopper Jr.	1 (4.6 oz)	330	—	40

FOOD	PORTION	CALS.	FIB.	CHOL.
Whopper Jr. With Cheese	1 (5.1 oz)	380	—	50
Whopper With Cheese	1 (10.3 oz)	720	—	115
SALAD DRESSINGS				
Bleu Cheese	1 serving (1.1 fl oz)	150	—	29
French	1 serving (1.1 fl oz)	145	—	0
Italian Reduced Calorie Light	1 serving (1.1 fl oz)	15	—	0
Ranch	1 serving (1.1 fl oz)	175	—	10
Thousand Island	1 serving (1.1 fl oz)	145	—	18
SALADS AND SALAD BARS				
Chef Salad w/o Dressing	1 (9.6 oz)	178	—	103
Chunky Chicken Salad w/o Dressing	1 (9.1 oz)	142	—	49
Dinner Side Salad	1 (3.5 oz)	20	—	0
Garden Salad w/o Dressing	1 (7.8 oz)	95	—	15

CAPTAIN D'S
DESSERTS

FOOD	PORTION	CALS.	FIB.	CHOL.
Carrot Cake	1 piece (4 oz)	434	0	32
Cheesecake	1 piece (4 oz)	420	0	141
Chocolate Cake	1 piece (4 oz)	303	0	20
Lemon Pie	1 piece (4 oz)	351	0	45
Pecan Pie	1 piece (4 oz)	458	4	4
MAIN MENU SELECTIONS				
Baked Fish Dinner w/ Slaw	1 dinner	451	4	105
Baked Potato	1 (9 oz)	277	—	0
Breadstick	1 (1.3 oz)	91	0	0
Breadsticks	6 (7.5 oz)	545	0	0
Broiled Chicken Sandwich	1 (8.2 oz)	451	—	105
Cheese	1 slice (0.5 oz)	54	0	14
Chicken Dinner w/ Salad	1 dinner	414	4	71
Cob Corn	1 serving (9.5 oz)	251	—	0
Cocktail Sauce	1 lg serving (4 fl oz)	137	0	0
Cocktail Sauce	1 lg serving (4 fl oz)	137	0	0
Cole Slaw	1 pt (16 oz)	633	8	66
Cole Slaw	1 serving (4 oz)	158	2	16
Crackers	4	50	tr	3
Cracklins	1 serving (1 oz)	218	0	0
Creamer	1 serving (0.4 fl oz)	14	0	0
Dinner Salad w/o Dressing	1 (2.5 oz)	27	1	1
French Fried Potatoes	1 serving (3.5 oz)	302	0	0
Fried Okra	1 serving (4 oz)	300	0	0
Green Beans Seasoned	1 serving (4 oz)	46	1	4
Hushpuppies	6 (6.7 oz)	756	1	0
Hushpuppy	1 (1.1 oz)	126	tr	0

FOOD	PORTION	CALS.	FIB.	CHOL.
Orange Roughy Dinner w/ Salad	1 dinner	537	4	39
Rice	1 serving (4 oz)	124	1	0
Shrimp Dinner w/ Salad	1 dinner	457	4	191
Sugar	1 pkg	18	0	0
Sweet & Sour Sauce	1 serving (1 fl oz)	52	0	0
Sweet & Sour Sauce	1 lg serving (4 fl oz)	206	0	0
Tartar Sauce	1 lg serving (4 fl oz)	298	0	41
Tartar Sauce	1 serving (1 fl oz)	75	0	10
White Beans	1 serving (4 oz)	126	3	2
SALAD DRESSINGS				
Blue Cheese	1 pkg (1 fl oz)	105	0	14
French	1 pkg (1 fl oz)	111	0	7
Italian Lo Cal	1 pkg (1 fl oz)	9	0	0
Ranch	1 pkg (1 fl oz)	92	0	15

CARL'S JR.

FOOD	PORTION	CALS.	FIB.	CHOL.
BAKED SELECTIONS				
Cheese Danish	1 (4 oz)	520	—	0
Cheesecake	1 serving (3.5 oz)	310	—	60
Chocolate Cake	1 serving (3 oz)	300	—	25
Chocolate Chip Cookie	1 (2.5 oz)	330	—	5
Cinnamon Roll	1 (4 oz)	460	—	0
Fudge Moussecake	1 slice (4 oz)	400	—	110
Muffin Blueberry	1 (4.2 oz)	340	—	45
Muffin Bran	1 (4.7 oz)	310	—	60
BEVERAGES				
Iced Tea	1 reg (21 fl oz)	2	—	0
Milk 1%	1 (11 fl oz)	150	—	13
Orange Juice	1 sm (3.2 fl oz)	90	—	0
Shake	1 reg (11.6 fl oz)	350	—	15
Soda	1 reg (21 fl oz)	240	—	0
Soda Diet	1 reg (21 fl oz)	2	—	0
BREAKFAST SELECTIONS				
Bacon	2 strips (0.3 oz)	45	—	5
Breakfast Burrito	1 (5.3 oz)	430	—	285
English Muffin w/ Margarine	1 (2.2 oz)	190	—	0
French Toast Dips w/o Syrup	1 serving (5.4 oz)	450	—	40
Hash Brown Nuggets	1 serving (3.3 oz)	270	—	5
Hot Cakes w/ Margarine w/o Syrup	1 serving (6.6 oz)	510	—	10
Sausage	1 patty (1.6 oz)	190	—	30
Scrambled Eggs	1 serving (2.4 oz)	120	—	245
Sunrise Sandwich	1 (4.1 oz)	300	—	160
MAIN MENU SELECTIONS				
American Cheese	1 serving (0.6 oz)	60	—	15

FOOD	PORTION	CALS.	FIB.	CHOL.
Carl's Catch Fish Sandwich	1 (7.4 oz)	560	—	5
Carl's Original Hamburger	1 (6.8 oz)	460	—	50
Charbroiled Chicken Club Sandwich	1 (8.8 oz)	570	—	60
Charbroiled BBQ Chicken Sandwich	1 (6.7 oz)	310	—	30
Chicken Strips	6 pieces (3.7 oz)	260	—	25
Double Western Bacon Cheeseburger	1 (11.5 oz)	1030	—	145
Famous Star Hamburger	1 (8.6 oz)	610	—	50
French Fries	1 reg (4.4 oz)	420	—	0
Great Stuff Potato Broccoli & Cheese	1 (15 oz)	590	—	25
Great Stuffs Potato Bacon & Cheese	1 (14.9 oz)	730	—	45
Great Stuffs Potato Cheese	1 (14.6 oz)	690	—	40
Great Stuffs Potato Chili	1 (14.3 oz)	500	—	50
Great Stuffs Potato Lite	1 (10 oz)	290	—	0
Great Stuffs Potato Sour Cream & Chives	1 (12.3 oz)	470	—	20
Hamburger	1 (4.2 oz)	320	—	35
Onion Rings	1 serving (5.3 oz)	520	—	0
Roast Beef Deluxe Sandwich	1 (9.3 oz)	540	—	40
Salsa	1 oz	8	—	0
Sante Fe Chicken Sandwich	1 (7.9 oz)	530	—	85
Super Star Hamburger	1 (11.2 oz)	820	—	105
Swiss Cheese	1 serving (0.6 oz)	60	—	15
Turkey Club Sandwich	1 (9.3 oz)	530	—	60
Western Bacon Cheeseburger	1 (8.1 oz)	730	—	90
Zucchini	1 serving (5.9 oz)	390	—	0
SALAD DRESSINGS				
1000 Island	1 fl oz	110	—	5
Blue Cheese	1 fl oz	150	—	20
French Reduced Calorie	1 fl oz	40	—	0
House	1 fl oz	110	—	10
Italian Reduced Calorie	1 fl oz	40	—	0
SALADS AND SALAD BARS				
Salad-To-Go Chicken	1 (12 oz)	200	—	70
Salad-To-Go Garden	1 (4.8 oz)	50	—	5
CARVEL				
FROZEN YOGURT				
Vanilla No Sugar Added	4 fl oz	100	—	10
ICE CREAM				
Brown Bonnet Cone	1	380	—	40

FOOD	PORTION	CALS.	FIB.	CHOL.
Chipsters	1	380	—	30
Chocolate	4 fl oz	180	—	40
Chocolate No Fat	4 fl oz	90	—	0
Flying Saucers	1	240	—	40
Ice Cream Cupcakes	1	210	—	30
Ice Cream Cake	1 piece (4 oz)	230	—	35
Vanilla	4 fl oz	190	—	50
Vanilla No Fat	4 fl oz	120	—	5
SHERBET				
Assorted Flavors	4 oz	150	—	5

CHICK-FIL-A
BEVERAGES

FOOD	PORTION	CALS.	FIB.	CHOL.
Iced Tea Unsweetened	1 reg (9 fl oz)	3	—	0
Lemonade	1 sm (10 fl oz)	138	—	tr
Lemonade Diet	1 sm (10 fl oz)	32	—	0
DESSERTS				
Cheesecake	1 slice (3.2 oz)	299	—	13
Cheesecake w/ Blueberry Topping	1 slice (4.3 oz)	350	—	13
Cheesecake w/ Strawberry Topping	1 slice (4.3 oz)	343	—	13
Fudge Brownie w/ Nuts	1 (2.78 oz)	369	—	31
Lemon Pie	1 slice (4.1 oz)	329	—	7
ICE CREAM				
Icedream	1 sm (4.5 oz)	134	—	24
MAIN MENU SELECTIONS				
Carrot & Raisin Salad	1 serving (2.67 oz)	116	—	6
Chargrilled Chicken Deluxe Sandwich	1 (7.15 oz)	266	—	40
Chargrilled Chicken Garden Salad	1 serving (10.4 oz)	126	—	28
Chargrilled Chicken Sandwich	1 (5.46 oz)	258	—	40
Chargrilled Chicken w/o Bun	1 piece (3.6 oz)	128	—	32
Chick-N-Q Sandwich	1 (6.8 oz)	409	—	10
Chicken Sandwich	1 (5.76 oz)	360	—	66
Chicken Deluxe Sandwich	1 (7.45 oz)	368	—	66
Chicken Salad Plate	1 serving (12.6 oz)	291	—	7
Chicken Salad Sandwich On Whole Wheat	1 (5.7 oz)	365	—	8
Chicken w/o Bun	1 piece (3.6 oz)	219	—	42
Cole Slaw	1 serving (3.72 oz)	175	—	13
Grilled 'n Lites	2 skewers (2.7 oz)	97	—	3
Hearty Breast of Chicken Soup	1 cup (8.5 fl oz)	152	—	46
Nuggets	8 pack (4 oz)	287	—	61
Potato Salad	1 serving (3.84 oz)	198	—	6
Waffle Potato Fries	1 sm (3 oz)	270	—	8

FOOD	PORTION	CALS.	FIB.	CHOL.
SALADS AND SALAD BARS				
Tossed Salad	1 serving (4.5 oz)	21	—	0
Tossed Salad w/ Blue Cheese Dressing	1 serving (6 oz)	243	—	38
Tossed Salad w/ Honey French Dressing	1 serving (6 oz)	277	—	0
Tossed Salad w/ Italian Lite Dressing	1 serving (6 oz)	43	—	0
Tossed Salad w/ Ranch Dressing	1 serving (6 oz)	298	—	5
Tossed Salad w/ Ranch Lite Dressing	1 serving (6 oz)	114	—	6
Tossed Salad w/ Thousand Island Dressing	1 serving (6 oz)	250	—	25
CHURCH'S FRIED CHICKEN				
Apple Pie	1 serving (3.1 oz)	280	1	<5
Biscuit	1 serving (2.1 oz)	250	1	<5
Breast	1 serving (2.8 oz)	200	0	65
Cajun Rice	1 serving (3.1 oz)	130	tr	5
Cole Slaw	1 serving (3 oz)	92	2	0
Corn On The Cob	1 serving (5.7 oz)	190	4	0
French Fries	1 serving (2.7 oz)	210	—	0
Leg	1 serving (2 oz)	140	0	45
Okra	1 serving (2.8 oz)	210	4	0
Potatoes & Gravy	1 serving (3.7 oz)	90	1	0
Thigh	1 serving (2.8 oz)	230	0	80
Wing	1 serving (3.1 oz)	250	0	60
COLOMBO FROZEN YOGURT				
Alpine Strawberry Nonfat	4 fl oz	100	0	0
Banana Strawberry Nonfat	4 fl oz	50	—	0
Brazlian Banana Nonfat	4 fl oz	100	0	0
Butter Pecan Nonfat	4 fl oz	100	0	0
Cappuccino Nonfat	4 fl oz	100	0	0
Cherry Amaretto Nonfat	4 fl oz	50	—	0
Cherry Vanilla Nonfat	4 fl oz	100	0	0
Chocolate Nonfat	4 fl oz	50	—	0
Coconut Cooler Nonfat	4 fl oz	100	0	0
Cool Berry Blue Nonfat	4 fl oz	100	0	0
Country Pumpkin Nonfat	4 fl oz	100	0	0
Double Dutch Chocolate Nonfat	4 fl oz	100	0	0
Egg Nog Nonfat	4 fl oz	100	0	0
French Vanilla Lowfat	4 fl oz	110	0	5
French Vanilla Nonfat	4 fl oz	100	0	0
Georgia Peach Nonfat	4 fl oz	100	0	0

FOOD	PORTION	CALS.	FIB.	CHOL.
German Fudge Chocolate Nonfat	4 fl oz	100	0	0
Hawaiian Pineapple Nonfat	4 fl oz	100	0	0
Hazelnut Amaretto Nonfat	4 fl oz	100	0	0
Honey Almond Nonfat	4 fl oz	100	0	0
Irish Cream Nonfat	4 fl oz	100	0	0
New York Cheesecake Nonfat	4 fl oz	100	0	0
Old World Chocolate Lowfat	4 fl oz	110	0	5
Orange Bavarian Creme Nonfat	4 fl oz	100	0	0
Peanut Butter Lowfat	4 fl oz	110	0	5
Pecan Praline Nonfat	4 fl oz	100	0	0
Pina Colada Nonfat	4 fl oz	100	0	0
Raspberry Nonfat	4 fl oz	50	—	0
Rockin' Raspberry Nonfat	4 fl oz	100	0	0
Simply Vanilla Lowfat	4 fl oz	110	0	5
Simply Vanilla Nonfat	4 fl oz	100	0	0
Strawberry Nonfat	4 fl oz	50	—	0
Tropical Tango Nonfat	4 fl oz	100	0	0
Vanilla Nonfat	4 fl oz	50	—	0
White Chocolate Almond Nonfat	4 fl oz	100	0	0
Wild Strawberry Lowfat	4 fl oz	110	0	5

D'ANGELO SANDWICH SHOPS
ICE CREAM

FOOD	PORTION	CALS.	FIB.	CHOL.
Frozen Yogurt Banana	5 oz	125	—	32
Frozen Yogurt Banana w/ Cone	5 oz	215	—	32
Frozen Yogurt Peach	5 oz	130	—	31
Frozen Yogurt Peach w/ Cone	5 oz	220	—	31

SALADS AND SALAD BARS

FOOD	PORTION	CALS.	FIB.	CHOL.
Beef	1 serving	350	—	63
Chicken	1 serving	325	—	49
Tuna	1 serving	305	—	32
Turkey	1 serving	375	—	64

SANDWICHES AND FILLINGS

FOOD	PORTION	CALS.	FIB.	CHOL.
D'Lite Pocket Chicken Stir Fry	1	340	—	60
D'Lite Pocket Roast Beef	1	325	—	63
D'Lite Pocket Steak	1	415	—	91
D'Lite Pocket Steak & Mushroom	1	420	—	91
D'Lite Pocket Steak & Pepper	1	420	—	91
D'Lite Pocket Turkey	1	350	—	64
D'Lite Pocket Vegetarian	1	350	—	26
D'Lite Small Sub Roast Beef	1	365	—	63
D'Lite Small Sub Turkey	1	390	—	64

DAIRY QUEEN/BRAZIER
FOOD SELECTION

FOOD	PORTION	CALS.	FIB.	CHOL.
¼lb. Super Dog	1	590	—	60

FOOD	PORTION	CALS.	FIB.	CHOL.
BBQ Beef Sandwich	1	225	—	20
Breaded Chicken Fillet Sandwich	1	430	—	55
Breaded Chicken Fillet Sandwich w/ Cheese	1	480	—	70
DQ Homestyle Ultimate Burger	1	700	—	140
Double Hamburger	1	460	—	95
Double Hamburger w/ Cheese	1	570	—	120
Fish Fillet Sandwich	1	370	—	45
Fish Fillet Sandwich w/ Cheese	1	420	—	60
French Dressing Reduced Calorie	2 oz	90	—	0
French Fries	1 sm	210	—	0
French Fries	1 lg	390	—	0
French Fries	1 reg	300	—	0
Garden Salad w/o dressing	1	200	—	0
Grilled Chicken Fillet Sandwich	1	300	—	50
Hot Dog	1	280	—	25
Hot Dog w/ Cheese	1	330	—	35
Hot Dog w/ Chili	1	320	—	30
Lettuce	0.5 oz	2	—	0
Onion Rings	1 reg	240	—	0
Side Salad w/o dressing	1	25	—	0
Single Hamburger	1	310	—	45
Single Hamburger w/ Cheese	1	365	—	60
Thousand Island Dressing	2 oz	225	—	25
Tomato	0.5 oz	3	—	0
ICE CREAM				
Banana Split	1	510	—	30
Blizzard Strawberry	1 reg	740	—	50
Blizzard Strawberry	1 sm	500	—	35
Breeze Strawberry	1 sm	400	—	5
Breeze Strawberry	1 reg	590	—	5
Buster Bar	1	450	—	15
Cone Chocolate	1 reg	230	—	20
Cone Chocolate	1 lg	350	—	30
Cone Vanilla	1 lg	340	—	30
Cone Vanilla	1 sm	140	—	15
Cone Vanilla	1 reg	230	—	20
Cone Dipped Chocolate	1 reg	330	—	20
Cone Yogurt	1 reg	180	—	<5
Cone Yogurt	1 lg	260	—	5
Cup Yogurt	1 lg	230	—	<5
Cup Yogurt	1 reg	170	—	<5
DQ Frozen Cake Slice Undecorated	1	380	—	20

FOOD	PORTION	CALS.	FIB.	CHOL.
DQ Sandwich	1	140	—	5
Dilly Bar	1	210	—	10
Heath Blizzard	1 reg	820	—	60
Heath Blizzard	1 sm	560	—	40
Heath Breeze	1 reg	680	—	15
Heath Breeze	1 sm	450	—	10
Hot Fudge Brownie Delight	1	710	—	35
Malt Vanilla	1 reg	610	—	45
Mr. Misty	1 reg	250	—	0
Nutty Double Fudge	1	580	—	35
Peanut Buster Parfait	1	710	—	30
QC Big Scoop Chocolate	1	310	—	35
QC Big Scoop Vanilla	1	300	—	35
Shake Chocolate	1 reg	540	—	45
Shake Vanilla	1 lg	600	—	50
Shake Vanilla	1 reg	520	—	45
Sundae Chocolate	1 reg	300	—	20
Sundae Waffle Cone Strawberry	1	350	—	20
Sundae Yogurt Strawberry	1 reg	200	—	<5

DELTACO
BEVERAGES
FOOD	PORTION	CALS.	FIB.	CHOL.
Coffee	1 serving	6	—	0
Coke Classic	1 sm	144	—	0
Coke Classic	1 lg	287	—	0
Coke Classic	1 med	198	—	0
Coke Classic Best Value	1 serving	395	—	0
Diet Coke	1 sm	1	—	0
Diet Coke	1 med	1	—	0
Diet Coke	1 lg	2	—	0
Diet Coke Best Value	1 serving	2	—	0
Iced Tea	1 sm	3	—	0
Iced Tea	1 lg	6	—	0
Iced Tea	1 med	4	—	0
Iced Tea Best Value	1 serving	8	—	0
Milk	1	126	—	12
Mr Pibb	1 lg	283	—	0
Mr Pibb	1 med	195	—	0
Mr Pibb	1 sm	142	—	0
Mr Pibb Best Value	1 serving	390	—	0
Orange Juice	1	83	—	0
Shake Chocolate	1 sm	549	—	40
Shake Chocolate	1 med	755	—	55
Shake Orange	1 sm	609	—	40

FOOD	PORTION	CALS.	FIB.	CHOL.
Shake Orange	1 med	837	—	55
Shake Strawberry	1 sm	486	—	40
Shake Strawberry	1 med	668	—	55
Shake Vanilla	1 med	707	—	63
Shake Vanilla	1 sm	514	—	46
Sprite	1 lg	287	—	0
Sprite	1 med	198	—	0
Sprite	1 sm	144	—	0
Sprite Best Value	1 serving	395	—	0
BREAKFAST SELECTIONS				
Burrito Beef And Egg	1	529	—	328
Burrito Breakfast	1	256	—	90
Burrito Egg And Cheese	1	443	—	305
Burrito Egg and Bean	1	470	—	305
Burrito Steak And Egg	1	500	—	337
CHILDREN'S MENU SELECTIONS				
Kid's Meal Hamburger	1	617	—	29
Kid's Meal Taco	1	532	—	16
ICE CREAM				
M&M's Toppers	1	256	—	19
Oreos Toppers	1	257	—	19
Snickers Toppers	1	254	—	18
MAIN MENU SELECTIONS				
American Cheese	1 slice	53	—	14
Beans And Cheese	1	122	—	9
Burrito Chicken	1	264	—	36
Burrito Combination	1	413	—	49
Burrito Del Beef	1	440	—	63
Burrito Deluxe Chicken	1	549	—	83
Burrito Deluxe Combo	1	453	—	59
Burrito Deluxe Del Beef	1	479	—	73
Burrito Green	1	229	—	15
Burrito Green Regular	1	330	—	22
Burrito Macho Beef	1	893	—	139
Burrito Macho Combo	1	774	—	100
Burrito Red	1	235	—	17
Burrito Red Regular	1	324	—	26
Cheeseburger	1	284	—	42
Chicken Salad	1	254	—	58
Chicken Salad Deluxe	1	716	—	98
Del Burger	1	385	—	42
Del Cheeseburger	1	439	—	55
Double Del Cheeseburger	1	618	—	108
French Fries	1 sm	242	—	0

FOOD	PORTION	CALS.	FIB.	CHOL.
French Fries	1 reg	404	—	0
French Fries	1 lg	566	—	0
Fries Chili Cheese	1 serving	562	—	38
Fries Deluxe Chili Cheese	1 serving	600	—	48
Fries Nacho	1 serving	669	—	2
Guacamole	1 oz	60	—	0
Hamburger	1	231	—	29
Hot Sauce	1 pkg	2	—	0
Nacho Cheese Sauce Side Order	1 serving	100	—	2
Nachos	1	390	—	2
Nachos Super Deluxe	1	684	—	46
Quesadilla	1	257	—	30
Quesadilla Chicken	1	544	—	113
Quesadilla Regular	1	483	—	75
Salsa	2 oz	14	—	tr
Salsa Dressing	1 oz	33	—	10
Sour Cream	1 oz	60	—	20
Taco	1	140	—	16
Taco Chicken	1	186	—	35
Taco Deluxe Double Beef	1	205	—	35
Taco Double Beef	1	172	—	25
Taco Soft	1	146	—	16
Taco Salad	1	235	—	31
Taco Salad Deluxe	1	741	—	83
Taco Soft Chicken	1	197	—	35
Taco Soft Deluxe Double Beef	1	211	—	35
Taco Soft Double Beef	1	178	—	25
Tostada	1	140	—	15

DENNY'S
BREAKFAST SELECTIONS

Harvest Slam	1 serving	1050	—	44
Harvest Slam w/ Eggbeaters	1 serving	960	—	33
Omelette Chili Cheese	1 serving	490	—	230
Omelette Denver	1 serving	720	—	650
Omelette Ham 'N'Cheddar	1 serving	480	—	240
Omelette Mexican	1 serving	540	—	245
Omelette Senior	1 serving	640	—	470
Omelette Ultimate	1 serving	850	—	670
Omelette Vegetable	1 serving	590	—	630
Omelette Vegetable w/ Eggbeaters	1 serving	450	—	15

DESSERTS
Apple Pie Regular	1 slice	480	—	4
Apple Pie w/ Equal	1 slice	460	—	0

FOOD	PORTION	CALS.	FIB.	CHOL.
MAIN MENU SELECTIONS				
BLT	1	620	—	40
Bacon Swiss w/o Lettuce And Tomato	1	750	—	130
Baked Potato	1 med	90	—	0
Catfish	2 pieces (8 oz)	640	—	107
Chicken Fried Steak w/o Gravy	2 pieces	500	—	90
Chicken Stir Fry w/ Rice	1 serving	420	—	60
Club Sandwich	1	590	—	90
Denny Burger	1	490	—	70
Grilled Cheese	1	710	—	100
Grilled Chicken	1	520	—	60
Grilled Chicken Breast	1 serving	125	—	70
Ham & Swiss Sandwich	1	500	—	76
Liver w/ Bacon & Onions	2 pieces	370	—	530
Patty Melt	1	775	—	120
Quesadila Beef	1	730	—	100
Quesadila Chicken	1	620	—	105
Quesadila Denny's	1	510	—	45
Senior Roast Beef Dinnner w/o Vegetable	1 serving	280	—	80
Senior Spaghetti Dinner	1 serving	580	—	80
Super Bird	1	750	—	110
Top Sirloin Steak	1 serving	270	—	90
Tuna Sandwich	1	400	—	22
Turkey Sandwich	1	340	—	70
Turkey w/o Gravy	6 slices	200	—	120
Veggie Cheese	1	560	—	70
Veggie Cheese Melt	1	560	—	70
Works Burger w/o Lettuce And Tomato	1	950	—	130
SALADS AND SALAD BARS				
Chef Salad	1	370	—	320
Garden Salad	1	110	—	75
Grilled Chicken Salad	1	290	—	80
Taco Salad	1	910	—	50
SOUPS				
Cheese	1 serving	406	—	38
Chicken Noodle	1 serving	120	—	20
Vegetable Beef	1 serving	159	—	9

DOMINO'S PIZZA
12 INCH PIZZA

FOOD	PORTION	CALS.	FIB.	CHOL.
Pepperoni	1 slice	219	1	14
Veggie	1 slice	204	2	9

FOOD	PORTION	CALS.	FIB.	CHOL.
15 INCH PIZZA				
Deluxe	2 slices	498	7	40
16 INCH PIZZA				
Cheese	2 slices	376	6	19
Double Cheese Pepperoni	2 slices	545	8	48
Ham	2 slices	417	2	26
Pepperoni	2 slices	460	4	28
Sausage Mushroom	2 slices	430	8	28
Veggie	2 slices	498	8	36
DUNKIN' DONUTS				
COOKIES				
Chocolate Chunk	1 (1.6 oz)	200	1	30
Chocolate Chunk w/ Nuts	1 (1.5 oz)	210	2	30
CROISSANTS				
Almond	1 (3.7 oz)	420	3	0
Chocolate	1 (3.3 oz)	440	3	0
Plain	1 (2.5 oz)	310	2	0
DOUGHNUTS				
Apple Crumb	1 (3 oz)	250	2	0
Apple Filled w/ Cinnamon Sugar	1 (2.8 oz)	250	1	0
Blueberry Filled	1 (2.4 oz)	210	2	0
Boston Kreme	1 (2.8 oz)	240	2	0
Butternut Cake Ring	1 (3.5 oz)	410	3	0
Chocolate Frosted Yeast Ring	1 (1.9 oz)	200	1	0
Chocolate Frosted Cake Ring	1 (2.3 oz)	280	1	0
Chocolate Glazed Ring	1 (3.4 oz)	420	3	0
Chocolate Kreme	1 (2.4 oz)	250	2	0
Cinnamon Cake Ring	1 (2.2 oz)	260	1	0
Coconut Coated Cake Ring	1 (3.1 oz)	360	5	0
Dunkin' Donut	1 (2.1 oz)	240	2	0
Glazed Buttermilk Ring	1 (2.6 oz)	290	1	10
Glazed Chocolate Ring	1 (2.7 oz)	320	1	0
Glazed Coffee Roll	1 (2.8 oz)	280	2	0
Glazed Cruller	1 (2.4 oz)	260	1	0
Glazed French Cruller	1 (1.4 oz)	140	0	30
Glazed Whole Wheat Ring	1 (2.5 oz)	280	2	0
Glazed Yeast Ring	1 (1.9 oz)	200	1	0
Jelly Filled	1 (2.4 oz)	220	1	0
Lemon Filled	1 (2.8 oz)	260	1	0
Mini Cake	1 (0.9 oz)	100	tr	0
Mini Chocolate Glazed	1 (1.1 oz)	122	1	0
Mini Cinnamon Cake	1 (1 oz)	116	1	0
Mini Coconut	1 (1.2 oz)	140	2	0

FOOD	PORTION	CALS.	FIB.	CHOL.
Mini Coffee Roll	1 (0.8 oz)	78	1	0
Mini Eclairs	1 (1.3 oz)	114	1	0
Munchkin Butternut Cake	1 (0.6 oz)	70	0	0
Munchkin Coconut Cake	1 (0.6 oz)	70	1	0
Munchkin Glazed Cake	1 (0.6 oz)	60	0	0
Munchkin Glazed Chocolate	1 (0.7 oz)	70	0	0
Munchkin Glazed Yeast	1 (0.5 oz)	50	0	0
Munchkin Jelly Filled Yeast	1 (0.5 oz)	50	0	0
Munchkin Plain Cake	1 (0.5 oz)	50	0	0
Munchkin Powdered Cake	1 (0.5 oz)	50	0	0
Peanut	1 (3.7 oz)	480	3	0
Plain Cake Ring	1 (2 oz)	262	1	0
Powdered Cake Ring	1 (2.2 oz)	270	2	0
Sugared Cake Ring	1 (2.1 oz)	270	2	0
Sugared Jelly Stick	1 (3 oz)	310	1	0
Vanilla Frosted Yeast Ring	1 (2 oz)	200	1	0
Vanilla Kreme	1 (2.4 oz)	250	3	0
MUFFINS				
Apple N'Spice	1 (3.4 oz)	300	2	25
Banana Nut	1 (3.3 oz)	310	3	30
Blueberry	1 (3.6 oz)	280	2	30
Bran w/ Raisins	1 (3.68 oz)	310	4	15
Corn	1 (3.4 oz)	340	1	40
Cranberry Nut	1 (3.4 oz)	290	2	25
Oat Bran	1 (3.3 oz)	330	3	0
Lowfat Apple n'Spice	1 (3.3 oz)	220	1	0
Lowfat Banana	1 (3.3 oz)	240	1	0
Lowfat Blueberry	1 (3.3 oz)	220	1	0
Lowfat Cherry	1 (3.3 oz)	230	1	0
Lowfat Cranberry Orange	1 (3.3 oz)	230	1	0

EL POLLO LOCO

DESSERTS

FOOD	PORTION	CALS.	FIB.	CHOL.
Cheesecake	1 serving (3.5 oz)	160	0	60
Churros	1 serving (1.5 oz)	140	0	4
Orange Bang	1 serving (7 oz)	110	0	0
Pina Colada Bang	1 serving (7 oz)	110	0	0
MAIN MENU SELECTIONS				
Beans	1 serving (4 oz)	100	8	0
Burrito Chicken	1 (7 oz)	310	4	65
Burrito Steak	1 (6 oz)	450	4	70
Burrito Vegetarian	1 (6 oz)	340	7	20
Cheddar Cheese	1 serving (1 oz)	90	0	27
Chicken Breast	1 piece (3 oz)	160	0	110

FOOD	PORTION	CALS.	FIB.	CHOL.
Chicken Leg	1 piece (1.75 oz)	90	0	75
Chicken Thigh	1 piece (2 oz)	180	0	130
Chicken Wing	1 (1.5 oz)	110	0	80
Chicken Fajita Meal	1 (17.5 oz)	780	17	58
Coleslaw	1 serving (3 oz)	70	1	0
Corn	1 serving (3 oz)	110	1	0
Guacamole	1 serving (1 oz)	60	0	0
Potato Salad	1 serving (4 oz)	180	1	10
Rice	1 serving (2 oz)	110	0	0
Salsa	2 oz	10	0	0
Sour Cream	1 serving (1 oz)	60	0	13
Steak Fajita Meal	1 (17.5 oz)	1040	17	100
Taco Chicken	1 (5 oz)	180	2	35
Taco Steak	1 (4.5 oz)	250	2	40
Tortillas Corn	1 (1 oz)	60	tr	0
Tortillas Flour	1 (1 oz)	90	tr	0
SALAD DRESSINGS				
Blue Cheese	1 fl oz	80	0	5
Deluxe French	1 fl oz	60	0	0
Honey Dijon Mustard	1 fl oz	50	0	0
Italian Reduced Calorie	1 fl oz	25	0	0
Ranch	1 fl oz	75	0	0
Thousand Island	1 fl oz	110	0	5
SALADS AND SALAD BARS				
Chicken Salad	1 (12 oz)	160	4	45
Side Salad	1 (9 oz)	50	4	0
FRIENDLY'S				
Fudge Nut Brownie	½ cup	200	0	25
Heath English Toffee	½ cup (2.7 oz)	190	0	30
Purely Pistachio	½ cup	160	0	35
Vanilla	½ cup	150	0	35
Vienna Mocha Chunk	½ cup	180	0	30
GODFATHER'S PIZZA				
Golden Crust Cheese	⅒ lg (3.5 oz)	261	—	23
Golden Crust Cheese	⅛ med (3.1 oz)	229	—	19
Golden Crust Cheese	⅙ sm (3 oz)	213	—	19
Golden Crust Combo	⅙ sm (4.5 oz)	273	—	31
Golden Crust Combo	⅛ med (4.5 oz)	283	—	29
Golden Crust Combo	⅒ lg (5.1 oz)	322	—	34
Original Crust Cheese	⅙ sm (3.5 oz)	239	—	25
Original Crust Cheese	⅒ lg (4 oz)	271	—	28
Original Crust Cheese	⅛ med (3.5 oz)	242	—	22
Original Crust Cheese	¼ mini (2 oz)	138	—	13

FOOD	PORTION	CALS.	FIB.	CHOL.
Original Crust Combo	1/10 lg (5.5 oz)	332	—	39
Original Crust Combo	1/6 sm (5 oz)	299	—	37
Original Crust Combo	1/4 mini (2.8 oz)	164	—	17
Original Crust Combo	1/8 med (5.2 oz)	318	—	38

GODIVA

Almond Butter Dome	3 pieces (1.5 oz)	240	0	5
Bouchee Au Chocolat	1 piece (1.5 oz)	210	0	5
Bouchee Ivory Raspberry	1 pieces (1 oz)	160	0	5
Gold Ballotin	3 pieces (1.5 oz)	210	0	5
Truffle Amaretto Di Saronno	2 pieces (1.5 oz)	210	0	5
Truffle Deluxe Liqueur	2 pieces (1.5 oz)	210	0	5

H.SALT SEAFOOD

Chicken	3 oz	108	—	69
Cod	3 oz	62	—	18
Hamburger	3 oz	228	—	65
Pork Loin	3 oz	254	—	55
Sirloin Steak	3 oz	239	—	58

HAAGEN-DAZS
FROZEN YOGURT

Chocolate	3 oz	130	—	25
Nonfat Soft Banana	1 oz	25	—	0
Nonfat Soft Chocolate	1 oz	30	—	0
Nonfat Soft Strawberry	1 oz	25	—	0
Peach	3 oz	120	—	31
Soft Chocolate	1 oz	30	—	3
Soft Coffee	1 oz	28	—	3
Soft Raspberry	1 oz	30	—	3
Soft Vanilla	1 oz	28	—	3
Strawberry	3 oz	120	—	30
Vanilla	3 oz	130	—	40
Vanilla Almond Crunch	3 oz	150	—	33

ICE CREAM

Butter Pecan	4 oz	390	—	115
Caramel Almond Crunch Bar	1	240	—	40
Chocolate	4 oz	270	—	120
Chocolate Chocolate Chip	4 oz	290	—	105
Coffee	4 oz	270	—	120
Honey Vanilla	4 oz	250	—	135
Peanut Butter Crunch Bar	1 (6.3 fl oz)	270	—	35
Rum Raisin	4 oz	250	—	110
Strawberry	4 oz	250	—	95
Vanilla	4 oz	260	—	120

FOOD	PORTION	CALS.	FIB.	CHOL.
Vanilla Crunch Bar	1	220	—	40
Vanilla Peanut Butter Swirl	4 oz	280	—	110

HARDEE'S

BAKED SELECTIONS

Big Cookie	1 (2.0 oz)	280	—	15
Blueberry Muffin	1 (4 oz)	400	—	65

BEVERAGES

Orange Juice	1 serving (11 oz)	140	—	0
Shake Chocolate	1 (11.4 fl oz)	390	—	30
Shake Peach	1 (11.4 fl oz)	530	—	45
Shake Strawberry	1 (11.4 fl oz)	390	—	30
Shake Vanilla	1 (11.4 fl oz)	370	—	25

BREAKFAST SELECTIONS

Bacon And Egg Biscuit	1 (4.4 oz)	490	—	155
Bacon, Egg And Cheese Biscuit	1 (4.8 oz)	530	—	155
Big Country Breakfast Bacon	1 (7.6 oz)	740	—	305
Big Country Breakfast Sausage	1 (9.6 oz)	930	—	340
Biscuit 'N' Gravy	1 (7.8 oz)	510	—	15
Canadian Rise 'N' Shine Biscuit	1 (5.8 oz)	570	—	175
Chicken Biscuit	1 (5.1 oz)	510	—	45
Cinnamon 'N' Raisin Biscuit	1 (2.8 oz)	370	—	0
Country Ham Biscuit	1 (3.8 oz)	430	—	25
Frisco Breakfast Sandwich Ham	1 (6.5 oz)	460	—	175
Ham Biscuit	1 (4 oz)	400	—	15
Ham, Egg And Cheese Biscuit	1 (5.6 oz)	500	—	170
Hash Rounds	1 serving (2.8 oz)	230	—	0
Rise 'N' Shine Biscuit	1 (2.9 oz)	390	—	0
Sausage And Egg Biscuit	1 (5.2 oz)	560	—	170
Sausage Biscuit	1 (4.1 oz)	510	—	25
Steak Biscuit	1 (5.2 oz)	580	—	30
Three Pancakes	1 serving (4.8 oz)	280	—	15
Three Pancakes w/ 1 Sausage Pattie	1 serving (6.2 oz)	430	—	40
Three Pancakes w/ 2 Bacon Strips	1 serving (5.3 oz)	350	—	25

ICE CREAM

Cool Twist Sundae Hot Fudge	1 (5.9 oz)	320	—	25
Cool Twist Sundae Strawberry	1 (5.8 oz)	260	—	15
Cool Twist Cone Chocolate	1 (4.1 oz)	180	—	15
Cool Twist Cone Vanilla	1 (4.1 oz)	180	—	15
Cool Twist Cone Vanilla/ Chocolate	1 (4.1 oz)	170	—	15

MAIN MENU SELECTIONS

Bacon Cheeseburger	1 (7.9 oz)	600	—	50

FOOD	PORTION	CALS.	FIB.	CHOL.
Big Deluxe Burger	1 (8.5 oz)	530	—	40
Big Roast Beef Sandwich	1 (5.9 oz)	370	—	40
Cheeseburger	1 (4.2 oz)	300	—	25
Chef Salad	1 (9.4 oz)	200	—	45
Chicken Fillet Sandwich	1 (6.6 oz)	400	—	55
Cole Slaw	1 serving (4 oz)	240	—	10
Crispy Curls	1 serving (3.0 oz)	300	—	0
Fisherman's Fillet Sandwich	1 (7.6 oz)	500	—	60
French Fries	1 sm (3.4 oz)	240	—	0
French Fries	1 med (5.0 oz)	350	—	0
French Fries	1 lg (6.1 oz)	430	—	0
Fried Chicken Breast	1 piece (5.2 oz)	370	—	75
Fried Chicken Leg	1 piece (2.4 oz)	170	—	45
Fried Chicken Thigh	1 piece (4.2 oz)	330	—	60
Fried Chicken Wing	1 piece (2.3 oz)	200	—	30
Frisco Burger	1 (8.5 oz)	760	—	70
Friso Grilled Chicken Sandwich	1 (8.6 oz)	620	—	95
Garden Salad	1 (9.3 oz)	190	—	40
Gravy	1 serving (1.5 fl oz)	20	—	0
Grilled Chicken Salad	1 (9.8 oz)	120	—	60
Hamburger	1 (3.6 oz)	260	—	20
Hot Dog	1 (6.8 oz)	450	—	35
Hot Ham 'N' Cheese Sandwich	1 (7.1 oz)	530	—	65
Mashed Potatoes	1 serving (4 oz)	70	—	0
Mushroom 'N' Swiss Burger	1 (7.1 oz)	520	—	45
Quarter-Pound Cheeseburger	1 (6.5 oz)	490	—	35
Regular Roast Beef Sandwich	1 (4.4 oz)	270	—	25
Side Salad	1 (4.9 oz)	20	—	0

IHOP

Pancake Buckwheat	1 (2.5 oz)	134	1	61
Pancake Buttermilk	1 (2 oz)	108	tr	31
Pancake Egg	1 (2 oz)	102	tr	66
Pancake Harvest Grain 'N Nut	1 (2.25 oz)	160	1	38
Waffle	1 (4 oz)	305	1	70
Waffle Belgian	1 (6 oz)	408	1	146
Waffle Belgian Harvest Grain 'N Nut	1 (6 oz)	445	3	147

JACK IN THE BOX
BEVERAGES

Coca-Cola Classic	1 sm (16 fl oz)	190	0	0
Coffee	1 cup (8 fl oz)	5	0	0
Diet Coke	1 sm (16 fl oz)	0	—	0
Dr Pepper	1 sm (16 fl oz)	190	0	0

FOOD	PORTION	CALS.	FIB.	CHOL.
Iced Tea	1 sm (16 fl oz)	0	0	0
Lowfat Milk 2%	1 serv (8 fl oz)	120	0	20
Milk Shake Chocolate	1 reg (11 fl oz)	390	tr	25
Milk Shake Strawberry	1 reg (11 fl oz)	330	0	30
Milk Shake Vanilla	1 reg (11 fl oz)	350	0	30
Orange Juice	1 serv (6 fl oz)	80	tr	0
Ramblin' Root Beer	1 sm (16 fl oz)	240	0	0
Sprite	1 sm (16 fl oz)	190	0	0
BREAKAST SELECTIONS				
Breakfast Jack	1 (4.3 oz)	300	0	185
Country Crock Spread	1 pat (5 g)	25	0	0
Grape Jelly	1 serving (0.5 oz)	40	0	0
Hash Brown	1 serving (2 oz)	160	1	0
Pancake Platter	1 serv (8.1 oz)	610	0	100
Pancake Syrup	1 serving (1.5 fl oz)	120	0	0
Sausage Crescent	1 (5.5 oz)	580	0	185
Scrambled Egg Platter	1 (7.5 oz)	560	0	380
Scrambled Egg Pocket	1 (6.4 oz)	430	0	355
Sourdough Breakfast Sandwich	1 (5.2 oz)	380	0	235
Supreme Crescent	1 (5.4 oz)	530	0	210
Ultimate Breakfast Sandwich	1 (8.5 oz)	620	tr	455
DESSERTS				
Cheesecake	1 serv (3.5 oz)	310	2	65
Cheesecake Chocolate Chip Cookie Dough	1 serv (3.6 oz)	360	1	45
Cinnamon Churritos	1 serving (2.6 oz)	330	3	20
Hot Apple Turnover	1 (3.9 oz)	350	0	0
MAIN MENU SELECTIONS				
¼ lb. Burger	1 (6 oz)	510	0	65
Bacon Bacon Cheeseburger	1 (8.5 oz)	710	0	110
Barbeque Sauce	1 serv (1 fl oz)	45	0	0
Cheeseburger	1 (3.9 oz)	330	0	35
Chicken Caesar Sandwich	1 (8.3 oz)	520	4	55
Chicken Fajita Pita	1 (6.6 oz)	290	3	35
Chicken Sandwich	1 (5.6 oz)	400	0	45
Chicken Strips Breaded	4 pieces (3.9 oz)	290	0	50
Chicken Strips Breaded	6 pieces (6.2 oz)	450	0	80
Chicken Supreme	1 (8.6 oz)	620	0	75
Chicken Taquitos	5 pieces (4.8 oz)	350	4	40
Chicken Taquitos	8 pieces (7.7 oz)	560	6	65
Country Fried Steak Sandwich	1 (5.4 oz)	450	0	35
Double Cheeseburger	1 (5.3 oz)	450	0	75
Egg Rolls	5 pieces (10 oz)	750	7	50
Egg Rolls	3 pieces (5.8 oz)	440	4	30

FOOD	PORTION	CALS.	FIB.	CHOL.
Fish Supreme	1 (8.6 oz)	590	0	60
French Fries	1 sm (2.4 oz)	220	3	0
French Fries	1 reg (3.8 oz)	350	—	0
Grilled Chicken Fillet	1 (7.4 oz)	430	0	65
Grilled Sourdough Burger	1 (7.8 oz)	670	0	110
Guacamole	1 serv (0.9 oz)	50	0	0
Hamburger	1 (3.4 oz)	280	0	25
Hot Sauce	1 serv (0.5 fl oz)	5	0	0
Jumbo Fries	1 serv (4.3 oz)	400	4	0
Jumbo Jack	1 (8 oz)	560	0	65
Jumbo Jack With Cheese	1 (8.5 oz)	610	0	80
Monterey Roast Beef Sandwich	1 (8.4 oz)	540	3	75
Onion Rings	1 serv (3.6 oz)	380	0	0
Salsa	1 serv (1 fl oz)	10	0	0
Seasoned Curly Fries	1 serv (3.8 oz)	360	4	0
Smoked Chicken Cheddar & Bacon Sandwich	1 (7.8 oz)	540	9	80
Sourdough Ranch Chicken Sandwich	1 (7.9 oz)	490	1	65
Soy Sauce	1 serv (0.3 oz)	9	0	0
Spicy Crispy Chicken Sandwich	1 (7.9 oz)	560	0	50
Super Scoop French Fries	1 serv (6.5 oz)	590	6	0
Super Taco	1 (4.4 oz)	280	3	30
Sweet & Sour Sauce	1 serv (1 fl oz)	40	0	0
Taco	1 (2.7 oz)	190	2	20
Teriyaki Bowl Beef	1 serving (15.4 oz)	640	7	25
Teriyaki Bowl Chicken	1 serv (15.4 oz)	580	6	30
The Colossus Burger	1 (9.5 oz)	940	0	165
Ultimate Cheeseburger	1 (9.8 oz)	830	0	130
SALAD DRESSINGS				
Bleu Cheese	1 serv (2 fl oz)	210	0	15
Buttermilk House	1 serv (2 fl oz)	290	0	20
Buttermilk House Sauce	1 serv (0.9 fl oz)	130	tr	10
Italian Low Calorie	1 serv (2 fl oz)	25	0	0
Thousand Island	1 serv (2 fl oz)	250	0	20
SALADS AND SALAD BARS				
Croutons	1 serv (0.4 oz)	50	0	0
Garden Chicken Salad	1 serv (8.9 oz)	200	3	65
Side Salad	1 (4 oz)	70	2	10

KENTUCKY FRIED CHICKEN
BAKED SELECTIONS

Biscuit	1 (2.2 oz)	220	—	<5
Breadstick	1 (1.2 oz)	110	0	0

FOOD	PORTION	CALS.	FIB.	CHOL.
Cornbread	1 (2 oz)	228	1	42
Sourdough Roll	1 (1.7 oz)	128	1	0
MAIN MENU SELECTIONS				
BBQ Baked Beans	1 serving (3.9 oz)	132	2	3
Chicken Littles Sandwich	1 (1.7 oz)	169	—	18
Cole Slaw	1 serving (3.2 oz)	114	—	<5
Colonel's Chicken Sandwich	1 (5.9 oz)	482	—	47
Colonel's Rotisserie Gold Dark Quarter	1 serving (5.1 oz)	333	—	163
Colonel's Rotisserie Gold Dark Quarter Skin Removed	1 serving (4.1 oz)	217	—	128
Colonel's Rotisserie Gold White Quarter	1 serving (6.2 oz)	335	—	157
Colonel's Rotisserie Gold White Quarter Skin Removed	1 serving (4.1 oz)	199	—	97
Corn On The Cob	1 ear (5.3 oz)	222	8	0
Crispy Fries	1 serving (2.5 oz)	210	3	4
Extra Crispy Tasty Side Breast	1 (4.1 oz)	400	—	75
Extra Tasty Crispy Center Breast	1 (4.1 oz)	330	—	75
Extra Tasty Crispy Drumstick	1 (2.3 oz)	190	—	65
Extra Tasty Crispy Thigh	1 (3.8 oz)	380	—	90
Extra Tasty Crispy Whole Wing	1 (2.1 oz)	240	—	65
Garden Rice	1 serving (3.8 oz)	75	1	0
Green Beans	1 serving (3.6 oz)	36	2	3
Hot & Spicy Center Breast	1 (4.3 oz)	360	—	80
Hot & Spicy Drumstick	1 (2.4 oz)	180	—	55
Hot & Spicy Side Breast	1 (4.2 oz)	400	—	80
Hot & Spicy Thigh	1 (4.2 oz)	370	—	100
Hot & Spicy Whole Wing	1 (2.1 oz)	220	—	65
Hot Wings	6 (4.8 oz)	471	—	150
Kentucky Nuggets	6 (3.4 oz)	284	—	66
Macaroni & Cheese	1 serving (4 oz)	162	0	16
Mashed Potatoes With Gravy	1 serving (4.2 oz)	70	—	<5
Mean Greens	1 serving (3.9 oz)	52	3	6
Original Center Breast	1 (3.6 oz)	260	—	92
Original Drumstick	1 (2 oz)	152	—	75
Original Side Breast	1 (2.9 oz)	245	—	78
Original Thigh	1 (3.4 oz)	287	—	112
Original Whole Wing	1 (1.9 oz)	172	—	59
Potato Wedges	1 serving (3.3 oz)	192	3	3
Red Beans & Rice	1 serving (3.9 oz)	114	3	4
Vegetable Medley Salad	1 serving (4 oz)	126	3	0
SALAD DRESSINGS				
Italian	1 serving (1 fl oz)	15	0	0
Ranch	1 serving (1 oz)	170	0	10

FOOD	PORTION	CALS.	FIB.	CHOL.
SALADS AND SALAD BARS				
Garden Salad	1 (3.1 oz)	16	1	0
Macaroni	1 serving (3.8 oz)	248	1	12
Pasta Salad	1 serving (3.8 oz)	135	1	1
Potato	1 serving (4.4 oz)	180	2	11
KRYSTAL				
BEVERAGES				
Chocolate Shake	1 (12.8 fl oz)	271	—	32
BREAKFAST SELECTIONS				
Biscuit	1 (3.2 oz)	289	—	1
Biscuit Bacon	1 (3.6 oz)	355	—	14
Biscuit Country Ham	1 (4.5 oz)	379	—	23
Biscuit Egg	1 (4.8 oz)	372	—	133
Biscuit Gravy	1 (8.2 oz)	445	—	13
Biscuit Sausage	1 (4.3 oz)	429	—	29
Sunriser	1 (3.6 oz)	264	—	157
DESSERTS				
Apple Pie	1 serving (4.5 oz)	320	—	0
Donut	1 (1.3 oz)	100	—	6
Donut w/ Chocolate Icing	1 (1.8 oz)	162	—	6
Donut w/ Vanilla Icing	1 (1.8 oz)	148	—	6
Lemon Meringue Pie	1 serving (4 oz)	340	—	45
Pecan Pie	1 serving (4 oz)	450	—	55
MAIN MENU SELECTIONS				
Bacon Cheeseburger	1 (6.4 oz)	583	—	114
Big K	1 (7.3 oz)	608	—	125
Burger Plus	1 (6.4 oz)	488	—	90
Burger Plus w/ Cheese	1 (7 oz)	545	—	105
Cheese Krystal	1 (2.6 oz)	189	—	30
Chicken Sandwich	1 (6.4 oz)	392	—	33
Chili	1 lg (12 oz)	322	—	25
Chili	1 reg (8 oz)	214	—	16
Chili Cheese Pup	1 (2.6 oz)	203	—	24
Chili Pup	1 (2.5 oz)	184	—	19
Corn Pup	1 (2.3 oz)	214	—	24
Double Cheese Krystal	1 (4.6 oz)	341	—	60
Double Krystal	1 (4 oz)	276	—	43
Fries	1 lg (5 oz)	615	—	15
Fries	1 med (3.9 oz)	474	—	12
Fries	1 sm (2.8 oz)	338	—	8
Krys Kross Fries	1 serving (2.6 oz)	242	—	10
Krys Kross Fries w/ Cheese	1 serving (3.6 oz)	292	—	11
Krystal	1 (2.2 oz)	157	—	21
Plain Pup	1 (1.9 oz)	164	—	15

FOOD	PORTION	CALS.	FIB.	CHOL.

LITTLE CAESARS PIZZA
MAIN MENU SELECTIONS
Antipasto Salad	1 sm	96	2	10
Crazy Bread	1 piece	98	1	2
Crazy Sauce	1 serving	63	4	0
Greek Salad	1 sm	85	1	10
Ham & Cheese Sandwich	1	552	4	50
Italian Sandwich	1	615	4	55
Tossed Salad	1 sm	37	2	0
Tuna Sandwich	1	610	6	75
Turkey Sandwich	1	450	3	45
Veggie Sandwich	1	784	4	95

PIZZA
Baby Pan!Pan!	1 order	525	17	60
Cheese & Pepperoni Round Large	1 slice	185	3	20
Cheese & Pepperoni Round Medium	1 slice	168	3	20
Cheese & Pepperoni Round Small	1 slice	151	2	15
Cheese & Pepperoni Square Large	1 slice	204	3	25
Cheese & Pepperoni Square Medium	1 slice	201	3	23
Cheese & Pepperoni Square Small	1 slice	204	3	20
Cheese Round Large	1 slice	169	3	15
Cheese Round Medium	1 slice	154	3	15
Cheese Round Small	1 slice	138	2	15
Cheese Square Large	1 slice	188	3	20
Cheese Square Medium	1 slice	185	3	20
Cheese Square Small	1 slice	188	3	20
Slice!Slice!	1 order	756	12	90

LONG JOHN SILVER'S
CHILDREN'S MENU SELECTIONS
1 Fish, 1 Chicken & Fries	1 meal (8.9 oz)	620	—	45
1 Piece Fish & Fries	1 meal (7 oz)	500	—	50
2 Chicken Planks & Fries	1 meal (7.8 oz)	560	—	30

DESSERTS
Cherry Pie	1 slice (4.5 oz)	360	—	5
Chocolate Chip Cookie	1 (1.8 oz)	230	—	10
Lemon Pie	1 slice (4 oz)	340	—	45
Oatmeal Raisin Cookie	1 (1.8 oz)	160	—	15
Pineapple Cream Cheese Cake	1 slice (3.2 oz)	310	—	10
Walnut Brownie	1 (3.4 oz)	440	—	20

MAIN MENU SELECTIONS
1 Fish & 2 Chicken w/ Fries & Slaw	1 serving (15.2 oz)	950	—	75

FOOD	PORTION	CALS.	FIB.	CHOL.
1 Fish, 1 Chicken & Fries	1 serving (8.1 oz)	550	—	45
2 Fish, 4 Shrimp Clams w/ Fries & Slaw	1 serving (18.1 oz)	1240	—	140
2 Fish, 5 Shrimp 1 Chicken w/ Fries & Slaw	1 serving (18.1 oz)	1160	—	135
2 Fish, 8 Shrimp w/ Fries & Slaw	1 serving (17.2 oz)	1140	—	145
Baked Chicken Entree	1 dinner (15.9 oz)	590	—	75
Baked Chicken Light Herb	1 piece (3.5 oz)	120	—	60
Baked Fish w/ Lemon Crumb	3 pieces (5 oz)	150	—	110
Baked Fish w/ Lemon Crumb Entree 3 Pieces	1 dinner (17.4 oz)	610	—	125
Baked Light Fish w/ Lemon Crumb Entree 2 Pieces	1 dinner (11.8 oz)	330	—	46
Batter Dipped Fish	1 piece (3.1 oz)	180	—	30
Batter Dipped Shrimp	1 piece (0.4 oz)	30	—	10
Catsup	1 serving (.32 oz)	12	—	0
Chicken Plank	1 piece (2 oz)	120	—	15
Chicken Planks	2 pieces (4 oz)	240	—	30
Chicken Planks 2 Pieces & Fries	1 serving (6.9 oz)	490	—	30
Chicken Planks 3 Pieces w/ Fries & Slaw	1 serving (14.1 oz)	890	—	55
Clams w/ Fries & Slaw	1 serving (12.7 oz)	990	—	75
Cole Slaw	1 serving (3.4 oz)	140	—	15
Corn Cobbette	1 piece (3.3 oz)	140	—	0
Crispy Fish	1 piece (1.8 oz)	150	—	20
Crispy Fish & More 3 Pieces w/ Fries & Slaw	1 serving (13.5 oz)	980	—	70
Fish & Fries 2 Pieces	1 serving (9.2 oz)	610	—	52
Fish & More 2 Pieces w/ Fries & Slaw	1 serving (14.4 oz)	890	—	75
Fries	1 serving (3 oz)	250	—	0
Green Beans	1 serving (3.5 oz)	20	—	0
Honey Mustard Sauce	1 serving (0.42 fl oz)	20	—	0
Hushpuppies	1 (0.8 oz)	70	—	<5
Rice	1 serving (4 oz)	190	—	0
Roll	1 (1.5 oz)	110	—	0
Saltine Crackers	1 pkg (0.2 oz)	25	—	0
Sandwich Batter Dipped Chicken 1 Piece	1 (4.5 oz)	280	—	15
Sandwich Batter Dipped Fish 1 Piece	1 (5.6 oz)	340	—	30
Seafood Sauce	1 serving (0.42 fl oz)	14	—	0

FOOD	PORTION	CALS.	FIB.	CHOL.
Shrimp w/ Fries & Slaw	1 serving (11.7 oz)	840	—	100
Sweet'N Sour Sauce	1 serving	20	—	0
	(0.42 fl oz)			
Tartar Sauce	1 serving	50	—	0
	(0.42 fl oz)			
SALAD DRESSINGS				
Malt Vinegar	1 serving	1	—	0
	(0.28 fl oz)			
Ranch Dressing	1 serving (1 fl oz)	180	—	<5
Sea Salad Dressing	1 serving (1 fl oz)	140	—	<5
SALADS AND SALAD BARS				
Ocean Chef Salad	1 serving (8.3 oz)	110	—	40
Seafood Salad	1 serving (9.8 oz)	380	—	55
Side Salad	1 (4.4 oz)	25	—	0
SOUPS				
Seafood Chowder w/ Cod	1 serving (7 oz)	140	—	20
Seafood Gumbo w/ Cod	1 serving (7 oz)	120	—	25

MACHEEZMO MOUSE
CHILDREN'S MENU SELECTIONS

FOOD	PORTION	CALS.	FIB.	CHOL.
Kid's Plate	7 oz	279	4	20
Kid's Plate With Chicken	9 oz	349	4	80
MAIN MENU SELECTIONS				
Bean/Cheese Enchilada	12 oz	405	9	28
Bean/Cheese Enchilada Dinner	22 oz	670	17	28
Beans	6 oz	214	5	0
Boss Sauce	1 oz	30	0	0
Cheese	1 oz	81	—	20
Cheese Quesadilla	5 oz	337	2	42
Chicken	3 oz	105	1	90
Chicken Burrito	13 oz	543	5	110
Chicken Burrito Dinner	23 oz	808	13	110
Chicken Enchilada	10 oz	332	6	88
Chicken Enchilada Dinner	20 oz	597	14	88
Chicken Majita	18 oz	704	11	128
Chicken Quesadilla	9 oz	407	3	102
Chicken Salad Large	17 oz	612	7	122
Chicken Salad Small	10 oz	324	4	76
Chicken Tacos	6 oz	294	3	82
Chicken Tacos Dinner	16 oz	559	11	82
Chicken w/ Green Salad	13 oz	377	8	128
Chili	3 oz	135	1	66
Chili Tacos	6 oz	314	3	66
Chili Tacos Dinner	16 oz	579	11	66

FOOD	PORTION	CALS.	FIB.	CHOL.
Chips	3 oz	394	2	0
Combo Burrito	14 oz	598	6	124
Combo Burrito Dinner	24 oz	863	14	124
Enchilada Sauce	1 oz	6	1	0
Famouse #5	14 oz	583	9	20
Guacamole	2 oz	201	1	0
Mex Cheese	1 oz	100	0	24
Mixed Greens	4 oz	tr	2	0
Nacho Grande	8 oz	704	3	74
Rice	6 oz	274	4	0
Salad w/ Marinated Veggies Large	8 oz	54	7	2
Salad w/ Marinated Veggies Small	5 oz	32	4	2
Sour Cream Blend	1 oz	27	0	8
Tortilla Corn	2 oz	128	3	0
Tortilla Flour	2 oz	160	1	0
Tortilla Mini Corn	3 oz	160	3	0
Tortilla Whole Wheat	2 oz	160	3	0
Vegetables	4 oz	43	5	8
Vegetarian Burrito	14 oz	601	8	20
Vegetarian Burrito Dinner	24 oz	866	16	20
Vegetarian Plate	15 oz	531	11	0
Vegetarian Tacos	6 oz	295	5	22
Vegetarian Tacos Dinner	16 oz	560	12	22
Veggie Taco Salad Large	17 oz	647	11	20
Veggie Taco Salad Small	10 oz	379	6	10
Yogurt Nonfat	1 oz	15	0	1

MCDONALD'S
BAKED SELECTIONS

FOOD	PORTION	CALS.	FIB.	CHOL.
Apple Pie	1 (3 oz)	260	—	6
Cookies Chocolaty Chip	1 pkg (2 oz)	330	—	4
Cookies McDonaldland	1 pkg (2 oz)	290	—	0
Danish Apple	1	390	—	25
Danish Cinnamon Raisin	1	440	—	34
Danish Iced Cheese	1	390	—	47
Danish Raspberry	1	410	—	26

BEVERAGES

FOOD	PORTION	CALS.	FIB.	CHOL.
Apple Juice	6 oz	90	—	0
Coca-Cola Classic	16 fl oz	145	—	0
Diet Coke	16 fl oz	1	—	0
Grapefruit Juice	6 oz	80	—	0
Milk 1%	8 oz	110	—	10
Milk Shake Lowfat Strawberry	10.4 oz	320	—	10
Milk Shake Lowfat Chocolate	10.4 oz	320	—	10

FOOD	PORTION	CALS.	FIB.	CHOL.
Milk Shake Lowfat Vanilla	10.4 oz	290	—	10
Orange Drink	16 fl oz	130	—	0
Orange Juice	6 oz	80	—	0
Sprite	16 fl oz	145	—	0
BREAKFAST SELECTIONS				
Biscuit w/ Bacon Egg & Cheese	1	440	—	240
Biscuit w/ Sausage	1	420	—	44
Biscuit w/ Sausage & Egg	1	505	—	260
Biscuit w/ Spread	1	260	—	1
Breakfast Burrito	1	280	—	135
Cheerios	¾ cup	80	—	0
Egg McMuffin	1	280	—	235
English Muffin w/ Spread	1	170	—	0
Fat-Free Apple Bran Muffin	1	180	—	0
Hash Brown Potatoes	1 serving	130	—	0
Hotcakes w/ Margarine & Syrup	1 portion	440	—	8
Sausage	1	160	—	43
Sausage McMuffin	1	345	—	57
Sausage McMuffin w/ Egg	1	430	—	270
Scrambled Eggs	1 portion	140	—	425
Wheaties	¾ cup	90	—	0
ICE CREAM				
Cone Lowfat Frozen Yogurt Vanilla	1 (3 oz)	105	—	3
Sundae Lowfat Frozen Yogurt Hot Caramel	1 (6 oz)	270	—	13
Sundae Lowfat Frozen Yogurt Hot Fudge	1 (6 oz)	240	—	6
Sundae Lowfat Frozen Yogurt Strawberry	1 (6 oz)	210	—	5
MAIN MENU SELECTIONS				
Big Mac	1	500	—	100
Cheeseburger	1	305	—	50
Chicken Fajita	1 (2.9 oz)	190	—	35
Chicken McNuggets	4 pieces (2.6 oz)	180	—	35
Chicken McNuggets	6	270	—	55
Chicken McNuggets	9 pieces (5.6 oz)	405	—	85
Filet-O-Fish	1	370	—	50
French Fries	1 lg	400	—	0
French Fries	1 med	320	—	0
French Fries	1 sm	220	—	0
Hamburger	1	255	—	37
McChicken	1	415	—	50
McLean Deluxe	1	320	—	60
McLean Deluxe w/ Cheese	1	370	—	75

FOOD	PORTION	CALS.	FIB.	CHOL.
McNuggets Sauce Barbeque	1.12 fl oz	50	—	0
McNuggets Sauce Honey	0.5 fl oz	45	—	0
McNuggets Sauce Hot Mustard	1.05 fl oz	70	—	5
McNuggets Sauce Sweet 'N Sour	1.12 fl oz	60	—	0
Quarter Pounder	1	410	—	85
Quarter Pounder w/ Cheese	1	510	—	115
SALAD DRESSINGS				
1000 Island	1 pkg	225	—	40
Bleu Cheese	1 pkg	250	—	35
Lite Vinaigrette	1 pkg	48	—	0
Ranch	1 pkg	220	—	20
Red French Reduced Calorie	1 pkg	160	—	0
SALADS AND SALAD BARS				
Bacon Bits	0.1 oz	15	—	1
Chef Salad	1 serving	170	—	111
Chunky Chicken Salad	1 serving	150	—	78
Croutons	0.3 oz	50	—	0
Garden Salad	1	50	—	65
Side Salad	1 serving	30	—	33

NATHAN'S

MAIN MENU SELECTIONS

FOOD	PORTION	CALS.	FIB.	CHOL.
Breaded Chicken Sandwich	1 (7.2 oz)	510	—	56
Charbroiled Chicken Sandwich	1 (4.5 oz)	288	—	53
Cheese Steak Sandwich	1 (6.1 oz)	485	—	73
Chicken 2 Pieces	1 serving (7.1 oz)	693	—	211
Chicken 4 Pieces	1 serving (14.2 oz)	1382	—	422
Chicken Platter 2 Pieces	1 serving (14.8 oz)	1096	—	212
Chicken Platter 4 Pieces	1 serving (21.9 oz)	1788	—	425
Chicken Salad	1 serving (12.7 oz)	154	—	49
Double Burger	1 (7.3 oz)	671	—	154
Filet of Fish Platter	1 serving (22 oz)	1455	—	147
Filet of Fish Sandwich	1 (5.2 oz)	403	—	32
Frank Nuggets	15 pieces (6.9 oz)	764	—	99
Frank Nuggets	11 pieces (5.1 oz)	563	—	73
Frank Nuggets	7 pieces (3.2 oz)	357	—	46
Frankfurter	1 (3.2 oz)	310	—	45
French Fries	1 serving (8.6 oz)	514	—	0
Fried Clam Platter	1 serving (13.1 oz)	1024	—	49
Fried Clam Sandwich	1 (5.4 oz)	620	—	44
Fried Shrimp	1 serving (4.4 oz)	348	—	71
Fried Shrimp Platter	1 serving (12.6 oz)	796	—	83
Hamburger	1 (4.7 oz)	434	—	77
Knish	1 (5.9 oz)	318	—	2

FOOD	PORTION	CALS.	FIB.	CHOL.
Pastrami Sandwich	1 (4.1 oz)	325	—	48
Sauteed Onions	1 serving (3.5 oz)	39	—	0
Super Burger	1 (7.6 oz)	533	—	86
Turkey Sandwich	1 (4.9 oz)	270	—	27
SALADS AND SALAD BARS				
Garden Salad	1 serving (10.9 oz)	193	—	36

OLIVE GARDEN

Baked Lasagna	1 lunch serving	330	—	60
Breadstick	1	70	—	0
Breadstick w/o margarine	1	30	—	0
Breadstick w/o margarine & garlic salt	1	30	—	0
Eggplant Parmigiana	1 lunch serving	220	—	45
Fettuccine Alfredo	1 lunch serving	790	—	160
Garden Salad	1 serving	230	—	4
Minestrone Soup	6 fl oz	45	—	0
Pasta e Fagioli	6 fl oz	140	—	15
Salad Dressing	1 tbsp	60	—	2
Spaghetti w/ Marinara Sauce	1 lunch serving	315	—	tr
Spaghetti w/ Tomato Sauce	1 lunch serving	400	—	75
Veal Marsala	1 dinner serving	330	—	100
Veal Parmigiana	1 dinner serving	590	—	150
Veal Piccata	1 dinner serving	230	—	45
Venetian Grilled Chicken w/o pasta or vegetable	1 dinner serving	320	—	140

PIZZA HUT

Beef Medium Hand Tossed	1 slice	261	—	25
Beef Medium Pan	1 slice	288	3	25
Beef Medium Thin 'N Crispy	1 slice	231	2	25
Cheese Big Foot	1 slice	179	2	14
Cheese Medium Hand Tossed	1 slice	253	2	25
Cheese Medium Pan	1 slice	279	2	25
Cheese Medium Thin 'N Crispy	1 slice	223	2	25
Chunky Combo Hand Tossed	1 slice	280	3	29
Chunky Combo Pan	1 slice	306	3	29
Chunky Combo Thin 'N Crispy	1 slice	250	2	29
Chunky Meat Hand Tossed	1 slice	325	3	40
Chunky Meat Pan	1 slice	352	3	40
Chunky Meat Thin 'N Crispy	1 slice	295	2	40
Chunky Veggie Hand Tossed	1 slice	224	3	17
Chunky Veggie Pan	1 slice	251	3	17
Chunky Veggie Thin 'N Crispy	1 slice	193	3	17
Italian Sausage Medium Hand Tossed	1 slice	313	2	38

FOOD	PORTION	CALS.	FIB.	CHOL.
Italian Sausage Medium Pan	1 slice	399	2	38
Italian Sausage Medium Thin 'N Crispy	1 slice	282	2	38
Meat Lovers Medium Hand Tossed	1 slice	321	3	42
Meat Lovers Medium Pan	1 slice	347	3	42
Meat Lovers Medium Thin 'N Crispy	1 slice	297	2	44
Pepperoni Big Foot	1 slice	195	2	17
Pepperoni Italian Sausage And Mushroom Big Foot	1 slice	213	2	21
Pepperoni Medium Hand Tossed	1 slice	253	2	25
Pepperoni Medium Pan	1 slice	280	2	25
Pepperoni Medium Thin 'N Crispy	1 slice	230	2	27
Pepperoni Personal Pan	1 pie	675	8	53
Pepperoni Lovers Medium Hand Tossed	1 slice	335	3	43
Pepperoni Lovers Medium Pan	1 slice	362	3	34
Pepperoni Lovers Medium Thin 'N Crispy	1 slice	320	3	46
Pork Medium Hand Tossed	1 slice	270	3	25
Pork Medium Pan	1 slice	296	3	25
Pork Medium Thin 'N Crispy	1 slice	240	2	25
Super Supreme Medium Hand Tossed	1 slice	276	3	32
Super Supreme Medium Pan	1 slice	302	3	32
Super Supreme Medium Thin 'N Crispy	1 slice	253	2	35
Supreme Medium Hand Tossed	1 slice	289	3	29
Supreme Medium Pan	1 slice	315	3	29
Supreme Medium Thin 'N Crispy	1 slice	262	3	31
Supreme Personal Pan	1 pie	647	9	53
Veggie Lovers Medium Hand Tossed	1 slice	222	3	17
Veggie Lovers Medium Pan	1 slice	249	3	17
Veggie Lovers Medium Thin 'N Crispy	1 slice	192	3	17

PONDEROSA

BEVERAGES

FOOD	PORTION	CALS.	FIB.	CHOL.
Cherry Coke	6 oz	77	—	0
Chocolate Milk	8 oz	208	—	33
Coca-Cola	6 oz	72	—	0
Coffee Black	6 oz	2	—	0

FOOD	PORTION	CALS.	FIB.	CHOL.
Diet Coke	6 oz	tr	—	0
Diet Coke Caffeine Free	6 oz	tr	—	0
Diet Sprite	6 oz	2	—	0
Dr Pepper	6 oz	72	—	0
Lemonade	6 oz	68	—	0
Milk	8 oz	159	—	34
Mr. Pibb	6 oz	71	—	0
Orange Soda	6 oz	82	—	0
Root Beer	6 oz	80	—	0
Sprite	6 oz	72	—	0
Tea	6 oz	2	—	0
ICE CREAM				
Ice Milk Chocolate	3.5 oz	152	—	22
Ice Milk Vanilla	3.5 oz	150	—	20
Topping Caramel	1 oz	100	—	2
Topping Chocolate	1 oz	89	—	0
Topping Strawberry	1 oz	71	—	0
Topping Whippped	1 oz	80	—	0
MAIN MENU SELECTIONS				
BBQ Sauce	1 tbsp	25	—	0
Bake 'R Broil Fish	1 serving (5.2 oz)	230	—	50
Baked Potato	1 (7.2 oz)	145	—	0
Beans Baked	1 serving (4 oz)	170	—	0
Beans Green	1 serving (3.5 oz)	20	—	0
Breaded Cauliflower	1 serving (4 oz)	115	—	1
Breaded Okra	1 serving (4 oz)	124	—	1
Breaded Onion Rings	1 serving (4 oz)	213	—	2
Breaded Zucchini	1 serving (4 oz)	102	—	1
Carrots	1 serving (3.5 oz)	31	—	0
Cheese Herb Garlic Spread	1 tbsp	100	—	0
Cheese Sauce	2 oz	52	—	4
Chicken Breast	1 serving (5.5 oz)	90	—	54
Chicken Wings	2	213	—	75
Chopped Steak	5.3 oz	296	—	105
Chopped Steak	4 oz	225	—	80
Corn	1 serving (3.5 oz)	90	—	0
Fish Fried	1 serving (3.2 oz)	190	—	15
Fish Nuggets	1	31	—	8
French Fries	1 serving (3 oz)	120	—	3
Gravy Brown	2 oz	25	—	0
Gravy Turkey	2 oz	25	—	0
Hot Dog	1	144	—	27
Italian Breadsticks	1	100	—	0
Kansas City Strip	5 oz	138	—	76

FOOD	PORTION	CALS.	FIB.	CHOL.
Macaroni And Cheese	4 oz	67	—	4
Margarine Liquid	1 tbsp	100	—	0
Mashed Potatoes	1 serving (4 oz)	62	—	20
Meatballs	1	58	—	11
Mini Shrimp	6	47	—	22
New York Strip Choice	10 oz	314	—	50
New York Strip Choice	8 oz	384	—	62
Pasta Shells Plain	2 oz	78	—	0
Peas	1 serving (3.5 oz)	67	—	0
Porterhouse	13 oz	441	—	67
Porterhouse Choice	16 oz	640	—	82
Ribeye	5 oz	219	—	75
Ribeye Choice	6 oz	281	—	60
Rice Pilaf	1 serving (4 oz)	160	—	22
Roll Dinner	1	184	—	0
Roll Sourdough	1	110	—	0
Roughy Broiled	1 serving (5 oz)	139	—	28
Salmon Broiled	1 serving (6 oz)	192	—	60
Sandwich Steak	4 oz	408	—	62
Scrod Baked	1 serving (7 oz)	120	—	65
Shrimp Fried	7 pieces	231	—	105
Sirloin Choice	7 oz	241	—	63
Sirloin Tips Choice	5 oz	473	—	72
Spaghetti Plain	2 oz	78	—	0
Spaghetti Sauce	4 oz	110	—	0
Steak Kabobs Meat Only	3 oz	153	—	67
Stuffing	4 oz	230	—	22
Sweet/Sour Sauce	1 oz	37	—	0
Swordfish Broiled	1 serving (6 oz)	271	—	85
T-Bone	8 oz	176	—	71
T-Bone Choice	10 oz	444	—	80
Teriyaki Steak	5 oz	174	—	64
Tortilla Chips	1 oz	150	—	0
Trout Broiled	1 serving (5 oz)	228	—	110
Winter Mix	1 serving (3.5 oz)	25	—	0
SALAD DRESSINGS				
Blue Cheese	1 oz	130	—	27
Cole Slaw	1 oz	150	—	31
Creamy Italian	1 oz	103	—	0
Cucumber Reduced Calorie	1 oz	69	—	tr
Italian Reduced Calorie	1 oz	31	—	0
Parmesan Pepper	1 oz	150	—	9
Ranch	1 oz	147	—	3
Salad Oil	1 tbsp	120	—	0

FOOD	PORTION	CALS.	FIB.	CHOL.
Sour Cream	1 tbsp	26	—	5
Sweet-N-Tangy	1 oz	122	—	1
Thousand Island	1 oz	113	—	1
SALADS AND SALAD BARS				
Alfalfa Sprouts	1 oz	10	—	0
Apple	1	80	—	0
Apples Canned	4 oz	90	—	0
Applesauce	4 oz	80	—	0
Banana	1	87	—	0
Banana Chips	0.2 oz	25	—	0
Banana Pudding	1 oz	52	—	0
Bean Sprouts	1 oz	10	—	0
Beets Diced	4 oz	55	—	0
Breadsticks Sesame	2	35	—	0
Broccoli	1 oz	9	—	0
Cabbage Green	1 oz	9	—	0
Cabbage Red	1 oz	1	—	0
Cantaloupe	1 wedge	13	—	0
Carrots	1 oz	12	—	0
Cauliflower	1 oz	8	—	0
Celery	1 oz	4	—	0
Cheese Imitation Shredded	1 oz	90	—	5
Cheese Spread	1 oz	98	—	26
Cherry Peppers	2 pieces	7	—	0
Chicken Salad	3.5 oz	212	—	42
Chow Mein Noodles	0.2 oz	25	—	0
Cocktail Sauce	1 oz	34	—	0
Coconut Shredded	0.2 oz	25	—	0
Cottage Cheese	4 oz	120	—	17
Croutons	1 oz	115	—	0
Cucumber	1 oz	4	—	0
Eggs Diced	2 oz	94	—	260
Fruit Cocktail	4 oz	97	—	0
Garbanzo Beans	1 oz	102	—	0
Gelatin Plain	4 oz	71	—	0
Granola	0.2 oz	24	—	0
Grapes	10	34	—	0
Green Onion	1	7	—	0
Green Pepper	1 oz	6	—	0
Ham Diced	2 oz	120	—	76
Honeydew	1 wedge	24	—	0
Lemon	1 wedge	3	—	0
Lettuce	1 oz	5	—	0
Macaroni Salad	3.5 oz	335	—	9

FOOD	PORTION	CALS.	FIB.	CHOL.
Margarine Whipped	1 tbsp	34	—	0
Meal Mates Sesame Crackers	2	45	—	0
Melba Snacks	2	18	—	0
Mousse Chocolate	1 oz	78	—	0
Mousse Strawberry	1 oz	74	—	0
Mushrooms	1 oz	8	—	0
Olives Black	1	4	—	0
Olives Green	1	3	—	0
Onions Red & Yellow	1 oz	11	—	3
Orange	1	45	—	0
Pasta Salad	3.5 oz	269	—	tr
Peaches Canned	4 oz	70	—	0
Peanuts Chopped	0.2 oz	30	—	0
Pears Canned	4 oz	98	—	0
Pickles Dill Spears	0.14 oz	tr	—	0
Pickles Sweet Chips	0.14 oz	4	—	0
Pineapple Tidbits	4 oz	95	—	0
Pineapple Fresh	1 wedge	11	—	0
Potato Salad	3.5 oz	126	—	7
Radishes	1 oz	4	—	0
Ritz	2	40	—	0
Saltine Crackers	2	25	—	0
Spiced Apple Rings	4 oz	100	—	0
Spinach	1 oz	7	—	0
Sunflower Seeds	0.2 oz	31	—	0
Tartar Sauce	1 oz	85	—	9
Tomatoes	1 oz	6	—	0
Turkey Ham Salad	3.5 oz	186	—	12
Turkey Julienne	1 oz	29	—	15
Vanilla Wafer	2	35	—	5
Watermelon	1 wedge	111	—	0
Yogurt Fruit	4 oz	115	—	5
Yogurt Vanilla	4 oz	110	—	6
Zucchini	1 oz	5	—	0

POPEYE

FOOD	PORTION	CALS.	FIB.	CHOL.
Apple Pie	1 serving (3.1 oz)	290	2	10
Biscuit	1 serving (2.3 oz)	250	1	<5
Cajun Rice	1 serving (3.9 oz)	150	3	25
Chicken Breast Mild	1 (3.7 oz)	270	2	60
Chicken Breast Spicy	1 (3.7 oz)	270	2	60
Chicken Leg Mild	1 (1.7 oz)	120	0	40
Chicken Leg Spicy	1 (1.7 oz)	120	0	40
Chicken Thigh Mild	1 (3.1 oz)	300	tr	70

FOOD	PORTION	CALS.	FIB.	CHOL.
Chicken Thigh Spicy	1 (3.1 oz)	300	tr	70
Chicken Wing Mild	1 (1.6 oz)	160	0	40
Chicken Wing Spicy	1 (1.6 oz)	160	0	40
Cole Slaw	1 serving (4 oz)	149	3	3
Corn On The Cob	1 serving (5.2 oz)	90	9	0
French Fries	1 serving (3 oz)	240	3	10
Nuggets	1 serving (4.2 oz)	410	3	55
Onion Rings	1 serving (3.1 oz)	310	2	25
Potatoes & Gravy	1 serving (3.8 fl oz)	100	3	<5
Red Beans & Rice	1 serving (5.9 oz)	270	7	10
Shrimp	1 serving (2.8 oz)	250	3	110

PUDGIE'S FAMOUS CHICKEN

Fried Chicken	3.5 oz	233		81

QUINCY'S FAMILY STEAKHOUSE

Rice Pilaf	1 serving (4 oz)	180	1	0
Stir Fry Beef	1 serving (16 oz)	950	5	130
Stir Fry Chicken	1 serving (16 oz)	790	5	80

RAX
BEVERAGES

Chocolate Shake	1 (11 fl oz)	445	—	35
Coke	16 fl oz	205	—	0
Diet Coke	16 fl oz	1	—	0

DESSERTS

Chocolate Chip Cookie	1 (2 oz)	262	—	6

MAIN MENU SELECTIONS

Bacon	1 slice (0.1 oz)	14	—	2
Baked Potato	1 (10 oz)	264	—	0
Baked Potato w/ 1 Tbsp Margarine	1 (10.5 oz)	364	—	0
Barbecue Sauce	1 pkg (0.4 oz)	11	—	0
Beef Bacon 'N Cheddar	1 (6.7 oz)	523	—	42
Cheddar Cheese Sauce	1 fl oz	29	—	0
Country Fried Chicken Breast Sandwich	1 (7.4 oz)	618	—	45
Deluxe Roast Beef	1 (7.9 oz)	498	—	36
French Fries	1 serving (3.25 oz)	282	—	3
Grilled Chicken Breast Sandwich	1 (6.9 oz)	402	—	69
Grilled Chicken Garden Salad w/ French Dressing	1 serving (12.7 oz)	477	—	32
Grilled Chicken Garden Salad w/ Lite Italian Dressing	1 serving (12.7 oz)	264	—	32
Mushroom Sauce	1 fl oz	16	—	0
Philly Melt	1 (8.2 oz)	396	—	27

FOOD	PORTION	CALS.	FIB.	CHOL.
Regular Rax	1 (4.7 oz)	262	—	15
Swiss Slice	1 slice (0.4 oz)	42	—	10
SALAD DRESSINGS				
French	2 fl oz	275	—	0
Lite Italian	2 fl oz	63	—	0
SALADS AND SALAD BARS				
Gourmet Garden Salad w/ French Dressing	1 serving (10.7 oz)	409	—	10
Gourmet Garden Salad w/ Lite Italian Dressing	1 serving (10.7 oz)	305	—	2
Gourmet Garden Salad w/o Dressing	1 serving (8.7 oz)	134	—	2
Grilled Chicken Garden Salad w/o Dressing	1 serving (10.7 oz)	202	—	32

RED LOBSTER

(All of the following are for a cooked portion unless otherwise noted.)

FOOD	PORTION	CALS.	FIB.	CHOL.
Atlantic Cod	1 lunch serving	100	—	70
Atlantic Ocean Perch	1 lunch serving	130	—	75
Blacktip Shark	1 lunch serving	150	—	60
Calamari, breaded & fried	1 lunch serving	360	—	140
Catfish	1 lunch serving	170	—	85
Chicken Breast Skinless	4 oz	140	—	70
Flounder	1 lunch serving	100	—	70
Grouper	1 lunch serving	110	—	65
Haddock	1 lunch serving	110	—	85
Halibut	1 lunch serving	110	—	60
Hamburger	5 oz	410	—	130
King Crab Legs	1 lb	170	—	100
Langostino	1 lunch serving	120	—	210
Lemon Sole	1 lunch serving	120	—	65
Mackerel	1 lunch serving	190	—	100
Maine Lobster	18 oz	240	—	310
Mako Shark	1 lunch serving	140	—	100
Monkfish	1 lunch serving	110	—	80
Norwegian Salmon	1 lunch serving	230	—	80
Pollack	1 lunch serving	120	—	90
Rainbow Trout	1 lunch serving	170	—	90
Red Rockfish	1 lunch serving	90	—	85
Red Snapper	1 lunch serving	110	—	70
Rib Eye Steak	12 oz	980	—	220
Rock Lobster	1 tail (13 oz)	230	—	200
Sirloin Steak	8 oz	350	—	150

FOOD	PORTION	CALS.	FIB.	CHOL.
Snow Crab Legs	1 lb	150	—	130
Sockeye Salmon	1 lunch serving	160	—	50
Strip Steak	9 oz	560	—	150
Swordfish	1 lunch serving	100	—	100
Tilefish	1 lunch serving	100	—	80
Yellowfin Tuna	1 lunch serving	180	—	70

ROY ROGERS
BEVERAGES
Orange Juice	11 fl oz	140	—	0

BREAKFAST SELECTIONS
3 Pancakes	1 serving (4.8 oz)	280	—	15
3 Pancakes w/ 1 Sausage	1 serving (6.2 oz)	430	—	40
3 Pancakes w/ 2 Bacon	1 serving (5.3 oz)	350	—	25
Bagel Cinnamon Raisin	1 (4 oz)	300	—	0
Bagel Plain	1 (4 oz)	300	—	0
Big Country Platters w/ Bacon	1 serving (7.6 oz)	740	—	305
Big Country Platters w/ Ham	1 serving (9.4 oz)	710	—	330
Big Country Platters w/ Sausage	1 serving (9.6 oz)	920	—	340
Biscuit	1 (2.9 oz)	390	—	0
Biscuit Bacon	1 (3.1 oz)	420	—	5
Biscuit Bacon & Egg	1 (4.2 oz)	470	—	150
Biscuit Cinnamon 'N' Raisin	1 (2.8 oz)	370	—	0
Biscuit Ham & Cheese	1 (4.5 oz)	450	—	25
Biscuit Ham & Egg	1 (5.1 oz)	460	—	165
Biscuit Ham, Egg & Cheese	1 (5.6 oz)	500	—	170
Biscuit Sausage	1 (4.1 oz)	510	—	25
Biscuit Sausage & Egg	1 (5.2 oz)	560	—	170
Hashrounds	1 serving (2.8 oz)	230	—	0
Sourdough Ham, Egg & Cheese	1 (6.8 oz)	480	—	185

DESSERTS
Strawberry Shortcake	1 serving (6.6 oz)	480	—	40

ICE CREAM
Ice Cream Cone	1 (4.1 oz)	180	—	15
Sundae Hot Fudge	1 (6 oz)	320	—	25
Sundae Strawberry	1 (5.5 oz)	260	—	15

MAIN MENU SELECTIONS
¼ Roaster Dark Meat	7.4 oz	490	—	225
¼ Roaster Dark Meat w/ Skin Off	4 oz	190	—	110
¼ Roaster White Meat	8.6 oz	500	—	240
¼ Roaster White Meat w/ Skin Off	4.7 oz	190	—	100
Baked Beans	1 serving (5 oz)	160	—	10
Baked Potato	1 (3.9 oz)	130	—	0
Baked Potato w/ Margarine	1 (4.4 oz)	240	—	0

FOOD	PORTION	CALS.	FIB.	CHOL.
Baked Potato w/ Margarine & Sour Cream	1 (5.4 oz)	300	—	15
Cheeseburger	1 (4.2 oz)	300	—	25
Chicken Fillet Sandwich	1 (8.3 oz)	500	—	20
Cole Slaw	1 serving (5 oz)	295	—	15
Cornbread	1 serving (2.7 oz)	310	—	30
Fisherman's Fillet	1 (6.5 oz)	490	—	15
Fried Chicken Breast	1 (5.2 oz)	370	—	75
Fried Chicken Leg	1 (2.4 oz)	170	—	45
Fried Chicken Thigh	1 (4.2 oz)	330	—	60
Fried Chicken Wing	1 (2.3 oz)	200	—	30
Fry	1 lg (6.1 oz)	430	—	0
Fry	1 reg (5 oz)	350	—	0
Gravy	1 serving (1.5 fl oz)	20	—	0
Grilled Chicken Sandwich	1 (8.3 oz)	340	—	30
Hamburger	1 (3.8 oz)	260	—	20
Mashed Potatoes	1 serving (5 oz)	92	—	0
Nuggets	9 (6.2 oz)	460	—	25
Nuggets	6 (4 oz)	290	—	15
Pizza	1 serving (4.75 oz)	282	1	14
Roast Beef Sandwich	1 (5.7 oz)	260	—	60
Sourdough Grilled Chicken	1 (10.1 oz)	500	—	45
SALADS AND SALAD BARS				
Garden Salad	1 (9.3 oz)	190	—	40
Grilled Chicken Salad	1 serving (9.8 oz)	120	—	60
Side Salad	1 (4.9 oz)	20	—	0

SHAKEY'S

(*see also* DOMINO'S PIZZA, GODFATHER'S, PIZZA, PIZZA HUT)

PIZZA				
Homestyle Crust Cheese	1 slice	303	—	21
Homestyle Crust Onion, Green Pepper, Black Olives, Mushrooms	1 slice	320	—	21
Homestyle Crust Pepperoni	1 slice	343	—	27
Homestyle Crust Sausage, Mushroom	1 slice	343	—	24
Homestyle Crust Sausage, Pepperoni	1 slice	374	—	24
Homestyle Crust Shakey's Special	1 slice	384	—	29
Thick Crust Cheese	1 slice	170	—	13
Thick Crust Green Pepper, Black Olives, Mushrooms	1 slice	162	—	13
Thick Crust Pepperoni	1 slice	185	—	17

FOOD	PORTION	CALS.	FIB.	CHOL.
Thick Crust Sausage, Mushrooms	1 slice	179	—	15
Thick Crust Sausage, Pepperoni	1 slice	177	—	19
Thick Crust Shakey's Special	1 slice	208	—	18
Thin Crust Cheese	1 slice	133	—	14
Thin Crust Onion, Green Pepper, Black Olives, Mushrooms	1 slice	125	—	11
Thin Crust Pepperoni	1 slice	148	—	14
Thin Crust Sausage, Mushroom	1 slice	141	—	13
Thin Crust Sausage, Pepperoni	1 slice	166	—	17
Thin Crust Shakey's Special	1 slice	171	—	16

SHONEY'S
BEVERAGES

FOOD	PORTION	CALS.	FIB.	CHOL.
Clear Soda	1 lg	105	0	0
Clear Soda	1 sm	52	0	0
Coffee Regular & Decaf	1 cup	8	0	0
Cola	1 lg	139	0	0
Cola	1 sm	69	0	0
Creamer	⅜ oz	14	0	0
Hot Chocolate	1 cup	110	0	154
Hot Tea	1 cup	0	0	0
Milk 2%	1 cup	121	0	18
Orange Juice	4 oz	54	0	0
Sugar	1 pkg	13	0	0

BREAKFAST SELECTIONS

FOOD	PORTION	CALS.	FIB.	CHOL.
100% Natural	½ cup	244	2	0
Ambrosia Salad	¼ cup	75	1	0
Apple	1	81	3	0
Apple Butter	1 tbsp	37	0	0
Apple Grape Surprise	¼ cup	19	tr	0
Apple Ring	1	15	0	0
Apple sliced	1 slice	13	1	0
Bacon	1 strip	36	0	5
Biscuit	1	170	1	0
Blueberries	¼ cup	21	1	0
Blueberry Muffin	1	107	1	17
Bread Pudding	1 sq	305	0	80
Breakfast Ham	1 slice	26	0	14
Brunch Cake Apple	1 sq	160	0	0
Brunch Cake Banana	1 sq	152	0	0
Brunch Cake Carrot	1 sq	150	0	0
Brunch Cake Pineapple	1 sq	147	0	0
Brunch Cake Sour Cream	1 sq	160	0	0
Buttered Toast	2 slices	163	1	0

FOOD	PORTION	CALS.	FIB.	CHOL.
Cantaloupe Diced	½ cup	28	tr	0
Cantaloupe Sliced	1 slice	8	tr	0
Captain Crunch Berry	½ cup	73	tr	0
Cheese Sauce	1 ladle	26	0	0
Chocolate Pudding	¼ cup	81	0	7
Cinnamon Honey Bun	1	344	0	0
Cottage Cheese	1 tbsp	12	0	1
Cottage Fries	¼ cup	62	0	0
Country Gravy	¼ cup	82	0	1
Croissant	1	260	0	2
Donut Mini Cinnamon	1 (14 g)	56	0	0
DoughNugget	1	157	0	0
Egg Fried	1	159	0	274
Egg Scrambled	¼ cup	95	0	248
English Muffin w/ margarine	1	140	1	0
Fluff	¼ cup	16	0	0
French Toast	1 slice	69	0	0
Fruit Delight	¼ cup	54	1	0
Fruit Topping All Flavors	1 tbsp	24	tr	0
Glaced Fruit	¼ cup	51	1	0
Golden Pound Cake	1 slice	134	0	13
Grape Jelly	1 tbsp	60	0	0
Grapefruit Canned	¼ cup	24	tr	0
Grapes	25	57	1	0
Grits	¼ cup	57	1	0
Hashbrowns	¼ cup	43	0	0
Home Fries	¼ cup	53	0	0
Honey Bun	1	265	0	3
Honeydew Sliced	1 slice	13	tr	0
Jelly Packet	1	40	0	0
Jr. Bun Chocolate	1	141	0	0
Jr. Bun Honey	1	141	0	0
Jr. Bun Maple	1	141	0	0
Kiwi Sliced	1 slice	11	tr	0
Marble Cake w/ Icing	1 slice	136	0	0
Mixed Fruit	¼ cup	37	tr	0
Mushroom Topping	1 oz	25	tr	0
Oleo Whipped	1 tbsp	70	0	0
Omelette Topping	1 spoonful	23	tr	3
Orange	1 med	65	tr	0
Orange Sections	1 section	7	tr	0
Oriental Salad	¼ cup	79	1	1
Pancake	1	41	0	0
Pear	1	98	4	0

FOOD	PORTION	CALS.	FIB.	CHOL.
Pineapple Bits	1 tbsp	9	0	0
Pineapple Fresh Sliced	1 slice	10	tr	0
Pistachio Pineapple Salad	¼ cup	98	0	3
Prunes	1 tbsp	19	1	0
Raisin Bran	½ cup	87	3	0
Raisin English Muffin w/ Margarine	1	158	0	0
Sausage Link	1	91	0	13
Sausage Patty	1	136	0	2
Sausage Rice	¼ cup	110	tr	8
Shortcake	1	60	0	0
Sirloin Steak Charbroiled	6 oz	357	0	99
Smoked Sausage	1	103	0	13
Snow Salad	¼ cup	72	tr	0
Strawberries	5	23	1	0
Syrup Light	1 ladle	60	0	0
Syrup Low-Cal	2.2 oz	98	0	0
Tangerine	1	37	tr	0
Trix	½ cup	54	tr	0
Waldorf Salad	¼ cup	81	1	2
Watermelon Sliced	1 slice	9	tr	0
Watermelon Diced	½ cup	50	tr	0
Whipped Topping	1 scoop	10	0	0
CHILDREN'S MENU SELECTIONS				
Jr. Burger All-American	1 serving	234	0	30
Kid's Chicken Dinner (fried)	1 serving	244	0	40
Kid's Fish N' Chips (includes fries)	1 serving	337	2	41
Kid's Fried Shrimp	1 serving	194	0	70
Kid's Spaghetti	1 serving	247	1	27
DESSERTS				
Apple Pie A La Mode	1 slice	492	—	35
Carrot Cake	1 slice	500	0	37
Strawberry Pie	1 slice	332	2	0
Walnut Brownie A La Mode	1	576	0	35
ICE CREAM				
Hot Fudge Cake	1 slice	522	0	27
Hot Fudge Sundae	1	451	0	60
Strawberry Sundae	1	380	tr	69
MAIN MENU SELECTIONS				
All-American Burger	1	501	1	86
BBQ Sauce	1 souffle cup	41	0	0
Bacon Burger	1	591	1	86
Baked Fish	1 serving	170	0	83

FOOD	PORTION	CALS.	FIB.	CHOL.
Baked Fish Light	1 serving	170	0	83
Baked Ham Sandwich	1	290	2	42
Baked Potato	10 oz	264	7	0
Beef Patty Light	1 serving	289	0	82
Charbroiled Chicken	1 serving	239	0	85
Charbroiled Chicken Sandwich	1	451	1	90
Chicken Fillet Sandwich	1	464	1	51
Chicken Tenders	1 serving	388	0	64
Cocktail Sauce	1 souffle cup	36	0	0
Country Fried Sandwich	1	588	1	29
Country Fried Steak	1 serving	449	1	27
Fish N' Chips (includes fries)	1 serving	639	3	103
Fish N' Shrimp	1 serving	487	tr	127
Fish Sandwich	1	323	tr	21
French Fries	4 oz	252	4	0
French Fries	3 oz	189	3	0
Fried Fish Light	1 serving	297	tr	65
Grecian Bread	1 slice	80	0	0
Grilled Bacon & Cheese Sandwich	1	440	1	36
Grilled Cheese Sandwich	1	302	1	36
Half O'Pound	1 serving	435	0	123
Ham Club On Whole Wheat	1	642	10	78
Hawaiian Chicken	1 serving	262	tr	85
Italian Feast	1 serving	500	1	74
Lasagna	1 serving	297	3	26
Liver N' Onions	1 serving	411	1	529
Mushroom Swiss Burger	1	616	1	106
Old-Fashioned Burger	1	470	1	82
Onion Rings	1	52	tr	2
Patty Melt	1	640	7	171
Philly Steak Sandwich	1	673	tr	103
Reuben Sandwich	1	596	6	138
Ribeye	6 oz	605	0	141
Rice	3.5 oz	137	tr	1
Sauteed Mushrooms	3 oz	75	1	0
Sauteed Onions	2.5 oz	37	1	0
Seafood Platter	1 serving	566	tr	127
Shoney Burger	1	498	tr	79
Shrimp Charbroiled	1 serving	138	0	162
Shrimp Bite-Size	1 serving	387	0	140
Shrimp Broiled	1 serving	93	0	182
Shrimp Sampler	1 serving	412	tr	217
Shrimper's Feast	1 serving	383	tr	125
Shrimper's Feast Large	1 serving	575	tr	188

FOOD	PORTION	CALS.	FIB.	CHOL.
Sirloin	6 oz	357	0	99
Slim Jim Sandwich	1	484	1	57
Spaghetti	1 serving	496	2	55
Steak N' Shrimp (charbroiled shrimp)	1 serving	361	0	141
Steak N' Shrimp (fried shrimp)	1 serving	507	tr	150
Sweet N' Sour Sauce	1 souffle cup	58	0	0
Tartar Sauce	1 souffle cup	84	0	11
Turkey Club On Whole Wheat	1	635	10	100
SALAD DRESSINGS				
Biscayne Lo-Cal	2 tbsp	62	0	0
Blue Cheese	2 tbsp	113	0	15
Creamy Italian	2 tbsp	135	0	0
French	2 tbsp	124	0	12
Golden Italian	2 tbsp	141	0	0
Honey Mustard	2 tbsp	165	0	18
Ranch	2 tbsp	95	0	15
Rue French	2 tbsp	122	0	0
Thousand Island	2 tbsp	130	0	12
W.W. Italian	2 tbsp	10	0	0
SALADS AND SALAD BARS				
Ambrosia Salad	¼ cup	75	1	0
Apple Grape Surprise	¼ cup	19	tr	0
Apple Ring	1	15	—	0
Beet Onion Salad	¼ cup	25	1	0
Broccoli	¼ cup	4	tr	0
Broccoli Cauliflower Carrot Salad	¼ cup	53	1	1
Broccoli Cauliflower Ranch	¼ cup	65	1	9
Broccoli & Cauliflower	¼ cup	98	1	0
Carrot	¼ cup	10	1	0
Carrot Apple Salad	¼ cup	99	1	8
Cauliflower	¼ cup	8	1	0
Celery	1 tbsp	5	tr	0
Cheese Shredded	1 tbsp	21	0	2
Chocolate Pudding	¼ cup	81	0	7
Chow Mein Noodles	1 spoonful	13	tr	0
Cole Slaw	¼ cup	69	1	7
Cottage Cheese	1 tbsp	12	0	1
Croutons	1 spoonful	13	0	0
Cucumber	1 tbsp	1	tr	0
Cucumber Lite	¼ cup	12	tr	0
Don's Pasta	¼ cup	82	tr	0
Egg Diced	1 tbsp	15	0	54
Fruit Delight	¼ cup	54	1	0

FOOD	PORTION	CALS.	FIB.	CHOL.
Fruit Topping All Flavors	¼ cup	64	tr	0
Glaced Fruit	¼ cup	51	1	0
Granola	1 spoonful	25	—	0
Grapefruit	¼ cup	24	tr	0
Green Pepper	1 tbsp	1	tr	0
Italian Vegetable	¼ cup	11	1	0
Jello	¼ cup	40	0	0
Jello Fluff	¼ cup	16	0	0
Kidney Bean Salad	¼ cup	55	2	2
Lettuce	1.8 oz	7	tr	0
Macaroni Salad	¼ cup	207	tr	14
Margarine Whipped	1 tsp	23	0	0
Melba Toast	2	20	0	0
Mixed Fruit Salad	¼ cup	37	tr	0
Mixed Squash	¼ cup	49	tr	0
Mushrooms	1 tbsp	1	tr	0
Oil	1 tsp	45	0	0
Olives Black	2	10	0	0
Olives Green	2	8	0	0
Onion Sliced	1 tbsp	1	tr	0
Oriental Salad	¼ cup	79	1	1
Pea Salad	¼ cup	73	2	42
Pickle Chips	1 slice	5	tr	0
Pickle Spear	1 spear	2	0	0
Pineapple Bits	1 tbsp	9	—	0
Pistachio Pineapple Salad	¼ cup	98	0	0
Prunes	1 tbsp	19	1	0
Radish	1 tbsp	1	tr	0
Raisins	1 spoonful	26	1	0
Rotelli Pasta	¼ cup	78	tr	0
Seign Salad	¼ cup	72	1	5
Snow Delight	¼ cup	72	tr	0
Spaghetti Salad	¼ cup	81	tr	0
Spinach	¼ cup	1	tr	0
Spring Pasta	¼ cup	38	1	0
Summer Salad	¼ cup	114	1	0
Sunflower Seeds	1 spoonful	40	0	0
Three Bean Salad	¼ cup	96	1	0
Trail Mix	1 spoonful	30	tr	0
Turkey Ham	1 tbsp	12	0	1
Waldorf	¼ cup	81	1	2
Wheat Bread	1 slice	71	1	0
SOUPS				
Bean	6 fl oz	63	1	4

FOOD	PORTION	CALS.	FIB.	CHOL.
Beef Cabbage	6 fl oz	86	2	13
Broccoli Cauliflower	6 fl oz	124	1	12
Cheese Florentine Ham	6 fl oz	110	1	11
Chicken Noodle	6 fl oz	62	—	14
Chicken Rice	6 fl oz	72	1	6
Clam Chowder	6 fl oz	94	0	0
Cream Of Broccoli	6 fl oz	75	tr	1
Cream Of Chicken	6 fl oz	136	tr	11
Onion	6 fl oz	29	tr	1
Potato	6 fl oz	102	2	0
Tomato Florentine	6 fl oz	63	0	0
Tomato Vegetable	6 fl oz	46	tr	0
Vegetable Beef	6 fl oz	82	tr	5

SKIPPER'S
BEVERAGES

Coke Classic	1 (12 fl oz)	144	—	0
Coke Diet	1 (12 fl oz)	2	—	0
Milk Lowfat	1 (12 fl oz)	181	—	0
Root Beer	1 (12 fl oz)	154	—	0
Root Beer Float	1 (12 oz)	302	—	10
Sprite	1 (12 fl oz)	142	—	0

DESSERTS

Jell-O	1 serving (2.75 oz)	55	—	0

MAIN MENU SELECTIONS

Baked Fish With Margarine & Seas	1 serving (4.4 oz)	147	—	85
Baked Potato	1 (6 oz)	145	—	0
Captain's Cut	1 piece (2.6 oz)	160	—	29
Cocktail Sauce	1 tbsp	20	—	0
Coleslaw	1 serving (5 oz)	289	—	50
Corn Muffin	1 (2 oz)	91	—	16
French Fries	1 serving (3.5 oz)	239	—	3
Green Salad (no dressing)	1 serving (4 oz)	24	—	0
Ketchup	1 tbsp	17	—	0
Margarine	1 serving (0.5 oz)	50	—	0
Shrimp Fried Cajun	1 serving (4 oz)	342	—	64
Shrimp Fried Jumbo	1 piece (.65 oz)	51	—	9
Shrimp Fried Original	1 serving (4 oz)	266	—	54
Tartar Original	1 tbsp	65	—	4

SOUPS

Clam Chowder	1 pint (12 fl oz)	200	—	24
Clam Chowder	1 cup (6 fl oz)	100	—	12

SONIC DRIVE-IN

#1 Hamburger	1 (6.6 oz)	409	—	58

FOOD	PORTION	CALS.	FIB.	CHOL.
#2 Hamburger	1 (6.6 oz)	323	—	50
B-L-T Sandwich	1 (6.1 oz)	327	—	9
Bacon Cheeseburger	1 (7.2 oz)	548	—	87
Chicken Sandwich Breaded	1 (7.4 oz)	455	—	42
Chili Pie	1 (3.7 oz)	327	—	28
Corn Dog	1 (3 oz)	280	—	35
Extra Long Cheese Coney w/ Onions	1 (9.4 oz)	640	—	65
Extra-Long Cheese Coney	1 (8.9 oz)	635	—	65
Fish Sandwich	1 (6.1 oz)	277	—	6
French Fries	1 lg (6.7 oz)	315	—	11
French Fries	1 reg (5 oz)	233	—	8
French Fries w/ Cheese	1 lg (7.7 oz)	219	—	38
Grilled Cheese Sandwich	1 (2.8 oz)	288	—	36
Grilled Chicken Sandwich w/o Dressing	1 (6.4 oz)	215	—	4
Hickory Burger	1 (5.1 oz)	314	—	50
Jalapeno Burger Double Meat & Cheese	1 (9.1 oz)	638	—	136
Mini Cheeseburger	1 (3.9 oz)	281	—	45
Mini Burger	1 (3.5 oz)	246	—	36
Regular Cheese Coney	1 (5 oz)	358	—	40
Regular Cheese Coney w/ Onions	1 (5.3 oz)	361	—	40
Regular Hot Dog	1 (3.5 oz)	258	—	23
Steak Sandwich Breaded	1 (3.9 oz)	631	—	50
Super Sonic Burger w/ Mustard Double Meat & Cheese	1 (10.1 oz)	644	—	136
Super Sonic Burger w/ Mayo Double Meat & Cheese	1 (10.1 oz)	730	—	144
Tater Tots	1 serving (3 oz)	150	—	10
Tater Tots w/ Cheese	1 serving (3.6 oz)	220	—	28

STARBUCKS

FOOD	PORTION	CALS.	FIB.	CHOL.
Americano Grande	1 serv	10	—	0
Americano Short	1 serv	5	—	0
Americano Tall	1 serv	5	—	0
Cappuccino Grande Lowfat Milk	1 serv	110	—	15
Cappuccino Grande Nonfat Milk	1 serv	80	—	5
Cappuccino Grande Whole Milk	1 serv	140	—	30
Cappuccino Short Lowfat Milk	1 serv	60	—	10
Cappuccino Short Nonfat Milk	1 serv	40	—	0
Cappuccino Short Whole Milk	1 serv	70	—	15
Cappuccino Tall Lowfat Milk	1 serv	80	—	15
Cappuccino Tall Nonfat Milk	1 serv	60	—	5

FOOD	PORTION	CALS.	FIB.	CHOL.
Cappuccino Tall Whole Milk	1 serv	110	—	25
Cocoa w/ Whipping Cream Grande Lowfat Milk	1 serv	350	—	70
Cocoa w/ Whipping Cream Grande Whole Milk	1 serv	400	—	90
Cocoa w/ Whipping Cream Grande Nonfat Milk	1 serv	310	—	50
Cocoa w/ Whipping Cream Short Nonfat Milk	1 serv	160	—	30
Cocoa w/ Whipping Cream Short Lowfat Milk	1 serv	180	—	40
Cocoa w/ Whipping Cream Short Whole Milk	1 serv	210	—	45
Cocoa w/ Whipping Cream Tall Whole Milk	1 serv	300	—	70
Cocoa w/ Whipping Cream Tall Nonfat Milk	1 serv	230	—	35
Cocoa w/ Whipping Cream Tall Lowfat Milk	1 serv	270	—	55
Drip Coffee Grande	1 serv	10	—	0
Drip Coffee Short	1 serv	5	—	0
Drip Coffee Tall	1 serv	10	—	0
Espresso Doppio	1 serv	5	—	0
Espresso Macchiato Doppio Lowfat Milk	1 serv	15	—	0
Espresso Macchiato Doppio Nonfat Milk	1 serv	15	—	0
Espresso Macchiato Doppio Whole Milk	1 serv	15	—	0
Espresso Macchiato Solo Lowfat Milk	1 serv	10	—	0
Espresso Macchiato Solo Nonfat Milk	1 serv	10	—	0
Espresso Macchiato Solo Whole Milk	1 serv	15	—	0
Espresso Solo	1 serv	5	—	0
Espresso Con Panna Doppio	1 serv	45	—	15
Espresso Con Panna Solo	1 serv	40	—	15
Latte Grande Lowfat Milk	1 serv	170	—	25
Latte Grande Nonfat Milk	1 serv	130	—	5
Latte Grande Whole Milk	1 serv	220	—	45
Latte Short Lowfat Milk	1 serv	80	—	10
Latte Short Nonfat Milk	1 serv	60	—	5
Latte Short Whole Milk	1 serv	100	—	20

FOOD	PORTION	CALS.	FIB.	CHOL.
Latte Tall Lowfat Milk	1 serv	140	—	20
Latte Tall Nonfat Milk	1 serv	110	—	5
Latte Tall Whole Milk	1 serv	180	—	40
Latte Iced Grande Lowfat Milk	1 serv	170	—	25
Latte Iced Grande Nonfat Milk	1 serv	130	—	5
Latte Iced Grande Whole Milk	1 serv	210	—	45
Latte Iced Short Lowfat Milk	1 serv	90	—	15
Latte Iced Short Nonfat Milk	1 serv	70	—	5
Latte Iced Short Whole Milk	1 serv	120	—	25
Latte Iced Tall Lowfat Milk	1 serv	120	—	20
Latte Iced Tall Nonfat Milk	1 serv	90	—	5
Latte Iced Tall Whole Milk	1 serv	150	—	35
Mocha w/ Whipping Cream Grande Nonfat Milk	1 serv	310	—	50
Mocha w/ Whipping Cream Grande Lowfat Milk	1 serv	350	—	70
Mocha w/ Whipping Cream Grande Whole Milk	1 serv	390	—	85
Mocha w/ Whipping Cream Short Nonfat Milk	1 serv	150	—	30
Mocha w/ Whipping Cream Short Lowfat Milk	1 serv	170	—	35
Mocha w/ Whipping Cream Short Whole Milk	1 serv	180	—	45
Mocha w/ Whipping Cream Tall Nonfat Milk	1 serv	230	—	35
Mocha w/ Whipping Cream Tall Whole Milk	1 serv	290	—	65
Mocha w/ Whipping Cream Tall Lowfat Milk	1 serv	260	—	50
Mocha w/o Whipping Cream Grande Lowfat Milk	1 serv	230	—	20
Mocha w/o Whipping Cream Grande Nonfat Milk	1 serv	190	—	5
Mocha w/o Whipping Cream Grande Whole Milk	1 serv	260	—	40
Mocha w/o Whipping Cream Short Whole Milk	1 serv	150	—	25
Mocha w/o Whipping Cream Short Lowfat Milk	1 serv	120	—	15
Mocha w/o Whipping Cream Short Nonfat Milk	1 serv	100	—	5
Mocha w/o Whipping Cream Tall Whole Milk	1 serv	190	—	30

FOOD	PORTION	CALS.	FIB.	CHOL.
Mocha w/o Whipping Cream Tall Nonfat Milk	1 serv	140	—	5
Mocha w/o Whipping Cream Tall Lowfat Milk	1 serv	170	—	15
Mocha Syrup Grande	1 serv (2 oz)	80	—	0
Mocha Syrup Short	1 serv (1 oz)	40	—	0
Mocha Syrup Tall	1 serv (1.5 oz)	60	—	0
Steamed Lowfat Milk Grande	1 serv	180	—	30
Steamed Lowfat Milk Short	1 serv	90	—	15
Steamed Lowfat Milk Tall	1 serv	140	—	20
Steamed Nonfat Milk Grande	1 serv	130	—	5
Steamed Nonfat Milk Short	1 serv	60	—	5
Steamed Nonfat Milk Tall	1 serv	100	—	5
Steamed Whole Milk Grande	1 serv	230	—	50
Steamed Whole Milk Short	1 serv	110	—	25
Steamed Whole Milk Tall	1 serv	180	—	40
Whipping Cream Grande	1 serv (1.1 oz)	110	—	45
Whipping Cream Short	1 serv (0.7 oz)	70	—	25
Whipping Cream Tall	1 serv (0.8 oz)	80	—	35

SUBWAY

FOOD	PORTION	CALS.	FIB.	CHOL.
Ham Sandwich Round	1 (4 in)	317	—	13
Roast Beef Sandwich Round	1 (4 in)	326	—	17
Roast Turkey Breast Salad	1 serving	154	—	31
Roast Turkey Breast Sub White Bread	1 (6 in)	312	—	31
Subway Club Salad	1 serving	165	—	38
Veggies & Cheese Sub Wheat Bread	1 (6 in)	258	—	10

T.J. CINNAMONS

FOOD	PORTION	CALS.	FIB.	CHOL.
Doughnuts Cake	2	454	tr	98
Doughnuts Raised	2	352	tr	98
Mini-Cinn Plain	1	75	tr	3
Mini-Cinn With Icing	1	80	tr	3
Original Gourmet Cinnamon Roll Plain	1	630	1	38
Original Gourmet Cinnamon Roll With Icing	1	686	1	38
Petite Cinnamon Roll Plain	1	185	tr	11
Petite Cinnamon Roll With Icing	1	202	tr	11
Sticky Bun Cinnamon Pecan	1	607	tr	29
Sticky Bun Petite Cinnamon Pecan	1	255	tr	11
Triple Chocolate Classic Roll Plain	1	412	tr	28
Triple Chocolate Classic Roll With Icing	1	462	tr	28

FOOD	PORTION	CALS.	FIB.	CHOL.
TCBY				
Nonfat All Flavors	1 super (15.2 fl oz)	418	—	<5
Nonfat All Flavors	1 giant (31.6 fl oz)	869	—	<5
Nonfat All Flavors	1 lg (10.5 fl oz)	289	—	<5
Nonfat All Flavors	1 reg (8.2 fl oz)	226	—	<5
Nonfat All Flavors	1 sm (5.9 fl oz)	162	—	<5
Nonfat All Flavors	1 kiddie (3.2 fl oz)	88	—	<5
Regular All Flavors	1 super (15.2 fl oz)	494	—	38
Regular All Flavors	1 lg (10.5 fl oz)	341	—	26
Regular All Flavors	1 sm (5.9 fl oz)	192	—	15
Regular All Flavors	1 giant (31.6 fl oz)	1027	—	79
Regular All Flavors	1 kiddie (3.2 fl oz)	104	—	8
Sugar Free All Flavors	1 super (15.2 fl oz)	304	—	<5
Sugar Free All Flavors	1 giant (31.6 fl oz)	632	—	<5
Sugar Free All Flavors	1 sm (5.9 fl oz)	118	—	<5
Sugar Free All Flavors	1 reg (8.2 fl oz)	164	—	<5
Sugar Free All Flavors	1 lg (10.5 fl oz)	210	—	<5
Sugar Free All Flavors	1 kiddie (3.2 fl oz)	64	—	<5
TGI FRIDAY'S				
Charbroiled Chicken Sandwich	1 (7.58 oz)	320	—	35
Garden Burger	1 (7.58 oz)	410	—	10
Herb Grilled Chicken	1 (17.72 oz)	550	—	110
Manicotti	1 serving (15.44 oz)	680	—	160
P&E Shrimp	1 serving (4.38 oz)	120	—	200
P.C. Tuna	1 (16.33 oz)	280	—	25
Pea Salsa	1 (6.35 oz)	170	—	0
Spinach Salad	1 (8.67 oz)	240	—	205
Turkey Burger	1 (9.81 oz)	410	—	95
Vegetable Bagette	1 (16.1 oz)	440	—	tr
Vegetable Medley	1 serving (13.8 oz)	140	—	5
TACO BELL				
Burrito Bean	1	381	3	9
Burrito Beef	1	431	2	57
Burrito Chicken	1	334	—	52
Burrito Combo	1	407	3	33
Burrito Supreme	1	440	3	33
Chilito	1	383	2	47
Cinnamon Twists	1 serving	171	1	0
Green Sauce	1 oz	4	tr	0
Guacamole	0.6 oz	34	5	0
Jalapeno Peppers	3.5 oz	20	tr	0
MexiMelt Beef	1	266	2	38

FOOD	PORTION	CALS.	FIB.	CHOL.
MexiMelt Chicken	1	257	2	48
Mexican Pizza	1	575	3	52
Nacho Cheese Sauce	2 oz	103	tr	9
Nachos	1 serving	346	1	9
Nachos Bellgrande	1	649	4	36
Nachos Supreme Bell	1	367	2	18
Pico De Gallo	1 oz	6	tr	1
Pintos 'N Cheese	1	190	2	16
Ranch Dressing	2.5 oz	236	tr	35
Red Sauce	1 oz	10	tr	0
Salsa	0.3 oz	18	4	0
Sour Cream	0.66 oz	46	tr	0
Taco	1	183	1	32
Taco Salad	1	905	4	80
Taco Salad w/o Shell	1	484	3	80
Taco Sauce	1 pkg	2	tr	0
Taco Sauce Hot	1 pkg	3	tr	0
Taco Soft	1	225	2	32
Taco Soft Chicken	1	213	2	52
Taco Soft Supreme	1	272	2	32
Taco Supreme	1	230	1	32
Tostada	1	243	2	16

TACO JOHN'S
CHILDREN'S MENU SELECTIONS

Kid's Meal Softshell Taco	1 serv (8.5 oz)	623	—	32
Kid's Meal Taco Burger	1 serv (8.75 oz)	668	—	35
Kids's Meal Crispy Taco	1 serv (8 oz)	575	—	31

DESSERTS

Choco Taco	1 serv (3.5 oz)	320	—	20
Churro	1 serv (1.5 oz)	147	—	4
Flauta Apple	1 serv (2 oz)	84	—	0
Flauta Cherry	1 serv (2 oz)	143	—	0
Flauta Cream Cheese	1 serv (2 oz)	181	—	10

MAIN MENU SELECTIONS

Bean Burrito	1 (6 oz)	340	—	15
Beans Refried	1 serv (9.25 oz)	301	—	8
Beef Burrito	1 (6 oz)	415	—	43
Chicken Fajita Burrito	1 (8 oz)	360	—	49
Chicken Fajita Salad w/o dressing	1 serv (12.25 oz)	561	—	55
Chicken Fajita Softshell	1 (4.25 oz)	216	—	33
Chili Texas Style w/ 2 Saltines	1 serv (9.25 oz)	297	—	47
Chimichanga Platter	1 serv (18.5 oz)	922	—	50
Combination Burrito	1 (6 oz)	378	—	30

FOOD	PORTION	CALS.	FIB.	CHOL.
Crispy Tacos	1 serv (3 oz)	178	—	22
Double Enchilada Platter	1 serv (18.5 oz)	901	—	73
Mexi Rolls w/ Guacamole	1 serv (9.75 oz)	839	—	46
Mexi Rolls w/ Nacho Cheese	1 serv (9.75 oz)	813	—	46
Mexi Rolls w/ Salsa	1 serv	754	—	46
Mexi Rolls w/ Sour Cream	1 serv	854	—	46
Mexican Pizza	1 (9.75 oz)	636	—	55
Mexican Rice	1 serv (8 oz)	567	—	0
Nachos	1 serv (3.5 oz)	294	—	6
Potato Oles w/ Nacho Cheese	1 serv (7.55 oz)	523	—	6
Salad Dressing House	1 serv (2 oz)	114	—	tr
Sample Platter	1 serv (25 oz)	1276	—	97
Sierra Chicken Fillet Sandwich	1 (8.5 oz)	500	—	41
Smothered Burrito Platter	1 serv (19 oz)	972	—	61
Super Burrito	1 (8.5 oz)	424	—	35

UNO RESTAURANT

FOOD	PORTION	CALS.	FIB.	CHOL.
DeepDish Pizza	1 serving	770	6	45

VILLAGE INN

FOOD	PORTION	CALS.	FIB.	CHOL.
French Toast Cinnamon Raisin	1 serving	809	—	9
Fruit & Nut Pancakes Low Cholesterol	1 serving	936	—	2
Omelette Chicken & Cheese	1 serving	721	—	120
Omelette Fresh Veggie	1 serving	704	—	102
Omelette Mushroom & Cheese	1 serving	680	—	102
Turkey & Vegetable Scrambled Sensation	1 serving	726	—	124

WENDY'S
BEVERAGES

FOOD	PORTION	CALS.	FIB.	CHOL.
Coffee Decaffeinated Black	1 cup (6 fl oz)	0	0	0
Coffee Black	1 cup (6 fl oz)	0	0	0
Cola	1 sm (8 fl oz)	90	0	0
Diet Cola	1 sm (8 fl oz)	0	0	0
Hot Chocolate	1 cup (6 fl oz)	92	2	0
Lemon-Lime	1 sm (8 fl oz)	90	0	0
Lemonade	1 sm (8 fl oz)	90	0	0
Milk 2%	1 (8 fl oz)	110	0	15
Tea Hot	1 cup (6 fl oz)	0	0	0
Tea Iced	1 cup (6 fl oz)	0	0	0

CHILDREN'S MENU SELECTIONS

FOOD	PORTION	CALS.	FIB.	CHOL.
Kid's Meal Cheeseburger	1 (4.3 oz)	310	2	45
Kid's Meal Hamburger	1 (3.9 oz)	270	2	35

DESSERTS

FOOD	PORTION	CALS.	FIB.	CHOL.
Chocolate Chip Cookie	1 (2.2 oz)	280	1	15

FOOD	PORTION	CALS.	FIB.	CHOL.
Frosty Dairy Dessert	1 sm (12 fl oz)	340	3	40
Frosty Dairy Dessert	1 med (16 fl oz)	460	4	55
Frosty Dairy Dessert	1 lg (20 fl oz)	570	5	70
MAIN MENU SELECTIONS				
¼ lb Hamburger Patty, no bun	1 (2.3 oz)	190	0	70
American Cheese	1 slice (0.6 oz)	70	0	15
American Cheese Jr.	1 slice (0.4 oz)	45	0	10
Bacon	1 strip (0.2 oz)	30	0	5
Baked Potato	1 sm (8 oz)	190	5	40
Baked Potato	1 lg (12 oz)	290	7	60
Baked Potato Bacon & Cheese	1 (13.3 oz)	530	7	20
Baked Potato Broccoli & Cheese	1 (14.4 oz)	460	9	0
Baked Potato Cheese	1 (13.4 oz)	560	7	30
Baked Potato Chili & Cheese	1 (4.8 oz)	610	9	45
Baked Potato Plain	1 (10 oz)	310	7	0
Baked Potato Sour Cream & Chives	1 (11 oz)	380	8	15
Big Bacon Classic	1 (10.1 oz)	640	3	110
Breaded Chicken Fillet, no bun	1 (3.5 oz)	220	0	55
Breaded Chicken Sandwich	1 (7.3 oz)	450	2	60
Cheddar Cheese Shredded	2 tbsp (0.6 oz)	70	0	15
Chicken Club Sandwich	1 (7.7 oz)	520	2	75
Chicken Nuggets	6 pieces (3.3 oz)	280	0	50
French Fries	1 Biggie (6 oz)	450	6	0
French Fries	1 med (4.8 oz)	360	4	0
French Fries	1 sm (3.2 oz)	240	3	0
Grilled Chicken Breast, no bun	1 (2.5 oz)	100	0	50
Grilled Chicken Sandwich	1 (6.2 oz)	290	2	55
Honey Mustard Reduced Calorie	1 tsp (0.2 oz)	25	0	0
Jr. Bacon Cheeseburger	1 (6 oz)	440	2	65
Jr. Cheeseburger	1 (4.5 oz)	320	2	45
Jr. Cheeseburger Deluxe	1 (6.3 oz)	390	3	50
Jr. Hamburger	1 (4.1 oz)	270	2	35
Jr. Hamburger Patty, no bun	1 (1.3 oz)	90	0	35
Kaiser Bun	1 (2.4 oz)	190	2	0
Ketchup	1 tsp (0.2 fl oz)	10	0	0
Lettuce	1 leaf (0.5 oz)	0	0	0
Mayonnaise	1½ tsp (0.3 oz)	70	0	5
Mustard	½ tsp (0.2 oz)	5	0	0
Nuggets Sauce Barbeque	1 pkg (1 oz)	50	—	0
Nuggets Sauce Honey	1 pkg (0.5 oz)	45	0	0
Nuggets Sauce Sweet & Sour	1 pkg (1 oz)	45	—	0
Nuggets Sauce Sweet Mustard	1 pkg (1 oz)	50	—	0
Onion	4 rings (0.5 oz)	0	0	0

FOOD	PORTION	CALS.	FIB.	CHOL.
Pickles	4 slices (0.4 oz)	0	0	0
Plain Single	1 (4.7 oz)	350	2	70
Saltines	2 (0.2 oz)	25	0	0
Sandwich Bun	1 (2 oz)	160	2	0
Single With Everything	1 (7.7 oz)	440	3	75
Sour Cream	1 pkt (1 oz)	60	0	10
Tomatoes	1 slice (0.9 oz)	5	0	0
Whipped Margarine	1 pkg (0.5 oz)	60	0	0
SALAD DRESSINGS				
Blue Cheese	2 tbsp (1 fl oz)	180	0	15
Blue Cheese Reduced Calorie Reduced Fat	2 tbsp (1 fl oz)	70	0	15
Celery Seed	2 tbsp (1 fl oz)	60	0	10
French	2 tbsp (1 fl oz)	120	0	0
French Fat Free	2 tbsp (1 fl oz)	35	0	0
French Sweet Red	2 tbsp (1 fl oz)	130	0	0
Hidden Valley Ranch	2 tbsp (1 fl oz)	90	0	10
Italian Caesar	2 tbsp (1 fl oz)	150	0	15
Italian Golden	2 tbsp (1 fl oz)	90	0	0
Italian Reduced Calorie Reduced Fat	2 tbsp (1 fl oz)	40	0	0
Salad Oil	1 tbsp (0.5 fl oz)	130	0	0
Thousand Island	2 tbsp (1 fl oz)	130	0	10
Wine Vinegar	1 tbsp (0.5 fl oz)	0	0	0
SALADS AND SALAD BARS				
Alfredo Sauce	¼ cup (1.4 oz)	30	0	0
Applesauce Chunky	2 tbsp (1.4 oz)	30	0	0
Bacon Bits	2 tbsp (0.5 oz)	40	0	5
Breadstick Sesame	1 (3 g)	15	0	0
Broccoli	¼ cup (0.5 oz)	0	0	0
Cantaloupe	1 piece (1.6 oz)	15	0	0
Carrots	¼ cup (0.6 oz)	5	0	0
Cauliflower	¼ cup (0.6 g)	0	0	0
Ceasar Side Salad	1 (3.1 oz)	110	2	15
Cheddar Chips	2 tbsp (0.4 oz)	70	0	0
Cheese Sauce	1.4 cup (1.2 oz)	25	—	0
Cheese Shredded Imitation	2 tbsp (0.6 oz)	50	0	0
Chicken Salad	2 tbsp (1.2 oz)	70	0	0
Chives	1 tbsp (1 g)	0	0	0
Chow Mein Noodles	¼ cup (0.2 oz)	35	0	0
Cole Slaw	2 tbsp (1.3 oz)	45	1	5
Cottage Cheese	2 tbsp (1.1 oz)	30	0	5
Croutons	2 tbsp (0.2 oz)	30	0	0
Cucumbers	2 slices (0.5 oz)	0	0	0

FOOD	PORTION	CALS.	FIB.	CHOL.
Deluxe Garden Salad	1 (9.5 oz)	110	4	0
Eggs hard cooked	2 tbsp (0.9 oz)	40	0	110
Green Peas	2 tbsp (0.7 oz)	15	1	0
Green Peppers	2 pieces (0.3 oz)	8	0	0
Grilled Chicken Salad	1 (11.9 oz)	200	4	50
Honeydew Melon	1 piece (1.8 oz)	20	0	0
Jalapeno Peppers	1 tbsp (0.4 oz)	8	0	0
Lettuce Iceberg/Romaine	1 cup (2.6 oz)	10	1	0
Macaroni & Cheese	½ cup (3.2 oz)	130	0	5
Mushrooms	¼ cup (0.5 oz)	0	0	0
Olives Black	2 tbsp (0.5 oz)	15	0	0
Orange Sections	1 piece (1.1 oz)	10	1	0
Parmesan Cheese	2 tbsp (0.5 oz)	70	0	15
Pasta Salad	2 tbsp (1.2 oz)	35	1	0
Peaches Sliced	1 piece (1 oz)	15	0	0
Pepperoni Sliced	6 slices (0.2 oz)	30	0	5
Picante Sauce	2 tbsp (1 oz)	10	0	0
Pineapple Chunks	4 pieces (1.1 oz)	20	0	0
Potato Salad	2 tbsp (1.3 oz)	80	0	5
Pudding Chocolate	¼ cup (1.8 oz)	70	0	0
Pudding Vanilla	¼ cup (1.8 oz)	70	0	0
Red Onions	3 rings (0.5 oz)	0	0	0
Red Peppers Crushed	1 tbsp (0.2 oz)	15	1	0
Refried Beans	¼ cup (1.9 oz)	80	5	0
Rotini	½ cup (1.9 oz)	90	1	0
Seafood Salad	¼ cup (1.3 oz)	70	0	0
Side Salad	1 (5.4 oz)	60	2	0
Soft Breadstick	1 (1.5 oz)	130	1	5
Sour Topping	2 tbsp (1 oz)	60	0	0
Spaghetti Meat Sauce	¼ cup (1.4 oz)	45	1	5
Spaghetti Sauce	1.4 cup (1.5 oz)	30	0	0
Spanish Rice	¼ cup (1.8 oz)	60	1	0
Strawberries	1 (0.9 oz)	10	1	0
Strawberry Banana Dessert	¼ cup (1.6 oz)	30	1	0
Sunflower Seeds & Raisins	2 tbsp (0.5 oz)	80	1	0
Taco Chips	8 (0.9 oz)	120	2	0
Taco Meat	2 tbsp (1.3 oz)	80	—	15
Taco Salad	1 (17.9 oz)	580	11	75
Taco Sauce	2 tbsp (0.8 oz)	10	0	0
Taco Shell	1 (0.4 oz)	60	1	0
Tomatoes Wedged	1 piece (0.9 oz)	5	0	0
Tortilla Flour	1 (1.2 oz)	110	1	0
Turkey Ham Diced	2 tbsp (0.8 oz)	50	0	25
Watermelon	1 piece (2.2 oz)	20	0	0

FOOD	PORTION	CALS.	FIB.	CHOL.
WHATABURGER				
BAKED SELECTIONS				
Apple Turnover	1	215	—	0
Blueberry Muffin	1	239	—	0
Buttermilk Biscuit	1	280	—	3
Cookie Chocolate Chunk	1	247	—	28
Cookie Macadamia Nut	1	269	—	34
Cookie Oatmeal Raisin	1	222	—	28
Cookie Peanut Butter	1	262	—	39
Pecan Danish	1	270	—	11
BEVERAGES				
Coffee	1 sm	5	—	0
Coke Cherry	16 fl oz	151	—	0
Coke Classic	16 fl oz	141	—	0
Creamer	1 pkg	10	—	0
Diet Coke	16 fl oz	1	—	0
Dr Pepper	16 fl oz	138	—	0
Iced Tea	16 fl oz	3	—	0
Lemon Juice	1 pkg	1	—	0
Milk 2%	1 serving	113	—	18
Orange Juice	1 serving	77	—	0
Root Beer	16 fl oz	158	—	0
Shake Chocolate	1 (12 fl oz)	364	—	36
Shake Strawberry	1 (12 fl oz)	352	—	35
Shake Vanilla	1 (12 fl oz)	325	—	37
Sprite	16 fl oz	141	—	0
Sugar	1 pkg	15	—	0
Sweet And Low	1 pkg	4	—	0
BREAKFAST SELECTIONS				
Biscuit With Bacon	1	359	—	15
Biscuit With Egg And Cheese	1	434	—	202
Biscuit With Egg, Cheese And Bacon	1	511	—	213
Biscuit With Egg, Cheese And Sausage	1	601	—	236
Biscuit With Gravy	1	479	—	20
Biscuit With Sausage	1	446	—	37
Breakfast Platter With Bacon	1 serving	695	—	389
Breakfast Platter With Sausage	1 serving	785	—	412
Breakfast On A Bun	1	455	—	232
Breakfast On A Bun Bacon	1	365	—	210
Butter	1 pkg	36	—	11
Egg Omelette Sandwich	1	288	—	198

FOOD	PORTION	CALS.	FIB.	CHOL.
Grape Jelly	1 pkg	38	—	0
Hash Brown	1	150	—	0
Honey	1 pkg	27	—	0
Margarine	1 pkg	25	—	0
Pancake Syrup	1 pkg	169	—	0
Pancakes	3	259	—	0
Pancakes w/ Sausage	1 serving	426	—	34
Scrambled Eggs	2 eggs	189	—	374
Strawberry Jam	1 pkg	37	—	0
MAIN MENU SELECTIONS				
Bacon	1 slice	38	—	6
Baked Potato	1	310	—	0
Baked Potato w/ Broccoli Cheese Topping	1	453	—	17
Baked Potato w/ Cheese Topping	1	510	—	22
Baked Potato w/ Mushroom Topping	1	360	—	0
Cheese Large	1 serving	89	—	22
Cheese Small	1 serving	46	—	12
Chicken Sandwich Grilled	1	442	—	66
Chicken Sandwich Grilled w/o Dressing	1	385	—	66
Club Crackers	1 pkg	31	—	0
Croutons	1 serving	29	—	0
Fajita Taco Beef	1	326	—	28
Fajita Taco Chicken	1	272	—	33
French Fries	1 junior	221	—	0
French Fries	1 reg	332	—	0
French Fries	1 lg	442	—	0
Garden Salad w/o dressing	1	56	—	0
Grilled Chicken Salad	1 serving	150	—	49
Jalapeno Pepper	1	3	—	0
Justaburger	1	276	—	34
Onion Rings	1 reg	329	—	0
Onion Rings	1 lg	493	—	0
Picante Sauce	1 pkg	5	—	0
Sour Cream	1 serving (2 oz)	121	—	25
Steak Sandwich	1	387	—	61
Taquito Bacon	1 serving	335	—	286
Taquito Potato	1 serving	446	—	281
Taquito Sausage	1 serving	443	—	315
Turkey Sandwich Grilled	1	439	—	46
Whataburger	1	598	—	84
Whataburger Double Meat	1	823	—	168

FOOD	PORTION	CALS.	FIB.	CHOL.
Whataburger Jr.	1	300	—	34
Whatacatch	1	475	—	32
Whatachick'n Deluxe	1	573	—	56
Whatachick'n Sandwich	1	501	—	40
SALAD DRESSINGS				
French	1 pkg	249	—	5
Ranch	1 pkg	364	—	5
Thousand Island	1 pkg	280	—	0
Vinaigrette Lite	1 pkg	36	—	0

NOTES

NOTES